# Basic ICD-10-CM/PCS and ICD-9-CM Coding

## 2015 Edition

**Lou Ann Schraffenberger, MBA, RHIA, CCS, CCS-P, FAHIMA**

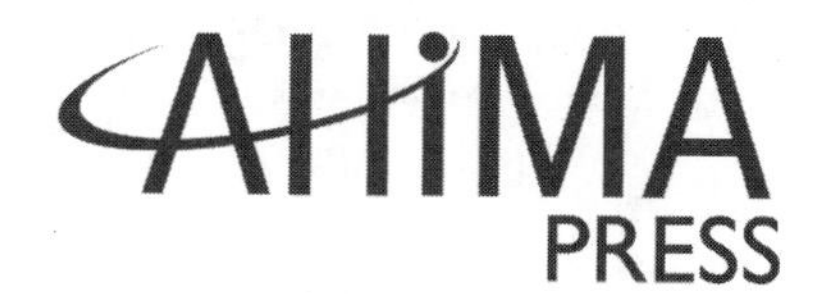
PRESS

This textbook includes ICD-9-CM changes announced in the Centers for Medicare and Medicaid Services (CMS) Hospital Inpatient Prospective Payment Systems (IPPS) Proposed Rules, as originally published in the May 5, 2011 *Federal Register*, available online from http://www.gpo.gov/fdsys/pkg/FR-2011-05-05/html/2011-9644.htm.

The last revision of ICD-9-CM occurred in 2011 to become effective for the Federal Government's fiscal year 2012 starting on October 1, 2011.

The 2011 ICD-9-CM files are available by FTP or rich text files on the website of http://www.cdc.gov/nchs/icd/icd9cm.htm.

The 2011 addenda and errata, which provide complete information on changes to the diagnosis part of ICD-9-CM is posted on CDC's webpage at: http://www.cdc.gov/nchs/icd/icd9cm.htm or at http://www.cdc.gov/nchs/icd/icd9cm_addenda_guidelines.htm#addenda.

Material quoted in this book from the *ICD-9-CM Official Guidelines for Coding and Reporting* is taken from the October 2011 updated version. Material quoted in this book from the *ICD-10-CM Official Guidelines for Coding and Reporting* is taken from the 2014 updated version.



First edition 1993, revised annually

ISBN 978-1-58426-503-0

AHIMA Product No. AC200514

Caitlin Wilson, Assistant Editor
Jason O. Malley, Vice President, Business and Innovation
Ashley R. Latta, Production Development Editor
Pamela Woolf, Director of Publications
Ann Zeisset, RHIT, CCS, CCS-P, Technical Review

Illustrator: Jason Isley



American Health Information Management Association
233 North Michigan Avenue, 21st Floor
Chicago, Illinois 60601-5809

ahima.org

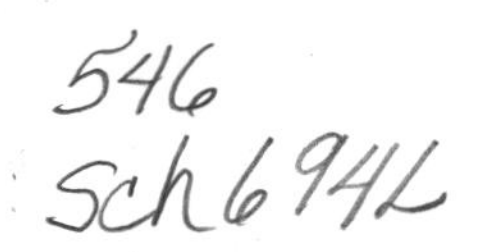

# Contents

## Online Contents

# About the Author

Lou Ann Schraffenberger, MBA, RHIA, CCS, CCS-P, FAHIMA, is employed by Advocate Health Care as the manager of clinical data in their Center for Health Information Services. Advocate Health Care is an integrated healthcare delivery system of 11 hospitals and other healthcare entities, based in Downers Grove, Illinois. Her position is dedicated to systemwide health information management (HIM) and clinical data projects, clinical coding education, and coding compliance issues. Prior to her current position, Lou Ann served as director of hospital health record departments, director of the Professional Practice Division of the American Health Information Management Association (AHIMA), and a faculty member at the University of Illinois at Chicago. An experienced seminar leader, Lou Ann serves as part-time faculty and a continuing education instructor in the health information technology and coding certificate program at Moraine Valley Community College in Illinois. She has also contributed her knowledge and skills as a consultant for clinical coding projects with hospitals, ambulatory care facilities, physicians, and medical group practices. Lou Ann is active in national, state, and local HIM associations. She served as chair of the Society for Clinical Coding (2000). She is a commissioner on the Commission on Certification for Health Informatics and Information Management (CCHIIM) for 2012 through 2014, and former chair of the Certified Coding Specialist (CCS) Examination Construction Committee (1997–1999). In 1997, Lou Ann was awarded the first AHIMA Volunteer Award. Lou Ann received the Legacy Award from the AHIMA Foundation in 2008 in recognition of her significant contribution to the HIM knowledge base through her authorship of this publication and two other coding books published by AHIMA.

# Acknowledgments

This book was originally published in 1993 under the authorship of Toula Nicholas, RHIT, CCS, and Linda Ertl Bank, RHIA, CCS. Earlier ICD-9-CM instructional material authored by Rita M. Finnegan, MA, RHIA, was the foundation for the original book. Therese M. Jorwic, MPH, RHIA, CCS, FAHIMA, updated several chapters in the 2012 edition of this book; her authorship is acknowledged and appreciated.

AHIMA Press would like to thank Ann Zeisset, RHIT, CCS, CCS-P for her review and feedback on this publication.

# Preface

The coding process requires a range of skills that combine knowledge and practice. *Basic ICD-10-CM/PCS and ICD-9-CM Coding* was designed to be a comprehensive text for students. It introduces the basic principles and conventions of ICD-9-CM coding and illustrates the application of coding principles with examples and exercises based on actual case documentation. To address the implementation of ICD-10-CM/PCS that is expected to occur on October 1, 2015, new information about ICD-10-CM/PCS has been added to the individual chapters in the textbook. Each chapter of the textbook includes information on the applicable portion of ICD-10-CM. Chapter 2, Procedures, includes information on ICD-10-PCS. These chapters are not intended to provide the reader with all the training they will need to code with ICD-10-CM/PCS, but rather to give the student a basic level of understanding of ICD-10-CM/PCS that will allow them to begin the education process of transitioning to coding with ICD-10-CM/PCS and be prepared to use the system beginning October 1, 2015.

## Organization of the Book

The chapters of *Basic ICD-10-CM/PCS and ICD-9-CM Coding* are organized to cover each section of ICD-9-CM; each chapter includes information about the applicable sections of ICD-10-CM or ICD-10-PCS. The coding self-test, appendices, and index at the back of the book make information readily accessible and provide additional resources for students. The website accompanying this book contains 11 appendices of valuable material for coding students, including the full text of the official coding guidelines for both ICD-9-CM and ICD-10-CM.

## Information Updates

This book must be used with the 2012 edition of *ICD-9-CM* (code changes effective October 1, 2011). It includes the code updates that are available on the Centers for Disease Control and Prevention (CDC), International Classification of Diseases, Ninth Revision, Clinical Modification: http://www.cdc.gov/nchs/icd/icd9cm.htm. This was the last update to ICD-9-CM.

It includes the code updates listed in the Centers for Medicare and Medicaid Services (CMS) hospital Inpatient Prospective Payment System (IPPS) Proposed Rules, May 5, 2011 *Federal Register* available online from http://www.gpo.gov/fdsys/pkg/FR-2011-05-05/html/2011-9644.htm. A direct link to the proposed rule for Medicare's hospital IPPS for acute care hospitals for Fiscal Year 2012 can be found at http://www.cms.gov/AcuteInpatientPPS/IPPS2012/list.asp.

## Coding Guidelines

The last edition of the *ICD-9-CM Official Guidelines for Coding and Reporting*, became effective October 2011. The guidelines are included as appendix H on the website accompanying this book. Additional information and updates to the current (last) edition of the ICD-9-CM coding guidelines http://www.cdc.gov/nchs/icd/icd9cm_addenda_guidelines.htm.

The 2014 *ICD-10-CM Official Guidelines* for Coding and Reporting are available at the website: http://www.cdc.gov/nchs/icd/icd10cm.htm. The same website will likely contain the 2015 version when available in the third or fourth quarter of 2014.

## ICD-9-CM Procedure Codes

CMS provides a current set of the *ICD-9-CM* diagnosis and procedure codes with abbreviated and full code titles on their website: http://www.cms.gov/Medicare/Coding/ICD9ProviderDiagnosticCodes/codes.html
Downloadable files of diagnosis and procedure codes and their full and abbreviated titles are available in the "Downloads" and "Related Links" portion of this webpage.

## ICD-10-CM and ICD-10-PCS Updated Codes

CMS provides the following website for information concerning the transition from ICD-9-CM to ICD-10-CM and ICD-10-PCS with various resources available: http://www.cms.gov/Medicare/Coding/ICD10/index.html.

On the left side of the page, the reader can find the 2014 ICD-10-CM and general equivalence mappings (GEMs) with another site for the 2014 ICD-10-PCS and GEMs for reference. Of particular interest are the ICD-10-PCS resources available at http://www.cms.gov/Medicare/Coding/ICD10/2014-ICD-10-PCS.html, including the ICD-10-PCS Coding Guidelines and the ICD-10-PCS Reference Manual. This site is expected to be updated with 2015 materials when they become available.

## Partial Code Freeze for ICD-9-CM and ICD-10-CM and ICD-10-PCS

The ICD-10 Coordination and Maintenance Committee (formerly the ICD-9-CM Coordination and Maintenance Committee) implemented a partial freeze of the ICD-9-CM and ICD-10 (ICD-10-CM and ICD-10-PCS) codes prior to the implementation of ICD-10 which would end one year after the implementation of ICD-10.

However, on April 1, 2014, the Protecting Access to Medicare Act of 2014 (PAMA) (Pub. L. No. 113-93) was enacted, which stated that the Secretary of Health and Human Services may not adopt ICD-10 prior to October 1, 2015. This required the partial code freeze process to be reexamined.

The US Department of Health and Human Services (HHS) is expected to release an interim final rule that will include a new compliance date that would require the use of ICD-10 beginning October 1, 2015. The rule will also require Health Insurance Portability and Accountability Act (HIPAA)-covered entities to continue to use ICD-9-CM through September 30, 2015. When published, links are expected to be provided at http://www.cms.gov/Medicare/Coding/ICD10/Statute_Regulations.html.

The partial freeze is expected to follow the following process:

- The last regular, annual updates to both ICD-9-CM and ICD-10 code sets were made on October 1, 2011.

- On October 1, 2012, October 1, 2013, and October 1, 2014 there were only limited code updates to both the ICD-9-CM and ICD-10 code sets to capture new technologies and diseases as required by section 503(a) of Pub. L. 108-173.
- On October 1, 2015, there will be only limited code updates to ICD-10 code sets to capture new technologies and diagnoses as required by section 503(a) of Pub. L. 108-173. There will be no updates to ICD-9-CM, as it will no longer be used for reporting.
- On October 1, 2016 (one year after implementation of ICD-10), regular updates to ICD-10 will begin.

The ICD-10 Coordination and Maintenance Committee is expected to meet twice a year during the partial freeze time period through 2015. At these meetings, public comment will be invited on whether or not requests for new diagnosis or procedure codes should be created based on the criteria of the need to capture a new technology or disease. Any requests that do not meet the criteria for new codes will be evaluated for implementation within ICD-10 on and after October 1, 2016 once the partial freeze has ended (AHIMA 2012).

## Additional Practice

In addition to the student review exercises throughout and at the end of each chapter, a companion student workbook, also by Lou Ann Schraffenberger, is available. *Basic ICD-10-CM/PCS and ICD-9-CM Coding Exercises,* contains ICD-9-CM and ICD-10-CM/PCS coding exercises related to each chapter of *Basic ICD-10-CM/PCS and ICD-9-CM Coding*. *Basic ICD-10-CM/PCS and ICD-9-CM Coding Exercises* provides the student with the next level of coding practice—that is, coding from case studies or scenarios instead of one-line diagnostic or procedural statements. The *ICD-10-CM/PCS and Basic ICD-9-CM Coding* student workbook can be used in conjunction with this textbook for the "lab" portion of a coding course, a text for a coding practicum or lab course, or can be used for independent study for skill building.

The answer key to *Basic ICD-9-Coding Exercises,* 3rd edition, has been updated online and is available electronically at ahimapress.org.

AHIMA's publication *Clinical Coding Workout* is an excellent follow-up resource after the coder completes *Basic ICD-10-CM/PCS and ICD-9-CM Coding*. Containing beginning, intermediate, and advanced exercises, it is also a perfect teaching tool for coders wanting to sharpen their ability to make critical coding decisions. The book is made up entirely of case studies that help students and coders alike understand what they need to know when it comes to correct coding practices and procedures. The case studies in the book require users to make the kinds of decisions that coding professionals must make every day on the job.

### Instructor Materials and Answer Key

AHIMA provides supplementary materials for educators who use this book in their classes. Materials include lesson plans, PowerPoint slides, and other useful instructional tips, reminders, and resources. Visit http://www.ahimapress.org/Schraffenberger5030/ and click the link to download the files. Please do not enter the scratch-off code from the interior front cover, as this will invalidate your access to the instructor materials. If you have any questions regarding the instructor materials, contact AHIMA Customer Relations at (800) 335-5535 or submit a customer support request at https://secure.ahima.org/contact/contact.aspx.

# Introduction to Coding

## What Is Coding?

In its simplest form, **coding** is the transformation of verbal descriptions into numbers. We are all very familiar with this task because we use codes every day to carry out simple business and personal transactions. For example, when we use a zip code in addressing a letter, we are transforming a street address into numbers.

In the healthcare arena, specific codes describe diagnoses and procedures. A **diagnosis** is a word or phrase used by a physician to identify a disease from which an individual suffers or a condition for which the patient needs, seeks, or receives medical care. A surgical or therapeutic **procedure** is any single, separate, systematic process upon or within the body that can be complete in itself. A procedure is normally performed by a physician, dentist, or other licensed practitioner. A procedure can be performed with or without instrumentation. It is performed to restore disunited or deficient parts, remove diseased or injured tissues, extract foreign matter, assist in obstetrical delivery, or aid in diagnosis. Whereas assigning a zip code is a rather simple activity, the assignment of diagnostic and procedural codes requires a detailed thought process that is supported by a thorough knowledge of medical terminology, anatomy, and pathophysiology.

## How Are Codes Assigned, and What Systems Are Used?

Hospitals and other healthcare facilities index healthcare data by referring and adhering to a classification system maintained by the National Center for Health Statistics (NCHS) and CMS. A **classification system** is a grouping of similar diseases and procedures, and organizing related information for easy retrieval. This type of system is used for assigning numeric or alphanumeric code numbers to represent specific diseases or procedures. Currently in the United States, that system expected to be implemented October 1, 2015 is the International Classification of Diseases, Tenth Revision, Clinical Modification (ICD-10-CM).

### ICD-9-CM

The notion of **classification** originated at the time of the ancient Greeks. In the 17th century, English statistician John Graunt developed the London Bills of Mortality, which provided the first documentation of the proportion of children who died before reaching age six years. In 1838, William Farr, the registrar general of England, developed a system to classify deaths. In 1893, a French physician, Jacques Bertillon, introduced the Bertillon Classification of Causes of Death at the International Statistical Institute in Chicago.

Several countries subsequently adopted Dr. Bertillon's system and in 1898, the American Public Health Association (APHA) recommended that the registrars of Canada, Mexico, and the United States also adopt it. In addition, APHA recommended revising the system every ten years to remain current with medical practice. As a result, the first international conference to revise the International Classification of Causes of Death convened in 1900; subsequent revisions occurred every 10 years. At that time, the classification system was contained in one book, which included an Alphabetic Index as well as a Tabular List. The book was quite small compared with current coding texts.

The revisions that followed contained minor changes; however, the sixth revision of the classification system brought drastic changes, as well as an expansion into two volumes. The sixth revision included morbidity and mortality conditions, and HHS changed its title to reflect these changes: *Manual of International Statistical Classification of Diseases, Injuries and Causes of Death (ICD).* Prior to the sixth revision, responsibility for ICD revisions fell to the Mixed Commission, a group composed of representatives from the International Statistical Institute and the Health Organization of the League of Nations. In 1948, the **World Health Organization (WHO)**, with headquarters in Geneva, Switzerland, assumed responsibility for preparing and publishing the revisions to ICD every 10 years. WHO sponsored the seventh and eighth revisions in 1957 and 1968, respectively.

The entire history of coding emphasizes the determination of many people to provide an international classification system for compiling and presenting statistical data. ICD has now become the most widely used statistical classification system in the world. Although some countries found ICD sufficient for hospital indexing purposes, many others believed that it did not provide adequate detail for diagnostic indexing. In addition, the original revisions of ICD did not provide for classification of operative and diagnostic procedures. As a result, interested persons in the United States began to develop their own adaptation of ICD for use in this country.

In 1959, the US Public Health Service published *The International Classification of Diseases, Adapted for Indexing of Hospital Records and Operation Classification (ICDA).* Completed in 1962, a revision of this adaptation—considered to be the seventh revision of ICD—expanded a number of areas to more completely meet the indexing needs of hospitals. The US Public Health Service later published the *Eighth Revision, International Classification of Diseases, Adapted for Use in the United States.* Commonly referred to as ICDA-8, this classification system fulfilled its purpose to code diagnostic and operative procedural data for official morbidity and mortality statistics in the United States.

In 1978, WHO published the ninth revision of ICD (ICD-9). The US Public Health Service modified ICD-9 to meet the needs of American hospitals and called it International Classification of Diseases, Ninth Revision, Clinical Modification (ICD-9-CM). The ninth revision expanded the book to three volumes and introduced a fifth-digit subclassification. ICD-9-CM was the coding and classification system used in the United States to report diagnoses in all healthcare settings, inpatient procedures, and services for morbidity and mortality reporting starting in 1979. The ICD-9-CM system is slated to be discontinued in the United States on September 30, 2015.

## ICD-10-CM and ICD-10-PCS

WHO published the 10th revision of ICD in 1990, and a number of countries subsequently adopted the system in either the original or an adapted form. The international version of the

ICD-10 system has been used in the United States since January 1, 1999 for death certificate coding. This allows for collection of international mortality data.

A US clinical modification of the ICD-10 system was initiated in 1994 by **NCHS**. NCHS is the federal agency responsible for collecting and disseminating information on health services utilization and the health status of the population in the United States. NCHS is responsible for developing the clinical modifications for the United States to the ICD for the reporting of diseases. NCHS is also responsible for the development and the use of ICD-10 in the United States. The result, ICD-10-CM, was released in 1998 and updated several times since the initial version. ICD-10-CM is expected to be used for the reporting of diseases and conditions of patients treated in all settings in the United States healthcare system effective October 1, 2015.

The ICD-10-CM system is more specific and contains significantly more codes than ICD-9-CM. It has the same hierarchical structure as ICD-9-CM, but the codes are alphanumeric with all letters except U used. The codes can extend to up to seven characters.

The 2015 version of ICD-10-CM is available on the NCHS website, at the Classifications of Diseases, Functioning, and Disability home page at http://www.cdc.gov/nchs/icd/icd10cm.htm. Although this release of ICD-10-CM is now available for public viewing, the codes in ICD-10-CM are not currently valid for any purpose or use pending the official implementation of ICD-10-CM and ICD-10-PCS in the United States. This version has been created by NCHS, under authorization by WHO.

On January 16, 2009, HHS published a final rule adopting ICD-10-CM (and ICD-10-PCS) to replace ICD-9-CM in HIPAA transactions, with an effective implementation date of October 1, 2013. The October 1, 2013 implementation date for ICD-10-CM/PCS was established in the original Final Rule of the HIPAA Administrative Simplification: Modifications to the Medical Data Code Set Standards to adopt ICD-10-CM and ICD-10-PCS, which was published in the *Federal Register* on January 16, 2009 (http://www.access.gpo.gov/su_docs/fedreg/a090116c.html). The ***Federal Register*** is the daily publication of the federal government printed by the US Government Printing Office that announces all changes in regulations and federally mandated standards, including rules concerning prospective payment systems and code sets.

**HIPAA** was federal legislation enacted to provide continuing health coverage, control fraud and abuse in healthcare, reduce healthcare costs, and guarantee the security and privacy of health information. HIPAA limits exclusions for preexisting medical conditions, prohibits discrimination against employees and dependents based on health status, guarantees availability of health insurance to small employers, and guarantees renewability of insurance to all employees regardless of size. The law is also known as Public Law 104-191 and the Kassebaum-Kennedy Law.

On April 17, 2012, the Secretary of HHS issued a proposed rule to change the compliance date for the ICD-10-CM and ICD-10-PCS code sets from October 1, 2013 to October 1, 2014. The comment period for the proposed rule closed in June 2012. The Final Rule published in the *Federal Register* on September 5, 2012 set the implementation date of October 1, 2014. On April 1, 2014, PAMA (Pub. L. No. 113-93) was enacted, which said that the Secretary may not adopt ICD-10 prior to October 1, 2015. Accordingly, HHS release a final rule on July 31, 2014 that will require a new compliance date for the use of ICD-10 beginning October 1, 2015. The rule will also require HIPAA-covered entities to continue to use ICD-9-CM through September 30, 2015.

The Final Rule adopts modifications to two of the code set standards adopted in the Transactions and Code Sets Final Rule published in the *Federal Register* pursuant to certain provisions of the Administrative Simplification subtitle of HIPAA. Specifically, this Final Rule modifies the standard medical data code sets for coding diagnoses and inpatient hospital procedures by concurrently adopting the ICD-10-CM for diagnosis coding, including the *Official ICD-10-CM Guidelines for Coding and Reporting*, as maintained by the National Center for Health Statistics, and ICD-10-PCS for inpatient hospital procedure coding, including the *Official ICD-10-PCS Guidelines for Coding and Reporting*, as maintained and distributed by HHS. These new codes replace ICD-9-CM, volumes 1, 2, and 3, including the *Official Guidelines for Coding and Reporting*.

ICD-10-PCS was developed by 3M Health Information Systems under contract with **CMS**. CMS is a division of HHS that is responsible for developing healthcare policy in the United States, administering the Medicare program and the federal portion of the Medicaid program, and maintaining the procedure portion of the ICD. On October 1, 2014, ICD-10-PCS will replace ICD-9-CM, volume 3, for the reporting of hospital inpatient procedures. It is a significant improvement over ICD-9-CM, volume 3, in terms of its comprehensiveness and expandability. ICD-10-PCS is discussed in further detail in Chapter 2.

## HIPAA Electronic Transactions and Coding Standards Rule

On August 17, 2000, the DHHS published the final regulations for electronic transactions and coding standards as established under HIPAA in the *Federal Register* (65 FR 50312). The final rule designated five medical code standards to be used initially under the HIPAA rule. These included:

- ***International Classification of Diseases, 9th Edition, Clinical Modification (ICD-9-CM),* volumes 1 and 2**
- ***International Classification of Diseases, 9th Edition, Clinical Modification (ICD-9-CM),* volume 3**
- ***Current Procedural Terminology (CPT), 4th Edition (CPT-4)***
- ***Healthcare Common Procedure Coding System (HCPCS)***
- ***Code on Dental Procedures and Nomenclatures, 2nd Edition (CDT-2)***
- ***National Drug Codes (NDC)***

On February 20, 2003, the DHHS published a final rule in the *Federal Register* (68 FR 8381) that repealed the adoption of the *National Drug Codes* (NDC) for institutional and professional claims. It did allow NDC to remain the standard medical data code set for reporting drugs and biologics for retail pharmacy claims. The intent of this decision was to give covered entities the choice in determining which code set to use with respect to payment of claims, including HCPCS and NDC codes. Hospitals and physicians are likely to continue using HCPCS. As a result of this repeal, there is no identified standard medical data code set in place for reporting drugs and biologics on nonretail pharmacy transactions. Covered entities could use HCPCS or NDC as the preferred and agreed-upon code set with their trading partners.

The ***ICD-9-CM Official Guidelines for Coding and Reporting*** were named as a required component of the ICD-9-CM code set in the final rule for electronic transactions and coding standards (65 FR 50323). This makes adherence to the ICD-9-CM guidelines a requirement for compliance with the rule. No other set of coding guidelines was specified in the coding standards.

The original deadline for compliance with the electronic transactions rule was October 16, 2002, for all covered entities except small health plans, which by law had an additional year. However, in January 2002, in the Administrative Simplification Compliance Act, Congress authorized a one-year extension, to October 16, 2003, for those covered entities required to comply in 2002.

As noted previously, the final rule identified five medical code sets. Although it is true that most of the code sets adopted are in current use, some changes were made regarding their use and context. It is important to note that, upon implementation, these medical code sets became the rule for nearly all insurance payers.

ICD-9-CM volumes 1 and 2 cover diseases, injuries, impairments, and other health problems and their manifestations, as well as causes of injury and disease impairment. Essentially, this part of the rule maintains the status quo.

ICD-9-CM volume 3, Procedures, has been limited to procedures or other actions taken for diseases, injuries, and impairments of hospital inpatients reported by hospitals and related to prevention, diagnosis, treatment, and management. This means that nonacute facilities do not use ICD-9-CM volume 3 to report procedures but instead use HCPCS Level I (CPT® codes published by the American Medical Association) or HCPCS level II codes as appropriate.

The CPT/HCPCS codes are used for physicians and other healthcare services, such as hospital outpatient services. These services include, but are not limited to: physician services, physical and occupational therapy services, radiological services, clinical laboratory tests, other medical diagnostic procedures, hearing and vision services, and transportation services, including ambulances.

The rule makes it clear that the use of ICD-9-CM procedure codes is restricted to the reporting of inpatient procedures by hospitals. Physicians and other healthcare providers use the combination of CPT and HCPCS Level II codes to report procedures and services provided.

More information about the medical code sets and other facts about the HIPAA transactions and code sets final rule can be found on AHIMA's website (www.ahima.org) or in the published final rule in the August 17, 2000, *Federal Register* (65 FR 50312). The *Federal Register* may be accessed from the Government Printing Office website at http://www.gpo.gov/fdsys/browse/collection.action?collectionCode=FR.

## Medicare Prescription Drug, Improvement, and Modernization Act of 2003

The **Medicare Prescription Drug, Improvement, and Modernization Act (MMA)** was signed into law on December 8, 2003. Section 503 of the bill includes language that opened up the possibility for code changes two times a year, on April 1 as well as October 1. Since this legislation took effect in 2005, there have not been any April 1 code changes. However, the potential for code changes twice a year still exists if a strong and convincing case is made by the requestor that the new code is needed to describe new technologies. Otherwise, the codes will be considered for the next October 1 implementation.

## Official Addendum to ICD-9-CM and ICD-9-CM Coordination and Maintenance Committee

ICD-9-CM represents the most current and comprehensive statistical classification system of its kind. In contrast to international ICD updates that occur less frequently, ICD-9-CM undergoes annual updates in the United States to remain current. Codes may be added, revised, or deleted. An ***Official Authorized Addendum*** documents the changes, which are effective April 1 and October 1 of each year. The addendum may be found at the NCHS website http://www.cdc.gov/nchs/icd/icd9cm.htm for the ICD-9-CM system. The website of http://www.cdc.gov/nchs/icd/icd10cm.htm contains the updated materials for the ICD-10-CM system.

CMS and NCHS publish the addenda with the approval of WHO. NCHS is responsible for maintaining the diagnosis classification—volumes 1 and 2; CMS is responsible for maintaining the procedure classification—volume 3. AHIMA and the American Hospital Association (AHA) give advice and assistance, as do HIM practitioners, physicians, and other users of ICD-9-CM.

The **ICD-9-CM Coordination and Maintenance Committee** is composed of representatives from NCHS and CMS and is responsible for maintaining the United States' clinical modification version of the ICD-9-CM code sets. The Coordination and Maintenance Committee holds two open meetings each year that serve as a public forum for discussing (but not making decisions about) proposed revisions to ICD-9-CM. Information about the ICD-9-CM and ICD-10-CM Coordination and Maintenance Committee, including meetings minutes, can be found at the CDC website: http://www.cdc.gov/nchs/icd/icd9cm_maintenance.htm.

Additional information about the Coordination and Maintenance Committee can be found on the CMS website: http://www.cms.gov/Medicare/Coding/ICD9ProviderDiagnosticCodes/meetings.html.

**A point to remember:** To ensure accurate coding, all ICD-9-CM coding books and the ICD-10-CM and ICD-10-PCS code books in the future must be updated yearly with revisions. In addition, all coding software (encoders) must be updated. As a general rule, new codes are effective October 1 of each year.

# Chapter 1

# Characteristics of ICD-9-CM and ICD-10-CM

## Learning Objectives

At the conclusion of this chapter, you should be able to:

1. Identify the characteristics of the ICD-9-CM and ICD-10-CM classification system
2. Describe the format of the Tabular List of Diseases and Injuries
3. Identify and define the sections, categories, subcategories, residual subcategories, and fifth-digit subclassifications used in ICD-9-CM
4. Identify and define the chapters and subchapters or blocks used in ICD-10-CM
5. Identify and define the main terms, subterms, carryover lines, nonessential modifiers, and eponyms used in ICD-10-CM
6. Identify the two supplementary classifications within ICD-9-CM
7. Identify the contents of the Appendices of ICD-9-CM and ICD-10-CM
8. Describe the format of the Alphabetic Index to Diseases in ICD-9-CM and ICD-10-CM
9. Identify and define the main terms, subterms, carryover lines, nonessential modifiers, and eponyms used in ICD-9-CM and ICD-10-CM
10. Explain how to accommodate the fact that all terms located in the Alphabetic Index are not included in the Tabular List
11. Identify and define the cross-reference terms and instructional notes used in ICD-9-CM and ICD-10-CM
12. Describe the rules for multiple coding
13. Explain how connecting words are used in the Alphabetic Index
14. Define the symbols, punctuations, and abbreviations used in ICD-9-CM and ICD-10-CM
15. List the basic steps in ICD-9-CM and ICD-10-CM coding
16. Assign diagnosis codes using the Alphabetic Index and Tabular List
17. Identify the main differences between the ICD-9-CM and ICD-10-CM systems for diagnosis coding

## Introduction to ICD-9-CM

The official ICD-9-CM code set currently comprises three volumes:

**Volume 1**: Tabular List of Diseases and Injuries
**Volume 2**: Alphabetic Index to Diseases
**Volume 3**: Tabular List and Alphabetic Index to Procedures

The official ICD-9-CM is available by download from the National Center for Health Statistics (NCHS) website. Downloading information can be found at http://www.cdc.gov/nchs/icd/icd9cm.htm. The last edition available is for 2011.

Since ICD-9-CM is not under copyright, many versions of the codebook appear on the market. Although each book may offer special features, the ICD-9-CM codes themselves remain the same. This workbook, *Basic ICD-10-CM/PCS and ICD-9-CM Coding,* refers to the official ICD-9-CM codebook throughout its text.

Because ICD-9-CM was reviewed annually, it is important to remember that all ICD-9-CM codebooks used must be the most current to reflect the revisions, deletions, and additions of codes that were generally implemented in the United States on October 1 of each year, the last edition available is 2011.

## ICD-9-CM Volume 1: Tabular List of Diseases and Injuries

The Tabular List of Diseases and Injuries (volume 1) contains the following major subdivisions:

Classification of Diseases and Injuries
Supplementary Classifications (V Codes and E Codes)
Appendices

### Classification of Diseases and Injuries

**Volume 1**, Classification of Diseases and Injuries, contains 17 chapters that classify conditions according to etiology (cause of disease) or by specific anatomical (body) system.

**EXAMPLE:** Chapter 1, Infectious and Parasitic Diseases, represents classification by etiology or cause of disease.

Chapter 7, Diseases of the Circulatory System, represents classification by anatomical system.

The Tabular List contains the following 17 chapters:

| | Chapter Titles | Categories |
|---|---|---|
| 1. | Infectious and Parasitic Diseases | 001–139 |
| 2. | Neoplasms | 140–239 |
| 3. | Endocrine, Nutritional and Metabolic Diseases, and Immunity Disorders | 240–279 |

| | | |
|---|---|---|
| 4. | Diseases of the Blood and Blood-Forming Organs | 280–289 |
| 5. | Mental, Behavioral and Neurodevelopmental Disorders | 290–319 |
| 6. | Diseases of the Nervous System and Sense Organs | 320–389 |
| 7. | Diseases of the Circulatory System | 390–459 |
| 8. | Diseases of the Respiratory System | 460–519 |
| 9. | Diseases of the Digestive System | 520–579 |
| 10. | Diseases of the Genitourinary System | 580–629 |
| 11. | Complications of Pregnancy, Childbirth, and the Puerperium | 630–679 |
| 12. | Diseases of the Skin and Subcutaneous Tissue | 680–709 |
| 13. | Diseases of the Musculoskeletal System and Connective Tissue | 710–739 |
| 14. | Congenital Anomalies | 740–759 |
| 15. | Certain Conditions Originating in the Perinatal Period | 760–779 |
| 16. | Symptoms, Signs, and Ill-Defined Conditions | 780–799 |
| 17. | Injury and Poisoning | 800–999 |

## Format

Each chapter of volume 1 is structured into the following subdivisions: **sections, categories,** and **subcategories.**

### Sections

A **section** consists of a group of three-digit categories that represent a single disease entity or a group of similar or closely related conditions.

**DISORDERS OF THYROID GLAND (240–246)**

### Categories

A three-digit **category** represents a single disease entity or a group of similar or closely related conditions.

**520 Disorders of tooth development and eruption**

### Subcategories

The fourth-digit **subcategory** provides more specificity or information regarding the etiology (cause of a disease or illness), site (location), or manifestation (display of characteristic signs, symptoms, or secondary processes of a disease or illness). Fourth-digit subcategories are collapsible to the three-digit level.

A three-digit code cannot be assigned if a category has been subdivided and fourth digits are available.

**476 Chronic laryngitis and laryngotracheitis**

**476.0 Chronic laryngitis**
Laryngitis:
catarrhal
hypertrophic
sicca

**476.1 Chronic laryngotracheitis**
Laryngitis, chronic, with tracheitis (chronic)
Tracheitis, chronic, with laryngitis

## Exercise 1.1

Turn to code 055, Measles, in volume 1, ICD-9-CM (Tabular List) to answer the following questions:

1. Are the subcategories manifestations, sites, or causes of the disease?

2. In what chapter and section is code 055 located?

3. What do the subcategory codes represent?

4. Is code 055 a category or a subcategory?

5. What is the subcategory code for measles without complications?

### Fifth-Digit Subclassifications

In some cases, fourth-digit subcategories have been expanded to the fifth-digit level or **fifth-digit subclassifications** to provide even greater specificity. Fifth-digit assignments and instructions can appear at the beginning of a chapter, a section, a three-digit category, or a fourth-digit category, as illustrated below.

**At the chapter level:** An instruction at the beginning of Chapter 13, Diseases of the Musculoskeletal System and Connective Tissue (710–739), states that certain categories must be assigned a fifth digit to describe the affected body site. Fifth-digit assignments and instructions appearing at the beginning of this chapter are shown in the following illustration:

**13. DISEASES OF THE MUSCULOSKELETAL SYSTEM AND CONNECTIVE TISSUE (710–739)**

The following fifth-digit subclassification is for use with categories 711–712, 715–716, 718–719, and 730:

**0 site unspecified**

**1 shoulder region**

Acromioclavicular, joint(s)
Clavicle
Glenohumeral, joint(s)
Scapula
Sternoclavicular, joint(s)

**2 upper arm**

Elbow joint
Humerus

**3 forearm**

Radius
Ulna
Wrist joint

**4 hand**

Carpus
Metacarpus
Phalanges [fingers]

**5 pelvic region and thigh**

Buttock
Femur
Hip (joint)

**6 lower leg**

Fibula
Knee joint
Patella
Tibia

**7 ankle and foot**

Ankle joint
Digits [toes]
Metatarsus
Phalanges, foot
Tarsus
Other joints in foot

**8 other specified sites**

Head
Neck
Ribs
Skull
Trunk
Vertebral column

**9 multiple sites**

**At the section level:** Information at the beginning of section 200–208, Malignant Neoplasm of Lymphatic and Hematopoietic Tissue, notes that a fifth digit must be assigned to categories 200 through 202 to describe the site of the lymph nodes involved. Fifth-digit assignments and instructions appearing at the beginning of this section are shown in the following illustration:

**MALIGNANT NEOPLASM OF LYMPHATIC AND HEMATOPOIETIC TISSUE (200–208)**

Excludes: *autoimmune lymphoproliferative syndrome (279.41)*
*secondary and unspecified neoplasm of lymph nodes (196.0–196.9)*
*secondary neoplasm of:*
*bone marrow (198.5)*
*spleen (197.8)*

The following fifth-digit subclassification is for use with categories 200–202:

**0 unspecified site, extranodal and solid organ sites**
**1 lymph nodes of head, face, and neck**
**2 intrathoracic lymph nodes**
**3 intra-abdominal lymph nodes**
**4 lymph nodes of axilla and upper limb**
**5 lymph nodes of inguinal region and lower limb**
**6 intrapelvic lymph nodes**
**7 spleen**
**8 lymph nodes of multiple sites**

**At the three-digit category level:** An instruction from the beginning of category 250, Diabetes mellitus, states that a fifth digit should be assigned to describe the type of diabetes mellitus. Fifth-digit assignments and instructions appearing at the beginning of this three-digit category are shown in the following illustration:

**250 Diabetes mellitus**

Excludes: *gestational diabetes (648.8)*
*hyperglycemia, NOS (790.29)*
*neonatal diabetes mellitus (775.1)*
*nonclinical diabetes (790.29)*
*secondary diabetes (249.0–249.9)*

The following fifth-digit subclassification is for use with category 250:

**0 type II or unspecified type, not stated as uncontrolled**

Fifth-digit 0 is for use for type II patients, even if the patient requires insulin

Use additional code, if applicable, for associated long-term (current) insulin use, V58.67

**1 type I [juvenile type], not stated as uncontrolled**

**2 type II or unspecified type, uncontrolled**

Fifth-digit 2 is for use for type II patients, even if the patient requires insulin

Use additional code, if applicable, for associated long-term (current) insulin use, V58.67

**3 type I [juvenile type], uncontrolled**

**At the fourth-digit subcategory level:** The fourth-digit subcategory 786.5, Chest pain, is further subdivided to the fifth-digit level to describe specific types of chest pain. Fifth-digit assignments and instructions appearing at the beginning of this fourth-digit subcategory are shown in the following illustration:

**786.5 Chest pain**

**786.50 Chest pain, unspecified**

**786.51 Precordial pain**

**786.52 Painful respiration**

Pain:

anterior chest wall

pleuritic

Pleurodynia

*Excludes:* *epidemic pleurodynia (074.1)*

**786.59 Other**

Discomfort in chest

Pressure in chest

Tightness in chest

*Excludes:* *pain in breast (611.71)*

**A point to remember:** When applicable, the use of fifth digits is required. Fifth digits can be quite easy to overlook. To remember to assign fifth digits, it is helpful to highlight all the fourth-digit subcategories requiring a fifth-digit subclassification in volume 1 of ICD-9-CM. Many publishers include special symbols and/or color highlighting to identify codes requiring fourth and/or fifth digits.

## Exercise 1.2

In volume 1 (Tabular List) of ICD-9-CM, turn to the section titled "Malignant Neoplasm of Lymphatic and Hematopoietic Tissue," which begins with category 200, to answer questions 1 through 3. Then turn to category 820, Fracture of neck of femur, to answer questions 4 and 5.

1. Identify the correct fifth digit for a patient with Hodgkin's sarcoma (201.2) with involvement of the intrapelvic lymph nodes.

   ______________________________

2. Identify the correct fifth digit for a patient with nodular lymphoma (202.0) with involvement of lymph nodes of multiple sites.

   ______________________________

3. Identify the correct fifth digit for a patient with Burkitt's tumor (200.2) of the intra-abdominal lymph nodes.

   ______________________________

4. Identify the code for a patient with a closed transcervical fracture of the epiphysis.

   ______________________________

5. Identify the code for a patient with an open fracture of the neck of the femur, with the actual site unspecified.

   ______________________________

### Residual Subcategories

**Residual subcategories** are codes with titles of "other" and "unspecified." They were developed to classify conditions not assigned a separate subcategory, thus ensuring that every disease always has a code. Residual subcategories titled "other" are easily distinguished because the fourth digit is often the number 8. Those codes describing "unspecified" conditions are usually assigned a fourth digit of 9.

**003.8 Other specified *Salmonella* infections**
**003.9 *Salmonella* infection, unspecified**

In the preceding example, code 003.8 would include all other specified types of *Salmonella* infections, excluding those listed in codes 003.0 through 003.29. But code 003.9 is assigned when the physician documents a diagnosis of *Salmonella* infection without further specification.

However, in a few instances, fourth digit 9 is assigned for both "other" and "unspecified" because digits 0 through 8 have been used.

**478.9 Other and unspecified diseases of upper respiratory tract**

Abscess } of trachea
Cicatrix }

Codes 478.0 through 478.8 are used to describe specific upper respiratory tract diseases. However, code 478.9 includes both unspecified diseases and other diseases not classified in subcategories 478.0 through 478.8.

## Supplementary Classifications

Two **supplementary classifications** exist in addition to the main classification for diseases and injuries. Unlike the numeric codes in the disease classification, the supplementary classifications contain alphanumeric codes.

### Supplementary Classification of Factors Influencing Health Status and Contact with Health Services (V01–V91)—V Codes

V codes consist of the alphabetic character V followed by two numeric digits, a decimal point, a fourth digit, and, where applicable, a fifth digit.

**V64 Persons encountering health services for specific procedures, not carried out**

V64.0 Vaccination not carried out
V64.00 Vaccination not carried out, unspecified reason
V64.01 Vaccination not carried out because of acute illness
V64.02 Vaccination not carried out because of chronic illness or condition
V64.03 Vaccination not carried out because of immune compromised state
V64.04 Vaccination not carried out because of allergy to vaccine or component
V64.05 Vaccination not carried out because of caregiver refusal

| | |
|---|---|
| V64.06 | Vaccination not carried out because of patient refusal |
| V64.07 | Vaccination not carried out for religious reasons |
| V64.08 | Vaccination not carried out because patient had disease being vaccinated against |
| V64.09 | Vaccination not carried out for other reasons |
| V64.1 | Surgical or other procedure not carried out because of contraindication |
| V64.2 | Surgical or other procedure not carried out because of patient's decision |
| V64.3 | Procedure not carried out for other reasons |
| V64.4 | Closed surgical procedure converted to open procedure |
| V64.41 | Laparoscopic surgical procedure converted to open procedure |
| V64.42 | Thoracoscopic surgical procedure converted to open procedure |
| V64.43 | Arthroscopic surgical procedure converted to open procedure |

### Supplementary Classification of External Causes of Injury and Poisoning (E000–E999)—E Codes

E codes consist of the alphabetic character E followed by three numeric digits, a decimal point, and a fourth digit.

| | | |
|---|---|---|
| **E953** | **Suicide and self-inflicted injury by hanging, strangulation, and suffocation** | |
| | **E953.0** | **Hanging** |
| | **E953.1** | **Suffocation by plastic bag** |
| | **E953.8** | **Other specified means** |
| | **E953.9** | **Unspecified means** |

Both supplementary classifications (E codes and V codes) are discussed in detail later in this book. E codes are discussed in Chapter 21; V codes are discussed in chapter 23.

## Appendices

Volume 1 of ICD-9-CM originally included five **appendices**. Changes in the mental disorders codes resulted in the deletion of Appendix B, Glossary of Mental Disorders in October 2004 and subsequent publications. Coders should refer to the *Diagnostic and Statistical Manual of Mental Disorders, Fifth Edition (DSM-5),* published by the American Psychiatric Association (APA), for definitions of the mental disorders classified in Chapter 5 of ICD-9-CM. DMS-5 was released by the APA at their 2013 Annual Meeting. Many ICD-9-CM book publishers have eliminated the appendices from the printed versions of the books sold. However, the appendices available on the NCHS website in the ICD-9-CM FTP files for the 2011 edition are:

### Appendix A: Morphology of Neoplasms

Appendix A includes a listing of all morphology types with the appropriate morphology, or M, code. Chapter 5 of this book describes morphology codes, or M codes, in greater detail.

### Appendix C: Classification of Drugs by the American Hospital Formulary Service List Number and Their ICD-9-CM Equivalents

The classification of drugs list by the American Hospital Formulary Service (AHFS) is published by the American Society of Hospital Pharmacists. It categorizes drugs into family-related groups. When coders must locate the category of a new drug or cannot find a new drug in the Table of Drugs and Chemicals, they turn to the AHFS list as a helpful reference. The Table of Drugs and Chemicals lists the AHFS number under the main term "Drug." Appendix C of ICD-9-CM includes a listing of the AHFS categories and the appropriate ICD-9-CM code.

### Appendix D: Classification of Industrial Accidents According to Agency

Appendix D is taken from Annex B to the Resolution concerning Statistics of Employment Injuries adopted by the Tenth International Conference of Labor Statisticians on 12 October 1962. The coding scheme identifies the type of machinery, means of transport, equipment, material, substances, radiations, and working environment involved in an industrial accident.

### Appendix E: List of Three-Digit Categories

Appendix E includes a listing of each three-digit category in ICD-9-CM, along with the appropriate title of each.

# Volume 2: Alphabetic Index to Diseases

**Volume 2** contains the following major sections:

Index to Diseases and Injuries
Table of Drugs and Chemicals
Alphabetic Index to External Causes of Injury and Poisoning (E Codes)

## Index to Diseases and Injuries

The Index to Diseases and Injuries includes the terminology for all the codes appearing in volume 1 (Tabular List) of ICD-9-CM. The Alphabetic Index employs three levels of indentations:

**Main terms**
**Subterms**
**Carryover lines**

### Main Terms

Printed in boldface type, **main terms** are set flush with the left margin of each column for easy reference. They may represent the following:

- Diseases such as influenza, bronchitis
- Conditions such as fatigue, fracture, injury
- Nouns such as disease, disturbance, syndrome
- Adjectives such as double, large, kink

Instead of a listing of subterms or codes, ICD-9-CM provides anatomical terms with a cross-reference that directs the coder to reference the condition. For example, bronchial asthma is found under the disease term "asthma" rather than the site "bronchial."

**A point to remember:** Many conditions are found in more than one place in the Alphabetic Index. For example:

- Complications of medical or surgical care are indexed under the name of the condition, as well as under the main term "Complications."
- Obstetrical conditions are found under the name of the condition and/or under main terms such as "Delivery," "Labor," "Pregnancy," and "Puerperal" (after delivery).
- Conditions that include the term *disease* or *syndrome* in their titles or descriptions may be found under "Disease" or "Syndrome," as well as under the disease or syndrome's name. For example, chronic obstructive lung disease may be found in the Alphabetic Index under "Obstructive," as well as under "Disease."

## Exercise 1.3

Using the Alphabetic Index, underline the main term in each of the following:

1. Arteriosclerotic heart disease
2. Primary hydronephrosis
3. Deviation of nasal septum
4. Inguinal adenopathy
5. Breast mass

### Subterms

Some main terms are followed by a list of indented **subterms** (modifiers) that affect the selection of an appropriate code for a given diagnosis. The subterms form individual line entries arranged in alphabetical order and printed in regular type beginning with a lowercase letter. Subterms are indented one standard indentation to the right under the main term. They describe essential differences in site, cause, or clinical type. More specific subterms are indented farther to the right as needed, indented one standard indentation after the preceding subterm, and listed in alphabetical order.

Prior to selecting a code, all subentries following the main term should be reviewed to determine the appropriate code. Note that the terms *with* and *without* are listed at the beginning of all the subterms, rather than in alphabetical order.

**Incontinence** 788.30 ← **Main Term**
  without sensory awareness 788.34
  anal sphincter 787.60 ← **Site**
  continuous leakage 788.37
  feces, fecal 787.60
    due to hysteria 300.11
    nonorganic origin 307.7
  hysterical 300.11
  mixed (male) (female) (urge and stress) 788.33

overflow 788.38
paradoxical 788.39
rectal 787.60
specified NEC 788.39
stress (female) 625.6 ← **Cause**
  male NEC 788.32
urethral sphincter 599.84
urge 788.31
  and stress (male) (female) 788.33
urine 788.30
  active 788.30 ← **Clinical Type**
  due to
    cognitive impairment 788.91
    severe physical disability 788.91
    immobility 788.91
  functional 788.91
  male 788.30
    stress 788.32
      and urge 788.33
  neurogenic 788.39
  nonorganic origin 307.6
  stress (female) 625.6
    male NEC 788.32
  urge 788.31
    and stress 788.33

### Carryover Lines

**Carryover lines** are needed because the number of words that can fit on a single line of print in the Alphabetic Index is limited. They are two indents from the preceding line. Coders must be careful to avoid confusing carryover lines with subterm entries. Careful reading is essential.

**Rubella** (German measles) 056.9
  complicating pregnancy, childbirth,
    or puerperium 647.5

## Exercise 1.4

Using the Alphabetic Index only, assign codes to the following:

1. Suppurative pancreatitis

   ______________________

2. Infectious endocarditis

   ______________________

3. Neonatal tooth eruption

   ______________________

4. Tension headache

   ______________________

5. Mitral endocarditis with active aortic disease

   ______________________

### Nonessential Modifiers

**Nonessential modifiers** are a series of terms in parentheses that sometimes directly follow main terms, as well as subterms. The presence or absence of these parenthetical terms in the diagnosis has no effect on the selection of the code listed for that main term or subterm.

**Pneumonia** (acute) (Alpenstich) (benign) (bilateral) (brain) (cerebral) (circumscribed) (congestive) (creeping) (delayed resolution) (double) (epidemic) (fever) (flash) (fulminant) (fungoid) (granulomatous) (hemorrhagic) (incipient) (infantile) (infectious) (infiltration) (insular) (intermittent) (latent) (lobe) (migratory) (newborn) (organized) (overwhelming) (primary) (progressive) (pseudolobar) (purulent) (resolved) (secondary) (senile) (septic) (suppurative) (terminal) (true) (unresolved) (vesicular) **486**

**EXAMPLE:**

1. Mike Rogers was seen by Dr. Moore and a diagnosis of congestive pneumonia was made. The appropriate code assignment is 486. ("Congestive" is a nonessential modifier.)
2. Cindy Stevens was seen by Dr. Smith and a diagnosis of pneumonia was made. The appropriate code assignment is 486. (Nonessential modifier is not stated.)

In the preceding patient examples, the presence or absence of a nonessential modifier in the diagnostic statement did not affect the code that was selected.

## Exercise 1.5

Using the Alphabetic Index only, underline the term that is the nonessential modifier in each of the following diagnostic statements and then assign a code to each condition:

1. Congenital distortion of chest wall
2. Ruptured diverticula of cecum
3. Bleeding external hemorrhoids of rectum
4. Acute urethritis
5. Surgical menopausal syndrome

### Eponyms

Many diseases and operations carry the name of a person, or an eponym. An **eponym** is defined by *Stedman's Medical Dictionary* as: "The name of a disease, structure, operation, or procedure, usually derived from the name of the person who discovered or described it first" (Stedman 2000, 611). The main terms for eponyms are located in the Alphabetic Index as follows:

1. Under the eponym itself

> **Alzheimer's**
> disease or sclerosis 331.0

2. Under main terms such as disease, syndrome, and disorder

> **Disease . . .**
> Alzheimer's—*see* Alzheimer's

3. With a description of the disease or syndrome, usually enclosed in parentheses, but sometimes following the eponym

> **Chiari's**
> disease or syndrome (hepatic vein thrombosis) 453.0

## Exercise 1.6

Using the Alphabetic Index only, assign codes to the following:

1. Lou Gehrig's disease

   ______________________

2. Sprengel's deformity

   ______________________

3. Stokes-Adams syndrome

   ______________________

4. Briquet's disorder

   ______________________

5. Erb's disease

   ______________________

## Terms Not Listed in the Tabular List

Occasionally, a diagnostic or procedure term located in the Alphabetic Index is not included in the Tabular List. In these situations, only similar terms are listed and the guidance of the Alphabetic Index should be trusted.

**EXAMPLE:** The condition ***listlessness*** is included in the Alphabetic Index with a code assignment of 780.79. In reviewing the Tabular List to verify the accuracy of the code, the following is noted:

**780.7 Malaise and fatigue**

*Excludes:* *debility, unspecified (799.3)*
*fatigue (during):*
*combat (308.0–308.9)*
*heat (992.6)*
*pregnancy (646.8)*
*neurasthenia (300.5)*
*senile asthenia (797)*

**780.71 Chronic fatigue syndrome**

**780.72 Functional quadriplegia**

Complete immobility due to severe physical disability or frailty

**780.79 Other malaise and fatigue**

Asthenia NOS
Lethargy
Postviral (asthenic) syndrome
Tiredness

Although the Alphabetic Index assigns 780.79 as the code for listlessness, that particular term is not included in the Tabular List description, but similar terms are given. Always trust the guidance of the Alphabetic Index in such cases.

### Index Tables

The following main entries in the Alphabetic Index to Diseases have subterms arranged in tables:

- Hypertension
- Neoplasm

Using tables for these terms simplifies access to complex combinations of subterms. These index tables are discussed in detail in other chapters of this book.

## Conventions in ICD-9-CM

To assign diagnostic and procedure codes accurately, a thorough understanding of ICD-9-CM conventions is necessary. All three volumes of ICD-9-CM adhere to most of the conventions addressed in the following sections, with the exception of volume 3, where slight variations occur. (Chapter 2 in this book discusses these variations.)

### Cross-Reference Terms

Cross-reference terms are used in the Alphabetic Index as directions to look elsewhere in the codebook before assigning a code. Three types of cross-reference terms appear in the Alphabetic Index: *see*, *see also*, and *see category*.

### See

The ***see*** cross-reference points to an alternative term. This mandatory instruction must be followed to ensure accurate ICD-9-CM code assignment.

> **Hemorrhage . . .**
> ulcer—*see* Ulcer, by site, with hemorrhage

In the preceding example, a code cannot be assigned until the instruction that has been provided is followed. The codes under the main term "Ulcer" must be reviewed.

Often the cross-reference *see* is found under the anatomical site, directing the coder to the condition or disease affecting that site.

> **Aorta, aortic**—*see* condition

In the preceding example, the main term "Aorta" offers the instruction to "*see* condition." Therefore, a condition affecting the aorta, such as arteriosclerosis, should be sought out. The *see* instruction also is used when a condition is indexed under more than one main term.

> **Metrorrhexis**—*see* Rupture, uterus

In the preceding example, the direction is to "*see* Rupture, uterus," for a listing of codes.

### See Also

The second type of cross-reference direction is ***see also***. This instruction requires the review of another main term in the index if all the needed information cannot be found under the first main term.

**EXAMPLE:** Patient's diagnosis is osteoarthritis, localized to the hip.

> **Osteoarthritis** (*see also* Osteoarthrosis) 715.9
> distal interphalangeal 715.9
> hyperplastic 731.2
> interspinalis (*see also* Spondylosis) 721.90
> spine, spinal NEC (*see also* Spondylosis) 721.90
> **Osteoarthrosis** (degenerative) (hypertrophic)
> (rheumatoid) 715.9
>
> *Note—Use the following fifth-digit subclassification with category 715:*
>
> *0 site unspecified*
> *1 shoulder region*
> *2 upper arm*
> *3 forearm*
> *4 hand*
> *5 pelvic region and thigh*
> *6 lower leg*
> *7 ankle and foot*
> *8 other specified sites except spine*
> *9 multiple sites*

deformans alkaptonuria 270.2
generalized 715.09
juvenilis (Kohler's) 732.5
localized 715.3
  idiopathic 715.1
  primary 715.1
  secondary 715.2

In the preceding example, the coder is instructed to "*see also* Osteoarthrosis." But first, the subterms under osteoarthritis would have to be reviewed to find an entry titled "localized." If that subterm were found, the code provided after it would be assigned. When the subterm is not found—as is the case in the preceding example—the next step is to turn to the main term "Osteoarthrosis" in the index and review its subterms to find an entry of "localized." When that entry is found, code 715.3 can be selected. The boxed note appearing under the main term "Osteoarthrosis" reminds the coder that a fifth digit is required. The final code assignment is 715.35.

### See Category

The ***see category*** is the least-used cross-reference in the Alphabetic Index. It is an instruction to consult a specific category in volume 1 (Tabular List).

**Late**—*see also* condition
  effect(s) (of)—*see also* condition
    abscess
      intracranial or intraspinal (conditions
        classifiable to 324)—*see* category 326

The *see category* instruction in the preceding example refers to category 326, which provides additional information on the coding of late effects of intracranial abscess or pyogenic infection.

## Exercise 1.7

Review each diagnostic statement and underline the appropriate main term. Locate the main term in the Alphabetic Index and follow all cross-references. Confirm the code in the Tabular List and enter it on the line provided.

1. Acute endomyometritis

2. Metrorrhexis, nontraumatic

3. Cervical intervertebral disc prolapse

4. Localized osteoarthritis, shoulder

5. Stenosis of endocervical os

## Instructional Notations

Occasionally, instructional notations appear throughout the Tabular List to clarify information or provide additional information. The following subsections describe the various types of instructional notes.

### Includes Notes

**Inclusion (or includes) notes** are used throughout the Tabular List to further define or provide an example of a category or section. The conditions may be synonyms or similar conditions that may be classifiable to the same code. It is important to note that inclusion notes are not exhaustive; that is, not every synonym or similar condition may be listed. The notes usually list other common phrases used to describe the same condition.

Inclusion notes can appear at the beginning of a chapter or section, or directly below a category or subcategory code.

**At the beginning of a chapter or section:** The instructions apply to all the codes within that chapter or section.

The following inclusion note appears at the beginning of a chapter:

> **INFECTIOUS AND PARASITIC DISEASES (001–139)**
> Includes: diseases generally recognized as communicable or transmissible
> as well as a few diseases of unknown, but possibly infectious, origin

The following inclusion note appears at the beginning of a section:

> **ISCHEMIC HEART DISEASE (410–414)**
> Includes: that with mention of hypertension

**Directly below a category or a subcategory code:** The instructions in the inclusion note apply to all codes within that range.

The following inclusion note appears below a category:

> **461 Acute sinusitis**
> Includes: abscess, acute, of sinus (accessory) (nasal)
> empyema, acute, of sinus (accessory) (nasal)
> infection, acute, of sinus (accessory) (nasal)
> inflammation, acute, of sinus (accessory) (nasal)
> suppuration, acute, of sinus (accessory) (nasal)

**A point to remember:** Because the inclusion note is not repeated, the coder must look back to the beginning of the subcategory, category, section, or chapter to ensure that important instructions are not missed.

### Excludes Notes

**The exclusion (or excludes) notes** found in the Tabular List are hard to miss on review because the word *Excludes* appears in italicized print with a box around it. Exclusion notes can appear at the beginning of a chapter or section, or below a category, subcategory, or subclassification.

Essentially, exclusion notes should be interpreted as a direction to code the particular condition listed elsewhere, usually with the code listed in the exclusion note.

Exclusion terms have three different meanings:

1. The most common exclusion note indicates that the code under consideration cannot be assigned if the associated condition specified in the exclusion note is present. Rather, the code specified in the exclusion note is assigned to fully identify the condition.

> **424.3 Pulmonary valve disorders**
>
> Pulmonic:
> incompetence NOS
> insufficiency NOS
>
> Pulmonic:
> regurgitation NOS
> stenosis NOS
>
> *Excludes:* *that specified as rheumatic (397.1)*

The exclusion note indicates that code 397.1, rather than code 424.3, should be assigned if the pulmonary valve disorder is specified as rheumatic.

2. The second type of exclusion note indicates that the condition may have to be coded elsewhere. The etiology of the condition determines whether the code under review or the code suggested in the exclusion note should be assigned. One or the other code is used, but not both.

> **603 Hydrocele**
>
> Includes: hydrocele of spermatic cord, testis, or tunica vaginalis
>
> *Excludes:* *congenital (778.6)*

The exclusion note indicates that a code from category 603, Hydrocele, should not be assigned if the hydrocele is congenital. Instead, code 778.6, Congenital hydrocele, is assigned.

3. The third type of exclusion note indicates that an additional code may be required to fully explain the condition. This note specifies conditions that are not included in the code under review. Should the condition specified in the exclusion note be present, the additional code should be assigned.

> **4. DISEASES OF THE BLOOD AND BLOOD-FORMING ORGANS (280–289)**
>
> *Excludes:* *anemia complicating pregnancy or the puerperium (648.2)*

The exclusion note indicates that two codes should be assigned to code an anemia that occurs during pregnancy or the puerperium: code 648.2x, Anemia in the mother classifiable elsewhere but complicating pregnancy, childbirth, or the puerperium, to indicate that the anemia is occurring during pregnancy; and a code from Chapter 4, Diseases of the Blood and Blood-Forming Organs (280–289), to indicate the specific type of anemia.

## Exercise 1.8

Answer the following questions:

1. According to the inclusion note in category 056, what condition is included in codes 056.0–056.9?

   ___

2. According to the inclusion note in category 555, what conditions are included in codes 555.0–555.9?

   ___

3. According to the exclusion note in category 558, what condition is assigned codes 009.2–009.3?

   ___

4. Which site is excluded from code 213.0?

   ___

5. According to the exclusion note in category 056, what condition is assigned code 771.0?

   ___

### Notes

**Notes** appear in the Tabular List and the Alphabetic Index in all three volumes of ICD-9-CM. Some notes carry an instruction to assign a fifth digit.

In the Tabular List:

**831 Dislocation of shoulder**

*Excludes:* *sternoclavicular joint (839.61, 839.71)*
*sternum (839.61, 839.71)*

The following fifth-digit subclassification is for use with category 831:

**0 shoulder, unspecified**
Humerus NOS
**1 anterior dislocation of humerus**
**2 posterior dislocation of humerus**
**3 inferior dislocation of humerus**
**4 acromioclavicular (joint)**
Clavicle
**9 other**
Scapula

Other notes provide additional coding instruction and also define terms.
In the Alphabetic Index:

**Injury** 959.9

*Note—For abrasion, insect bite (nonvenomous), blister, or scratch, see Injury, superficial.*

*For laceration, traumatic rupture, tear, or penetrating wound of internal organs, such as heart, lung, liver, kidney, pelvic organs, whether or not accompanied by open wound in the same region, see Injury, internal.*

*For nerve injury, see Injury, nerve.*

*For late effect of injuries, classifiable to 850–854, 860–869, 900–919, 950–959, see Late, effect, injury, by type.*

In the Tabular List:

**326 Late effects of intracranial abscess or pyogenic infection**

Note: This category is to be used to indicate conditions whose primary classification is to 320–325 [excluding 320.7, 321.0–321.8, 323.01–323.42, 323.61–323.72] as the cause of late effects, themselves classifiable elsewhere. The "late effects" include conditions specified as such, or as sequelae, which may occur at any time after the resolution of the causal condition.

Use additional code to identify condition, as:
hydrocephalus (331.4)
paralysis (342.0–342.9, 344.0–344.9)

In the Tabular List:

**765.0 Extreme immaturity**

Note: Usually implies a birth weight of less than 1,000 g. Use additional code for weeks of gestation (765.20–765.29).

**A point to remember:** The appearance of a note differs depending on the volume of ICD-9-CM in which it is located. Alphabetic Index notes are boxed and set in italic type. Tabular List notes are located at various levels of the classification system and are not boxed.

## Exercise 1.9

Use the Tabular List and Alphabetic Index to answer the following questions:

1. According to the note under code 766.0, what is considered an exceptionally large baby?

2. What do the fifth digits in category 832 indicate?

3. Use the Alphabetic Index and the note following the main term "Injury" to answer this question: What main term and subterm should be indexed to code the diagnosis of nonvenomous insect bite?

4. Turn to category 250, Diabetes mellitus. What is the appropriate fifth digit for uncontrolled type I diabetes?

5. Use the Alphabetic Index and the note following the main term "Fracture" to answer this question: Is a greenstick fracture open or closed?

## Multiple Coding

In ICD-9-CM, it often is necessary to use more than one code number to fully identify a given condition. A diagnostic statement that includes phrases such as "due to," "secondary to," or "with" may require multiple codes. The coder should follow the directions in the Tabular List for the use of additional codes. The Alphabetic Index may refer the coder to a **combination code** through the use of connecting terms. When no combination codes are available, multiple codes should be assigned to fully describe the condition.

### *Mandatory Multiple Coding*

Certain conditions require **mandatory multiple coding**. In such cases, one code describes the underlying condition (cause or etiology of the condition) and the other identifies the manifestation(s). Mandatory multiple coding is identified in the Alphabetic Index with the second code listed in brackets. The first code identifies the underlying condition, and the second code identifies the manifestations or other conditions that occur as a result of the underlying condition. In such cases, both codes must be assigned and sequenced in the order listed in the Alphabetic Index.

In the Tabular List, mandatory multiple coding is indicated by the phrase "use additional code" and the code for the underlying condition. The manifestation code acknowledges the need for multiple codes with the phrase "code first underlying condition." The manifestation codes and the titles are listed in italic print. The codes in italic print can never be designated as principal diagnoses and always require a code for the underlying condition to be listed first.

**EXAMPLE:** Type I diabetes (not stated as uncontrolled) with diabetic retinopathy
Alphabetic Index:
Diabetes, diabetic
Retinopathy 250.5 *[362.01]*

In this example the diabetes is the underlying condition, and the retinopathy is the condition that occurs as a result of the diabetes. Referring to the Tabular List and category 250, Diabetes mellitus, the coder would assign as the diagnosis codes:

1. Diabetes with ophthalmic manifestations, Type I, 250.51
2. Diabetic retinopathy, 362.01

### Indiscriminate Multiple Coding

Multiple codes should not be used to code irrelevant medical information, such as certain signs and symptoms that are integral to a condition. The signs and symptoms that are characteristic of an illness are not coded when the causes of the signs or symptoms are known. For example, abdominal pain is integral to acute appendicitis and thus is not coded.

**Indiscriminate coding** of conditions listed in diagnostic test reports should be avoided. When a laboratory test, x-ray, EKG (electrocardiogram), or other diagnostic test includes a finding, that condition is not coded unless the diagnosis is confirmed by the physician.

Coders should follow the Uniform Hospital Discharge Data Set (UHDDS) criteria when reporting additional diagnoses. Often diagnostic reports mention conditions such as atelectasis, hiatal hernias, or nonspecific cardiac arrhythmias with no other information in the record as to treatment or evaluation. Assigning a code for such conditions would be inappropriate without first consulting with the physician.

Finally, coding both an unspecified and a specified type of condition is usually not done to describe the same general condition. For example, a patient with chronic maxillary sinusitis would not be identified with both codes 473.0, Chronic sinusitis, maxillary, and 473.9, Unspecified sinusitis (chronic). Code 473.0 is more specific, fully describing the patient's condition, and should be assigned.

### Use Additional Code

The instructional notation "**Use additional code**" is found in the Tabular List of ICD-9-CM. This notation indicates that use of an additional code may provide a more complete picture of the diagnosis or procedure. The additional code should always be assigned if the health record provides supportive documentation.

If this instruction appears at the beginning of a chapter, it applies to all the codes in that chapter.

**8. DISEASES OF THE RESPIRATORY SYSTEM (460–519)**

Use additional code to identify infectious organism.

Sometimes it appears at the beginning of a section.

**INFLAMMATORY DISEASE OF FEMALE PELVIC ORGANS (614–616)**

Use additional code to identify organism such as *Staphylococcus* (041.1), or *Streptococcus* (041.0).

Finally, it also may appear in a subcategory.

**530.2 Ulcer of esophagus**

Ulcer of esophagus:
fungal
peptic

Ulcer of esophagus due to ingestion of:
aspirin
chemicals
medicines

Use additional E code to identify cause, if induced by chemical or drug

## Code First Underlying Disease

The instruction "**Code first underlying disease**" is found in the Tabular List for categories in which primary tabulation (listing the code first) is *not* intended. (See the subsection on mandatory multiple coding.) The code, title, and instructions are set in italic type to serve as a red flag not to assign that code as a principal diagnosis. The note requires listing the code for the underlying disease (etiology) first and the code for the manifestation second. Although the note will suggest underlying diseases in most instances, it is not all-inclusive because the physician may identify other causes not included in the list.

**366.4 Cataract associated with other disorders**

***366.41 Diabetic cataract***
*Code first diabetes (249.5, 250.5)*

***366.42 Tetanic cataract***
*Code first underlying disease, as:*
calcinosis (275.40)
hypoparathyroidism (252.1)

***366.43 Myotonic cataract***
*Code first underlying disorder (359.21, 359.23)*

***366.44 Cataract associated with other syndromes***
*Code first underlying condition, as:*
craniofacial dysostosis (756.0)
galactosemia (271.1)

**366.45 Toxic cataract**
Drug-induced cataract
Use additional E code to identify drug or other toxic substance

**366.46 Cataract associated with radiation and other physical influences**
Use additional E code to identify cause

## Connecting Words

**Connecting words or connecting terms** are subterms that indicate a relationship between the main term and an associated condition or etiology in the Alphabetic Index. Following are examples of these subterms:

| | | |
|---|---|---|
| Associated with | During | Secondary to |
| Complicated (by) | Following | With |
| Due to | In | With mention of |
| Of | Without | |

**A point to remember:** The connecting words "with" and "without" are sequenced before all other subterms. Other connecting words are listed in alphabetical order.

ICD-9-CM assumes a causal relationship between some combinations of conditions, even though the diagnostic statement may not make such a distinction.

**EXAMPLE:** Mitral valve stenosis is assumed to be rheumatic in origin and is assigned code 394.0, Mitral stenosis, from the chronic rheumatic heart disease section.

For cases where conditions often occur together, ICD-9-CM developed combination codes to identify both the etiology and the manifestation.

**EXAMPLE:** Streptococcal infection occurs often in the throat resulting in streptococcal sore throat. Therefore, code 034.0, Streptococcal sore throat, incorporates both the underlying disease, the streptococcal infection, and the manifestation—the sore throat.

## Exercise 1.10

Using the Tabular List and Alphabetic Index, assign codes to the following:

1. Rheumatic chorea without mention of heart involvement

   ______

2. Bleeding esophageal varices in liver cirrhosis

   ______

3. Acute duodenal ulcer with hemorrhage and obstruction

   ______

4. Anemia of prematurity

   ______

5. Urinary tract infection due to *Escherichia coli*

   ______

## Abbreviations and Punctuation Marks

ICD-9-CM uses abbreviations and punctuation marks to facilitate the coding process.

## Abbreviations

Two abbreviations are used in ICD-9-CM:

- **NEC: Not elsewhere classifiable**
- **NOS: Not otherwise specified**

### NEC: Not Elsewhere Classifiable

**NEC** serves two purposes. First, it can be used with ill-defined terms listed in the Tabular List to warn the user that specified forms of the condition are classified differently. The codes given for such terms should be used only if more precise information is unavailable.

> **459.0 Hemorrhage, unspecified**
> Rupture of blood vessel, not otherwise specified (NOS)
> Spontaneous hemorrhage, not elsewhere classified (NEC)
>
> *Excludes:* *hemorrhage:*
> *gastrointestinal NOS (578.9)*
> *in newborn NOS (772.9)*
> *nontraumatic hematoma of soft tissue (729.92)*
> *secondary or recurrent following trauma (958.2)*
> *traumatic rupture of blood vessel (900.0–904.9)*

The material in the preceding example advises to assign code 459.0 only if no other information is available. Furthermore, the exclusion note indicates that other forms of hemorrhage, such as gastrointestinal hemorrhage, NOS (578.9), are classified elsewhere.

Second, NEC can be used with terms for which a more specific code is unavailable, even though the diagnostic statement is very specific.

> **008.67 Enteritis due to Enterovirus NEC**
> Coxsackie virus
> Echovirus
>
> *Excludes:* *poliovirus (045.0–045.9)*

In this example, code 008.67 is reported even if a specific enterovirus such as echovirus has been identified because ICD-9-CM does not provide a specific code for it.

### NOS: Not Otherwise Specified

**NOS** is the equivalent of "unspecified." It is used only in the Tabular Lists for both diseases and procedures. Codes describing "not otherwise specified" conditions or procedures are assigned only when the diagnostic or procedural statement, as well as the health record, does not provide enough information.

> **382.9 Unspecified otitis media**
> Otitis media:
> NOS
> acute NOS
> chronic NOS

In the preceding example, code 382.9 is the appropriate code assignment because the diagnostic statement and/or the health record lack(s) additional information, such as purulent or serous.

## Punctuation Marks

ICD-9-CM contains five punctuation marks with specialized meanings.

### Parentheses ( )

**Parentheses** enclose supplementary words or explanatory information that may or may not be present in the statement of a diagnosis or procedure. They do not affect the code number assigned to the case. Terms in parentheses are considered **nonessential modifiers**, and all three volumes of ICD-9-CM use them.

**494 Bronchiectasis**
Bronchiectasis (fusiform) (postinfectious) (recurrent)
Bronchiolectasis
*Excludes:* *congenital (748.61)*
*tuberculous bronchiectasis (current disease) (011.5)*

In the preceding example, category 494 includes three nonessential modifiers enclosed in parentheses: fusiform, postinfectious, and recurrent. The presence or absence of these modifiers in the diagnostic statement has no bearing on the assignment of code 494.

### Square Brackets [ ]

**Square brackets** are used to enclose synonyms, alternative wordings, abbreviations, and explanatory phrases. In effect, they are similar to parentheses in that they are not required as part of the diagnostic or procedural statement. Square brackets are used for both diseases and procedures, but only in the Tabular Lists.

**427.0 Paroxysmal supraventricular tachycardia**
Paroxysmal tachycardia:
atrial [PAT]
atrioventricular [AV]
junctional
nodal

Because they are abbreviations, PAT (paroxysmal atrial tachycardia) and AV (atrioventricular) are enclosed in brackets.

**460 Acute nasopharyngitis [common cold]**
Coryza (acute)
Nasal catarrh, acute
Nasopharyngitis:
NOS
Acute
Infective, NOS
Rhinitis:
acute
infective

In the preceding example, the phrase "common cold" is a synonym for acute nasopharyngitis and is enclosed in brackets.

### Slanted Brackets *[ ]*

**Slanted, or italicized, brackets** are found only in the Alphabetic Index. They enclose a code number that must be used in conjunction with a code immediately preceding it. Thus, the code in the slanted brackets is always sequenced second.

In the Alphabetic Index to Diseases, the first code represents the underlying condition and the second code, enclosed in italicized brackets, is the manifestation.

**Nephritis, nephritic**
due to systemic lupus erythematosus 710.0 *[583.81]*

The coding and sequencing of the preceding example is as follows:

1. Systemic lupus erythematosus, 710.0
2. Nephritis and nephropathy, not specified as acute or chronic, in disease classified elsewhere, 583.81

### Colon :

The **colon** is used in the Tabular List after an incomplete term that needs one or more modifiers in order to be assigned to a given category or code.

**204 Lymphoid leukemia**

| Includes: | leukemia: | leukemia: |
|---|---|---|
| | lymphatic | lymphocytic |
| | lymphoblastic | lymphogenous |

In the preceding example, the colon indicates that the type of leukemia must be lymphatic, lymphoblastic, lymphocytic, or lymphogenous to be assigned a code from category 204.

### Exercise 1.11

Using the Tabular List and Alphabetic Index, assign codes to the following:

1. Anterolateral wall myocardial infarction, initial episode

2. Angiodysplasia of stomach and duodenum, no hemorrhage noted

3. Primary malignant neoplasm of the spleen

4. Tuberculous iritis

5. Fifth disease

## Basic Steps in ICD-9-CM Coding

To code each disease or condition completely and accurately, the coder should:

1. Identify all main terms included in the diagnostic statement
2. Locate each main term in the Alphabetic Index
3. Refer to any subterms indented under the main term. The subterms form individual line entries and describe essential differences by site, etiology, or clinical type
4. Follow cross-reference instructions if the needed code is not located under the first main entry consulted
5. Verify the code selected in the Tabular List
6. Read and be guided by any instructional terms in the Tabular List
7. Assign codes to their highest level of specificity
    - Assign three-digit codes only when no four-digit codes appear within the category
    - Assign a fifth digit for any subcategory where a fifth-digit subclassification is provided
8. Continue coding the diagnostic statement until all the component elements are fully identified

## Review Exercises: Chapter 1

Using the instructions and conventions introduced in this chapter, assign the appropriate codes to the following:

1. Carotid artery occlusion with cerebral infarction; essential hypertension
2. Streptococcal pneumonia
3. Acute appendicitis with perforation
4. Acute cor pulmonale
5. Chest pain, originating in chest wall
6. Toxic nodular goiter with crisis
7. Osteoarthrosis, localized, primary of ankle
8. Angiodysplasia of the colon with hemorrhage
9. Extra thyroid gland
10. Arteriosclerotic heart disease of native coronary artery with stable angina
11. Acute tracheobronchitis with bronchospasm
12. Prenatal care, normal first pregnancy
13. Nephrotic syndrome secondary to systemic lupus erythematosus
14. Prostatitis due to *Trichomonas*
15. Comminuted fracture of femur involving the subtrochanteric section

# Introduction to ICD-10-CM

ICD-10-CM is a classification system that depends on its users understanding the system's organization and rules. Two essential documents are required reading each year by all coders: the *ICD-10-CM Official Guidelines for Coding and Reporting* and the Official Addendum for ICD-10-CM. Members of the Cooperating Parties for the ICD-10-CM develop these documents and participate in the ICD-10-CM Coordination and Maintenance Committees meetings twice a year. The following sections explain the content and structure of ICD-10-CM.

## ICD-10-CM Official Guidelines for Coding and Reporting

*ICD-10-CM Official Guidelines for Coding and Reporting* should be used in conjunction with the official version of the ICD-10-CM as published on the NCHS website. These guidelines have been approved by the **Cooperating Parties for the ICD-10-CM** that includes representatives from the American Hospital Association (AHA), the American Health Information Management Association (AHIMA), the Centers for Medicare and Medicaid Services (CMS), and NCHS.

These guidelines are a set of coding rules that accompany and complement the official conventions and instructions provided within the ICD-10-CM code set. The instructions and conventions in the ICD-10-CM classification take precedence over the guidelines. The guidelines provide additional instruction for the coder and are based on the coding and sequencing instructions in the Tabular List and Alphabetic Index of ICD-10-CM.

The Health Insurance Portability and Accountability Act (HIPAA) requires all coders adhere to these guidelines when assigning ICD-10-CM diagnosis codes. The diagnosis codes have been adopted under HIPAA for all healthcare settings.

The guidelines have been developed to identify the diagnoses and procedures that are to be reported. The importance of consistent, complete documentation in the health record cannot be overemphasized.

The conventions, general guidelines, and chapter-specific ICD-10-CM guidelines are applicable to all healthcare settings unless otherwise indicated. The guidelines for the principal and additional diagnoses are only applicable to the inpatient settings.

The *ICD-10-CM Official Guidelines for Coding and Reporting* is referenced throughout this chapter. You can find the complete document in Appendix I.

## Official Addendum to ICD-10-CM and ICD-10-PCS

In contrast to international ICD updates that occur less frequently, ICD-10-CM/PCS undergoes annual updates in the United States to remain current. Codes may be added, revised, or deleted. An ***Official Addendum*** documents the changes, which are effective April 1 and October 1 of each year. The addendum may be found at the NCHS's website (http://www.cdc.gov/nchs/icd/icd10cm.htm). CMS and NCHS publish the addenda with the approval of the World Health Organization (WHO). NCHS is responsible for maintaining the diagnosis classification; CMS is responsible for maintaining the procedure classification. AHIMA and AHA give advice and assistance, as do health information management (HIM) practitioners, physicians, and other users of ICD-10-CM/PCS.

### *Coordination and Maintenance Committee*

The **ICD-10-CM Coordination and Maintenance (C&M) Committee** is chaired by a representative from the NCHS and a representative from CMS. The committee is responsible for maintaining the United States' clinical modification version of the ICD-10-CM/PCS code sets. The Coordination and Maintenance Committee holds two open meetings each year that serve as a public forum for discussing (but not making decisions about) proposed revisions to ICD-10-CM/PCS. Information about the ICD-10-CM/PCS Coordination and Maintenance Committee, including meeting minutes, can be found at http://www.cdc.gov/nchs/icd/icd9cm.htm and at http://www.cms.gov/Medicare/Coding/ICD9ProviderDiagnosticCodes/meetings.html.

## Characteristics of ICD-10-CM

The ICD-10-CM system is expected to be used for all diagnosis coding beginning on October 1, 2015. The system is more extensive and specific than ICD-9-CM, but much of the hierarchical structure and conventions are similar. ICD-10-CM is divided into the Alphabetic Index, which is an alphabetic listing of terms and codes, and the Tabular List, which is a numerical list of the codes divided by chapters.

## Conventions for ICD-10-CM

To assign ICD-10-CM codes accurately, a thorough understanding of the ICD-10-CM conventions is necessary. These coding conventions address the structure and format of the coding system, including how to use the Alphabetic Index and the Tabular List, as well as the rules and instructions that the coder must follow.

### *Alphabetic Index*

The **Alphabetic Index** is divided into two parts—the Index to Diseases and Injury and the Index to External Causes of Injury. Within the Index of Diseases and Injury there is a Neoplasm Table and a Table of Drugs and Chemicals.

The Alphabetic Index in ICD-10-CM is formatted with main terms set in boldface and listed in alphabetical order. **Main terms** are entries printed in boldface type and flush with the left margin of each column in the Alphabetic Index. Main terms represent diseases, conditions, nouns, and adjectives. This is the first place the coder uses to locate the ICD-10-CM code for the patient's disease or condition. Indented beneath the main term, any applicable subterm or essential modifier is shown in their own alphabetic list. The indented subterm is always read in combination with the main term. The dash ( - ) at the end of an Index entry indicates that additional characters are required.

#### Nonessential Modifiers

A term or a series of terms that appear in parentheses following a main term or subterm are known as **nonessential modifiers**. The presence or absence of these parenthetical terms in the diagnosis statement has no effect on the selection of the codes listed for that main term or subterm.

#### "See" and "See Also" Instructions

The Alphabetic Index in ICD-10-CM includes both "see" and "see also" instructions following a main term to indicate that another term should be referenced.

The **"see" note** is a cross-reference term in the Alphabetic Index to Diseases and Injuries that provides direction to the coder to look elsewhere in the Index before assigning a code. The "see" cross-reference points to an alternative term. This is a mandatory instruction that must be followed to ensure accurate ICD-10-CM code assignment.

The **"see also" note** in the Alphabetic Index to Disease and Injuries provides direction to the coder to look elsewhere in the Index. It requires the review of another term in the Index if all the needed information cannot be found under the first main term. However, it is not necessary to follow the *see also* note when the original main term provides the necessary code.

**EXAMPLE:** **Aberrant (congenital)—see also Malposition, congenital**
-adrenal gland Q89.1
-artery (peripheral) Q27.8
---basilar NEC Q28.1
---cerebral Q28.3

### "Code Also" Note

The **"code also" note** appears in ICD-10-CM, meaning that two codes may be required to fully describe a condition, but this note does not provide sequencing direction.

The ICD-10-CM Alphabetic Index includes manifestation of disease codes by including the manifestation code as the second code, shown in brackets, directly after the underlying or etiology code, which should always be reported first.

**EXAMPLES:** **Dementia**
-with
---Parkinson's disease G20 *[F02.80]*
**Retinitis**
-renal N18.9 *[H32]*
-syphilitic
--congenital (early) A50.01 *[H32]*

### Default Code

ICD-10-CM refers to the code listed next to a main term in the Alphabetic Index as a **default code**. The default code represents the condition that is most commonly associated with the main term, or is the unspecified code for the condition. If a condition is documented in the medical record without any additional information, such as whether it is acute or chronic, the default code should be assigned.

### Tabular List

The ICD-10-CM **Tabular List** is a numerical listing of all the codes. The Tabular List is divided into 21 chapters. For some chapters, the body or organ system is the axis of the classification. Other chapters, such as Chapter 1, Certain Infectious and Parasitic Diseases, group together conditions by etiology or nature of the disease process.

The 21 chapters of the ICD-10-CM classification system are as follows:

1. Certain infectious and parasitic diseases (A00–B99)
2. Neoplasms (C00–D49)
3. Diseases of the blood and blood-forming organs and certain disorders involving the immune mechanism (D50–D89)
4. Endocrine, nutritional and metabolic disorders (E00–E89)
5. Mental, behavioral and neurodevelopmental disorders (F01–F99)
6. Diseases of the nervous system (G00–G99)

7. Diseases of the eye and adnexa (H00–H59)
8. Diseases of the ear and mastoid process (H60–H95)
9. Diseases of the circulatory system (I00–I99)
10. Diseases of the respiratory system (J00–J99)
11. Diseases of the digestive system (K00–K95)
12. Diseases of the skin and subcutaneous tissue (L00–L99)
13. Diseases of the musculoskeletal system and connective tissue (M00–M99)
14. Diseases of the genitourinary system (N00–N99)
15. Pregnancy, childbirth and the puerperium (O00–O9A)
16. Certain conditions originating in the perinatal period (P00–P96)
17. Congenital malformations, deformations and chromosomal abnormalities (Q00–Q99)
18. Symptoms, signs and abnormal clinical and laboratory findings, not elsewhere classified (R00–R99)
19. Injury, poisoning and certain other consequences of external causes (S00–T88)
20. External causes of morbidity (V00–Y99)
21. Factors influencing health status and contact with health services (Z00–Z99)

Each chapter in the Tabular List of ICD-10-CM begins with a summary of the blocks to provide an overview of the categories within the chapter.

## Code Format and Structure

The ICD-10-CM Coding Guidelines state the ICD-10-CM contains chapters, categories, subcategories, and codes. Chapters are further subdivided into subchapters (blocks) and subcategories that contain three character categories and form the foundation of the code.

### Categories, Subcategories, and Codes

The characters for categories, subcategories, and codes may contain either letters or numbers. All categories are three characters. A three-character category that has no further subdivision is equivalent to a code.

Most three-character categories are further subdivided into four- or five-character subcategories. Codes can be three, four, five, six, or seven characters. Each level of subdivision after a category is a subcategory. Five- and six-character codes provide greater specificity or additional information about the condition being coded.

The final level of subdivision of a category is a code. Certain categories have an additional seventh character. The seventh character must always be the final character of the code. When the code contains fewer than seven characters, the placeholder X must be used to fill the empty character(s).

The fourth character 8, when placed after a decimal point (.8), is used to indicate some "other" specified category. The fourth character 9, when placed after a decimal point (.9), is usually reserved for an unspecified condition. In ICD-10-CM, the "other specified" and "unspecified" conditions each have their own code and are not combined into one code.

### First Character

The first character of an ICD-10-CM code is always an alphabetic letter. All the letters of the alphabet are utilized with the exception of the letter U. The letter U has been reserved by WHO for the provisional assignment of new diseases of uncertain etiology (U00–U49) and for bacterial agents resistant to antibiotics (U80–U89.) ICD-10-CM codes may consist of up to seven characters and are formatted as shown in figure 1.1.

**Figure 1.1.** ICD-10-CM code format

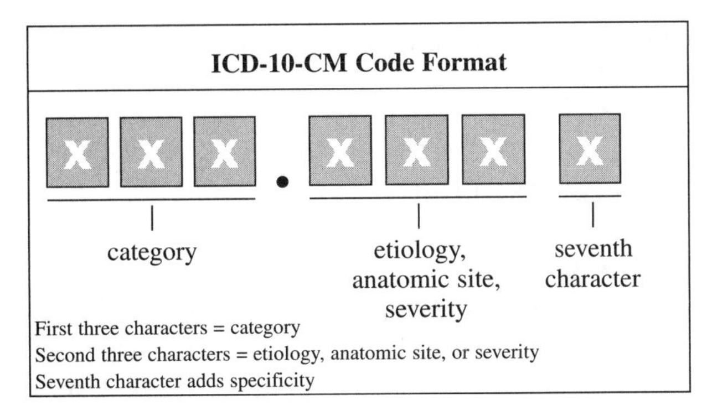


### Placeholder Character

ICD-10-CM utilizes a placeholder character, which is always the letter X, and it has two uses:

1. The X provides for future expansion without disturbing the overall code structure.

   **EXAMPLE:** T42.3X1A, Poisoning by barbiturates, accidental, initial encounter

2. It is also used when a code has less than six characters and a seventh character extension is required. The X is assigned for all characters less than six in order to meet the requirement of coding to the highest level of specificity.

   **EXAMPLE:** T58.11XA, Toxic effect of carbon monoxide from utility gas, accidental, initial encounter

### Seventh Character

Certain ICD-10-CM categories have applicable seventh characters. The applicable seventh character is required for all codes within the category, or as the notes in the Tabular List instruct. The seventh character must always be the seventh character in the data field. If a code that requires a seventh character does not contain six characters, a placeholder X must be used to fill in the empty characters.

**EXAMPLES:** O40.1XXA, Polyhydramnios, first trimester, fetus 1
S02.65XA, Fracture of angle of mandible

To summarize the code format and structure of ICD-10-CM, the following facts are presented:

- ICD-10-CM codes consist of three to seven characters
- The first character of an ICD-10-CM code is always an alphabetic character
- All letters are used except U in the ICD-10-CM codes

- The second character of the ICD-10-CM code is always numeric
- Characters 3 through 7 of ICD-10-CM can be alphabetic or numeric
- A decimal is placed after the first three characters of an ICD-10-CM code
- Alpha characters used in the ICD-10-CM codes are not case-sensitive
- Only complete ICD-10-CM codes are used for reporting purposes, not categories or subcategories
- When a seventh character is required but there is less than six characters, the X must be used as a placeholder for the ICD-10-CM code to be valid

## Abbreviations

Two abbreviations are used in ICD-10-CM:

### NEC: Not Elsewhere Classifiable

An abbreviation of **not elsewhere classifiable (NEC)** is used in ICD-10-CM. This abbreviation appears in the Alphabetic Index. When NEC appears in the Alphabetic Index, it will direct the coder to the Tabular List showing an "other specified" codes description. The NEC entry appears when a specific code is not available. The NEC code usually directs the coder to an "other specified" code in the Tabular List that includes the number 8 after the decimal point.

**EXAMPLES:** K65.8, Other peritonitis
N30.80, Other cystitis without hematuria

### NOS: Not Otherwise Specified

The abbreviation of **not otherwise specified (NOS)** is the equivalent of unspecified. The abbreviation "NOS" appears in the Alphabetic Index and the Tabular List. The unspecified or NOS codes are available for use when the documentation of the condition identified by the provider in the health record does not provide enough information to assign a more specific code.

**EXAMPLES:** I50.9, Heart failure, unspecified
L02.93, Carbuncle, unspecified

## Punctuation

The punctuation used in ICD-10-CM is brackets, parentheses, and colons.

### Brackets [ ]

**Square brackets [ ]** are a punctuation mark used in the Tabular List to enclose synonyms, abbreviations, alternative wording, or explanatory phrases. The terms within the brackets are presented for informational purposes. The words within the square brackets are not required to be part of the diagnostic statement to use the code. **Slanted brackets *[ ]*** are used in the Alphabetic Index to identify manifestation codes. Manifestation codes represent the secondary condition that is present in addition to the underlying or primary disease that caused the secondary condition. Two codes are required when the patient has both the underlying disease and the secondary condition. The use of the slanted bracket in the Alphabetic Index provides sequencing direction. The code that appears in the slanted bracket is listed in the second position or follows the disease code listed directly after the diagnosis term in the Index. The diagnosis in the slanted brackets is not entered into a computer or data entry system in the italicized font. The italicized font is used to emphasize the presence of the second code that is required.

**EXAMPLES:** Tabular List:

B20, Human immunodeficiency virus [HIV] disease

The HIV that appears in the brackets is an abbreviation for human immunodeficiency virus.

Alphabetic Index:

Amyloid heart (disease) E85.4 *[I43]*

For amyloid heart disease, two codes are required in the following order or sequence:

E85.4 Organ-limited amyloidosis

*I43 Cardiomyopathy in diseases classified elsewhere*

### Parentheses ( )

**Parentheses** are a punctuation mark that encloses supplementary words or explanatory information that may or may not be present in the statement of a diagnosis. The words within the parentheses do not affect the code assigned to the condition. Terms in parentheses are considered nonessential modifiers and appear in both the Alphabetic Index and the Tabular List.

**EXAMPLES:** Alphabetic Index:

Amputee (bilateral) (old) Z89.9

The diagnosis statement could be amputee, bilateral amputee, old amputee or old bilateral amputee and the code would be the same for all: Z89.9.

Tabular List:

C83.5 Lymphoblastic (diffuse) lymphoma

The diagnosis statement could be lymphoblastic lymphoma or lymphoblastic diffuse lymphoma and the code would be the same for both: C83.5.

### Colon :

The **colon** is a punctuation term that is used in the Tabular List after an incomplete term that needs one or more additional terms in order to be assigned to a particular code.

In the official ICD-10-CM electronic version, the colon is used with "includes" and "excludes" notes, in which the words that precede the colon are not considered complete terms and must be appended by one of the modifiers indented under the statement before the condition can be assigned the correct code. Other publishers of the printed version of the ICD-10-CM codes have not used the colon punctuation with the "includes" and "excludes" notes.

**EXAMPLE:** F02 Dementia in other diseases classified elsewhere

Code first the underlying physiological condition, such as:

Alzheimer's (G30.-)

cerebral lipidosis (E75.4)

Creutzfeldt-Jakob disease (A81.0-)

## Instructional Notes

Instructional notes are included in the Tabular List to clarify information and provide additional directions for the coder. The following paragraphs describe the various types of instructional notes.

### Inclusion Terms

Inclusion terms are lists of medical diagnoses under some codes in the Tabular List. These are conditions for which that code is to be used. The terms may be synonyms of the code title or the terms are a list of various conditions assigned to "other specified" codes. The inclusion terms are not an exhaustive list of terms. Additional terms found only in the Alphabetic Index may also be assigned to a code.

**EXAMPLE:** I51.7 Cardiomegaly
Cardiac dilatation
Cardiac hypertrophy
Ventricular dilatation

### Includes Notes

Another type of inclusion term is the **includes note** used in the ICD-10-CM Tabular List. Includes notes appear immediately under a three-character code title to further define, or give examples of, the content of the category.

**EXAMPLE:** J44 Other chronic obstructive pulmonary disease Includes:
asthma with chronic obstructive pulmonary disease
chronic asthmatic (obstructive) bronchitis
chronic bronchitis with airways obstruction
chronic bronchitis with emphysema
chronic emphysematous bronchitis
chronic obstructive asthma
chronic obstructive bronchitis
chronic obstructive tracheobronchitis

### Excludes Notes

ICD-10-CM has two types of excludes notes. Each type of note has a different definition for use. However, they are similar in intent. The **excludes note** indicates that codes excluded from each other are independent of each other. In ICD-10-CM, there are two types of excludes notes designated either as Excludes1 or Excludes2 in their title. Either or both may appear under a category, subcategory, or code.

#### The Excludes1 Note

The Excludes1 note indicates that the conditions listed after it cannot ever be used at the same time as the code above the Excludes1 note. The conditions listed in the code and in the Excludes1 note are mutually exclusive. A patient cannot have both conditions at the same time. The coder must determine, based on the documentation in the health record, which condition the patient actually has in order to assign the correct code.

**EXAMPLE:** E06 Thyroiditis
Excludes1: postpartum thyroiditis (O90.5)

In this example, a patient who is in the postpartum period and has thyroiditis would have the diagnosis code O90.5 assigned. Other patients who have thyroiditis and are not in the postpartum period would have the disease coded as E06. This is an either/or situation. Both codes could not be used on the same patient during the same episode of care.

#### The Excludes2 Note

The Excludes2 note means that two codes are applied when both conditions are present. The conditions that appear as an Excludes2 note are not part of the code that is listed above it. A patient may have both conditions at the same time. One code does not include both conditions.

When both conditions are present, two codes are applied. A coder can think of it as "2" codes are required when there is documentation for a condition present in the Excludes"2" note.

**EXAMPLE:** G47 Sleep disorders
Excludes2: nightmares (F51.5)
nonorganic sleep disorders (F51.-)
sleep terrors (F51.4)

In this example, a patient can have sleep disorders and nightmares at the same time. The Excludes2 note means that code G47 for sleep disorders does not include the condition of nightmares. When the patient has both a sleep disorder and nightmares, two codes must be used: a code from the category G47 and the code F51.4.

## Etiology and Manifestation Convention

Some diseases produce another disease or a condition the patient would not have without the underlying disease. In ICD-10-CM, there is a coding convention that requires two codes for situations when one disease produces another condition. The first disease is considered the **etiology** and the second condition that it produces is called the **manifestation**. The etiology or the first disease must be coded first. The manifestation(s) are listed as additional codes.

### *"Code First" and "Use Additional Code" Notes*

The coding convention used in ICD-10-CM that directs the coder as to which condition is coded first is known as a "code first" note. The "code first" note appears in the Tabular List under the manifestation code. The title of the manifestation code usually includes the phrase "in diseases classified elsewhere" in the title. It is important to remember that the "in diseases classified elsewhere" or "in other specified diseases classified elsewhere" codes are never first-listed or principal diagnosis codes nor can these codes be listed as a single code. These manifestation codes also appear in *italicized fonts*. These instructions make sure the proper sequencing of codes is followed, that is, the etiology condition is coded first, followed by the manifestation code.

There are also diseases that require two codes to completely describe the condition because all the facts of the disease are not expressed in one code. When such a condition exists, the coding convention in ICD-10-CM will remind the coder to "use additional code" to fully describe the condition. This also indicates the sequencing required with the code identified as the "use additional code" listed as an additional code.

The etiology and manifestation conventions appear in both the Alphabetic Index and the Tabular List. In the Alphabetic Index, both conditions may be listed on one line with the etiology code listed first and the manifestation code appearing in slanted brackets after it. The code in the brackets is never listed first or used as a single code. The manifestation code must be listed second. In the Tabular List, there are notes the coder must read at the category or at the code level, that is, "code first" a certain condition or "use additional code" as an additional code to the code it appears with.

An example of the etiology or manifestation convention is dementia in Alzheimer's disease. The main term is disease, subterm is Alzheimer's, with an indent term for early onset.

**EXAMPLE:** Early onset Alzheimer's disease with dementia without behavioral disturbance
G30.0 Alzheimer's disease with early onset
F02.80 Dementia in other diseases classified elsewhere, without behavioral disturbance

In the above example, Alzheimer's disease with early onset is coded to G30.0. Under category G30, there is a directive to "use additional code to identify" dementia without behavioral disturbance (F02.80). If the patient had early onset Alzheimer's disease with dementia without behavioral disturbance, two codes would be required: G30.0 with F02.80. Under category F02, Dementia in other diseases classified elsewhere, there is a "code first the underlying physiological condition, such as" note directing the coder to first assign a code for the type of Alzheimer's disease present with a code from category G30.

## Multiple Coding for a Single Condition

Multiple codes may be required to code a disease that includes multiple disease processes or factors. As noted in the prior section, ICD-10-CM uses such conventions as "use additional code" in the Tabular List to identify a condition that is not part of the code it appears with. Another example when a "use additional code" note appears is with an infectious disease code that does not identify the specific bacterial or viral organism that caused it, but that organism can be identified with another code.

Other requirements for multiple coding of a single condition or a condition that includes multiple parts can be identified in ICD-10-CM with such notes as "code first," code, if applicable, a causal condition first, and "code also."

### *"Code First"*

"Code first" notes appear under certain codes that are not specifically manifestation codes. But certain conditions may be due to an underlying cause. When there is a "code first" note and an underlying condition present, the underlying condition should be sequenced first. In the following example, a patient with malignant ascites suffers from the ascites because the patient also has a malignant condition that should be coded first as it is the underlying cause of the ascites.

**EXAMPLE:** R18.0 Malignant ascites
Code first malignancy, such as:
malignant neoplasm of ovary (C56.-)
secondary malignant neoplasm of retroperitoneum and peritoneum (C78.6)

### *"Code, If Applicable, a Causal Condition First"*

"Code, if applicable, a causal condition first" note indicates that this code may be assigned as a first-listed or principal diagnosis when the causal condition is unknown or not applicable. If a causal condition is known, then the code for that condition should be sequenced as the principal or first-listed diagnosis. In the following example, if a patient has urinary retention and the cause of the urinary retention, such as an enlarged prostate, is known, the code for the enlarge prostate is coded first followed by a second code for the urinary retention.

**EXAMPLE:** R33.8 Other retention of urine
Code first, if applicable, any causal condition, such as:
Enlarged prostate (N40.1)

### *"Code Also"*

A "code also" note indicates that two codes may be required to fully describe a condition. This code does not provide sequencing direction, that is, either code may be listed first depending on the circumstances of the medical visit or admission. In the following example, a patient may be seen for the purpose of receiving renal dialysis. The fact that the patient has end stage renal disease that requires the patient to have renal dialysis is an important fact that is reported with an additional code.

**EXAMPLE:** Z49 Encounter for care involving renal dialysis
Code also associated end stage renal disease (N18.6)

## Cross-References and Other Terms Used in ICD-10-CM

Cross-references are used as directions for the coder to look elsewhere in the Alphabetic Index before assigning a code. Other terms are used to explain the relationships between the diagnoses and conditions included in both the Alphabetic Index and the Tabular List. To assign diagnosis codes accurately, a thorough understanding of the ICD-10-CM cross-references and other terms is essential.

### And

The term "and" is interpreted to mean "and" or "or" when it appears in a code title. The term "and" means the patient may have one or the other of the statements included in the code title. In the following example, code Z51.1 is used if the patient's encounter is for the purpose of receiving antineoplastic chemotherapy or for the purpose of receiving antineoplastic immunotherapy. If the patient is receiving both chemotherapy and immunotherapy, the code is also appropriate to use.

**EXAMPLE:** Z51.1 Encounter for antineoplastic chemotherapy and immunotherapy

### *With*

The term "with" may be used by the physician to acknowledge two conditions exist but the physician may also use other phrases such as "associated with" or "due to" and the ICD-10-CM phrase of "with" also applies in the Alphabetic Index or in the Tabular List in an instructional note.

In the Alphabetic Index, the term "with" will appear immediately following the main term. The term "with" does not appear necessarily with other subterms starting with the letter "W."

In the Tabular List, the term "with" appearing in a code title means that two conditions (condition A with condition B) must be present in the patient to use that particular code.

**EXAMPLES:** Tabular List:
B15.0 Hepatitis A with hepatic coma

In this example, code B15.0 presents the fact that the patient has two conditions: hepatitis A and hepatic coma. Here "with" means both conditions exist at the same time.

Alphabetic Index:
Bronchiolitis
with
bronchospasm or obstruction J21.9
influenza, flu, grippe - see Influenza, with, respiratory manifestations NEC
chemical (chronic) J68.4
acute J68.0
chronic (fibrosing)(obliterative) J44.9
due to
external agent - see Bronchitis, acute, due to

In this example, the condition of bronchiolitis with bronchospasm is found in the Alphabetic Index under the main term "bronchiolitis." The "with" connecting term, to identify that bronchospasm also exists, appears immediately under the main term and before the other terms that appear in alphabetic order such as chemical, chronic, or due to.

### "See" and "See Also"

In ICD-10-CM, the "see" direction is used to instruct the coder to reference another term in the Alphabetic Index that provides more complete information about the condition to be coded. The "see" note also appears with an anatomical site main term to direct the coder to locate the disease present at that anatomic site in the Alphabetic Index. For example, if the main term of "leg" is located in the Alphabetic Index, the same line includes the phrase "see condition."

**EXAMPLE:** Alphabetic Index:
Angina
with
atherosclerotic heart disease - see Arteriosclerosis, coronary (artery)

The cross-reference note "see also" in the Alphabetic Index follows a main term if the coder should reference another term in the Index for additional information. The instruction is intended to help the coder find the most information available in the Alphabetic Index when the coder may not identify all the options that could be used. However, it is not necessary to follow the "see also" note when the original main term provides all the necessary information to assign a complete code.

**EXAMPLE:** Alphabetic Index:
Bruise (skin surface intact) (see also Contusion)

In this example, no codes are available under the main term of bruise that occurs on the skin. The more appropriate medical term of contusion should be referenced to identify the many anatomic sites on which a bruise may be found.

### Connecting Words

**Connecting words** or connecting terms are subterms in the Alphabetic Index that appear after a main term to indicate a relationship between the main term and an associated condition or etiology.

Associated with
Complicated by
Due to
During
Following
In
Secondary to
With
With mention of
Without

The connecting words "with" and "without" appear in both the Alphabetic Index and in the Tabular List in code titles. "With and "without" connecting terms are sequenced before all other subterms in the Alphabetic Index but may also appear with the other subterms in alphabetic order.

## General Coding Guidelines

There are basic concepts and rules that a coder must understand in order to assign ICD-10-CM codes accurately and completely. These general coding guidelines describe how to locate a code in ICD-10-CM and how to apply all the necessary codes to fully describe a patient's condition and reason for health services.

### *Locating a Code in the ICD-10-CM*

The coder must use both the Alphabetic Index and Tabular List when locating and assigning a code. The first step in coding is to locate the main term and applicable subterms in the Alphabetic Index. Then the code found in the Alphabetic Index is verified in the Tabular List. The coder must read and be guided by the instructional notations that appear in both the Alphabetic Index and the Tabular List.

The Alphabetic Index does not always provide the complete code. Every code listed in the Alphabetic Index must be reviewed in the Tabular List. Selection of the complete code, including laterality and any applicable seventh character can only be done in the Tabular List. If additional characters are required, a dash ( - ) at the end of the Alphabetic Index entry is present. The coder then uses the Tabular List to identify what additional characters are necessary to complete the code to fully describe the patient's condition. Even if it appears that a complete code is included in the Alphabetic Index, it is mandatory for the coder to review the code in the Tabular List for all the instructional notes that may require additional coding.

### *Level of Detail in Coding*

Diagnosis codes are to be used and reported with the highest number of characters available. Codes with three characters are included in ICD-10-CM as the heading of a category of codes. A category may be further subdivided by the use of fourth, fifth, or sixth characters to provide greater detail. A seventh character may be applicable for certain codes. A three-character code is to be used only if it is not further subdivided, that is, there are no applicable fourth, fifth, sixth, or seventh characters to be used. A code is invalid if it is not coded to the full number of characters required for that code.

### Signs and Symptoms

Codes that describe symptoms and physical signs are perfectly acceptable for reporting when the sign or symptom is what the physician knows for certain about the patient. There are occasions when no definitive diagnosis can be made, even after investigation or study of the patient's presenting signs and symptoms. Signs and symptoms may be transient and disappear before the physician can identify their cause. A patient may come to a physician for treatment of a sign or symptom but fail to return for further investigation and it is not determined what caused the problem. Patients with certain signs and symptoms may be referred to another physician or treatment center for investigation before the physician can identify the cause of the symptom or sign. In all of these situations and the other scenarios described at the start of Chapter 18, Symptoms, Signs and Abnormal Clinical Findings, Not Elsewhere Classified (R00–R99), the assignment of a sign or symptom code is appropriate. Most but not all signs and symptoms appear in Chapter 18. Signs and symptoms applicable to certain body systems appear in the body system chapter of ICD-10-CM, for example, ear pain is assigned a code from ICD-10-CM Chapter 8, Diseases of the Ear and Mastoid Process.

### Conditions That Are an Integral Part of a Disease Process

Signs and symptoms that are associated routinely with a disease process should not be assigned as additional codes, unless other instructions exist. Once the reason for the signs and symptoms are known and these complaints routinely occur with that particular disease process, the signs and symptoms are not coded. For example, abdominal pain is a common symptom of acute appendicitis and is not coded when the reason for abdominal pain is attributed to the appendicitis. The coder's knowledge of disease processes is essential to coding, especially to avoid coding the unnecessary sign and symptoms codes.

### Conditions That Are Not an Integral Part of a Disease Process

Additional signs and symptoms that may not be associated routinely with a disease process should be coded when present. Again, the coder's knowledge of disease pathology is essential to coding. The coder needs to know when the physician describes accompanying signs and symptoms with a disease whether to code these conditions or not. For example, if a patient with a skull fracture is in a coma, the coma is assigned an additional code. Not every patient with a skull fracture will be in a coma.

### Acute and Chronic Conditions

If a patient has both the acute form and the chronic form of one disease, the coder must identify in the Alphabetic Index if there are separate entries at the same indentation level. If there are two separate lines in the Alphabetic Index for acute and chronic forms, then both codes are assigned. The acute or subacute code is sequenced first, followed by the chronic code for the disease. For example, the doctor may describe the patient's condition as acute and chronic pancreatitis. The Alphabetic Index has the following entries:

Pancreatitis
Acute K85.9
    alcoholic induced K85.2
    biliary K85.1
    drug induced K85.3

gallstone K85.1
idiopathic K85.0
specified NEC K85.8
Chronic (infectious) K86.1
alcohol induced K86.1
recurrent K86.1
relapsing K86.1

The code for acute pancreatitis, K85.9, is listed first with an additional code for chronic pancreatitis, K86.1, as both conditions are listed in the Alphabetic Index at the same indentation level.

### Combination Codes

A combination code is a single code used to classify two diagnoses. A combination code may also represent a diagnosis with an associated secondary process or manifestation. Finally, a combination code can be a diagnosis with an associated complication.

Combination codes are identified by referring to subterm entries in the Alphabetic Index that identify conditions that are associated with or due to each other. Combination codes are also identified by reading all the includes and excludes notes in the Tabular List. Combination codes are only assigned when the one code fully identifies the condition.

Multiple coding should not occur when the classification provides a combination code that clearly identifies all of the elements documented in the diagnosis. An additional code should be used as a secondary code only when the combination code lacks necessary specificity in describing the manifestation or complication. There may be a third condition that exists with two other conditions that requires an additional code. For example, a patient may have acute bronchitis with bronchiectasis and tobacco use. Two codes are required: J47.0, a combination code for bronchiectasis with acute bronchitis, and Z72.0, the code for tobacco use.

### Sequela or Late Effects

A condition that is produced by another illness or an injury and remains after the acute phase of the illness or injury is referred to as a **sequela**. There is no time period as to when a sequela must appear or be present. The condition can be identified at the same time as the original disease, such as dysphagia that occurs with a cerebral infarction. Other conditions may occur a period of time after the acute phase of the illness is over, for example, the scar that remains after a burn heals.

Two codes are required for coding sequela conditions. The first reported code is the condition that exists at present or the sequela. The second code is the original conditions identified as the cause of the present condition. However, the code for the acute phase of an illness that led to the sequela is never used with a code for the late effect.

There are exceptions to the above guideline:

1. The code for the sequela is followed by a manifestation code identified in the Tabular List and title.
2. The sequela code has been expanded at the fourth, fifth, or sixth character levels to include the manifestations.

The main term "sequela" must be referenced in the Alphabetic Index to identify if a combination code for the sequela and the underlying cause exists. In the Tabular List, an instructional note may appear under these category codes to "code first condition resulting from (sequela of)" that particular category. In the Alphabetic Index, following the main term "sequela," is the direction term "see also condition" to remind the coder that other entries in the Alphabetic Index are also applicable to coding of these conditions.

Below is a step-by-step example of how to accurately code a sequela and the underlying condition:

> A doctor documents the following condition: scar of the skin on the face due to previous third-degree burn of face. The coder must recognize the condition present today is the scar and the cause of the scar was the previous third-degree burn on the face.
>
> First the coder accesses the term "scar" in the Alphabetic Index as follows:
> Alphabetic Index:
> Scar, scarring (see also Cicatrix) L90.5
> Cicatrix, skin L90.5
>
> Then the coder must confirm the code in the Tabular List as L90.5. There are no further instructions in the Tabular List. The code does not include any anatomic locations so all scars are coded here. However, the coder must know to identify the cause of the scar having been stated as due to a previous burn on the face.
>
> The coder must translate that fact to the word "sequela" to identify the burn and use the Alphabetic Index again as follows:
> Alphabetic Index:
> Sequela, burn and corrosion—code to injury with seventh character S
> Burn, face—see Burn, head
> Burn, head, third degree, T20.30
>
> Again, the coder must access the Tabular List to review the entry of code T20.20 to determine if more characters are required to complete the coding assignment.
>
> T20.30 requires a seventh character of S for sequela; therefore, a placeholder character of X is needed in the sixth position, that is, T20.30XS.
>
> After following these steps, the coder concludes that the coding of scar of the skin of the face due to previous third-degree burn of the face is coded as L90.5 and T20.30XS

### Impending or Threatened Condition

According to the *ICD-10-CM Draft Official Guidelines for Coding and Reporting*, Guideline I.B.12, impending or threatened conditions are coded as follows:

> If a condition described at the time of discharge as "impending" or "threatened," it should be coded as follows:
>
> 1. If the condition did occur, code as a confirmed diagnosis
> 2. If the condition did not occur, reference the Alphabetic Index to determine if the condition has a subentry term for "impending" or "threatened" and also reference main term entries for "Impending" and for "Threatened"
>    a. If the subterms are listed, assign the given code
>    b. If the subterms are not listed, code the existing underlying condition(s) and not the condition described as impending or threatened.

### Reporting Same Diagnosis Code More Than Once

According to the *ICD-10-CM Draft Official Guidelines for Coding and Reporting*, Guideline I.B.13, "each unique ICD-10-CM diagnosis codes may be reported only once for an encounter. This applies to bilateral conditions when there are no distinct codes identifying laterality or two different conditions classified to the same ICD-10-CM diagnosis code."

### Laterality

Some ICD-10-CM diagnosis codes include laterality or whether the condition exists on the right or left side of the body. For bilateral sites, the final character of the code indicates laterality. An unspecified side code is available for use if the side of the body is not identified in the medical record. If no bilateral code is provided and the condition is bilateral, the coder must assign separate codes for both the left and right side.

### Documentation for BMI and Pressure Ulcer Stages

In the *ICD-10-CM Draft Official Guidelines for Coding and Reporting*, Guideline I.B.14 describes how to code according to the documentation of the body mass index and the pressure ulcer stages.

> For the body mass index (BMI) and pressure ulcer stage codes, the code assignment may be made based on the medical record documentation from clinicians who are not the patient's provider (such as a physician or other qualified healthcare practitioner legally accountable for establishing the patient's diagnosis). This information is typically documented by other clinicians involved in the care of the patient, for example, a dietitian documents the BMI and nurses often document the pressure ulcer stages. However, the associated diagnosis (such as overweight, obesity or pressure ulcer) must be documented by the patient's provider. If there is conflicting medical record documentation, either from the same clinician or different clinicians, the patient's attending provider should be queried for clarification.
>
> The BMI codes should only be reported as secondary diagnoses. As with all other secondary diagnosis codes, the BMI codes should only be assigned when they meet the definition of a reportable additional diagnosis.

### Syndromes

Guideline I.B.15 in the *ICD-10-CM Draft Official Guidelines for Coding and Reporting* describes the coding of named syndromes.

> The coder should follow the Alphabetic Index guidance when coding named syndromes. In the absence of Alphabetic Index guidance, the coder should assign codes for each of the documented individual manifestations or conditions identified as the syndrome when the multiple conditions exist at the same time.

### Documentation of Complications of Care

In Guideline I.B.16 of the *ICD-10-CM Draft Official Guidelines for Coding and Reporting*, the coder is given direction on how and when to assign complication codes.

> Code assignment is based on the provider's documentation of the relationship between the condition and the care or procedure. The guideline extends to any complication of care, regardless of the chapter the code is located in. It is important to note that not all conditions that occur during or

following medical care or surgery are classified as complications. There must be a cause-and-effect relationship between the care and the condition, and an indication in the documentation that it is a complication. The physician should be queried or asked for clarification if the complication is not clearly documented.

## Basic Steps in ICD-10-CM Coding

The basic steps described in this chapter should be followed when assigning a code in ICD-10-CM. To code each disease or condition completely and accurately, the coder should:

1. Identify all main terms included in the diagnostic statement
2. Locate each main term in the Alphabetic Index
3. Refer to any subterms indented under the main term. The subterms form individual line entries and describe essential differences by site, etiology, or clinical type
4. Follow the instructions (see, see also) provided in the Alphabetic Index if the needed code is not located under the first main entry consulted
5. Verify the code selected in the Tabular List
6. Read and be guided by any instructional terms in the Tabular List
7. Assign codes to their highest level of specificity, up to a total of seven characters if applicable
8. Continue coding the diagnostic statement until all the component elements are fully identified

## ICD-10-CM Review Exercises: Chapter 1

Assign the correct ICD-10-CM diagnosis codes to the following exercises.

1. Acute appendicitis with perforation

 ______________________________

2. Personal history of breast carcinoma (malignant neoplasm)

 ______________________________

3. Precordial chest pain

 ______________________________

4. Acute cor pulmonale

 ______________________________

5. Streptococcal pneumonia

 ______________________________

6. Toxic nodular goiter

 ______________________________

## ICD-10-CM Review Exercises: Chapter 1 (Continued)

7. Extra thyroid gland

8. Osteoarthrosis, primary of right ankle

9. Acute tracheobronchitis with bronchospasm (age 16)

10. Arteriosclerotic heart disease of native coronary artery with angina pectoris

11. Angiodysplasia of the colon with hemorrhage

12. Prenatal care, normal first pregnancy, second trimester

13. Traumatic comminuted fracture of left femur involving the intertrochanteric section, initial visit

14. Nephritis due to systemic lupus erythematosus

15. Carotid artery occlusion with cerebral infarction. Essential hypertension.

16. Acute hepatitis C with hepatic coma

17. Prostatitis due to Trichomonas

18. Benign carcinoid tumor of the appendix

19. Enlarged prostate with urinary obstruction

20. Acute lymphoblastic leukemia in remission

Chapter 2

# Procedure Coding in ICD-9-CM and ICD-10-PCS

## Learning Objectives

At the conclusion of this chapter, you should be able to:

1. Describe the content and purpose of volume 3 in ICD-9-CM
2. Identify the healthcare setting in which ICD-9-CM volume 3 codes are used
3. Explain the classification used to organize the chapters in ICD-9-CM volume 3
4. Describe the format of the ICD-9-CM Tabular List and the procedure codes
5. Describe the format of the ICD-9-CM Alphabetic Index
6. Identify and define the main terms, subterms, connecting words, and eponyms used in the Alphabetic Index of ICD-9-CM volume 3
7. Identify and define the conventions used in the Alphabetic Index of ICD-9-CM volume 3
8. Explain the basic instructions for ICD-9-CM procedural coding
9. Assign procedure codes using the Alphabetic Index and Tabular List of ICD-9-CM volume 3
10. Compare and contrast ICD-9-CM procedure codes with ICD-10-PCS codes
11. Explain the ICD-10-PCS code structure
12. Explain the overall organization of ICD-10-PCS
13. Identify ICD-10-PCS attributes, characteristics, and definitions
14. Describe the ICD-10-PCS components and table structure
15. Describe the Medical and Surgical Section
16. Explain the basic instructions for ICD-10-PCS coding
17. Assign ICD-10-PCS codes for procedural statements

## ICD-9-CM Volume 3

ICD-9-CM classifies procedures in **volume 3**, which includes both an Alphabetic Index and a Tabular List. The classification of procedures in volume 3 follow much of the same format, organization, and conventions as the classification of diseases in volumes 1 and 2 of ICD-9-CM. Specific procedures are discussed in other chapters of this book.

ICD-9-CM procedure classification is used to code hospital inpatient procedures. Hospital inpatient procedures are consistently coded when performed in the range of procedure code categories 00–86. ICD-9-CM, volume 3, Chapter 16, Miscellaneous Diagnostic and Therapeutic Procedures (87–99), may be used selectively for inpatient procedure coding. For example, subcategory 88.5, Angiocardiography using contrast material, would be assigned when the procedure was performed on an inpatient. However, diagnostic ultrasound, subcategory 88.7, is less likely to be used for any inpatient coding. Because facility policies may vary, coders should follow the hospital or facility coding policy concerning the coding of procedures in categories 87–99 for miscellaneous diagnostic and therapeutic procedures for inpatient services.

Hospital outpatient departments and other ambulatory facilities are required to use ***Current Procedural Terminology, Fourth Edition (CPT),*** as well as ***Healthcare Common Procedure Coding System (HCPCS)*** to report outpatient procedures on electronic healthcare transactions. Likewise, physician practices are required to use CPT and HCPCS to report services and procedures.

## Tabular List

Volume 3 contains the following 17 chapters:

| | Chapter Titles | Categories |
|---|---|---|
| 0. | Procedures and Interventions, Not Elsewhere Classified | 00 |
| 1. | Operations on the Nervous System | 01–05 |
| 2. | Operations on the Endocrine System | 06–07 |
| 3. | Operations on the Eye | 08–16 |
| 3A. | Other Miscellaneous Diagnostic and Therapeutic Procedures | 17 |
| 4. | Operations on the Ear | 18–20 |
| 5. | Operations on the Nose, Mouth, and Pharynx | 21–29 |
| 6. | Operations on the Respiratory System | 30–34 |
| 7. | Operations on the Cardiovascular System | 35–39 |
| 8. | Operations on the Hemic and Lymphatic System | 40–41 |
| 9. | Operations on the Digestive System | 42–54 |
| 10. | Operations on the Urinary System | 55–59 |
| 11. | Operations on the Male Genital Organs | 60–64 |
| 12. | Operations on the Female Genital Organs | 65–71 |
| 13. | Obstetrical Procedures | 72–75 |
| 14. | Operations on the Musculoskeletal System | 76–84 |
| 15. | Operations on the Integumentary System | 85–86 |
| 16. | Miscellaneous Diagnostic and Therapeutic Procedures | 87–99 |

Almost all of the chapters classify data by anatomical system. Chapter 13 classifies procedures performed for obstetrical purposes, and Chapter 16 classifies diagnostic and therapeutic procedures that are not generally considered surgical in nature. The first chapter titled Procedures and Interventions, Not Elsewhere Classified consists of codes that begin with digits 00. The codes in this chapter are intended to capture new technology.

### *Format of the Tabular List*

ICD-9-CM procedure codes consist of three or four digits, with two digits preceding a decimal point and one or two following it. Three-digit codes cannot be used if four-digit codes are available. The third and fourth digits provide further information about the site, procedure, or diagnosis.

**53 Repair of hernia**
Includes: hernioplasty
herniorrhaphy
herniotomy
Code also any application or administration of an adhesion barrier substance (99.77)

*Excludes:* *manual reduction of hernia (96.27)*

**53.0 Other unilateral repair of inguinal hernia**

*Excludes:* *laparoscopic unilateral repair of inguinal hernia (17.11–17.13)*

**53.00 Unilateral repair of inguinal hernia, not otherwise specified**
Inguinal herniorrhaphy NOS
**53.01 Other and open repair of direct inguinal hernia**
Direct and indirect inguinal hernia
**53.02 Other and open repair of indirect inguinal hernia**
**53.03 Other and open repair of direct inguinal hernia with graft or prosthesis**
**53.04 Other and open repair of indirect inguinal hernia with graft or prosthesis**
**53.05 Repair of inguinal hernia with graft or prosthesis, not otherwise specified**

In the preceding example, repair of hernia is assigned to category 53, unless it is a laparoscopic unilateral repair of inguinal hernia. At the third-digit level, the codes describe whether the hernia repair was unilateral or bilateral. At the fourth-digit level, they describe the clinical type of hernia, direct or indirect.

## Alphabetic Index

The Alphabetic Index to Procedures contains a listing of procedures, studies, tests, operations, surgeries, therapies, and so forth. It contains many procedures that the text of the Tabular List may not include.

**A point to remember:** Always trust the Alphabetic Index. The terms listed in the Tabular List are examples of the contents of the category, whereas the entries in the Alphabetic Index are much more comprehensive.

**EXAMPLE:** In Tabular List—**93.53 Application of other cast**
In Alphabetic Index—**Application**
Unna's paste boot 93.53

By trusting the Alphabetic Index, code 93.53 is assigned for Unna's paste boot because the narrative of the code in the Tabular List does not include Unna's paste boot.

### Main Terms

The structure of the Alphabetic Index to Procedures is similar to that of the Alphabetic Index to Diseases. The **main terms** are set in boldface type and identify the type of procedure performed, with the subterms indented in alphabetical order.

Main terms can include:

- Operations, such as cholecystectomy, duodenostomy, Dorrance operation
- Procedures or tests, such as bronchogram, audiometry, physical therapy, scan
- Nouns, such as examination, operation, pacemaker
- Verbs, such as clipping, cooling, repair

## Exercise 2.1

Using the Alphabetic Index, underline the main term(s) in the following statements. (Hint: Think of the procedures as "action" words instead of anatomic locations.)

1. Stomach anastomosis takedown
2. Bilateral repair of inguinal hernia
3. Removal of intrauterine contraceptive device
4. Anorectal myectomy
5. Dilation and curettage of uterus
6. Irwin operation
7. Transurethral biopsy of bladder
8. Chest wall suture
9. Activities of daily living (ADL) training
10. Mohs' chemosurgery

### Subterms

The **subterms** listed under the main term in the Alphabetic Index have a definitive effect on the selection of the appropriate code for a given procedure. They form individual line entries and describe essential differences in site, diagnosis, or surgical technique. Subterms can be indented farther to the right, with each indentation amounting to two spaces.

The appropriate main term should be located in the Alphabetic Index first, then the subterm that leads to the correct code. All entries must be verified in the Tabular List.

**EXAMPLE:** **Revision**
joint replacement
acetabular and femoral components (total) 00.70
acetabular component only 00.71
acetabular liner and/or femoral head only 00.73
ankle 81.59
elbow 81.97
and so on

### Connecting Words

Because they are considered **connecting words or terms**, subterms beginning with the words *as, by,* and *with* immediately follow the main term or subterm, instead of appearing in the usual alphabetical sequence.

**Laminectomy** (decompression) (for
 exploration) 03.09
 as operative approach—***omit code***
 with
  excision of herniated intervertebral
   disc (nucleus pulposus) 80.51
  excision of other intraspinal lesion
   (tumor) 03.4
 reopening of site 03.02

In this example, *as* and *with* are indented before the subterm "reopening of site," indicating that these terms are being used as connecting words.

### Exercise 2.2

Assign procedure codes to the following:

1. Phlebectomy with thoracic graft replacement
2. Percutaneous needle biopsy of breast
3. Arthrodesis of ankle
4. Myotomy of the hand with division
5. Control of epistaxis by anterior nasal packing

### Eponyms

Surgical procedures that are identified by **eponyms** (named for their originators) are indexed in the following three ways:

1. Under the eponym

**McDonald operation** (encirclement suture, cervix) 67.59

2. Under the main term "Operation" or "Procedure"

> **Operation** . . .
> McDonald (encirclement suture, cervix) 67.59

3. Under a main term or subterm describing the operation

> **Suture** . . .
> cervix . . .
> internal os, encirclement 67.59

## Exercise 2.3

Assign procedure codes to the following:

1. Marshall-Marchetti-Krantz operation

______________________

2. Mayo operation—bunionectomy

______________________

3. Shirodkar operation

______________________

4. Nissen's fundoplication

______________________

5. Maxillary sinusotomy, external approach (Caldwell-Luc)

______________________

## ICD-9-CM Conventions in Volume 3

Most of the principles concerning ICD-9-CM conventions discussed in chapter 1 of this book also apply to volume 3 of ICD-9-CM. The few exceptions are discussed below.

### *Code Also*

In volume 3, the phrase "**code also**" serves as a reminder to code additional procedures only when they have actually been performed. The instruction is used for two purposes:

1. To code each individual component of an operation or two procedures that are often performed together

> **46.2 Ileostomy**
> Code also any synchronous resection (45.34, 45.61–45.63)

In the above example, the "code also" statement serves as a reminder to assign an additional code for any synchronous resection performed in conjunction with an ileostomy.

> **13.5 Other extracapsular extraction of lens**
> Code also any synchronous insertion of pseudophakos (13.71)

This example directs the coder to assign a code for synchronous insertion of pseudophakos, along with the code for the extracapsular extraction of the lens.

2. To code the use of special adjunctive procedures or equipment

> **35.6 Repair of atrial and ventricular septa with tissue graft**
> Code also cardiopulmonary bypass [extracorporeal circulation] [heart-lung machine] (39.61)

Again, in this example, the reminder is to code also cardiopulmonary bypass, if performed with repair of atrial and ventricular septa with tissue graft.

### *Omit Code and Coding Operative Approach*

The convention ***omit code*** is found only in **volume 3** of ICD-9-CM, in both the Tabular List and the Alphabetic Index. This instruction indicates that no code is to be assigned and usually applies to the following procedures:

- An exploratory procedure incidental to the procedure carried out
- The usual surgical approaches of a given procedure
- Blunt, digital, manual, or mechanical lysis of adhesions
- The closure portion of a procedure

> **Laparotomy** NEC 54.19
> as operative approach—*omit code*
> exploratory (pelvic) 54.11
> reopening of recent operative site
> (for control of hemorrhage) (for exploration) (for incision of hematoma) 54.12

The Alphabetic Index advises the coder to omit the code if the laparotomy is the **operative approach** or the surgical entry into the body. For example, in an open appendectomy, the laparotomy would not be assigned because it is the operative approach. The abdominal wall must be incised to perform the removal.

When a definitive procedure (therapeutic or diagnostic) is performed, the operative approach is considered part of the procedure and is not coded. The Alphabetic Index and Tabular List frequently indicate when a code should be omitted. However, some procedures that constitute an operative approach are listed in the Alphabetic Index or Tabular List without the instruction to **omit code**. In such cases, the coder's knowledge of operative techniques is essential. Regardless of the presence or lack of instruction, if the procedure itself serves as the operative approach, it is not coded. For example, the title of the procedure describes an exploratory laparotomy and an open cholecystectomy. Only the definitive procedure—the open cholecystectomy, ICD-9-CM procedure code 51.22, Cholecystectomy—would be coded because the exploratory laparotomy is the approach, and the exploration is incidental to the definitive procedure. Therefore ICD-9-CM procedure code 54.11, Exploratory laparotomy, would not be coded.

When an exploratory procedure is performed along with a diagnostic procedure, both procedures are coded. For example, a surgeon performs an exploratory thoracotomy. In addition to the exploratory thoracotomy, the surgeon takes a biopsy of the mediastinum and closes the incision. In this case, the exploratory thoracotomy, ICD-9-CM procedure code 34.02, is sequenced first, with an additional code for the diagnostic procedure, open biopsy of mediastinum, ICD-9-CM procedure code 34.26.

### Codes for Procedures Involving a Laparoscope, Arthroscope, Bronchoscope, Thoracoscope, or Endoscope

An **endoscope**—such as a laparoscope, arthroscope, bronchoscope, or thoracoscope—allows the removal of organs or tissue through small incisions under videoscopic guidance. ICD-9-CM provides a unique code for many endoscopic procedures. When a separate code is unavailable, the open (incisional) procedure code is assigned. In this instance, no code is assigned for procedures using an endoscope such as a laparoscope, thoracoscope, arthroscope, or laryngoscope. For example, if a laparoscopic partial nephrectomy is performed, the ICD-9-CM procedure code 55.4 is assigned. Code 55.4 is an open procedure. The title of the code, "Partial Nephrectomy," does not include the term laparoscopic. However, this is the correct procedure code to use because a code does not exist for laparoscopic partial nephrectomy.

If the laparoscopic approach is unsuccessful, the surgeon may elect to perform an open approach to complete the procedure. When the procedure is converted to an open approach, only the open approach is coded.

- For example, if a laparoscopic appendectomy (ICD-9-CM procedure code 47.01) could not be completed on a patient, and the physician removed the appendix as an open procedure, the only ICD-9-CM procedure code that would be assigned is 47.09, other appendectomy.
- The fact that the laparoscopic approach was first used is indicated by the supplementary diagnosis V code, V64.41, Laparoscopic surgical procedure converted to open procedure. V codes are discussed in chapter 23 of this book.

In the Alphabetic Index to Diseases, the main term "Conversion" is used to locate the code that describes the conversion of a laparoscopic procedure to an open procedure.

The main term "Endoscopy" may be used in the Alphabetic Index to locate a variety of endoscopic procedures. More precise terms describing endoscopic procedures also may be referenced; for example, bronchoscopy, colonoscopy, or cystoscopy. When an endoscope is passed through more than one body cavity, the code for the endoscope should identify the most distant site. For example, an esophagogastroduodenoscopy is assigned code 45.13, Other endoscopy of small intestine, to reflect the fact that the duodenum or small bowel was visualized; this code indicates that the most distal site examined was the small intestine or the duodenum.

## Exercise 2.4

Assign procedure codes to the following:

1. Thoracotomy with total lobectomy of left lung

2. Craniotomy with excision of meningeal cyst

3. Arthroscopy of knee

4. Injection of cortisone into hip joint

5. Intracapsular extraction of lens by temporal inferior route with insertion of pseudophakos

6. Partial resection of colon with end-to-end anastomosis

7. Transpleural thoracoscopy

8. Cystoscopy with biopsy

9. Laparoscopic total cholecystectomy

10. Arthroscopic meniscectomy

### *Slanted Brackets [ ]*

The requirement to assign two codes for closely related procedures is indicated in the Alphabetic Index or the Tabular List by **slanted brackets** enclosing the second code. This convention means both codes must be used and sequenced as listed.

**Aneurysmectomy** . . . 38.60
  with
    graft replacement (interposition) 38.40
      aorta (arch) (ascending) (descending thoracic)
        abdominal 38.44
        thoracic 38.45
        thoracoabdominal 38.45 *[38.44]*

Therefore, to fully describe a thoracoabdominal aneurysmectomy, two codes are required: code 38.45 is sequenced first, followed by code 38.44.

## Coding Aborted or Incomplete Surgery or Procedure

ICD-9-CM generally does not include codes for procedures that are not completed (**incomplete procedures**). The one exception is code 73.3, Failed forceps, in Chapter 13, Obstetrical Procedures. When a planned procedure is started, but not completed, it is coded according to the following principles:

- When a cavity or space is entered, code exploration of the site.
- When an endoscopic approach is used, but the definitive procedure could not be carried out, code the endoscopy only.
- When only an incision is made, code the site of the incision.
- When the procedure does not involve an incision, no procedure code is assigned. Instead, a code from the V64 category is used to indicate why the planned procedure was not carried out.

An aborted surgery is a surgical procedure that was started but not completed due to unforeseen circumstances. In these cases, the coder should review the operative report carefully and code the procedure to the extent it was performed. For example:

- If a cavity or space was entered, assign a code describing the exploratory procedure for that site.

**EXAMPLE:** Cholecystectomy canceled secondary to tachycardia after the abdominal wall was incised. The patient's diagnosis and reason for surgery was acute cholecystitis with cholelithiasis.

The cholecystectomy is not coded because it was not performed; however, code 54.0, Incision of abdominal wall, is assigned to describe the extent of the procedure. Diagnosis codes include the reasons for the surgery and the tachycardia, and the appropriate V code for the planned procedure not carried out are:

- Acute cholecystitis with cholelithiasis, 574.00
- Tachycardia, 785.0
- Surgical or other procedure not carried out because of contraindication, V64.1

The procedure code for entering the abdomen:

- Incision of abdominal wall, 54.0

Although the procedure was not performed as planned, the principal diagnosis does not change.

- If a catheterization is performed, code to the extent that it was performed.

**EXAMPLE:** Patient admitted for cardiac catheterization for substernal chest pain. After the catheter was inserted into the right femoral artery to gain access for the cardiac catheterization procedure, the patient experienced an anxiety reaction, and blood pressure readings were noted to be elevated. Procedure was aborted and rescheduled for a later time. The diagnosis codes assigned would be:

- Substernal chest pain, 786.51
- Anxiety reaction, 300.00
- Elevated blood pressure, 796.2
- Surgical or other procedure not carried out because of contraindication, V64.1

The procedure code to describe the extent of the procedure performed would be:

- Code 38.91, Arterial catheterization, is assigned to describe the extent of the surgery.

- If a closed fracture reduction was attempted and aborted, no procedure code is available. A code from category V64 (V64.1, V64.2, or V64.3) should be assigned as an additional diagnostic code to describe the reason why the procedure was not carried out. In the Alphabetic Index to Diseases, the main term used to locate the V64 code is "Procedure (surgical) not done."
- In some cases, a procedure is canceled before it begins. Cancellation is often due to contraindications such as infections or other illnesses. Other reasons for canceled surgery include unavailability of the surgeon, patient's decision, or malfunctioning equipment. As an additional patient's diagnostic code, a code should be assigned from category V64, Persons encountering health services for specific procedures, not carried out.

**EXAMPLE:** Patient is admitted to outpatient surgery department with hypertrophy of tonsils and adenoids and is scheduled for tonsillectomy and adenoidectomy. The nurse notes the patient has a runny nose and cough, and a diagnosis of upper respiratory infection is made. The physician cancels the surgery until the infection has cleared.

The following codes are assigned: 474.10, Hypertrophy of tonsils with adenoids; 465.9, Acute upper respiratory infection; and V64.1, Surgical or other procedure not carried out because of contraindication. No procedure code is assigned.

### Coding Failed Procedures

Some procedures are completely performed but are considered to have failed. This means that not every objective of the procedure was secured or the procedure did not achieve the desired result. In such a situation, the **failed procedure** is coded as performed.

**EXAMPLE:** A patient underwent a percutaneous coronary angioplasty of a single vessel for total occlusion with coronary artery arteriosclerosis of a native vessel. Immediately after the procedure, the coronary artery became totally occluded again.

Because the procedure was performed, it should be coded 00.66, even though the desired result, an open coronary artery, was not achieved.

The diagnosis code would be:

- Coronary artery arteriosclerosis, native vessel, 414.01
- Total occlusion of coronary artery, 414.2

The procedure code would be:

- Percutaneous coronary angioplasty, 00.66
- Procedure on single vessel, 00.40

**EXAMPLE:** A patient suffering from a severe epistaxis came to the emergency department. Because the patient also needed treatment for accelerated hypertension, the patient was admitted to the hospital and a consultation with an ear, nose, and throat physician was requested to treat the epistaxis. The consultant performed an anterior nasal packing on the first hospital day. The next day, it appeared the nasal hemorrhage had continued and the consultant took the patient back to the operating room. The first packing was removed and another anterior nasal packing was performed.

Both the first and second anterior packing should be coded 21.01, even though the first packing seemed to have failed to control the hemorrhage.

The diagnosis codes would be:

- Epistaxis, 784.7
- Hypertension, accelerated, 401.0

The procedure codes would be:

- Anterior packing (first), 21.01
- Anterior packing (second), 21.01

## Codes for Biopsy with Extensive Surgical Procedure

When a biopsy is performed and then followed by a more extensive surgery, code the surgical procedure first, followed by the biopsy. Typically, these are open biopsies followed by definitive procedures. An open biopsy is performed by means of an incision with removal of tissue for microscopic examination. When an open biopsy is performed by incision, the incision is implicit in the code.

**EXAMPLE:** Open biopsy of the breast with frozen section and unilateral radical mastectomy

85.45, Unilateral radical mastectomy
85.12, Open biopsy of breast

**EXAMPLE:** Open biopsy of pancreas via laparotomy

52.12, Open biopsy of pancreas

## Codes for Closed-Biopsy Procedure

A closed biopsy may be performed percutaneously, endoscopically, or through use of a needle. When a needle or percutaneous biopsy is performed via an open procedure, such as a laparotomy, code both the open procedure and the needle biopsy. Another type of closed biopsy is a brush biopsy. In a brush biopsy, tissue is removed by using a brush or bristle-type instrument to collect cells for cytological examination.

The following guidelines apply for coding endoscopic biopsies:

1. When ICD-9-CM provides one code to identify both the biopsy and the endoscopy, assign that code.

**EXAMPLE:** 45.16, Esophagogastroduodenoscopy [EGD] with closed biopsy

2. When ICD-9-CM does not provide a code to identify both the biopsy and the endoscopy, assign two separate codes. The principal procedure is the endoscopy code.

   **EXAMPLE:** 34.22, Mediastinoscopy
   34.25, Closed [percutaneous] [needle] biopsy of mediastinum

### Bilateral Procedure Coding

In some cases, ICD-9-CM provides a single code to identify that a **bilateral procedure** was performed. In these cases, that procedure code is listed only once.

**EXAMPLE:** 53.10, Bilateral inguinal hernia repair

When the same procedure is performed bilaterally, and ICD-9-CM does not identify it as being performed bilaterally, assign the code of the procedure twice.

**EXAMPLE:** 79.04 and 79.04, Closed reduction of two finger fractures

## Using the Pathology Report for Inpatient Diagnosis Coding

The Official Guidelines for Coding and Reporting (Section III, B, Abnormal Findings) states:

> Abnormal findings (laboratory, x-ray, pathologic, and other diagnostic results) are not coded and reported unless the provider indicates their clinical significance. If the findings are outside the normal range and the provider has ordered other tests to evaluate the condition or prescribed treatment, it is appropriate to ask the provider whether the abnormal finding should be added (CDC 2011).

According to a question and answer published in Coding Clinic for ICD-9-CM, it is not appropriate to code (a diagnosis) directly from the pathology reports (AHA 2013, 24–25). A coder cannot code a pathological finding from the pathology report that has not been documented by the attending physician. It is not equivalent to the attending physician's documentation of the patient's diagnosis based on the patient's clinical picture. The pathologist's interpretation of a specimen is not the same as a diagnosis provided by a physician directly involved in the care of the patient. The attending physician should be queried if it appears a diagnosis that is stated on the pathology report is not included by the attending physician in the health record to determine if the information should be added. Note: this question and answer pertains to coding of inpatient records only. Outpatient guidelines are different and allow the coding of condition in documents written by physicians.

## Basic Instructions for ICD-9-CM Procedural Coding

To code procedures performed for a patient completely and accurately, the coder must:

1. Identify all main terms included in the procedural statement.
2. Locate each main term in the Alphabetic Index.
3. Refer to any subterms indented under the main term.
4. Follow cross-reference instructions when the needed code is not located under the first main entry consulted.

5. Verify the code selected from the index in the Tabular List.
6. Read and be guided by any instructional terms in the Tabular List.
7. Continue coding the procedural statement until all the component elements are fully identified.
8. Note: When the same procedure is performed bilaterally, and ICD-9-CM does not identify it as a bilateral procedure, assign the code of the procedure twice.

**A point to remember:** Each healthcare facility should specify the procedures that will be assigned codes in that particular facility in its coding policies. Some healthcare facilities do not assign codes to many diagnostic and nonsurgical procedures, such as radiology procedures, cardiovascular monitoring, blood transfusions, and suture removal.

## Selection of Principal Procedure

According to the Fourth Quarter 2012 issue of Coding Clinic for ICD-9-CM, the following instructions should be applied in the selection of principal procedure and clarification on the importance of the relation to the principal diagnosis when more than one procedure is performed:

1. Procedure performed for definitive treatment of both principal diagnosis and secondary diagnosis.
   a. Sequence procedure performed for definitive treatment most related to principal diagnosis as principal procedure.
2. Procedure performed for definitive treatment and diagnostic procedures performed for both principal diagnosis and secondary diagnosis.
   a. Sequence procedure performed for definitive treatment most related to principal diagnosis as principal procedure.
3. A diagnostic procedure was performed for the principal diagnosis and a procedure is performed for definitive treatment of a secondary diagnosis.
   a. Sequence diagnostic procedure as principal procedure, since the procedure most related to the principal diagnosis takes precedence.
4. No procedures performed that are related to principal diagnosis; procedures performed for definitive treatment and diagnostic procedure were performed for secondary diagnosis.
   a. Sequence procedure performed for definitive treatment of secondary diagnosis as principal procedure, since there are no procedures (definitive or nondefinitive treatment) related to principal diagnosis (AHA 2012, 80–81).

## Additional Exercises

Additional exercises for coding surgical and other procedures can be found in other chapters in this book. Chapters on individual body systems and the self-test contain other procedural statements to be coded. Answers can be found within the answer key. In addition, another American Health Information Management Association (AHIMA) publication offers more coding practice. Two student workbooks, *Basic ICD-9-CM Coding Exercises* and *Basic ICD-10-CM/PCS Coding Exercises* also written by Lou Ann Schraffenberger, complement this textbook with diagnosis and procedure coding exercises related to each chapter in this book. To challenge students to increase their coding skill and comprehension, the student workbook includes more complex coding scenarios rather than one-line diagnoses of procedure statements.

## ICD-9-CM Review Exercises: Chapter 2

Following the basic instructions for procedural coding, assign the appropriate procedure codes and diagnosis codes (for question 11 only) to the following:

1. Ventral herniorrhaphy canceled after beginning laparotomy
2. Appendectomy with drainage of appendiceal abscess
3. Removal of leg cast
4. Tarsoplasty with skin graft
5. Coronary artery bypass graft of three coronary arteries with cardiopulmonary bypass
6. Esophagoscopy with removal of chicken bone
7. Alcoholism counseling
8. Robotic-assisted laparoscopic total abdominal hysterectomy
9. Colostomy takedown
10. Gill arthrodesis, shoulder
11. Ovarian cyst; oophorectomy planned but cancelled due to the fact the patient also had an upper respiratory infection
12. Open reduction of femur fracture with internal fixation
13. Open biopsy of liver via laparotomy
14. Turbinectomy with frontal and maxillary sinusectomy
15. Percutaneous biopsy of the prostate

# Introduction to ICD-10-PCS

According to the Centers for Medicare and Medicaid Services (CMS) announcement on July 31, 2014, ICD-10-PCS will be implemented on October 1, 2015, ICD-10-PCS will be implemented for reporting inpatient procedures on electronic healthcare claims transactions, replacing volume 3 of ICD-9-CM. ICD-10-PCS stands for International Classification of Diseases, Tenth Revision, Procedure Coding System. ICD-10-PCS is unique to the United States, developed by CMS, under contract with 3M Health Information Systems. ICD-10-PCS was initially released in 1998 and updated many times since the first version. The most recent version of the ICD-10-PCS was released for October 1, 2014 on the CMS website. (http://www.cms.gov/Medicare/Coding/ICD10/2015-ICD-10-PCS-and-GEMs.html) Only limited code changes will be made yearly as needed until ICD-10-PCS is implemented.

Unlike ICD-10-CM for diagnoses, which is similar in structure and format as the ICD-9-CM volumes 1 and 2, ICD-10-PCS is a completely different system. ICD-10-PCS has a multiaxial seven-character alphanumeric code structure providing unique codes for procedures.

The following table presents a brief side-by-side comparison of ICD-9-CM and ICD-10-PCS.

| ICD-9-CM Volume 3 | ICD-10-PCS |
|---|---|
| Follows ICD structure (designed for diagnosis coding) | Designed and developed to meet healthcare needs for a procedure code system |
| Codes available as a fixed or finite set in list form | Codes constructed from flexible code components (values) using tables |
| Codes are numeric | Codes are alphanumeric |
| Codes are 3–4 digits long | All codes are seven characters long |

## The ICD-10-PCS Code

All codes in ICD-10-PCS have seven characters. Each character represents an aspect of the procedure. For example, in the first section of ICD-10-PCS, Medical and Surgical, the characters represent the following:

| 1 | 2 | 3 | 4 | 5 | 6 | 7 |
|---|---|---|---|---|---|---|
| Section | Body System | Root Operation | Body Part | Approach | Device | Qualifier |

Each of the characters has a defined meaning:

Character 1: Section—The first character of a code determines the broad procedure category, or section, where the code is located. The first section of ICD-10-PCS includes the vast majority of codes. Codes in the first section, the Medical and Surgical Section, all begin with the 0 character. Other sections will be covered in the next portion of this discussion.

Character 2: Body System—The second character defines the body system which is the general physiological system or anatomical region involved. Examples of body systems in the Medical and Surgical section include *central nervous system, upper arteries, respiratory system, tendons, muscles and upper joints.* Note that in some of the Sections of ICD-10-PCS, the second character may have an alternate meaning. For example, in the Physical Rehabilitation and Diagnostic Audiology section (F), the second character indicates whether this is Rehabilitation or Diagnostic Audiology.

Character 3: Root Operation—The third character defines the root operation, or the objective of the procedure being performed. Examples of root operations are *excision, bypass, division, and fragmentation.* In some sections, the root operation is known as the root type. For example, in the Imaging section (B), the third character indicates the root type, not the root operation.

Character 4: Body Part—The fourth character generally defines the body part or specific anatomical site where the procedure was performed. The body system, second character, provides only a general indication of the procedure site and the body part, fourth character, indicates the precise body part. This can vary in some sections of ICD-10-PCS. As in the Physical Rehabilitation and Diagnostic Audiology section example, in this section the fourth character represents the body system or region rather than the body part.

Character 5: Approach—The fifth character defines the approach, or the technique used to reach the operative site. Seven different approach values are used in the Medical and Surgical section of ICD-10-PCS. The meaning of the fifth character can vary in sections other than the Medical and Surgical section. For example, in the Imaging section (B), the fifth character indicates Contrast used in the Imaging Procedure.

Character 6: Device—The sixth character defines the device and depending on the procedure performed. There may or may not be a device left in place at the end of the procedure. Device values fall into four basic categories:

- Grafts and Prostheses
- Implants
- Simple or Mechanical Appliances
- Electronic Appliances

Again, not all sections in ICD-10-PCS include Device as the sixth character. For example, in the Radiation Therapy section (D), the sixth character represents the Isotope used, if applicable.

Character 7: Qualifier—The seventh character defines a qualifier for a particular code. A qualifier specifies an additional attribute of the procedure, if applicable

If a given character does not have a value assigned, the Z value is used. This is particularly frequent for the seventh character, qualifier and the sixth character, generally for the device.

## Overall Organization of ICD-10-PCS

ICD-10-PCS is composed of 16 sections, represented by the numbers 0–9 and the letters B–D and F–H. The broad procedure categories contained in these sections range from surgical procedures to substance abuse treatment. The 16 sections are contained in three main sections: Medical and Surgical section, Medical and Surgical-related sections and Ancillary sections.

The first section, Medical and Surgical section, contains the majority of procedures typically reported in an inpatient setting. All procedure codes in this section begin with the section value of 0.

| Section Value | Description |
|---|---|
| 0 | Medical and Surgical |

Sections 1–9 of ICD-10-PCS comprise the Medical and Surgical-related sections. These sections include the following:

| Section Value | Description |
|---|---|
| 1 | Obstetrics |
| 2 | Placement |
| 3 | Administration |
| 4 | Measurement and Monitoring |
| 5 | Extracorporeal Assistance and Performance |
| 6 | Extracorporeal Therapies |
| 7 | Osteopathic |
| 8 | Other Procedures |
| 9 | Chiropractic |

Codes in sections 1–9 are structured for the most part like their counterparts in the Medical and Surgical section, with a few exceptions. For example, in sections 5 and 6, the fifth character is defined as the duration instead of approach.

Additional differences include these uses of the sixth character:

- Section 3 defines the sixth character as substance
- Sections 4 and 5 define the sixth character as function
- Sections 7–9 define the sixth character as method

Sections B–D and F–H comprise the Ancillary sections of ICD-10-PCS which includes the following sections:

| Section Value | Description |
|---|---|
| B | Imaging |
| C | Nuclear Medicine |
| D | Radiation Therapy |
| F | Physical Rehabilitation and Diagnostic Audiology |
| G | Mental Health |
| H | Substance Abuse Treatment |

The definitions of some characters in the Ancillary sections also differ from those seen in the previous sections. For example, in the Imaging section, the third character is defined as the root type, and the fifth and sixth characters define contrast and contrast/qualifier, respectively.

# The Medical and Surgical Section (0)

The Medical and Surgical section is the largest in ICD-10-PCS. The second through seventh characters will be the concentration of this section.

## Body Systems

The meaning of the second character in the Medical and Surgical section is general body system. The way in which ICD-10-PCS defines a body system, however, is a bit different than the usual meaning of the term. A review of the following list shows how some customary body systems are given multiple body-system values. For example, note the circulatory system does not have a single value.

| Values | ICD-10-PCS Body Systems |
|---|---|
| 0 | Central Nervous System |
| 1 | Peripheral Nervous System |
| 2 | Heart and Great Vessels |
| 3 | Upper Arteries |
| 4 | Lower Arteries |
| 5 | Upper Veins |
| 6 | Lower Veins |
| 7 | Lymphatic and Hemic System |
| 8 | Eye |
| 9 | Ear, Nose, Sinus |
| B | Respiratory System |
| C | Mouth and Throat |
| D | Gastrointestinal System |
| F | Hepatobiliary System and Pancreas |
| G | Endocrine System |
| H | Skin and Breast |
| J | Subcutaneous Tissue and Fascia |
| K | Muscles |
| L | Tendons |
| M | Bursae and Ligaments |
| N | Head and Facial Bones |
| P | Upper Bones |
| Q | Lower Bones |
| R | Upper Joints |
| S | Lower Joints |
| T | Urinary System |
| U | Female Reproductive System |
| V | Male Reproductive System |
| W | Anatomic Regions, General |
| X | Anatomical Regions, Upper Extremities |
| Y | Anatomic Regions, Lower Extremities |

## Root Operations

The third character in the Medical and Surgical section is the root operation. There are a total of 31 root operations in the Medical and Surgical section, each representing the specific objective of the procedure. These 31 root operations are divided into nine groups that share similar attributes.

The nine groups are:

1. Root operations that take out some/all of a body part
2. Root operations that take out solids/fluids/gases from a body part
3. Root operations involving cutting or separation only
4. Root operations that put in/put back or move some/all of a body part
5. Root operations that alter the diameter/route of a tubular body part
6. Root operations that always involve a device
7. Root operations involving examination only
8. Root operations that define other repairs
9. Root operations that define other objectives

The following table is from the ICD-10-PCS Reference Manual and lists these nine groups and the root operations within each group.

| Root Operation | What Operation Does | Objective of Procedure | Procedure Site | Example |
|---|---|---|---|---|
| **Root operations that take out some/all of a body part** | | | | |
| Excision (B) | Takes out some/all of a body part | Cutting out/off without replacement | Some of a body part | Breast lumpectomy |
| Resection (T) | Takes out some/all of a body part | Cutting out/off without replacement | All of a body part | Total mastectomy |
| Detachment (6) | Takes out some/all of a body part | Cutting out/off without replacement | Extremity only, any level | Amputation above elbow |
| Destruction (5) | Takes out some/all of a body part | Eradicating without replacement | Some/all of a body part | Fulguration of endometrium |
| Extraction (D) | Takes out some/all of a body part | Pulling out or off without replacement | Some/all of a body part | Suction D&C |
| **Root operations that take out solids/fluids/gases from a body part** | | | | |
| Drainage (9) | Takes out solids/fluids/ gases from a body part | Taking/letting out fluids/ gases | Within a body part | Incision and drainage |
| Extirpation (C) | Takes out solids/fluids/ gases from a body part | Taking/cutting out solid matter | Within a body part | Thrombectomy |
| Fragmentation (F) | Takes out solids/fluids/ gases from a body part | Breaking solid matter into pieces | Within a body part | Lithotripsy |

| **Root operations involving cutting or separation only** | | | | |
|---|---|---|---|---|
| Division (8) | Involves cutting or separation only | Cutting into/separating a body part | Within a body part | Neurotomy |
| Release (N) | Involves cutting or separation only | Freeing a body part from constraint | Around a body part | Adhesiolysis |
| **Root operations that put in/put back or move some/all of a body part** | | | | |
| Transplantation (Y) | Puts in/puts back or moves some/all of a body part | Putting in a living body part from a person/animal | Some/all of a body part | Kidney transplant |
| Reattachment (M) | Puts in/puts back or moves some/all of a body part | Putting back a detached body part | Some/all of a body part | Reattach severed finger |
| Transfer (X) | Puts in/puts back or moves some/all of a body part | Moving, to function for a similar body part | Some/all of a body part | Skin tissue transfer |
| Reposition (S) | Puts in/puts back or moves some/all of a body part | Moving, to normal or other suitable location | Some/all of a body part | Move undescended testicle |
| **Root operations that alter the diameter/route of a tubular body part** | | | | |
| Restriction (V) | Alters the diameter/ route of a tubular body part | Partially closing orifice/ lumen | Tubular body part | Gastroesophageal fundoplication |
| Occlusion (L) | Alters the diameter/ route of a tubular body part | Completely closing orifice/ lumen | Tubular body part | Fallopian tube ligation |
| Dilation (7) | Alters the diameter/ route of a tubular body part | Expanding orifice/lumen | Tubular body part | Percutaneous transluminal coronary angioplasty (PTCA) |
| Bypass (1) | Alters the diameter/ route of a tubular body part | Altering route of passage | Tubular body part | Coronary artery bypass graft (CABG) |
| **Root operations that always involve a device** | | | | |
| Insertion (H) | Always involves a device | Putting in non-biological device | In/on a body part | Central line insertion |
| Replacement (R) | Always involves a device | Putting in device that replaces a body part | Some/all of a body part | Total hip replacement |
| Supplement (U) | Always involves a device | Putting in device that reinforces or augments a body part | In/on a body part | Abdominal wall herniorrhaphy using mesh |
| Change (2) | Always involves a device | Exchanging a device without cutting/puncturing | In/on a body part | Drainage tube change |
| Removal (P) | Always involves a device | Taking out device | In/on a body part | Central line removal |
| Revision (W) | Always involves a device | Correcting a malfunctioning/displaced device | In/on a body part | Revision of pacemaker insertion |

| Root operations involving examination only | | | | |
|---|---|---|---|---|
| Inspection (J) | Involves examination only | Visual/manual exploration | Some/all of a body part | Diagnostic cystoscopy |
| Map (K) | Involves examination only | Locating electrical impulses/ functional areas | Brain/ cardiac conduction mechanism | Cardiac mapping |
| **Root operations that include other repairs** | | | | |
| Repair (Q) | Includes other repairs | Restoring body part to its normal structure | Some/all of a body part | Suture laceration |
| Control (3) | Includes other repair | Stopping/attempting to stop post-procedural bleed | Anatomical region | Post-prostatectomy bleeding |
| **Root operations that include other objectives** | | | | |
| Fusion (G) | Includes other objectives | Rending joint immobile | Joint | Spinal fusion |
| Alteration (0) | Includes other objectives | Modifying body part for cosmetic purposes without affecting function | Some/all of a body part | Face lift |
| Creation (4) | Includes other objectives | Making new structure for sex change operation | Perineum | Artificial vagina/ penis |

Source: CMS 2015

## Objective of the Procedure

In ICD-10-PCS, each component of a procedure is defined separately. The seven characters together are intended to describe the procedure performed. The coder analyzes the operative report to identify the objective of the procedure.

The procedure is coded in ICD-10-PCS as the procedure that was actually performed. If the procedure performed was not what was intended when the procedure started, that does not matter. The intended procedure may not always be completed. When the intended or anticipated procedure is changed or discontinued, the root operation is coded based on the actual procedure that was performed.

## Multiple Procedures

If multiple procedures are performed that are defined by distinct objectives during a single operative episode, then multiple procedure codes are used. For example, obtaining a vein graft used for coronary artery bypass surgery is coded as a separate procedure from the bypass itself.

### *Multiple procedures are coded if:*

a. The same root operation is performed on different body parts that have distinct body part values in ICD-10-PCS. For example, a biopsy or diagnostic excision is performed on the duodenum and rectum.

b. The same root operation is repeated on different body sites that are included in the same body part value. For example, a biopsy is performed on the scalene muscle and the platysma muscle, which are both neck muscles, and neck muscle is the body part.

c. Distinctive procedures with multiple root operations are performed on the same body part. For example, biopsy of the pancreas and partial pancreatectomy is performed.

d. The intended procedure cannot be accomplished and is converted to a different approach. For example, a laparoscopic nephrectomy is attempted but must be converted to an open nephrectomy. The laparoscopic portion of the procedure is coded as an inspection and the open procedure is coded as an open resection for the nephretomy.

## Redo of Procedures

If the procedure performed is a complete or partial redo of a previous procedure, the root operation that identifies the "redo" procedure that was performed is what is coded rather than the root operation of revision. For example, a complete redo of a knee replacement procedure which requires putting in a new prosthesis is coded to the root operation Replacement instead of Revision. The physician is likely to describe this procedure as a "revision arthroplasty" but the coder must use the definitions of the root operations to identify the objective of a "Revision as actually a replacement procedure."

The correction of complications arising from the original procedure other than device complications as defined in the root operation Revision are also coded to the procedure performed. For example, a procedure to add mesh to the abdominal wall to repair a postoperative ventral hernia is coded to Supplement rather than Revision.

## Body Part

The meaning of the fourth character in the Medical and Surgical section is body part. The value chosen for this character represents the specific part of the body system (character 2) on which the surgery was performed. Body parts may specify laterality. Some examples of body parts and their body systems in ICD-10-PCS are:

| Body System | Body Part |
|---|---|
| Lower extremities | Left foot |
| Central nervous | Trigeminal nerve |
| Upper veins | Right cephalic vein |
| Gastrointestinal | Stomach |

ICD-10-PCS does not provide a specific value for every body part. In those instances the body part value selected would be either the whole body part value (for example, alveolar process is part of the mandible), or in the instance of nerves and vessels, the body part value is coded to the closest proximal branch.

ICD-10-PCS originally included an Appendix C titled the Body Part Key. The purpose of the Body Part Key was to translate specific anatomical sites that could be found in a health record or operative report, such as a specific muscle or tendon, to the body part term or PCS description used in ICD-10-PCS. For example, the adductor brevis muscle does not have its own body part value identified in ICD-10-PCS. The Body Part Key has an entry for the adductor brevis muscle that instructs the coder to use "upper leg muscle" as the equivalent for the body part in the ICD-10-PCS code. Since ICD-10-PCS was first published by CMS, yearly revisions have added the body part key entries to the Alphabetic Index of ICD-10-PCS for ease of reference. For this reason, if the coder is having difficulty identifying the body part value to use for a specific anatomical site, the coder should use the ICD-10-PCS and reference the anatomic site there. Using the example above, in the ICD-10-PCS Index there is an entry for "adductor brevis muscle" that states "use muscle, upper leg, left" or "use muscle, upper leg, right."

### Approach

ICD-10-PCS defines *approach* as the technique used to reach the site of the procedure. It is important to know the differences between the different approaches in order to correctly assign the fifth character value in the Medical and Surgical section.

There are seven different approaches, as shown in the table.

| Approach | Definition | Examples |
|---|---|---|
| Open (0) | Cutting through the skin or mucous membrane and any other body layers necessary to expose the site of the procedure | Open cholecystectomy, open appendectomy |
| Percutaneous (3) | Entry, by puncture or minor incision, of instrumentation through the skin or mucous membrane and/or any other body layers necessary to reach the site of the procedure | Needle biopsy of breast |
| Percutaneous Endoscopic (4) | Entry, by puncture or minor incision, of instrumentation through the skin or mucous membrane and/or any other body layers necessary to reach and visualize the site of the procedure | Laparoscopic cholecystectomy, laparoscopic appendectomy |
| Via Natural or Artificial Opening (7) | Entry of instrumentation through a natural or artificial external opening to reach the site of the procedure | Insertion of Foley urinary catheter, Endotracheal intubation |
| Via Natural or Artificial Opening Endoscopic (8) | Entry of instrumentation through a natural or artificial external opening to reach and visualize the site of the procedure | Colonoscopy, cystoscopy, esophagogastroduodenoscopy |
| Via Natural or Artificial Opening Endoscopic with Percutaneous Endoscopic Assistance (F) | Entry of instrumentation through a natural or artificial external opening to reach and visualize the site of the procedure, and entry, by puncture or minor incision, of instrumentation through the skin or mucous membrane and any other body layers necessary to aid in the performance of the procedure | Laparoscopic assisted vaginal hysterectomy |
| External (X) | Procedures performed directly on the skin or mucous membrane and procedures performed indirectly by the application of external force through the skin or mucous membrane | Closed reduction of fracture of radius, extraction of upper or lower teeth |

Source: CMS 2015

The approach is composed of three components: the access location, method, and type of instrumentation.

### Access Location

For procedures performed on an internal organ, the access location specifies the external site through which the internal organ is reached. There are two types of access locations: skin or mucous membrane and external orifices. Except for the external approach, every other approach value includes one of these two access locations. The skin or mucous membrane can be incised or punctured to reach the procedure site. All open and percutaneous approach values use skin or mucous membrane as the access location. The site of a procedure of a can also be reached through an external opening. External openings can be natural (for example, mouth) or artificial (for example, nephrostomy stoma).

### Method

The method specifies how the external access location is entered for procedures performed on an internal body part. An open method of an approach means there was cutting through the skin or mucous membrane and other body layers to expose the site of the procedure. An instrumental approach method specifies the entry of instrumentation through the access location to the internal procedure site. Instrumentation can be introduced by puncture or minor incision or through an external opening. The puncture or minor incision should not be interpreted as an open approach. An approach can define multiple methods. For example, the approach through a natural or artificial orifice with percutaneous endoscopic assistance uses both the orifice and the percutaneous endoscopic approach to reach the procedure site.

### Type of Instrumentation

Specialized equipment or instrumentation is used to perform a procedure on an internal body part. The instrumentation is used in all internal approaches other than the basic open approach. Instrumentation may or may not be used to visualize the procedure site. For example, the bronchoscope is the instrument used to perform a bronchoscopy that permits the internal site of the procedure to be visualized. Instrumentation used to perform a needle biopsy of the pancreas does not visualize the site The term "endoscopic" as used in approach values refers to instrumentation that permits a procedure site to be visualized.

### External Approaches

The external approach is used when procedures are performed directly on the skin or mucous membrane. External procedures may be performed indirectly by the application of external force. Examples of procedures using external approaches are skin lesion excision, closed reduction of a fracture, and tonsillectomy (because the tonsils can be reached through the mouth) (CMS 2015).

### Device and Qualifier

In the Medical and Surgical section, the sixth character specifies devices that remain after the procedure is completed. The seventh character, qualifier, is used with certain procedures to define an additional attribute of the procedure. The following lists illustrate examples of the sixth and seventh characters available in the urinary system.

**Device—Character 6**

0 Drainage Device
2 Monitoring Device
3 Infusion Device
7 Autologous Tissue Substitute
C Extraluminal Device
D Intraluminal Device
J Synthetic Substitute
K Nonautologous Tissue Substitute
L Artificial Sphincter
M Stimulator Lead
Y Other Device
Z No Device

**Qualifier—Character 7**

0 Allogeneic
1 Syngeneic
2 Zooplastic
3 Kidney Pelvis, Right
4 Kidney Pelvis, Left
6 Ureter, Right
7 Ureter, Left
8 Colon
9 Colocutaneous
A Ileum
B Bladder
C Ileocutaneous
D Cutaneous
X Diagnostic
Z No Qualifier

### Device

A device is specified in the sixth character and is only used to specify devices that remain after the procedure is completed. There are four general types of devices:

- Grafts and prostheses are biological or synthetic material that takes the place of all or a portion of a body part (that is, skin graft or joint prosthesis).
- Implants are therapeutic material that is not absorbed by, eliminated by, or incorporated into a body part (that is, radioactive implant). The therapeutic implants can be retained permanently in the body or removed when no longer needed. Examples of implants are internal fixation devices, an intramedullary nail, or a tissue expander implanted under the skin or muscle.

- Simple or mechanical appliances are biological or synthetic material that assists or prevents a physiological function. Examples of these appliances are a tracheostomy airway device, a monoplanar external fixation device, or an intraluminal device such as a vascular graft.
- Electronic appliances used to assist, monitor, take the place of or prevent a physiological function. Examples of electronic appliances are a cardiac pacemaker generator, cochlear implant hearing device, or a neurostimulator.

Instrumentation used to visualize the procedure site is not specified in the device value. This information is specified in the approach value.

If the objective of the procedure is to put in a device, then the root operation is Insertion. If the device is put in to meet an objective other than Insertion, the root operation defining the underlying objective of the procedure is used, with the device specified in the sixth character, device. For example, if a procedure to replace the hip joint is performed, the root operation Replacement is coded and the prosthetic device is specified as the sixth character. Materials incidental to a procedure such as clips, ligatures, and sutures are not specified in the device character.

## Device Key

ICD-10-PCS originally included an Appendix D: Device Key and Aggregation Table. Some publishers have kept Appendix D in the printed code books. The Device Key translates specific device terms to an equivalent PCS description for the sixth character of an ICD-9-PCS code. The device terms may be general device descriptions, such as non-tunneled central venous catheter, or a device by a specific trade name, such as Kirschner wire. Using the later example, if "Kirschner wire" is located in the Device Key, the coder is instructed to use "internal fixation device" in the bone or joint it is inserted.

As ICD-10-PCS has been updated by CMS over the past few years, the Device Key entries have been added to the Index for ICD-10-PCS for ease of reference. When the coder is uncertain what PCS description should be used for the sixth character of a code, the coder should access the Index to see if the device is located there. For example, in the ICD-10-PCS Index, an entry for Kirschner wire is included and instructs the coder to "use internal fixation device" as the description of the device in the ICD-10-PCS code.

## Root Operations and Devices

Devices can be removed from the body but some devices cannot be removed without being replace with another non-biological appliance or another substitute for the body part.

The following root operations **may or may not** have specific devices as part of the procedure:

Alteration
Bypass
Creation
Destruction
Dilation
Division
Drainage
Excision
Extirpation
Fragmentation
Fusion

Map
Occlusion
Release
Repair
Reposition
Resection
Restriction
Transfer

The following root operations **must** have specific devices coded with these procedures:

Change
Insertion
Removal
Replacement
Revision
Supplement

The approach includes the fact that instrumentation was used to visualize the procedure site. This information is not specified in the device value.

The root operation of "insertion" is used when the procedure's objective is to put in a device. If the device is put in to meet a procedure's objective other than insertion, then the root operation defining the underlying objective of the procedure is used. The device used is identified with the device specified in the device character. For example, if the procedure is to replace the shoulder joint, the root operation is "replacement" and the prosthetic device is specified in the device character. The device is being "inserted" to "replace" the joint so the objective of the procedure is "replacement."

Materials incidental to a procedure such as clips, ligatures, and sutures are not what is meant by a device and is not specified in the device character.

Because new devices can be developed at any time, the value "Other Device" is provided as an option for use until a specific device value may be added to the system. With this option, a procedure that involves a new device can be coded as soon as the device is available instead of waiting until the coding system is updated in the future.

The following lists illustrate examples of the sixth character available in the urinary system.

**Device—Character 6**

0 Drainage Device
2 Monitoring Device
3 Infusion Device
7 Autologous Tissue Substitute
C Extraluminal Device
D Intraluminal Device
J Synthetic Substitute
K Nonautologous Tissue Substitute
L Artificial Sphincter
M Stimulator Lead
Y Other Device
Z No Device

### Qualifier

The seventh character is the qualifier to add more information to describe the procedure. Individual procedures have unique values for the qualifier in the seventh character position. The qualifiers may have a narrow application to a specific root operation, body system or body part. For example, the qualifier can be used to identify the destination site in a bypass procedure. Other qualifiers identify the type of transplant performed such as allogeneic, syngeneic, and zooplastic. The more common qualifier that is expected to be used is the qualifier "X" for "diagnostic" to identify when a biopsy procedure is performed.

The following lists illustrate examples of the seventh character available in the heart and great vessels system.

**Qualifier—Character 7**

| | |
|---|---|
| 3 | Coronary Artery |
| 4 | Coronary Vein |
| 5 | Coronary Circulation |
| 7 | Atrium, Left |
| 8 | Internal Mammary, Right |
| 9 | Internal Mammary, Left |
| B | Subclavian |
| C | Thoracic Artery |
| D | Carotid |
| F | Abdominal Artery |
| P | Pulmonary Trunk |
| Q | Pulmonary Artery, Right |
| R | Pulmonary Artery, Left |
| W | Aorta |

## ICD-10-PCS Official Guidelines for Coding and Reporting

Two departments within the Federal Government's Department of Health and Human Services provide the ICD-10-PCS Official Guidelines for Coding and Reporting. This is a new reference for coders as the ICD-9-CM did not have a set of official coding guidelines for the procedures codes in volume 3. The guidelines were developed by CMS and the National Center for Health Statistics (NCHS). The guidelines were approved by the four organizations that comprise the "Cooperating Parties for ICD-10-PCS," that is American Hospital Association (AHA), AHIMA, CMS, and NCHS.

The guidelines are intended to accompany and assist in the interpretation of the official conventions and instructions within the ICD-10-PCS coding system. It is important to note that the conventions and instructions in the ICD-10-PCS coding system take precedence over the guidelines, that is, they are the most important rules for coding. The guidelines are based on the coding instructions and definitions found in ICD-10-PCS. Adherence to the guidelines is required under the Health Insurance Portability and Accountability Act (HIPAA) as the ICD-10-PCS codes are required for hospital inpatient healthcare settings under HIPAA.

The 2015 edition of the ICD-10-PCS Official Guidelines for Coding and Reporting can be located in Appendix J on the website provided by this publication. In addition, the guidelines can be accessed on the CMS website at http://www.cms.gov/Medicare/Coding/ICD10/, under the section titled "2015 ICD-10-PCS and GEMs."

The guidelines consist of four parts:

A. Conventions
B. Medical and Surgical Section Guidelines including directions for body system, root operations, body part, approach, and device characters in the ICD-10-PCS code
C. Obstetric Section Guidelines
D. Selection of the Principal Procedure

## Overview of the ICD-10-PCS Guidelines

The entire set of ICD-10-PCS Guidelines for Coding and Reporting is required reading for coders. This table is intended to be a synopsis of the information contained within the guidelines,

| Section | Summary of Instruction |
|---|---|
| Conventions | |
| A1 | All ICD-10-PCS codes are composed of seven characters. Each character provides specific information about the procedure performed. |
| A2 | One of 34 possible values can be assigned to each axis in the seven character code. Values are numbers 0–9 and letters A–Z without using letters I and O so not to confuse with numbers 1 and 0. |
| A3 | Values will be added over time to ICD-10-PCS as needed. |
| A4 | The meaning of a single value depends on the character it describes and the any preceding values upon which it may be dependent. One value, such as 0, does not mean the same in different body systems, for example. |
| A5 | As the system expands to add detail, more values will depend on preceding values for their meaning. |
| A6 | The purpose of the alphabetic index is to locate the appropriate table that contains all the information necessary to construct a code. The Tables must always be consulted to assign the valid code. |
| A7 | A valid code may be chosen directly from the PCS Tables without using the index. |
| A8 | All seven characters must be specified to be a valid code. |
| A9 | Valid codes include combinations of choices in characters 4–7 on the same row of the PCS Tables. |
| A10 | "And" should be read as "and/or." |
| A11 | It is the coder's responsibility to determine what documentation in the record equates to the PCS definitions. Physicians are not required to use PCS terminology. |
| Medical and Surgical Section Guidelines | |
| B2 Body System | |
| B2.1a Body System General Guidelines | Describes when to use general anatomical region body systems rather than a specific body part. |
| B2.1b Upper and Lower | Upper and lower body parts are located above and below the diaphragm. |
| B3 Root Operations | |
| B3.1a Root operations General Guidelines | Full definition of the root operation must be applied. |
| B3.1b Components of a Procedure | Procedural steps necessary to reach the operative site and close the operative site, including anastomosis of a tubular body part, are not coded separately. |

| | |
|---|---|
| B3.2 Multiple Procedures | Describes when to code multiple procedures:<br>1. Same root operation is performed on different body parts.<br>2. Same root operation is repeated at different body parts that are included in the same body part value.<br>3. Multiple root operations with distinct objectives are performed on the same body part.<br>4. The intended root operation is attempted using one approach, but is converted to a different approach. |
| B3.3 Discontinued Procedures | If the intended procedure is discontinued, code the procedure to the root operation performed. If the procedure is discontinued before any root operation is performed, code the root operation Inspection of the body part or anatomical region inspected. |
| B3.4a Biopsy Procedures | Biopsy procedures are coded with root operations Excision, Extraction, or Drainage and the qualifier Diagnostic. The qualifier Diagnostic is used only for biopsies. |
| B3.4b Biopsy Followed by More Definitive Treatment | If a diagnostic Excision, Extraction, or Drainage procedure (Biopsy) is followed by a more definitive procedure, such as Destruction, Excision, or Resection at the same procedure site, both the biopsy and the more definitive treatment are coded. |
| B3.5 Overlapping Body Layers | If the root operations Excision, Repair or Inspection are performed on overlapping layers of the musculoskeletal system, the body part specifying the deepest layer is coded. |
| B3.6a Bypass Procedures | Bypass procedures are coded by identifying the body part bypassed "from" and the body part bypassed "to." The fourth character body part specifies the body part bypassed from, and the qualifier specifies the body part bypassed to. |
| B3.6b Coronary Arteries | Coronary arteries are classified by number of distinct sites treated, rather than the number of coronary arteries or the anatomic name of a coronary artery. The body part identifies the number of coronary artery sites bypassed to and the qualifier specifies the vessel bypassed from. |
| B3.6c Multiple Sites Bypassed | If multiple coronary artery sites are bypassed, a separate procedure is coded for each coronary artery site that uses a different device and/or qualifier. |
| B3.7 Control as Root Operation | The root operation Control is defined as "Stopping, or attempting to stop, postprocedural bleeding." If any definitive root operation such as Bypass, Detachment, Excision, Extraction, Reposition, Replacement, or Resection are performed to stop the postprocedural bleeding, then that root operation is coded instead of Control. |
| B3.8 Excision versus Resection as Root Operation | PCS contains specific body parts for anatomical divisions of a body part. Resection is coded whenever all of a body part is cut out or off. Excision is coded when a portion of a body part is cut out or off. |
| B3.9 Excision for Graft | If an autograft is obtained from a different body part in order to complete the objective of a procedure, a separate procedure is coded. |
| B3.10a Fusion Procedures for Spine-Body Parts | The body part coded for a spinal vertebral joint(s) rendered immobile by a spinal fusion procedure is classified by the level of the spine. |
| B3.10B Fusion Procedures Using Different Device and/ or Qualifier | If multiple vertebral joints are fused, a separate procedure is coded for each vertebral joint that uses a different device and/or qualifier. |
| B3.10c Fusion Procedures-Combinations of Devices and Materials Hierarchy | Combinations of devices and materials are often used on a vertebral joint to render the joint immobile. The guideline gives a hierarchy of how to select the device value when combinations of devices are used. |
| B3.11a Inspection procedures as Root Operation | Inspection of a body part(s) performed in order to achieve the objective of a procedure is not coded separately. |
| B3.11b Inspection of Most Distal Body Part | If multiple tubular body parts are inspected, the most distal body part inspected is coded. If multiple non-tubular body parts are inspected, the body part that specifies the entire area inspected is coded. |
| B3.11c Inspection Done by Different Approach | When both an Inspection procedure and another procedure are performed on the same body part during the same episode, if the Inspection procedure is performed using a different approach than the other procedure, the Inspection procedure is coded separately. |

| | |
|---|---|
| B3.12 Occlusion versus Restriction as Root Operation | If the objective of an embolization procedure is to completely close a vessel, the root operation Occlusion is coded. If the objective is to narrow the lumen of a vessel, the root operation Restriction is coded. |
| B3.13 Release Procedures as Root Operation | In the root operation Release, the body part value is the body part being freed and not the tissue being manipulated or cut to free the body part. |
| B3.14 Release versus Division Procedures as Root Operation | If the sole objective of the procedure is freeing a body part without cutting the body part, the root operation is Release. If the sole objective is separating or transecting a body part, the root operation is Division. |
| B3.15 Reposition for fracture treatment | Reduction of a displaced fracture is coded to the root operation Reposition and the application of a cast or splint with the reposition procedure is not coded separately. The treatment of a nondisplaced fracture is coded to the procedure performed. |
| B3.16 Transplantation versus Administration | Putting in a mature and functioning living body part taken from another individual or animal is coded to the root operation Transplantation. Putting in autologous or nonautologous cells is coded to the Administration section. |
| B4 Body Part | |
| B4.1a Portion of a Body Part | If the procedure is performed on a portion of a body part that does not have a separate body part value, code the body part value corresponding to the whole body part. |
| B4.1b Prefix "Peri" used with a Body part | If the prefix "peri" is combined with a body part to identify the site of the procedure, the procedure is coded to the body part named. |
| B4.2 Branches of a Body Part | When a specific branch of a body part does not have its own body part value, the body part is coded to the closest proximal branch that has a specific body part value. |
| B4.3 Bilateral Body Parts | If identical procedures are performed on contralateral body parts, and a bilateral body part value exists, a single procedure is coded using the bilateral body part value. If no bilateral body part value exists, each procedure is coded separately using the appropriate body part value. |
| B4.4 Coronary Arteries | The coronary arteries are classified as a single body part that is further specified by the number of sites treated and not by name or number of arteries. Separate body part values are used to specify the number of sites treated when the same procedure is performed on multiple sites in the coronary arteries. |
| B4.5 Tendons, Ligaments, Bursae and Fascia Near a Joint | Procedures performed on tendons, ligaments, bursae and fascia supporting a joint are coded to the body part in the respective body system that is the focus of the procedure. Procedures performed on joint structures are coded to the body part in the joint body systems. |
| B4.6 Skin, Subcutaneous Tissue and Fascia Overlying a Joint | If a procedure is performed on the skin, subcutaneous tissue and fascia overlying a joint, this guideline identifies the body part to be used, for example, shoulder is coded to upper arm. |
| B4.7 Fingers and Toes | If a body system does not contain a separate body part value for fingers or toes, the procedure performed should be coded to hand and foot respectively. |
| B4.8 Upper and Lower Gastrointestinal Tract | Contains the definition of Upper and Lower GI tract for root operations Change, Inspective, Removal and Revision. Upper GI is the portion of the GI tract from the esophagus down to and including the duodenum. Lower GI tract is the portion of the GI tract from the jejunum down to and including the rectum and anus. |
| B5 Approach | |
| B5.2 Open Approach with Percutaneous Endoscopic Assistance | Procedures performed using the open approach with percutaneous endoscopic assistance is coded to the approach Open. |
| B5.3a External Approach | Procedures performed within an orifice on structures that are visible without the aid of any instrumentation are coded to the approach External. |
| B5.3b External Approach through Body Layers | Procedures performed indirectly by the application of external force through intervening body layers are coded to the approach External. |
| B5.4 Percutaneous Procedure via a Device | Procedures performed percutaneously via a device placed for the procedure are coded to the approach percutaneous. |

| B6. Device | |
|---|---|
| B6.1a General Guidelines | A device is coded only if a device remains after a procedure is completed. If no device remains, the device value No Device is used. |
| B6.1b What is Not Considered a Device | Materials such as sutures, ligatures, radiological markers and temporary post-operative wound drains are considered integral to the performance of the procedure and not coded as devices. |
| B6.1c Procedures Performed on a Device Only | Procedures performed on a device only and not on a body part specified in the root operations Change, Irrigation, Removal and Revision and are coded to the procedure performed. |
| B6.2 Drainage Device | A separate procedure to put in a drainage device is coded to the root operation Drainage with the device value Drainage Device. |
| C. Obstetric Section Guidelines | |
| C1 Products of Conception | Procedures performed on the products of conception are coded to the Obstetrics section. Procedures performed on the pregnant female other than the products of conception are coded to the root operation in the Medical and Surgical section. |
| C2 Procedures Following Delivery or Abortion | Procedure performed following a delivery or abortion for curettage of the endometrium or evacuation of retained products of conception are all coded in the Obstetrics section, to the root operation Extraction and the body part Products of Conception, retained. Diagnostic or therapeutic D&C performed during times other than postpartum or post-abortion are coded to the Medical and Surgical section, to the root operation Extraction and the body part Endometrium. |
| Section of Principal Procedure | The following instructions should be applied in the selection of principal procedure and clarification on the importance of the relation to the principal diagnosis when more than one procedure is performed. |
| 1. Procedure performed for Definitive Treatment for Both Principal Diagnosis and Secondary Diagnosis | Sequence procedure performed for definitive treatment most related to principal diagnosis as principal procedure. |
| 2. Procedure performed for Definitive Treatment and Diagnostic Procedure performed for Both Principal Diagnosis and Secondary Diagnosis | Sequence procedure performed for definitive treatment most related to principal diagnosis as principal procedure. |
| 3. Diagnostic Procedure performed for the Principal Diagnosis and Procedure performed for Definitive Treatment of a Secondary Diagnosis | Sequence diagnostic procedure as principal procedure, since the procedure most related to the principal diagnosis takes precedence. |
| 4. No Procedure Performed for Principal Diagnosis. Procedure performed for Definitive Treatment and Diagnostic Procedure performed for Secondary Diagnosis. | Sequence procedure performed for definitive treatment of secondary diagnosis as principal procedure, since there are no procedures (definitive or nondefinitive treatment) related to principal diagnosis. |

Reference: CMS 2015

## Assigning an ICD-10-PCS Code

An ICD-10-PCS code is constructed by assigning values for each of the characters. The procedural term is referenced in the Index. The main terms listed in the Index can be either the root operation phrase, such as resection, with the subterm gallbladder, or occasionally a common procedure term, such as cholecystectomy.

According to the ICD-10-PCS Official Guidelines for Coding and Reporting, the purpose of the alphabetic index is to locate the appropriate table to construct an ICD-10-PCS procedure code. The PCS tables should also be consulted for the most appropriate valid code (guideline A6.) However, the coder does not have to use the Index before proceeding to the tables to construct a code. A coder may choose the appropriate code directly from the code tables (guideline A7). A coder experienced with ICD-10-PCS may perform ICD-10-PCS coding directly from the tables after becoming confident with the definitions of the root operations and the body systems. For new coders, the normal process would likely be to locate the procedure turn in the index and then move to the code tables as directed (CMS 2015).

As an example, to code a laparoscopic total cholecystectomy, the coder could access the root operation "Resection" in the Index and find:

> Resection
> Gallbladder, 0FT4

Alternatively, the coder could access the common procedure term "Cholecystectomy" in the Index and find:

> Cholecystectomy
> See Excision, Gallbladder 0FB4
> See Resection, Gallbladder 0FT4

It is important to note that in order to choose the appropriate cross reference, the coder must know the definitions of the root operations "excision" and "resection." *Excision* is defined as cutting out or off, without replacement, a portion of a body part. *Resection* is defined as cutting out or off, without replacement, all of a body part. A cholecystectomy would be a resection of the gallbladder, as the entire gallbladder is removed during a cholecystectomy.

The next step in the process is to access the 0FT code table. The remaining four characters are assigned based on this table. The values for each of the characters must be from the same row.

For example, using the table that follows, the code for a cholecystectomy performed through a laparoscopic approach would be 0FT44ZZ. Each of the seven characters of the procedure code describes the procedure of a laparoscopic total cholecystectomy:

0 = Medical and Surgical Section
F = Hepatobiliary system and pancreas body system
T = Resection
4 = Gallbladder body part
4 = Percutaneous endoscopic approach
**Z = No device**
**Z = No qualifier**

Table for OFT, first three characters for a surgical procedure in the hepatobiliary system and pancreas that is a resection.

| **0 Medical and Surgical**<br>**F Hepatobiliary System and Pancreas**<br>**T Resection—Cutting out or off, without replacement, all of a body part** | | | |
|---|---|---|---|
| **Body Part Character 4** | **Approach Character 5** | **Device Character 6** | **Qualifier Character 7** |
| **0** Liver<br>**1** Liver, Right Lobe<br>**2** Liver, Left Lobe<br>**4** **Gallbladder**<br>**G** Pancreas | **0** Open<br>**4** **Percutaneous Endoscopic** | **Z** **No Device** | **Z** **No Qualifier** |
| **5** Hepatic Duct, Right<br>**6** Hepatic Duct, Left<br>**8** Cystic Duct<br>**9** Common Bile Duct<br>**C** Ampulla of Vater<br>**D** Pancreatic Duct<br>**F** Pancreatic Duct, Accessory | **0** Open<br>**4** Percutaneous Endoscopic<br>**7** Via Natural or Artificial Opening<br>**8** Via Natural or Artificial Opening Endoscopic | **Z** No Device | **Z** No Qualifier |

## ICD-10-PCS Review Exercises:

Assign the appropriate ICD-10-PCS codes to the following statements:

1. Esophagogastroduodenoscopy (EGD)

2. Left partial mastectomy, open

3. Open left femoral-popliteal artery bypass using cadaver vein graft

4. Laparoscopy with lysis of adhesions of bilateral ovaries and bilateral fallopian tubes

5. Posterior spinal fusion of the posterior column at L2-L4 with Bak cage interbody fusion device, open

6. Cystoscopy with retrieval of right ureteral stent

7. Reattachment of severed right hand

8. Diagnostic percutaneous paracentesis for ascites

9. Transmetatarsal amputation of foot at right big toe

10. Transplant of left kidney from a living donor

11. Open repair of laceration of large intestine

12. Open reduction fracture of right tibia

13. Mitral valve replacement using porcine tissue, open

14. Percutaneous transluminal coronary angioplasty of right coronary artery

15. Endoscopic fulguration of sigmoid colon polyp

## ICD-10-PCS Review Exercises: (Continued)

16. Thrombectomy, by incision, arteriovenous dialysis graft, right upper arm, cephalic vein

17. Revision of left knee replacement with readjustment of prosthesis, open

18. Hysteroscopy with diagnostic D&C

19. Extracorporeal shockwave lithotripsy (EWSL) of right ureter

20. Esophagogastroduodenoscopy with esophagomyotomy of esophagogastric junction

21. Skin flap transfer, open wound, right lower leg

22. Thoracotomy with banding of left pulmonary artery with extraluminal device

23. Percutaneous embolization of right uterine artery using coils

24. Construction of a vagina in a male patient using tissue bank donor graft as part of a sex change operation

25. Bilateral breast augmentation with silicone implants, open, cosmetic

26. Percutaneous insertion of spinal neurostimulator lead, lumbar spinal cord

27. Open anterior colporrhaphy with polypropylene mesh reinforcement

28. Tracheostomy tube exchange (remove and replace with new tube)

29. Intraoperative whole brain mapping by craniotomy

30. Laparotomy for control of postoperative bleeding in peritoneal cavity

# Chapter 3

# Introduction to the Uniform Hospital Discharge Data Set and Official Coding Guidelines

## Learning Objectives

At the conclusion of this chapter for both ICD-9-CM and ICD-10-CM, you should be able to:

1. Describe the purpose of the Uniform Hospital Discharge Data Set and identify its data elements
2. Define the terms *principal diagnosis, other diagnoses, complication, comorbidity, significant procedure,* and *principal procedure*
3. Identify the number of ICD-9-CM diagnosis and procedure codes that can appear on the Uniform Bill-04
4. Explain the purpose of the "present on admission" indicator with diagnosis codes
5. Apply the ICD-9-CM Official Guidelines for Coding and Reporting for selecting the principal diagnosis for inpatient care and reporting of additional diagnoses
6. Apply the ICD-10-CM Official Guidelines for Coding and Reporting for selecting the principal diagnosis for inpatient care and reporting of additional diagnoses

## Uniform Hospital Discharge Data Set

As discussed in the Introduction to this text, there are many uses for the data that are created by the coding activity, including compiling statistical data. In order for these data to be useful, the same data must be collected the same way by everyone gathering the data. The **Uniform Hospital Discharge Data Set (UHDDS)** was promulgated by the US Department of Health, Education, and Welfare in 1974 as a minimum, common core of data on individual acute care short-term hospital discharges in Medicare and Medicaid programs. It sought to improve the uniformity and comparability of hospital discharge data.

In 1985, the data set was revised to improve the original version in light of timely needs and developments. These data elements and their definitions can be found in the July 31, 1985, *Federal Register* (50 FR 31038). Since that time, the application of the UHDDS definitions has been expanded to include all non-outpatient settings (acute care, short-term care, long-term care, and psychiatric hospitals; home health agencies; rehabilitation facilities; nursing homes; and so forth).

Part of the current UHDDS includes the following specific items pertaining to patients and their episodes of care:

- **Personal identification:** The unique number assigned to each patient that distinguishes the patient and his or her health record from all others
- **Date of birth**
- **Sex**
- **Race**
- **Ethnicity (Hispanic–Non Hispanic)**
- **Residence:** The zip code or code for foreign residence
- **Hospital identification:** The unique number assigned to each institution
- **Admission and discharge dates**
- **Physician identification:** The unique number assigned to each physician within the hospital (the attending physician and the operating physician [if applicable] are both to be identified)
- **Disposition of patient:** The way in which the patient left the hospital—discharged to home, left against medical advice, discharged to another short-term hospital, discharged to a long-term care institution, died, or other
- **Expected payer for most of the bill:** The single major source expected by the patient to pay for this bill (for example, Blue Cross/Blue Shield, Medicare, Medicaid, Workers' Compensation)

In keeping with UHDDS standards, medical data items for the following diagnoses and procedures also are reported:

- **Diagnoses:** All **diagnoses** affecting the current hospital stay must be reported as part of the UHDDS.
- **Principal diagnosis:** The **principal diagnosis** is designated and defined as the condition established after study to be chiefly responsible for occasioning the admission of the patient to the hospital for care.
- **Other diagnoses:** These are designated and defined as all conditions that coexist at the time of admission, that develop subsequently, or that affect the treatment received and/or the length of stay (LOS). Diagnoses are to be excluded that relate to an earlier episode that has no bearing on the current hospital stay. Within the Medicare Acute Care Inpatient Prospective Payment System (IPPS), ***other diagnoses*** may qualify as a major complication or comorbidity (MCC), or other **complication** or **comorbidity** (CC). The terms ***complication*** and ***comorbidity*** are not part of the UHDDS definition set but were developed as part of the diagnosis-related group (DRG) system. The presence of the complication or comorbidity may influence the MS-DRG assignment and produce a higher-valued DRG with a higher payment for the hospital.
- **Complication:** This is defined as an *additional* diagnosis that describes a condition arising after the beginning of hospital observation and treatment and then modifying the course of the patient's illness or the medical care required.

- **Comorbidity:** This is defined as a *preexisting* condition that, because of its presence with a specific principal diagnosis, will likely cause an increase in the patient's length of stay in the hospital.
- **Procedures and dates:** All **significant procedures** are to be reported. For significant procedures, both the identity (by unique number within the hospital) of the person performing the procedure and the date of the procedure must be reported.
- **Significant procedure:** A procedure is identified as significant when it:
  - Is surgical in nature
  - Carries a procedural risk
  - Carries an anesthetic risk
  - Requires specialized training
- **Principal procedure:** This type of procedure is performed for definitive treatment rather than for diagnostic or exploratory purposes, or when it is necessary to take care of a complication. If two procedures appear to be principal, the one most related to the principal diagnosis should be selected as the principal procedure.

## Uniform Bill-04

In 1975, the **National Uniform Billing Committee (NUBC)** was established with the goal of developing an acceptable, uniform bill that would consolidate the numerous billing forms hospitals were required to use. In 1982, the Uniform Bill-82 (UB-82), also known as the CMS-1450 form, was implemented for use in billing services to Medicare fiscal intermediaries and other third-party payers. In 1988, the NUBC began preparations for a revised uniform bill. The resulting Uniform Bill-92 (UB-92) was implemented in October 1993 and provided for the collection of additional statistical data, including clinical information.

The NUBC approved the Uniform Bill-04 (UB-04) as the replacement for the UB-92 at its February 2005 meeting. As of May 23, 2007, all institutional paper claims were submitted with the UB-04, as the UB-92 is no longer accepted. The UB-04 provides better alignment with the electronic Health Insurance Portability and Accountability Act of 1996 (HIPAA) 837 transaction standard or the electronic billing format. In addition, the electronic 837 transaction standard and UB-04 accommodate the national provider identifiers, the health plan identifiers, and migration to the ICD-10-CM and ICD-10-PCS coding systems when they are implemented. There is an increased emphasis on clinical codes.

Look at the sample UB-04 claim form in appendix F on the accompanying website to text. The UB-04 has expanded the number of diagnosis codes that can be reported by adding nine new fields for a total of 18. The 18 diagnosis codes are placed on form locator 67 and 67A–67Q. There is space for one admitting diagnosis for a patient who is admitted as an inpatient (form locator 69), as well as three "patient reason" diagnosis codes (form locator 70a–70c) to describe the patient's reason for visit at the time of outpatient registration. Additional space is allowed for reporting external cause of injury codes or E codes (form locator 72a–72c). There is room to report three E codes on the UB-04 paper and electronic claim forms. In addition, there is a "diagnosis indicator" field to identify whether a particular final inpatient diagnosis was present at the time of admission with a yes/no (Y/N) indicator. There is space for six ICD-9-CM procedure codes on the UB-04 (form locator 74 and 74a–74e). These details are summarized next.

**Inpatient claims:**

| | |
|---|---|
| Admitting diagnosis: | 1 ICD-9-CM diagnosis code |
| Final diagnosis: | 18 ICD-9-CM diagnosis codes |
| External cause of injury: | 3 ICD-9-CM diagnosis codes |
| **Total:** | **22 ICD-9-CM diagnosis codes** |
| Procedure: | 6 ICD-9-CM Volume 3 procedure codes |

**Outpatient claims:**

| | |
|---|---|
| Reason for visit: | 3 ICD-9-CM diagnosis codes |
| Final diagnosis: | 18 ICD-9-CM diagnosis codes |
| External cause of injury: | 3 ICD-9-CM diagnosis codes |
| **Total:** | **24 ICD-9-CM diagnosis codes** |

Effective January 1, 2011, the Centers for Medicare and Medicaid Services (CMS) expanded the number of ICD-9-CM diagnosis and procedure codes allowed to be processed on institutional claims through the implementation of version 5010/837I of the electronic claims transaction standards. The move to using more than the first nine ICD-9-CM diagnosis codes and the first six ICD-9-CM procedure codes for payment purposes was long awaited. This expansion allowed for 24 additional ICD-9-CM codes, including the associated Present on Admission indicator, and 24 secondary procedure codes. With this expansion, CMS processed a total of 25 ICD-9-CM diagnosis codes (one principal diagnosis and 24 additional diagnoses) and a total of 25 ICD-9-CM procedure codes for its institutional electronic claims processing. With version 4010 and the paper claims transaction, CMS does not process more than nine diagnosis codes and six procedure codes (CMS 2010b).

The UB-04 data elements also include the **present on admission (POA)** indicator. The POA reporting purpose is to differentiate between conditions present at admission and conditions that develop during an inpatient admission. The POA indicator applies to diagnosis codes for claims involving inpatient admissions to acute care hospitals or other facilities, as required by law or regulation for public health reporting. The **Cooperating Parties for ICD-9-CM** (AHIMA, the American Hospital Association, CMS, and the National Center for Health and Statistics (NCHS)) have developed comprehensive POA reporting guidelines that are included as a separate section of the ICD-9-CM Official Guidelines for Coding and Reporting and the ICD-10-CM Official Guidelines for Coding and Reporting.

## Selection of Principal Diagnosis

As the UHDDS definition states, a **principal diagnosis** is the condition "established after study to be chiefly responsible for occasioning the admission of the patient to the hospital for care." (50 FR 31038) Selecting the principal diagnosis depends on the circumstances of the admission, or why the patient was admitted. The admitting diagnosis has to be worked up through diagnostic tests and studies. Therefore, the words "after study" serve as an integral part of this definition. During the course of hospitalization, the admitting diagnosis, which may be a symptom or ill-defined condition, could change substantially based on the results of "further study."

**EXAMPLE:** Patient was admitted through the emergency department with an admitting diagnosis of seizure disorder. During hospitalization, diagnostic tests and studies revealed carcinoma of the brain, which explained the seizures.

The principal diagnosis was the carcinoma of the brain, which was the condition determined after study.

At times, however, it may be difficult to distinguish between the *principal* diagnosis and the *most significant* diagnosis. The most significant diagnosis is defined as the condition having the most impact on the patient's health, LOS, resource consumption, and the like. However, the most significant diagnosis may or may not be the principal diagnosis.

**EXAMPLE:** Patient was admitted with a fractured hip due to an accident. The fracture was reduced and the patient discharged home.

In this case, the principal diagnosis was fracture of the hip.

**EXAMPLE:** Patient was admitted with a fractured hip due to an accident. While hospitalized, the patient suffered a myocardial infarction.

In this case, the principal diagnosis was still the fracture of the hip, with the myocardial infarction coded as an additional diagnosis. Although the myocardial infarction may be the most significant diagnosis in terms of the patient's health and resource consumption, it was not the reason, after study, for the admission; therefore, it was not the principal diagnosis.

Another important consideration in determining principal diagnosis is the fact that the coding conventions in ICD-9-CM, volumes 1 and 2, take precedence over the Official Coding Guidelines. (See Section I.A. Conventions for the ICD-9-CM.)

## ICD-9-CM Official Guidelines for Coding and Reporting

The **ICD-9-CM Official Guidelines for Coding and Reporting** is available from the Centers for Disease Control and Prevention (CDC) (http://www.cdc.gov/nchs/icd/icd9cm.htm). All coding students are strongly encouraged to read the guidelines and become familiar with the rules in order to put them into practice. The application of the guidelines in everyday practice helps to ensure data accuracy in both coding and reporting for all healthcare encounters.

## Selecting Principal Diagnosis for Inpatient Care

The following information on selecting the principal diagnosis and additional diagnoses should be reviewed carefully to ensure appropriate coding and reporting of hospital claims.

The circumstances of inpatient admission always govern selection of the principal diagnosis in keeping with the UHDDS definition of the term as the condition determined after study to be chiefly responsible for bringing about the admission of the patient to the hospital for care. In determining the principal diagnosis, the coding directives in ICD-9-CM, volumes 1, 2, and 3, take precedence over all other guidelines. General guidelines related to the selection of the principal diagnosis follow. Disease-specific guidelines are discussed in later chapters. Guidelines throughout this section are titled and numbered as presented in the ICD-9-CM Official Guidelines for Coding and Reporting.

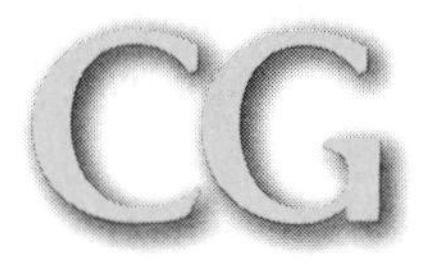

**Guideline II.A. Codes for symptoms, signs, and ill-defined conditions:** Codes for symptoms, signs, and ill-defined conditions from chapter 16 are not to be used as the principal diagnosis when a related definitive diagnosis has been established.

**EXAMPLE:** Patient was admitted to the hospital with chest pain to rule out myocardial infarction. After study, myocardial infarction was ruled out; the cause of the chest pain was undetermined.

Code 786.50, Chest pain, unspecified, was assigned. Although the code for chest pain (786.50) is located in chapter 16, a definitive diagnosis could not be made, so chest pain was coded as the principal diagnosis.

**EXAMPLE:** Patient was admitted to the hospital with dysphagia secondary to malignant neoplasm of the mouth. A PEG tube was inserted.

Code 145.9, Malignant neoplasm of the mouth, unspecified, was selected as the principal diagnosis, with code 787.20 as an additional diagnosis to describe the dysphagia. Because the dysphagia was related to the malignancy and code 787.20 is from chapter 16, the principal diagnosis was the definitive diagnosis rather than the symptom.

**Guideline II.B. Two or more interrelated conditions, each potentially meeting the definition for principal diagnosis:** When there are two or more interrelated conditions (such as diseases in the same ICD-9-CM chapter, or manifestations characteristically associated with a certain disease) potentially meeting the definition of principal diagnosis, either condition may be sequenced first, unless the circumstances of the admission, the therapy provided, the Tabular List, or the Alphabetic Index indicates otherwise.

**EXAMPLE:** Patient was admitted with closed fracture of the femur and tibia of the right leg. The fractures were reduced.

The following codes were assigned: 821.00, Fracture of unspecified part of femur, closed; 823.80, Fracture of unspecified part of tibia, closed; 79.05, Closed reduction of fracture of femur without internal fixation; and 79.06, Closed reduction of fracture of tibia and fibula without internal fixation. Both fractures potentially met the definition of principal diagnosis; therefore, either code 821.00 or code 823.80 could be sequenced first.

**Guideline II.C. Two or more diagnoses that equally meet the definition for principal diagnosis:** In the unusual instance when two or more diagnoses equally meet the criteria for principal diagnosis, as determined by the circumstances of admission, diagnostic workup, and/or the therapy provided, and the Alphabetic

Index, Tabular List, or another coding guideline does not provide sequencing direction in such cases, any one of the diagnoses may be sequenced first.

**EXAMPLE:** Patient was admitted for elective surgery. A lesion on the lip was excised and revealed squamous cell carcinoma. In addition, a right recurrent inguinal hernia was repaired.

The following codes were assigned: 140.9, Malignant neoplasm of lip, unspecified, vermilion border; 550.91, Inguinal hernia, without mention of obstruction or gangrene, unilateral or unspecified, recurrent; 27.43, Other excision of lesion or tissue of lip; 53.00, Unilateral repair of inguinal hernia, not otherwise specified. Both the squamous cell carcinoma of the lip and the right recurrent inguinal hernia met the criteria for principal diagnosis; therefore, either condition could be selected as the principal diagnosis.

**Guideline II.D. Two or more comparative or contrasting conditions:** In those rare instances when two or more contrasting or comparative diagnoses are documented as "either/or" (or similar terminology), they are coded as if confirmed and sequenced according to the circumstances of the admission. If no further determination can be made as to which diagnosis is principal, either diagnosis may be sequenced first.

**EXAMPLE:** Diverticulosis of colon versus angiodysplasia of intestine

Codes 562.10, Diverticulosis of colon (without mention of hemorrhage), and 569.84, Angiodysplasia of intestine (without mention of hemorrhage), are assigned.

Either unconfirmed diagnosis, diverticulosis of colon or angiodysplasia of intestine, may be sequenced as the principal diagnosis.

**Note:** Guidelines II.A through II.D reveal that designation of the principal diagnosis is not always an exact and easy task. At times, more than one condition may have occasioned the admission. In such cases, the actual circumstances of the case dictate designation of the principal diagnosis.

**Guideline II.E. A symptom(s) followed by contrasting or comparative diagnoses:** When a symptom(s) is (are) followed by contrasting or comparative diagnoses, the symptom code is sequenced first. All the contrasting or comparative diagnoses should be coded as additional diagnoses.

**EXAMPLE:** Patient was admitted with symptoms of periodic diarrhea and constipation during the previous 3 weeks. Following workup, physician documented the following diagnostic statement: Constipation and diarrhea due to either irritable bowel syndrome or diverticulitis.

*(Continued)*

(*Continued*)

The following codes were assigned: 564.00, Constipation; 787.91, Diarrhea; 564.1, Irritable bowel syndrome; and 562.11, Diverticulitis of colon (without mention of hemorrhage).

**Guideline II.F. Original treatment plan not carried out:** Sequence as the principal diagnosis the condition that after study occasioned the admission to the hospital, even if treatment may not have been carried out due to unforeseen circumstances.

**EXAMPLE:** Patient with ulcerated internal hemorrhoids was admitted for hemorrhoidectomy. Prior to the beginning of surgery, the patient developed bradycardia and the surgery was canceled.

The following codes were assigned: 455.2, Internal hemorrhoids with other complication; 427.89, Other specified cardiac dysrhythmias; and V64.1, Surgical or other procedure not carried out because of contraindication. The code for ulcerated internal hemorrhoids (455.2) was listed as the principal diagnosis because it was the reason for admission. An additional code for sinus bradycardia (427.89) was reported, as well as code V64.1, Surgical or other procedure not carried out because of contraindication, to indicate that the procedure was not carried out due to the complication of sinus bradycardia.

**Guideline II.G. Complications of surgery and other medical care:** When the admission is for treatment of a complication resulting from surgery or other medical care, the complication code is sequenced as the principal diagnosis. If the complication is classified to 996 through 999 series, and the code lacks the necessary specificity in describing the complication, an additional code for the specific complication should be assigned.

**EXAMPLE:** Patient was being treated for an atelectasis due to recent cardiovascular surgery. The diagnosis codes would include 997.39, Respiratory complications, and 518.0, Atelectasis

**Guideline II.H. Uncertain diagnosis:** If the diagnosis documented at the time of discharge is qualified as "probable," "suspected," "likely," "questionable," "possible," or "still to be ruled out," or other similar terms indicating uncertainty, code the condition as if it existed or was established. The bases for these guidelines are the diagnostic workup, arrangements for further workup or observation, and initial therapeutic approach that correspond most closely with the established diagnosis. Note: This guideline is applicable only to inpatient admissions to short-term, acute, and long-term care, and psychiatric hospitals.

Guideline II.I. Admission from observation unit:

1. Admission Following Medical Observation.
When a patient is admitted to an observation unit for a medical condition, which either worsens or does not improve, and is subsequently admitted as an inpatient of the same hospital for this same medical condition, the principal diagnosis would be the medical condition that led to the hospital admission.

2. Admission Following Postoperative Observation.
When a patient is admitted to an observation unit to monitor a condition (or complication) that develops following outpatient surgery, and then is subsequently admitted as an inpatient of the same hospital, hospitals should apply the UHDDS definition of principal diagnosis as "that condition established after study to be chiefly responsible for occasioning the admission of the patient to the hospital for care."

**Guideline II.J. Admission from outpatient surgery:** When a patient receives surgery in the hospital's outpatient surgery department and is subsequently admitted for continuing inpatient care at the same hospital, the following guidelines should be followed in selecting the principal diagnosis for the inpatient admission:

- When the reason for the inpatient admission is a complication, assign the complication as the principal diagnosis.
- When no complication, or other condition, is documented as the reason for the inpatient admission, assign the reason for the outpatient surgery as the principal diagnosis.
- When the reason for the inpatient admission is another condition unrelated to the surgery, assign the unrelated condition as the principal diagnosis.

## Reporting of Additional Diagnoses

The UHDDS item number 11-B defines other diagnoses as all conditions that coexist at the time of admission, that develop subsequently, or that affect the treatment received and/or the length of stay. Diagnoses that relate to an earlier episode that have no bearing on the current hospital stay are to be excluded (50 FR 31038).

Since 1985, when the UHDDS definitions were used by acute care short-term hospitals to report inpatient data elements in a standardized manner, the application of the UHDDS definitions has been expanded. Today, the UHDDS definitions are applicable to all nonoutpatient settings (acute care, short-term care, long-term care, and psychiatric hospitals; home health agencies; rehabilitation facilities; nursing homes; and so forth).

For reporting purposes, the general rule is that the definition for other diagnoses is interpreted to include additional conditions affecting patient care in terms of requiring:

- Clinical evaluation
- Therapeutic treatment
- Diagnostic procedures
- Extended length of hospital stay
- Increased nursing care and/or monitoring

Patients may have several chronic conditions that coexist at the time of their hospital admission and qualify as additional diagnoses. If there is documentation in the health record to indicate the patient has a chronic condition, it should be coded. Even if this condition is listed only by the physician in the history section with no contradictory information, the condition should be coded. Chronic conditions such as, but not limited to, hypertension, Parkinson's disease, chronic obstructive pulmonary disease (COPD), and diabetes mellitus are chronic systemic conditions that ordinarily should be coded even in the absence of documented intervention or further evaluation. Chronic conditions can affect the patient for the rest of their lives and usually require some form of evaluation, monitoring, or medication management. This applies to the coding of the patient in the inpatient setting. (See *Coding Clinic for ICD-9-CM,* 3rd Quarter, 2007, pp 13–14 for the discussion of coding chronic conditions.)

In an *outpatient* setting, the ICD-9-CM Official Guidelines for Coding and Reporting state that "Chronic diseases treated on an ongoing basis may be coded and reported as many times as the patient receives treatment and care for the condition(s)." (CDC 2011)

The following guidelines are to be applied in designating other diagnoses in the *inpatient* setting when neither the Alphabetic Index nor the Tabular List in ICD-9-CM provides direction.

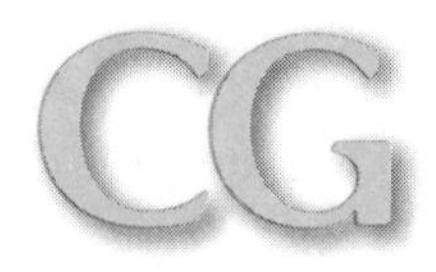


**Guideline III.A. Previous conditions:** If the provider has included a diagnosis in the final diagnostic statement, such as the discharge summary or the face sheet, the diagnosis should ordinarily be coded. Some providers include in the diagnostic statement resolved conditions or diagnoses and status post procedures from a previous admission that have no bearing on the current stay. Such conditions are not to be reported and are coded only if required by hospital policy.

However, history codes (V10–V19) may be used as secondary codes if the historical condition or family history has an impact on current care or influences treatment.

**EXAMPLE:** Face sheet states the following diagnoses: acute diverticulitis, congestive heart failure, status post cholecystectomy, status post hysterectomy.

All are coded except the status post cholecystectomy and hysterectomy. The heart failure and the diverticulitis affect the current hospitalization and thus are coded.

**Guideline III.B. Abnormal findings:** Abnormal findings (laboratory, x-ray, pathologic, and other diagnostic results) are not coded and reported unless the provider indicates their clinical significance. When the findings are outside the normal range and the attending provider has ordered other tests to evaluate the condition or prescribed treatment, the coder should ask the provider whether the abnormal findings should be added. For example, in the inpatient setting, coders should not assign codes for conditions described in a pathology report alone without the provider's input. The provider or physician should be asked for clarification of the pathological findings if the physician has not documented the same condition in the health record.

**Note:** This differs from the coding practices in the outpatient setting for coding encounters for diagnostic tests that have been interpreted by a provider. (See Coding Clinic for ICD-9-CM, First Quarter 2000, for information on Outpatient Laboratory, Pathology and Radiology Coding which allowed for the coding of diagnoses in outpatient reports that were authenticated by a physician, for example a pathologist or a radiologist.)

**Guideline III.C. Uncertain diagnosis:** If the diagnosis documented at the time of discharge is qualified as "probable," "suspected," "likely," "questionable," "possible," or "still to be ruled out," or other similar terms indicating uncertainty, code the condition as if it existed or was established. The bases for these guidelines are the diagnostic workup, arrangements for further workup or observation, and initial therapeutic approach that correspond most closely with the established diagnosis.

**Note:** This guideline is applicable only to inpatient admissions to short-term, acute, long-term care, and psychiatric hospitals.

In addition to Sections I and II of the ICD-9-CM Official Guidelines for Coding and Reporting, coders must also review Section IV Diagnostic Coding and Reporting Guidelines for Outpatient Services. Guidelines are different for the coding of outpatient records, for example, uncertain diagnoses are not coded as if it exists as is done when coding inpatient records. Chapter 18 in this textbook reviews Section IV for the outpatient coding guidelines.

## Review Exercise: Chapter 3

1. The physician's discharge summary includes the final diagnoses of (1) coronary artery disease, (2) hypertension, and (3) benign prostatic hypertrophy. The coder notes in the patient's laboratory reports that the patient has an elevated cholesterol and an elevated PSA positive finding.

2. What healthcare organizations collect UHDDS data?

3. What is the UHDDS definition of principal diagnosis?

4. What is the UHDDS definition of other diagnoses?

5. What is the purpose of the UHDDS?

6. What is the name of the organization that develops the billing form that hospitals are required to use?

7. What is the maximum number of diagnosis codes that can appear on a UB-04 claim form for a hospital inpatient?

8. What is the maximum number of procedure codes that can appear on a UB-04 claim form for a hospital inpatient?

Apply the ICD-9-CM Official Guidelines for Coding and Reporting of the Principal Diagnosis for Inpatient Care (Guidelines II A.–J.) to identify the principal diagnosis in the following scenarios:

9. Patient was admitted to the hospital after having a seizure at work. The admitting diagnosis was rule out epilepsy. After testing was performed, the cause of the seizure was not determined, as the physician stated the patient did not have epilepsy.

10. What is the difference between a "complication" and a "comorbidity?"

11. Patient was admitted to the hospital with acute exacerbation of chronic obstructive pulmonary disease and acute low back pain. Both conditions were evaluated and the patient received medical treatment. The patient was discharged home to continue to receive physical therapy for the back pain and pulmonary rehabilitation therapy for his chronic lung disease.

## Review Exercise: Chapter 3 (Continued)

12. The patient was admitted to the hospital with a multitude of gastrointestinal symptoms. After diagnostic tests were performed the physician was unable to determine exactly what was causing the patient's symptoms. The physician's final diagnosis was "Acute pancreatitis versus acute cholangitis."

13. The patient was admitted to the hospital for a total right knee replacement for osteoarthritis of the knee. During the patient's pre-operative preparation, the patient began having chest pain. The patient's knee surgery was cancelled, and the patient had extensive testing to determine the source of the chest pain, which was determined to be due to hypertensive heart disease.

14. The patient was admitted to the hospital with left lower quadrant abdominal pain. After study, the physician concluded the patient's abdominal pain could have been due to either of two conditions. Her final diagnosis was abdominal pain due to either a ruptured ovarian cyst or acute salpingitis.

15. Patient was admitted to the hospital with acute pyelonephritis and acute cystitis. Both infections were evaluated and treated with intravenous antibiotic therapy. The patient was discharged home to continue taking oral medications.

16. The patient was admitted to the hospital with fever, cough, and shortness of breath. After study, the physician could not identify the exact cause of these symptoms but felt the most likely cause was pneumonia. The physician's final diagnosis was "possible viral pneumonia now resolving."

17. The patient comes to the Emergency Department complaining of an asthma attack. The patient is placed into the observation unit to monitor his response to the asthma treatment. During the observation time the patient is determined to have status asthmaticus and is admitted for treatment of this condition. After a three-day hospital stay, the patient's asthma is better controlled, and he is discharged.

18. The patient was registered as an outpatient for a left-sided cataract extraction, which was performed successfully. While the patient was preparing to leave the hospital after surgery, the patient felt faint, and it was determined the patient's blood pressure was much lower than earlier in the day. The patient was admitted to the hospital to monitor the low blood pressure. The next day, the patient felt well again and was discharged. The physician described the patient's condition as "Orthostatic hypotension."

*(Continued on next page)*

## Review Exercise: Chapter 3 (Continued)

Apply the ICD-9-CM Official Guidelines for Coding and Reporting of the Principal Diagnosis for Inpatient Care (Guidelines III A.–C.) to identify the other diagnosis/diagnoses in the following scenarios:

19. The physician's discharge summary includes the final diagnoses of (1) acute cholecystitis, with additional diagnosis of (2) cholelithiasis, (3 ) type II diabetes, (4) history of pneumonia last year, and (5) status post bunionectomy three months ago.

 ___

20. The patient was re-admitted to the hospital for a postoperative wound infection. The patient had been discharged from the hospital five days ago, after having colon surgery for ruptured diverticulitis. During this hospital stay, the patient was treated for the wound infection and monitored for the remaining diverticulitis in his colon.

 ___

21. The physician's discharge summary includes the final diagnoses of (1) acute hemorrhagic gastritis, (2) acute duodenitis, and (3) possible acute pancreatitis.

 ___

22. The patient was admitted to the hospital with acute abdominal pain that was determined to be due to acute appendicitis, and the surgeon performed an open appendectomy on the patient. During the recovery period, the patient experienced two episodes of urinary retention that required the placement of a temporary urinary catheter. Would the second diagnosis of urinary retention be reported with a "yes" or a "no" as present on admission?

 ___

## ICD-10-CM Official Guidelines for Coding and Reporting

The *ICD-10-CM Official Guidelines for Coding and Reporting* is available from the CDC at http://www.cdc.gov/nchs/icd/icd10cm.htm. All coding students are strongly encouraged to read the guidelines and become familiar with the rules in order to put them into practice. The application of the guidelines in everyday practice helps to ensure data accuracy in both coding and reporting for all healthcare encounters. Reporting is the process of communicating the patient's diagnoses and procedures in codes to third party payers for reimbursement purposes and to other internal/facility databases and other external required databases for financial, quality measurement, public data, and other purposes.

The *ICD-10-CM Official Guidelines for Coding and Reporting* is referenced throughout this chapter. You can find the complete document in Appendix I. The following sections in this chapter from these guidelines (Sections II, III, IV) are included here to emphasize the connection between the UHDDS definitions and the related coding guidelines. The following information on selecting the principal diagnosis and additional diagnoses should be reviewed carefully to ensure appropriate coding and reporting of hospital claims.

## Section II. Selecting Principal Diagnosis for Inpatient Care

The circumstances of inpatient admission always govern selection of the principal diagnosis. The principal diagnosis is defined in the UHDDS as "that condition established after study to be chiefly responsible for occasioning the admission of the patient to the hospital for care."

The UHDDS definitions are used by hospitals to report inpatient data elements in a standardized manner. These data elements and their definitions can be found in the July 31, 1985 *Federal Register* (Vol. 50, No. 147, FR 31038, 31038–31040).

Since that time the application of the UHDDS definitions has been expanded to include all non-outpatient settings (acute care, short-term, long-term care and psychiatric hospitals; home health agencies; rehab facilities; nursing homes, and so on).

In determining the principal diagnosis, the coding convention in ICD-10-CM, the Tabular List and Alphabetic Index take precedence over all other guidelines. (See Section I.A. Conventions for the ICD-10-CM in the complete set of the Official Guidelines for Coding and Reporting.)

The importance of consistent, complete documentation In the medical record cannot be overemphasized. Without such documentation the application of all coding guidelines is a difficult, if not impossible, task.

The following is Section II of the ICD-10-CM Official Guidelines for Coding and Reporting written to address the selection of the principal diagnosis:

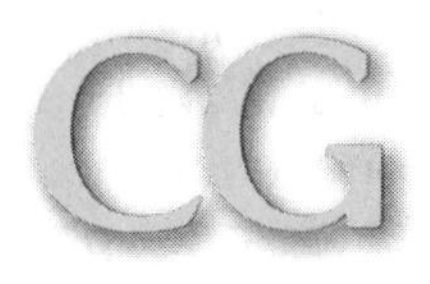


**Guideline II.A. Codes for symptoms, signs, and ill-defined conditions:** Codes for symptoms, signs, and ill-defined conditions from chapter 18 are not to be used as the principal diagnosis when a related definitive diagnosis has been established.

**EXAMPLE:** Patient was admitted to the hospital with chest pain to rule out myocardial infarction. After study, myocardial infarction was ruled out; the cause of the chest pain was undetermined.

Code R07.9, Chest pain, unspecified, was assigned. Although the code for chest pain (R07.9) is located in chapter 18, a definitive diagnosis could not be made, so chest pain was coded as the principal diagnosis.

**EXAMPLE:** Patient was admitted to the hospital with dysphagia secondary to malignant neoplasm of the esophagus. A PEG tube was inserted.

Code C15.9, Malignant neoplasm of the esophagus, unspecified, was selected as the principal diagnosis, with code R13.10 as an additional diagnosis to describe the dysphagia. Because the dysphagia was related to the malignancy and code R13.10 is from chapter 18, the principal diagnosis was the definitive diagnosis rather than the symptom.

(*Continued*)

*(Continued)*

**Guideline II.B. Two or more interrelated conditions, each potentially meeting the definition for principal diagnosis:** When there are two or more interrelated conditions (such as diseases in the same ICD-10-CM chapter, or manifestations characteristically associated with a certain disease) potentially meeting the definition of principal diagnosis, either condition may be sequenced first, unless the circumstances of the admission, the therapy provided, the Tabular List, or the Alphabetic Index indicates otherwise.

**EXAMPLE:** Patient was admitted for initial treatment for a closed fracture of the right femur lower end and fracture of the right tibia upper end.

The following diagnosis codes were assigned: S72.401A, Fracture of femur, right, lower end, closed; S82.101A, Fracture of tibia, right, upper end, closed. Both fractures potentially met the definition of principal diagnosis; therefore, either code could be sequenced first.

**Guideline II.C. Two or more diagnoses that equally meet the definition for principal diagnosis:** In the unusual instance when two or more diagnoses equally meet the criteria for principal diagnosis, as determined by the circumstances of admission, diagnostic workup, and/or the therapy provided, and the Alphabetic Index, Tabular List, or another coding guideline does not provide sequencing direction in such cases, any one of the diagnoses may be sequenced first.

**EXAMPLE:** Patient was admitted for elective surgery. A lesion on the left breast was excised and revealed fibroadenosis of breast. In addition, a right recurrent inguinal hernia was repaired.

The following diagnosis codes were assigned: N60.22, Fibroadenosis of left breast and K40.91, Unilateral inguinal hernia, without mention of obstruction or gangrene, recurrent. Both the fibroadenosis of left breast and the right recurrent inguinal hernia met the criteria for principal diagnosis. Therefore, either condition could be selected as the principal diagnosis.

**Guideline II.D. Two or more comparative or contrasting conditions:** In those rare instances when two or more contrasting or comparative diagnoses are documented as "either/or" (or similar terminology), they are coded as if confirmed and sequenced according to the circumstances of the admission. If no further determination can be made as to which diagnosis is principal, either diagnosis may be sequenced first.

**EXAMPLE:** Diverticulosis of large intestine versus angiodysplasia of colon

Codes K57.30, Diverticulosis of large intestine without perforation or abscess without bleeding and K55.20, Angiodysplasia of colon without hemorrhage are assigned.

Either unconfirmed diagnosis, diverticulosis or angiodysplaia of colon, may be sequenced as the principal diagnosis.

**Author Note:** Guidelines II.A through II.D reveal that designation of the principal diagnosis is not always an exact and easy task. At times, more than one condition may have occasioned the admission. In such cases, the actual circumstances of the case dictate designation of the principal diagnosis.

**Guideline II.E. A symptom(s) followed by contrasting or comparative diagnoses:** When a symptom(s) is (are) followed by contrasting or comparative diagnoses, the symptom code is sequenced first. However, if the symptom code is integral to the conditions listed, no code for the symptoms is reported. All the contrasting or comparative diagnoses should be coded as additional diagnoses (Author Note: this guideline is different than the same Section II.E. in the ICD-9-CM guidelines that does not mention the statement about the symptom code being integral to the condition is not coded).

**EXAMPLE:** Patient was admitted with symptoms of constipation and a possible bowel obstruction. The bowel obstruction was not present. Following workup, physician documented the following diagnostic statement: Constipation due to either irritable bowel syndrome or diverticulitis of large intestine. Since constipation is an integral condition to diverticulitis, it is not coded.

The following code is assigned: K57.32, Diverticulitis of large intestine (without mention of hemorrhage).

**Guideline II.F. Original treatment plan not carried out:** Sequence as the principal diagnosis the condition which after study occasioned the admission to the hospital, even though treatment may not have been carried out due to unforeseen circumstances.

**EXAMPLE:** Patient with ulcerated internal hemorrhoids was admitted for hemorrhoidectomy. Prior to the beginning of surgery, the patient developed bradycardia and the surgery was canceled.

The following codes were assigned: K64.8 Ulcerated internal hemorrhoids; R00.1, Bradycardia; and Z53.09, Procedure not carried out because of contraindication. The code for ulcerated internal hemorrhoids (R64.8) was listed as the principal diagnosis because it was the reason for admission. An additional code for bradycardia (R00.1) was reported, as well as code Z53.09, Procedure not carried out because of contraindication, to indicate that the procedure was not carried out due to the complication of bradycardia.

*(Continued)*

*(Continued)*

**Guideline II.G. Complications of surgery and other medical care:** When the admission is for treatment of a complication resulting from surgery or other medical care, the complication code is sequenced as the principal diagnosis. If the complication is classified to T80-T88 series, and the code lacks the necessary specificity in describing the complication, an additional code for the specific complication should be assigned.

EXAMPLE: Patient was being treated for an atelectasis due to recent cardiovascular surgery. The diagnosis codes would include J95.89, Other postprocedural complications and disorders of respiratory system, not elsewhere classified, and J98.11, Atelectasis.

**Guideline II.H. Uncertain diagnosis:** If the diagnosis documented at the time of discharge is qualified as "probable," "suspected," "likely," "questionable," "possible," or "still to be ruled out," or other similar terms indicating uncertainty, code the condition as if it existed or was established. The bases for these guidelines are the diagnostic workup, arrangements for further workup or observation, and initial therapeutic approach that correspond most closely with the established diagnosis. Note: This guideline is applicable only to inpatient admissions to short-term, acute, and long-term care, and psychiatric hospitals.

**Guideline II.I. Admission from observation unit:**

1. Admission Following Medical Observation.
   When a patient is admitted to an observation unit for a medical condition, which either worsens or does not improve, and is subsequently admitted as an inpatient of the same hospital for this same medical condition, the principal diagnosis would be the medical condition that led to the hospital admission.
2. Admission Following Postoperative Observation.
   When a patient is admitted to an observation unit to monitor a condition (or complication) that develops following outpatient surgery, and then is subsequently admitted as an inpatient of the same hospital, hospitals should apply the UHDDS definition of principal diagnosis as "that condition established after study to be chiefly responsible for occasioning the admission of the patient to the hospital for care."

**Guideline II.J. Admission from outpatient surgery:** When a patient receives surgery in the hospital's outpatient surgery department and is subsequently admitted for continuing inpatient care at the same hospital, the following guidelines should be followed in selecting the principal diagnosis for the inpatient admission:

- When the reason for the inpatient admission is a complication, assign the complication as the principal diagnosis.
- When no complication, or other condition, is documented as the reason for the inpatient admission, assign the reason for the outpatient surgery as the principal diagnosis.
- When the reason for the inpatient admission is another condition unrelated to the surgery, assign the unrelated condition as the principal diagnosis.

**Guideline II.K. Admissions/Encounters for Rehabilitation**

- When the purpose for the admission/encounter is rehabilitation, sequence first the code for the condition for which the service is being performed. For example, for an admission/encounter for rehabilitation for right-sided dominant hemiplegia following a cerebrovascular infarction, report code I69.351, Hemiplegia and hemiparesis following cerebral infarction affecting right dominant side, as the first listed or principal diagnosis.
- If the condition for which rehabilitation service is no longer present, report the appropriate aftercare code as the first-listed or principal diagnosis. For example, if a patient with severe degenerative osteoarthritis of the hip underwent hip replacement and the current encounter/admission is for rehabilitation, report code Z47.1, Aftercare following joint replacement surgery, as the first-listed or principal diagnosis.

(Author Note: This guideline is new to ICD-10-CM and not included in the ICD-9-CM guidelines)

## Section II. Reporting of Additional Diagnoses

Deciding what else to code can be a challenge for coders. Doctors write many facts about the patient in terms of diagnoses and conditions that are present in the patient. However, not everything a doctor includes in a record is something to be coded. The ICD-10-CM Official Guidelines help the coder decide what else to code in addition to the principal diagnosis.

In the definition of "other diagnoses," conditions that require clinical evaluation are to be coded. Clinical evaluation usually means the physician has taken the condition into consideration when examining the patient. An evaluation can mean the physician is considering testing of the condition and/or closely observing the condition to decide if new treatment is necessary or if the current treatment is sufficient. Frequently when a condition is being evaluated there also will be treatment or diagnostic procedures performed for it as well.

The sequencing of the additional diagnoses is not mandated by a particular coding guideline. Generally, the diagnoses that were more significant in terms of what received the most attention during the patient's hospital stay are listed first in the list of all additional diagnoses. This is a style that many coders follow but again, not a specific coding guideline.

**Section III, Reporting Additional Diagnoses, of the ICD-10-CM Official Guidelines for Coding and Reporting address the general rules for reporting other or additional diagnoses.**

For reporting purposes, the definition for "other diagnoses" is interpreted as additional conditions that affect patient care in terms of requiring:

- Clinical evaluation, or
- Therapeutic treatment, or
- Diagnostic procedures, or
- Extended length of hospital stay, or
- Increased nursing care and/or monitoring

The UHDDS item #11-B defines other diagnoses as "all conditions that coexist at the time of admission, that develop subsequently, or that affect the treatment received and/or the length of stay. Diagnoses that relate to an earlier episode that have no bearing on the current hospital stay are to be excluded." UHDDS definitions apply to inpatients in acute care, short-term, long-term care, and psychiatric hospital settings. The UHDDS definitions are used by acute care short-term hospitals to report inpatient data in a standardized manner. These data elements and their definitions can be found in the July 31, 1985 *Federal Register* (Vol. 50, No. 147), pp.31038-31040.

Since that time, the application of the UHDDS definitions have been expanded to include all non-outpatient settings (acute care, short-term, long-term care, and psychiatric hospitals; home health agencies; rehab facilities; nursing homes, and such).

The following guidelines are to be applied in designating "other diagnoses" when neither the Alphabetic Index nor the Tabular List in ICD-10-CM provide directions. The listing of the diagnoses in the patient record is the responsibility of the attending provider.

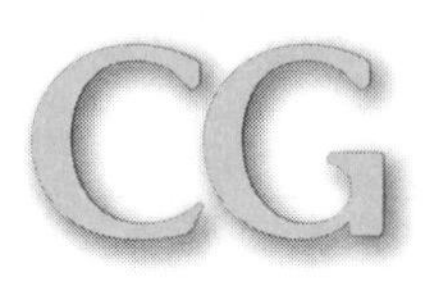


**Guideline III.A. Previous conditions:** If the provider has included a diagnosis in the final diagnostic statement, such as the discharge summary or the face sheet, it should ordinarily be coded. Some providers include in the diagnostic statement resolved conditions or diagnoses and status post procedures from a previous admission that have no bearing on the current stay. Such conditions are not to be reported and are coded only if required by hospital policy.

However, history codes (categories Z80-Z87) may be used as secondary codes if the historical condition or family history has an impact on current care or influences treatment.

**EXAMPLE:** Face sheet states the following diagnoses: acute diverticulitis, congestive heart failure, status post cholecystectomy, status post hysterectomy.

All are coded except the status post cholecystectomy and hysterectomy. The heart failure and the diverticulitis affect the current hospitalization and thus are coded.

**Guideline III.B. Abnormal findings:** Abnormal findings (laboratory, x-ray, pathologic, and other diagnostic results) are not coded and reported unless the provider indicates their clinical significance. If the findings are outside the normal range and the attending provider has ordered other tests to evaluate the condition or prescribed treatment, it is appropriate to ask the provider whether the abnormal finding should be added.

**EXAMPLE:** In the inpatient setting, coders should not assign codes for conditions described in a pathology report alone without the provider's input. The provider or physician should be asked for clarification of the pathological findings if the provider has not documented the same condition in the health record.

**Note:** This differs from the coding practices in the outpatient setting for coding encounters for diagnostic tests that have been interpreted by a provider.

**Guideline III.C. Uncertain diagnosis:** If the diagnosis documented at the time of discharge is qualified as "probable," "suspected," "likely," "questionable," "possible," or "still to be ruled out," or other similar terms indicating uncertainty, code the condition as if it existed or was established. The bases for these guidelines are the diagnostic workup, arrangements for further workup or observation, and initial therapeutic approach that correspond most closely with the established diagnosis.

**Note:** This guideline is applicable only to inpatient admissions to short-term, acute, long-term care, and psychiatric hospitals.

## Section IV: Diagnostic Coding and Reporting Guidelines for Outpatient Services

The coding of healthcare services in an outpatient setting is different from the coding of patient's diagnoses provided in an inpatient setting. Outpatient encounters are often short visits and there is not a lot of time to study the patient's condition in depth. For the outpatient visit, the goal of coding is to code what is known for certain about the patient's diagnosis, problem, or condition at that point in time and what was the focus of the healthcare attention at that time. The coding guidelines listed below direct the coder on how to code patient visits in a hospital, physician's office or other ambulatory care center.

**Section IV of the ICD-10-CM Official Guidelines for Coding and Reporting address the general rules for diagnostic coding and reporting guidelines for outpatient services.**

These coding guidelines for outpatient diagnoses have been approved for use by hospitals/providers in coding and reporting hospital-based outpatient services and provider-based office visits.

Information about the use of certain abbreviations, punctuation, symbols, and other conventions used in the ICD-10-CM Tabular List (code numbers and titles), can be found in

Section IA of these guidelines, under "Conventions Used in the Tabular List." Information about the correct sequence to use in finding a code is also described in Section I.

The terms encounter and visit are often used interchangeably in describing outpatient service contacts and, therefore, appear together in these guidelines without distinguishing one from the other.

Though the conventions and general guidelines apply to all settings, coding guidelines for outpatient and provider reporting of diagnoses will vary in a number of instances from those for inpatient diagnoses, recognizing that:

- The UHDDS definition of principal diagnosis applies only to inpatients in acute, short-term, long-term care and psychiatric hospitals.
- Coding guidelines for inconclusive diagnoses (probable, suspected, rule out, and so on) were developed for inpatient reporting and do not apply to outpatients.

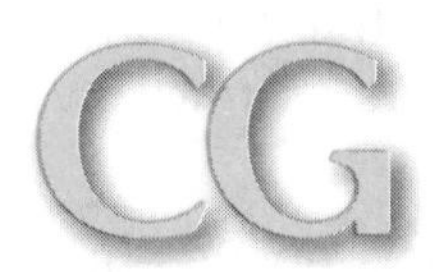


**A. Selection of first-listed condition**

In the outpatient setting, the term first-listed diagnosis is used in lieu of principal diagnosis.

In determining the first-listed diagnosis, the coding conventions of ICD-10-CM, as well as the general and disease specific guidelines take precedence over the outpatient guidelines.

Diagnoses often are not established at the time of the initial encounter/visit. It may take two or more visits before the diagnosis is confirmed.

The most critical rule involves beginning the search for the correct code assignment through the Alphabetic Index. Never begin searching initially in the Tabular List as this will lead to coding errors.

1. Outpatient Surgery
When a patient presents for outpatient surgery (same day surgery), code the reason for the surgery as the first-listed diagnosis (reason for the encounter), even if the surgery is not performed due to a contraindication.

2. Observation Stay
When a patient is admitted for observation for a medical condition, assign a code for the medical condition as the first-listed diagnosis.

When a patient presents for outpatient surgery and develops complications requiring admission to observation, code the reason for the surgery as the first reported diagnosis (reason for the encounter), followed by codes for the complications as secondary diagnoses.

**B. Codes from A00.0 through T88.9, Z00-Z99**
The appropriate code(s) from A00.0 through T88.9, Z00-Z99 must be used to identify diagnoses, symptoms, conditions, problems, complaints, or other reason(s) for the encounter/visit.

**C. Accurate reporting of ICD-10-CM diagnosis codes**
For accurate reporting of ICD-10-CM diagnosis codes, the documentation should describe the patient's condition, using terminology which includes specific diagnoses as well as symptoms, problems, or reasons for the encounter. There are ICD-10-CM codes to describe all of these.

**D. Codes that describe symptoms and signs**
Codes that describe symptoms and signs, as opposed to diagnoses, are acceptable for reporting purposes when a diagnosis has not been established (confirmed) by the provider. Chapter 18 of ICD-10-CM, Symptoms, Signs, and Abnormal Clinical and Laboratory Findings Not Elsewhere Classified (codes R00-R99) contain many, but not all codes for symptoms.

**E. Encounters for circumstances other than a disease or injury**
ICD-10-CM provides codes to deal with encounters for circumstances other than a disease or injury. The Factors Influencing Health Status and Contact with Health Services codes (Z00-Z99) are provided to deal with occasions when circumstances other than a disease or injury are recorded as diagnosis or problems. *See Section I.C.21. Factors influencing health status and contact with health services.*

**F. Level of Detail in Coding**

1. ICD-10-CM codes with 3, 4, 5, 6 or 7 characters
ICD-10-CM is composed of codes with 3, 4, 5, 6 or 7 characters. Codes with three characters are included in ICD-10-CM as the heading of a category of codes that may be further subdivided by the use of fourth, fifth, sixth or seventh characters to provide greater specificity.

2. Use of full number of characters required for a code.
A three-character code is to be used only if it is not further subdivided. A code is invalid if it has not been coded to the full number of characters required for that code, including the 7th character, if applicable.

**G. ICD-10-CM code for the diagnosis, condition, problem, or other reason for encounter/visit**
List first the ICD-10-CM code for the diagnosis, condition, problem, or other reason for encounter/visit shown in the medical record to be chiefly responsible for the services provided. List additional codes that describe any coexisting conditions. In some cases the first-listed diagnosis may be a symptom when a diagnosis has not been established (confirmed) by the physician.

(*Continued*)

(*Continued*)

**H. Uncertain diagnosis**
Do not code diagnoses documented as "probable", "suspected," "questionable," "rule out," or "working diagnosis" or other similar terms indicating uncertainty. Rather, code the condition(s) to the highest degree of certainty for that encounter/visit, such as symptoms, signs, abnormal test results, or other reason for the visit.

**Please note:** This differs from the coding practices used by short-term, acute care, long-term care and psychiatric hospitals.

**I. Chronic diseases**
Chronic diseases treated on an ongoing basis may be coded and reported as many times as the patient receives treatment and care for the condition(s).

**J. Code all documented conditions that coexist**
Code all documented conditions that coexist at the time of the encounter/visit, and require or affect patient care treatment or management. Do not code conditions that were previously treated and no longer exist. However, history codes (categories Z80-Z87) may be used as secondary codes if the historical condition or family history has an impact on current care or influences treatment.

**K. Patients receiving diagnostic services only**
For patients receiving diagnostic services only during an encounter/visit, sequence first the diagnosis, condition, problem, or other reason for encounter/visit shown in the medical record to be chiefly responsible for the outpatient services provided during the encounter/visit. Codes for other diagnoses (e.g., chronic conditions) may be sequenced as additional diagnoses.

For encounters for routine laboratory/radiology testing in the absence of any signs, symptoms, or associated diagnosis, assign Z01.89, Encounter for other specified special examinations. If routine testing is performed during the same encounter as a test to evaluate a sign, symptom, or diagnosis, it is appropriate to assign both the Z code and the code describing the reason for the non-routine test.

For outpatient encounters for diagnostic tests that have been interpreted by a physician, and the final report is available at the time of coding, code any confirmed or definitive diagnosis(es) documented in the interpretation. Do not code related signs and symptoms as additional diagnoses.

**Please note:** This differs from the coding practice in the hospital inpatient setting regarding abnormal findings on test results.

**L. Patients receiving therapeutic services only**
For patients receiving therapeutic services only during an encounter/visit, sequence first the diagnosis, condition, problem, or other reason for the encounter/visit shown in the medical record to be chiefly responsible for the outpatient services provided during the encounter/visit. Codes for other diagnoses (e.g., chronic conditions) may be sequenced as additional diagnoses.

The only exception to this rule is when the primary reason for the admission/encounter is chemotherapy or radiation therapy, the appropriate Z code for the service is listed first, and the diagnosis or problem for which the service is being performed listed second.

**M. Patients receiving preoperative evaluations only**
For patients receiving preoperative evaluations only, sequence first a code from subcategory Z01.81, Encounter for pre-procedural examinations, to describe the pre-op consultations. Assign a code for the condition to describe the reason for the surgery as an additional diagnosis. Code also any findings related to the pre-op evaluation.

**N. Ambulatory surgery**
For ambulatory surgery, code the diagnosis for which the surgery was performed. If the postoperative diagnosis is known to be different from the preoperative diagnosis at the time the diagnosis is confirmed, select the postoperative diagnosis for coding, since it is the most definitive.

**O. Routine outpatient prenatal visits**
*See Guidelines for Coding and Reporting Section I.C.15. Routine outpatient prenatal visits.*

**P. Encounters for general medical examinations with abnormal findings**
The subcategories for encounters for general medical examinations, Z00.0-, provide codes for with and without abnormal findings. Should a general medical examination result in an abnormal finding, the code for general medical examination with abnormal finding should be assigned as the first-listed diagnosis. A secondary code for the abnormal finding should also be coded.

**Q. Encounters for routine health screenings**
*See Guidelines for Coding and Reporting Section I.C.21. Factors influencing health status and contact with health services, Screening.*

**NOTE:** A complete version of the *ICD-10-CM Official Guidelines for Coding and Reporting* can be found at http://www.cdc.gov/nchs/icd/icd10cm.htm and are also included in Appendix I of the website related to this text.

# Chapter 4

# Infectious and Parasitic Diseases

## Learning Objectives

At the conclusion of this chapter, you should be able to:

1. Describe the organization of the conditions and codes included in Chapter 1 of ICD-9-CM, Infectious and Parasitic Diseases (001–139)
2. Describe the organization of the conditions and codes included in Chapter 1 of ICD-10-CM, Certain infectious and parasitic diseases (A00–B99)
3. Define the term *combination codes* as it pertains to ICD-9-CM and ICD-10-CM
4. Explain how the *etiology/manifestation convention* applies to Chapter 1 codes in both ICD-9-CM and ICD-10-CM
5. Explain the circumstances in which codes from ICD-9-CM categories 041 and 079 are used
6. Explain the circumstances in which codes from ICD-10-CM categories B95–B97 are used
7. Define and explain the differences among the following terms:
   - *Bandemia*
   - *Septicemia*
   - *Systemic Inflammatory Response Syndrome*
   - *Sepsis*
   - *Severe sepsis*
   - *Septic shock*
   - *Human immunodeficiency virus (HIV)*
8. Apply the coding guidelines for HIV disease reporting
9. Assign diagnosis codes for infectious and parasitic diseases

## ICD-9-CM Chapter 1, Infectious and Parasitic Diseases (001–139)

ICD-9-CM, volume 1, Chapter 1, Infectious and Parasitic Diseases, in the Tabular List, is based on the organism responsible for a disease or condition. Communicable diseases are classified in an inclusion note at the beginning of the chapter. Chapter 1 includes diseases of unknown, but possibly of infectious, origin. Noncommunicable diseases are classified by site in other chapters of ICD-9-CM.

Chapter 1 is subdivided into the following categories and section titles:

| Categories | Section Titles |
|---|---|
| 001–009 | Intestinal Infectious Diseases |
| 010–018 | Tuberculosis |
| 020–027 | Zoonotic Bacterial Diseases |
| 030–041 | Other Bacterial Diseases |
| 042 | Human Immunodeficiency Virus (HIV) Infection |
| 045–049 | Poliomyelitis and Other Non-arthropod-borne Viral Diseases and Prion Diseases of Central Nervous System |
| 050–059 | Viral Diseases Generally Accompanied by Exanthem |
| 060–066 | Arthropod-borne Viral Diseases |
| 070–079 | Other Diseases due to Virus and Chlamydiae |
| 080–088 | Rickettsioses and Other Arthropod-borne Diseases |
| 090–099 | Syphilis and Other Venereal Diseases |
| 100–104 | Other Spirochetal Diseases |
| 110–118 | Mycoses |
| 120–129 | Helminthiases |
| 130–136 | Other Infectious and Parasitic Diseases |
| 137–139 | Late Effects of Infectious and Parasitic Diseases |

Chapter 4 of this book introduces the coding instructions specific to tuberculosis, septicemia, late effects of infectious and parasitic diseases, and HIV. See Appendix C on the accompanying website for a listing of common bacteria and their associated diseases.

In coding infectious and parasitic diseases, the entire health record must be reviewed to identify:

- Body site: for example, intestine, kidney, or blood
- Severity of the disease: for example, acute versus chronic
- Specific organism: for example, *Candida,* bacteria, virus, or parasite
- Etiology of infection: for example, food poisoning
- Associated signs, symptoms, or manifestations: for example, gangrene, bleeding, or Kaposi's sarcoma

## Combination Codes and Multiple Coding

Chapter 1 of ICD-9-CM includes many combination codes to identify both the condition and the causative organism.

**EXAMPLE:**

112.0 Candidiasis of mouth
006.1 Chronic intestinal amebiasis without mention of abscess
130.1 Conjunctivitis due to toxoplasmosis

Mandatory multiple coding is required to describe etiology/manifestations when infections and parasitic diseases produce a manifestation within another body system. The Alphabetic Index to Diseases identifies when the etiology/manifestation convention or mandatory multiple coding is required by listing two codes after the main term with the second code listed in brackets. The first code identifies the underlying infectious or parasitic condition. The second code identifies the manifestation that occurs as a result of it.

**EXAMPLE:** Arthritis due to Lyme disease 088.81 *[711.8]*

The underlying cause and first-listed code is 088.81. The second code describes the arthritis associated with this tick-transmitted illness, 711.8, with a required fifth digit to identify the joint(s) involved.

### *ICD-9-CM Categories 041 and 079*

Typically, both categories 041 and 079 are assigned as an additional diagnosis to describe the causative organism in diseases that are classified elsewhere in ICD-9-CM. A code from Category 041, Bacterial infection in conditions classified elsewhere and of unspecified site, is assigned when the physician documents the bacterial organism causing the infection. A code from Category 079, Viral and chlamydial infection in conditions classified elsewhere and of unspecified site, is assigned when the organism is a virus or chlamydia. In both categories, the codes may be located using the main term "Infection" in the Alphabetic Index to Diseases.

Category 041 is further subdivided to identify specific bacteria such as *Streptococcus, Staphylococcus, Pneumococcus,* and so forth.

**EXAMPLE:** Urinary tract infection due to *E. coli*

599.0 Urinary tract infection, site not specified
041.49 Other and unspecified *Escherichia coli* [*E. coli*]

Two organisms identified in category 041 that occur frequently in patients are methicillin resistant Staphylococcus aureus (MRSA) (code 041.12) and methicillin susceptible Staphylococcus aureus (MSSA) (code 041.11). When a patient is diagnosed with an infection that is due to MRSA, and that infection has a combination code that includes the causal organism (such as septicemia or pneumonia due to Staphylococcus aureus), the appropriate combination code for that infection and its causal organism is assigned. The codes 041.11 or 041.12 are not assigned as additional codes.

When there is documentation of a current infection, such as a wound infection, that is due to MRSA or MSSA and that infection does not have a combination code that includes the causal organism, the appropriate code to identify the infection or condition is assigned, with an additional code for MRSA (041.12) or MSSA (041.11). The coder would not assign a code from subcategory V09.0, Infection with microorganisms resistant to penicillins, as an additional code.

The term "colonization" means that MRSA or MSSA is present on or in the body without necessarily causing illness. A positive colonization test may be documented as a "positive

MRSA screen" or "positive MSSA screen." Either code V02.54, Carrier or suspected carrier, methicillin resistant Staphylococcus aureus (MRSA) colonization, or V02.53, Carrier or suspected carrier, methicillin susceptible Staphylococcus aureus (MSSA) colonization, is assigned to identify the colonization or carrier status of the patient.

If a patient has both an MRSA colonization and infection during an episode of care, code V02.54, Carrier or suspected carrier, methicillin resistant Staphylococcus aureus (MRSA) colonization, and a code for the MRSA infection may both be assigned.

Category 079 is further subdivided to identify specific viruses, such as adenovirus; echovirus; Coxsackie virus; retrovirus; human T-cell lymphotropic virus, types I and II; HIV, type 2; and so forth.

**EXAMPLE:** Acute viral osteomyelitis of the hip

730.05 Acute osteomyelitis, pelvic region and thigh
079.99 Unspecified viral infection

### Tuberculosis (010–018)

Tuberculosis can develop anywhere in the body. This disease has category codes that identify the specific anatomical site involved, such as pulmonary, genitourinary, meninges, central nervous system, and so forth.

The fifth-digit subclassification for use with the tuberculosis codes is noted at the beginning of the section, "Tuberculosis." The fifth digit requires identification of the method used to establish the diagnosis of tuberculosis. The fifth digit 0 is assigned when the method of diagnosis is not documented. The fifth digit 2 is assigned when a bacteriological or histological examination is performed, but the results are not available in the health record.

### Septicemia, SIRS, Sepsis, Severe Sepsis, and Septic Shock

ICD-9-CM classifies septicemia by the underlying organism involved. Bacterial septicemia is classified to category 038, which is further subdivided to identify the specific bacteria, such as *Staphylococcus.* Without further specification, septicemia is reported with code 038.9. Septicemia due to *Candida albicans* is reported with code 112.5.

The terms *bandemia, septic shock, severe sepsis, sepsis,* and *septicemia* may be used interchangeably by physicians, but they are clinically distinct conditions and are not synonymous terms.

Bandemia is diagnosed in a patient when the white cell count is normal but there is an excess of immature white blood cells or band cells. Bandemia is frequently present in cases of bacterial infection. It is possible to identify bandemia before a diagnosis of a particular type of infection is made.

Septicemia is defined as a systemic disease associated with the presence of pathological organisms or toxins in the blood, which may include bacteria, fungi, viruses, or other organisms.

The condition "systemic inflammatory response syndrome" (SIRS) is the systemic response to infection or trauma or other insult such as cancer. A systemic inflammatory response to variety of severe clinical insults is manifested by two or more of the following clinical factors:

- Temperature less the 36° C or more than 38° C
- Heart rate >90 beats per minute

- Respiratory rate >20 breaths per minute or arterial blood carbon dioxide level <32 mmHg
- White blood cell count >12,000 or < 4000

Sepsis is defined as SIRS caused by an infection. This definition of sepsis replaces all previous coding advice that equated sepsis with septicemia. Finally, severe sepsis is defined as sepsis with associated acute organ dysfunction.

In ICD-9-CM, the term *sepsis* is indexed to code 995.91, Sepsis. An inclusion term under code 995.91 is systemic inflammatory response due to infectious process without acute organ dysfunction. A note appearing after code 995.91 in the Tabular List states "Code first underlying infection."

The term *severe sepsis* is indexed to code 995.92, Severe sepsis. An inclusion term under code 995.92 is SIRS due to infectious process with acute organ dysfunction. Other inclusion terms include sepsis with acute organ dysfunction and sepsis with multiple organ dysfunction (MOD). A note appearing after code 995.92 in the Tabular List states "Code first underlying infection." A second note reminds the coder to "Use additional code to specify acute organ dysfunction," with examples including septic shock. Patients with septic shock have sepsis with hypotension, a failure of the cardiovascular system.

The "code first" notes at codes 995.91, 995.92, 995.93 and 995.94 provides instruction that the underlying cause of the sepsis or SIRS should be coded first. The underlying condition for codes 995.91 and 995.92 is an infection. The underlying condition for codes 995.93 and 995.94 may be either trauma or a noninfectious condition. In the absence of a specified underlying condition, the default first code should be 038.9. If only the term sepsis is documented, codes 038.9 and 995.91 would be assigned in that sequence. Either sepsis or SIRS must be documented to assign a code from subcategory 995.9.

Only one code from subcategory 995.9 should be assigned. 995.91 and 995.92 identify sepsis or severe sepsis due to an infectious process. Codes 995.93 and 995.94 identify SIRS due to a noninfectious process with or without acute organ dysfunction. However, when a noninfectious condition leads to an infection resulting in sepsis or severe sepsis, only a code from either 995.91 or 995.92 is assigned—without an additional code from 995.93 or 995.94 to identify the noninfectious SIRS original condition.

If documentation is not clear whether the sepsis was present on admission, the provider should be queried. If the sepsis is determined at that point to have met the definition of principal diagnosis, the underlying systemic infection (038.xx, 112.5, and so forth) may be used as principal diagnosis with code 995.91, Sepsis as an additional code.

When the term *sepsis, severe sepsis,* or *SIRS* is used with an underlying infection other than septicemia, for example, pneumonia, cellulitis, or nonspecific urinary tract infection, a code for the systemic infection (such as a code from category 038) should be assigned first, then code 995.91, followed by a code for the initial infection, such as the pneumonia. The reason for this is that the term *sepsis* or *SIRS* indicates that the patient's infection has advanced to a systemic infection and the systemic infection code should be sequenced before the localized infection code.

To code patients with severe sepsis, the code for the systemic infection (038 category, 112.5, or other underlying systemic infection) should be sequenced first, followed by code 995.92, Severe sepsis. Codes for the underlying infection and the specific acute organ dysfunction should also be assigned.

These instructions refer to coding of sepsis in nongravid patients who are not newborns because separate codes exist for sepsis complicating a pregnancy and in newborns.

The ICD-9-CM Official Guidelines for Coding and Reporting contain guidelines for coding septicemia, SIRS, sepsis, severe sepsis, and septic shock. Please refer to appendix H on the accompanying website for a complete review.

## Late Effects of Infectious and Parasitic Diseases (137–139)

Three categories are identified for use in describing late effects of infectious and parasitic diseases:

**Category 137 Late effects of tuberculosis**
**Category 138 Late effects of acute poliomyelitis**
**Category 139 Late effects of other infectious and parasitic diseases**

Late effects are located under the main term "Late" with the subterm "effect." In sequencing, the first code listed is the residual condition that is currently present in the patient (arthritis, hemiplegia, and so forth) followed by the late effect code (137.0, 137.2, 138, and so forth) identifying the underlying cause, unless the Alphabetic Index directs otherwise.

**EXAMPLE:** Mental retardation due to old viral encephalitis

319 Unspecified intellectual disabilities
139.0 Late effects of viral encephalitis

## HIV Disease

HIV disease attacks the body's immune system and leads to associated infections and malignant tumors. HIV is the virus that leads to acquired immunodeficiency syndrome (AIDS). HIV destroys the body's ability to fight disease, so that common infections from which healthy people generally recover can prove fatal to people who have contracted the virus.

HIV infection is caused by one of two related retroviruses, HIV-1 and HIV-2, that produce a wide range of conditions varying from the presence of contagious infections with no apparent symptoms to disorders that are severely disabling and eventually fatal. HIV-1 is widespread throughout the world and causes AIDS. Found primarily in West Africa, HIV-2 seems to be less virulent and causes a different type of illness.

There is no cure for HIV infection and HIV treatment is complex. One major emphasis of treatment is to find effective combinations of antiviral medications that a person can tolerate over an indefinite period. Another is to prevent opportunistic infections that can prove fatal.

### HIV Classification

The HIV classification includes the following categories and codes:

- 042, Human immunodeficiency virus (HIV) disease: Patients with HIV-related illness should be coded to 042. Category 042 includes AIDS, AIDS-like syndrome, AIDS-related complex, and symptomatic HIV infection. This code is located under the Alphabetic Index entries of AIDS; Disease, human immunodeficiency; Human immunodeficiency virus; and Infection, human immunodeficiency, with symptoms, symptomatic
- V08, Asymptomatic human immunodeficiency virus (HIV) infection status: Patients with physician-documented asymptomatic HIV infection who have never had an HIV-related illness should be coded to V08. This code is located under the Alphabetic Index entries of Human immunodeficiency virus, infection or Infection, human immunodeficiency virus
- 795.71, Nonspecific serologic evidence of human immunodeficiency virus (HIV): Code 795.71 should be used for patients (including infants) with inconclusive HIV test results. This code is located under the Alphabetic Index entries of Findings,

abnormal, serological (for) human immunodeficiency virus, inconclusive and Positive, serology, AIDS virus, inconclusive or Positive, serology, HIV, inconclusive or Positive, serology, human immunodeficiency virus, inconclusive

Code only confirmed cases of HIV infection/illness. Health records with diagnostic statements of "suspected," "likely," "possible," or "questionable" HIV infection provide examples of diagnostic statements in which confirmation of HIV infection or illness is not documented. The instructions to code only confirmed cases of HIV infection/illness represent an exception to the general ICD-9-CM inpatient coding guidelines that state that diagnoses identified as "suspected" or "possible" should be coded as if they have been established. In this context, "confirmation" does not require documentation of positive serology or culture for HIV. The physician's diagnostic statement that the patient is HIV positive or has an HIV-related illness is sufficient.

### Coding Guidelines for HIV Disease

Official coding guidelines exist for the coding of HIV infections. See Section I, C. Chapter-Specific Coding Guidelines, 1. Chapter 1, Infectious and Parasitic Diseases (001–139) for the complete set of HIV coding guidelines.

The circumstances of admission for patients with HIV-related illness govern the selection of principal diagnosis in keeping with its Uniform Hospital Discharge Data Set (UHDDS) definition of that "condition established after study to be chiefly responsible for occasioning the admission of the patient to the hospital for care." (UHDDS 1985, 31038–31040)

Patients who are admitted for an HIV-related illness should be assigned a minimum of two codes in the following order:

1. Code 042 to identify the HIV disease
2. Additional codes to identify other diagnoses, such as Kaposi's sarcoma

**EXAMPLE:** Disseminated candidiasis secondary to AIDS

042 Human immunodeficiency virus [HIV] disease
112.5 Disseminated candidiasis

**EXAMPLE:** Acute lymphadenitis with HIV infection

042 Human immunodeficiency virus [HIV] disease
683 Acute lymphadenitis

During pregnancy, childbirth, or the puerperium, a patient admitted because of an HIV-related illness should receive a principal diagnosis of 647.6x, Other viral diseases in the mother classifiable elsewhere, but complicating the pregnancy, childbirth, or the puerperium, followed by 042 and the code(s) for the HIV-related illness(es). This is an exception to the sequencing rule discussed above.

**EXAMPLE:** Delivery of a liveborn male in mother with AIDS

647.61 Other viral diseases in the mother classifiable elsewhere, but complicating the pregnancy, childbirth, or the puerperium
042 Human immunodeficiency virus [HIV] disease
V27.0 Outcome of delivery, single liveborn

**EXAMPLE:** Patient is admitted for evaluation and treatment of pneumonia; workup reveals *Pneumocystis carinii* pneumonia. Patient is also 25 weeks pregnant and has AIDS.

| | |
|---|---|
| 647.63 | Other viral diseases in the mother classifiable elsewhere, but complicating the pregnancy, childbirth, or the puerperium |
| 042 | Human immunodeficiency virus [HIV] disease |
| 136.3 | Pneumocystosis |

If a patient with symptomatic HIV disease or AIDS is admitted for an unrelated condition, such as a traumatic injury, the code for the unrelated condition should be the principal diagnosis. An additional diagnosis would include code 042, as well as all other manifestations or conditions associated with the HIV disease.

**EXAMPLE:** Patient was admitted with a diagnosis of acute appendicitis and an appendectomy was performed. Patient also has AIDS.

| | |
|---|---|
| 540.9 | Acute appendicitis |
| 042 | Human immunodeficiency virus [HIV] disease |
| 47.09 | Other appendectomy |

Code V08, Asymptomatic HIV infection status, is applied when the patient without any documentation of symptoms is reported as being HIV positive, known HIV, HIV test positive, or similar terminology. Do not use this code if the term AIDS is used or if the patient is treated for any HIV-related illness or is described as having any condition(s) resulting from his or her HIV positive status. Use code 042 in these cases.

During pregnancy, childbirth, or the puerperium, a patient admitted with a diagnosis of asymptomatic HIV infection (or similar terminology as described above) should receive a principal diagnosis of 647.6x, Other viral diseases in the mother classifiable elsewhere, but complicating the pregnancy, childbirth, or the puerperium, followed by code V08, Asymptomatic human immunodeficiency virus (HIV) infection status. In addition, codes should be assigned to describe other complications of pregnancy, childbirth, or the puerperium, as appropriate. Codes from Chapter 15, Pregnancy, always take sequencing priority.

**EXAMPLE:** Normal delivery of liveborn female; patient has a diagnosis of HIV infection with no related symptoms.

| | |
|---|---|
| 647.61 | Other specified infectious and parasitic diseases in the mother |
| V27.0 | Outcome of delivery, single liveborn |
| V08 | Asymptomatic human immunodeficiency virus [HIV] infection status |

Code 795.71, Inconclusive serologic test for human immunodeficiency virus [HIV], is reported for patients with inconclusive HIV serology, but with no definitive diagnosis or manifestations of the illness.

**A point to remember:** Patients with any known prior diagnosis of an HIV-related illness should be assigned code 042. After a patient has developed an HIV-related illness, the patient should always be assigned code 042 on every subsequent admission. Patients previously diagnosed with any HIV illness (042) should never be assigned code 795.71 or V08.

## Testing for HIV

Patients requesting testing for HIV should be assigned code V73.89, Screening for other specified viral disease. In addition, code V69.8, Other problems related to lifestyle, may be assigned to identify patients who are in a known high-risk group for HIV. Code V65.44, HIV counseling, also may be assigned if these services are provided during the encounter.

If the results of the test are positive and the patient is asymptomatic, code V08, Asymptomatic HIV infection status, should be assigned. If the results are positive and the patient is symptomatic with an HIV-related illness, such as Kaposi's sarcoma, code 042, HIV disease, should be assigned.

## ICD-9-CM Review Exercises: Chapter 4

Assign ICD-9-CM codes to the following:

1. Dermatophytosis of the foot

2. Asymptomatic HIV infection

3. Sepsis due to *Staphylococcus aureus*

4. Syphilitic endocarditis involving the aortic valve

5. Fracture, right radius, shaft; AIDS

6. Nodular pulmonary tuberculosis; confirmed histologically

7. Acute poliomyelitis

8. Left lower extremity paralysis; late effect of poliomyelitis

9. Candidiasis of the mouth due to AIDS

10. Staphylococcal food poisoning

11. AIDS with encephalopathy, and esophageal candidiasis

*(Continued on next page)*

## ICD-9-CM Review Exercises: Chapter 4 (Continued)

12. Acute gonococcal cervicitis and gonococcal endometritis

13. Toxic shock syndrome due to group A streptococcus

14. Septic nasopharyngitis

15. Filarial orchitis

16. Osteitis due to yaws

17. Acute cystitis due to *E. coli*

18. Vaginitis due to *Candida albicans*

19. Tuberculous osteomyelitis of knee; confirmed by histology

20. Viral hepatitis A

21. Plantar wart

22. Septic shock, severe sepsis, Hemophilus influenza septicemia, acute renal failure

23. Creutzfeldt-Jakob Disease

24. Sarcoidosis with lung involvement

25. Acanthamoeba infection with keratitis

# ICD-10-CM Chapter 1, Certain Infectious and Parasitic Diseases (A00–B99)

Chapter 1 of ICD-10-CM classifies certain infectious and parasitic diseases and maintains many of the same rules for coding these conditions as in ICD-9-CM. For example, only confirmed cases of HIV infection are coded with code B20.

## Organization and Structure of ICD-10-CM Chapter 1

Chapter 1 of ICD-10-CM includes categories A00–B99 arranged in the following blocks:

| | |
|---|---|
| A00–A09 | Intestinal infectious diseases |
| A15–A19 | Tuberculosis |
| A20–A28 | Certain zoonotic bacterial diseases |
| A30–A49 | Other bacterial diseases |
| A50–A64 | Infections with a predominantly sexual mode of transmission |
| A65–A69 | Other spirochetal diseases |
| A70–A74 | Other diseases caused by Chlamydia |
| A75–A79 | Rickettsioses |
| A80–A89 | Viral and prion infections of the central nervous system |
| A90–A99 | Arthropod-borne viral fevers and viral hemorrhagic fevers |
| B00–B09 | Viral infections characterized by skin and mucous membrane lesions |
| B10 | Other human herpesviruses |
| B15–B19 | Viral hepatitis |
| B20 | Human immunodeficiency virus [HIV] disease |
| B25–B34 | Other viral diseases |
| B35–B49 | Mycoses |
| B50–B64 | Protozoal diseases |
| B65–B83 | Helminthiases |
| B85–B89 | Pediculosis, acariasis and other infestations |
| B90–B94 | Sequelae of infectious and parasitic diseases |
| B95–B97 | Bacterial, viral and other infectious agents |
| B99 | Other infectious diseases |

While overall, Chapter 1 of ICD-10-CM is organized similarly to ICD-9-CM, some category and subcategory titles have been changed.

**EXAMPLES:**

| | | |
|---|---|---|
| | ICD-9-CM: | 008, Intestinal infections due to other organisms |
| | ICD-10-CM: | A08, Viral and other specified intestinal infections |
| | ICD-9-CM: | 024, Glanders |
| | ICD-9-CM: | 025, Melioidosis |
| | ICD-10-CM: | A24, Glanders and melioidosis |
| | ICD-9-CM: | 036.4, Meningococcal carditis |
| | ICD-10-CM: | A39.5, Meningococcal heart disease |

In Chapter 1 of ICD-10-CM, a separate subchapter, or block, has been created and appropriate conditions grouped together for Infections with a predominantly sexual mode of transmission (A50–A64). Two additional examples of separate blocks being created with the appropriate conditions grouped together are viral hepatitis (B15–B19) and other viral diseases (B25–B34).

The term *sepsis* has replaced *septicemia* throughout Chapter 1. Additionally, *streptococcal sore throat* and its inclusion terms found in the Infectious and Parasitic Disease chapter of ICD-9-CM are reclassified in ICD-10-CM to Chapter 10, Diseases of the Respiratory System.

Many of the codes in Chapter 1 of ICD-10-CM have been expanded to reflect manifestations of the disease with the use of fourth or fifth characters allowing the infectious disease and manifestation to be captured in one code instead of two.

**EXAMPLE:** **A01.0** **Typhoid fever**
Infection due to Salmonella typhi
A01.00, Typhoid fever, unspecified
A01.01, Typhoid meningitis
A01.02, Typhoid fever with heart involvement
A01.03, Typhoid pneumonia
A01.04, Typhoid arthritis
A01.05, Typhoid osteomyelitis
A01.09, Typhoid fever with other complications

## Coding Guidelines and Instructional Notes for ICD-10-CM Chapter 1

The National Center for Health Statistics has published chapter-specific guidelines for Chapter 1 of ICD-10-CM. An outline of the Chapter 1 guidelines are as follows. The complete guidelines are provided in appendix I of the accompanying website, and are also available at http://www.cdc.gov/nchs/icd/icd10cm.htm under 2014 release of ICD-10-CM, ICD-10-CM Guidelines, or the most current version available.

- Guidelines I.C.1.a. Human Immunodeficiency Virus [HIV] Infections
  - 1) Code only confirmed cases
  - 2) Selection and sequencing of HIV codes (eight specific rules)
- Guideline I.C.1.b. Infectious agents as the cause of diseases classified to other chapters
  - Certain infections are classified in chapters other than Chapter 1, and no organism is identified as part of the infection code. In these instances, it is necessary to use an additional code from Chapter 1 to identify the organism (B95, Streptococcus, Staphylococcus, and Enterococcus; B96, Other bacterial agents; B97 Viral agents).
- Guideline I.C.1.c .Infections resistant to antibiotics
  - Many bacterial infections are resistant to current antibiotics. It is necessary to identify all infections documented as antibiotic resistant. Assign category Z16, Infection with drug resistant microorganisms, following the infection code for these cases.
- Guidelines I.C.1.d. Sepsis, Severe Sepsis, and Septic Shock
  - 1) Coding of sepsis and severe sepsis
  - 2) Septic shock
  - 3) Sequencing of severe sepsis
  - 4) Sepsis and severe sepsis with a localized infection

- 5) Sepsis due to a postprocedural infection
- 6) Sepsis and severe sepsis associated with a noninfectious process
- 7) Sepsis and septic shock complicating abortion, pregnancy, childbirth, and the puerperium
- 8) Newborn sepsis

- Guidelines I.C.1. Methicillin resistant *Staphylococcus aureus* (MRSA) condition
  1) Selection and sequencing of MRSA codes

## Coding Overview for ICD-10-CM Chapter 1

The following notes are available at the beginning of ICD-10-CM Chapter 1 in the Tabular List of Diseases and Injuries:

| *Includes:* | diseases generally recognized as communicable or transmissible<br>Use additional code for any associated drug resistance (Z16-). |
|---|---|

| *Excludes1:* | certain localized infections—see body system-related chapters |
|---|---|

| *Excludes2:* | carrier or suspected carrier of infectious disease (Z22.-)<br>infectious and parasitic diseases complicating pregnancy, childbirth and the puerperium (O98.-)<br>infectious and parasitic diseases specific to the perinatal period (P35–P39)<br>influenza and other acute respiratory infections (J00–J22) |
|---|---|

Chapter 1 of ICD-10-CM includes a new section called infections with a predominantly sexual mode of transmission (A50–A64). Many codes have been moved from other places in the classification to this section.

### Sepsis, Severe Sepsis, and Septic Shock

When coding sepsis, it is important to review the coding guidelines and the notes at the category level of ICD-10-CM. The coding of patients with sepsis in ICD-10-CM follows mostly the same pattern as in ICD-9-CM. An unspecified type of sepsis is coded A41.9, Sepsis, unspecified, in cases where a specific underlying systemic infection is not further specified. Severe sepsis requires the use of at least two ICD-10-CM diagnosis codes: first a code for the underlying systemic infection, followed by a code from subcategory R65.2, Severe sepsis, followed by the code for organ dysfunction. For patients with septic shock, two codes are used: the code for the underlying systemic infection is sequenced first, followed by code R65.21,

Severe sepsis with septic shock. Additional codes for any other acute organ dysfunctions are also assigned.

### HIV Disease

It is also important to review coding guidelines and notes at the category level of ICD-10-CM when coding HIV. Only confirmed cases of HIV infection/illness are coded, and codes are available for the different forms of HIV-related conditions. The diagnosis of AIDS is coded with B20, followed by additional codes for all reported HIV-related conditions. Asymptomatic HIV infection status is coded as Z21. However, once the diagnosis of AIDS is established, or if the HIV-positive patient is treated for any HIV-related illness or is described as having any conditions resulting from his or her HIV-positive status, the code B20 is used instead. Patients with inconclusive laboratory evidence of HIV are coded with code R75.

### Sequelae of Infectious and Parasitic Diseases

There is an important note in the Sequelae of Infectious and Parasitic Diseases (B90–B94) section. Categories B90–B94 are to be used to indicate conditions in categories A00–B89 as the cause of sequelae, which are themselves classified elsewhere. The "sequelae" include conditions specified as such; they also include residuals of diseases classifiable to the above categories if there is evidence that the disease itself is no longer present. Codes from these categories are not to be used for chronic infections. Code chronic current infections to active infectious disease as appropriate.

Code first condition resulting from (sequela) the infectious or parasitic disease.

### ICD-10-CM Categories B95–B97

Similar to categories 041 and 079 in ICD-9-CM, codes assigned as additional diagnoses to identify the causative organism in diseases classified elsewhere, ICD-10-CM contains a series of codes to identify the infective agents causing diseases:

- B95.0–B95.8, Streptococcus, Staphylococcus and Enterococcus, as the cause of diseases classified elsewhere; for example, Staphylococcus aureus with subcategory B95.6.
- B96.0–B96.89, Other bacterial agents, as the cause of diseases classified elsewhere; for example, *Escherichia coli* (*E. coli*) with subcategory B96.2.
- B97.0–B97.89, Viral agents, as the cause of diseases classified elsewhere; for example, respiratory syncytial virus with code B97.4.

Bacterial and viral infectious agents (B95–B97) also have a note that specifies that these categories are provided for use as supplementary or additional codes to identify the infectious agent(s) in diseases classified elsewhere. The following are examples of how to locate these conditions in the Alphabetic Index:

- Infection, infected, infective; bacterial as cause of disease classified elsewhere; Streptococcus group A—B95.0
- Streptococcus, streptococcal; group A, as cause of disease classified elsewhere—B95.0

### Infection with Drug Resistant Microorganisms

As in ICD-9-CM, ICD-10-CM allows for the coding of bacterial infections that are resistant to current antimicrobial drugs. This specificity is necessary to identify all infections documented as drug resistant. The ICD-10-CM category Z16, Infection with drug resistant microorganisms, is assigned following the infection code for such cases.

## ICD-10-CM Review Exercises: Chapter 4

Assign the correct ICD-10-CM diagnosis codes to the following exercises.

1. Candidal esophagitis

   ______

2. *Clostridium difficile* (c. diff) colitis. This organism was resistant to multiple antimicrobial drugs

   ______

3. Acute bacterial food poisoning due to Salmonella

   ______

4. Urinary tract infection due to *E. coli* bacteria

   ______

5. Pneumocystis pneumonia due to AIDS

   ______

6. *E. coli* sepsis

   ______

7. Pelvic inflammatory disease as the result of sexually transmitted Chlamydia

   ______

8. Septic shock due to acute meningococcal severe sepsis

   ______

9. Chronic viral hepatitis, type B

   ______

10. Gram-negative severe sepsis with acute respiratory failure

    ______

# Chapter 5

# Neoplasms

## Learning Objectives

At the conclusion of this chapter, you should be able to:

1. Describe the organization of the conditions and codes included in Chapter 2 of ICD-9-CM, Neoplasms (140–239)
2. Describe the organization of the conditions and codes included in Chapter 2 of ICD-10-CM, Neoplasms (C00–D49)
3. Define the term *neoplasm*
4. Identify the three criteria used to classify neoplasms
5. Define the seven specific types of neoplasm behavior
6. Describe the organization of the neoplasm table in ICD-9-CM and ICD-10-CM
7. Explain the purpose of morphology codes
8. Apply the guidelines for using ICD-9-CM V codes to describe patients with neoplasms
9. Apply the guidelines for using ICD-10-CM Z codes to describe patients with neoplasms
10. Describe how to use the Alphabetic Index and Tabular List to locate a neoplasm code
11. Define and explain the terms *primary site* and *secondary site* for a neoplasm
12. Identify the purpose of the asterisk (*) in the ICD-9-CM neoplasm table
13. Identify the purpose of the dash (-) in the ICD-10-CM neoplasm table
14. Define the term *contiguous sites in ICD-9-CM, and overlapping sites In ICD-10-CM,* and explain how ICD-9-CM and ICD-10-CM accommodate the coding of them
15. Describe how to code a primary malignant neoplasm according to its site
16. Describe how to code a secondary malignant neoplasm according to its site

17. Explain the differences among the following phrases and how they are coded:
    - *metastatic from*
    - *metastatic to*
    - *direct extension to*
    - *spread to*
    - *extension to*
18. Explain how to code a condition that describes a metastatic neoplasm of one site
19. Identify the ICD-9-CM codes for neoplasm-related pain
20. Assign ICD-9-CM diagnosis and procedure codes for neoplasms
21. Assign ICD-10-CM codes for neoplasms

# ICD-9-CM Chapter 2, Neoplasms (140–239)

The term *neoplasm* refers to any new or abnormal growth. Chapter 2 in the Tabular List in ICD-9-CM, volume 1, classifies *all* neoplasms. The following categories and section titles are included:

| Categories | Section Titles |
|---|---|
| 140–195 | Malignant Neoplasms, Stated or Presumed to Be Primary, of Specified Sites, Except of Lymphatic and Hematopoietic Tissue |
| 196–198 | Malignant Neoplasms, Stated or Presumed to Be Secondary, of Specified Sites |
| 199 | Malignant Neoplasms, without Specification of Site |
| 200–208 | Malignant Neoplasms, Stated or Presumed to Be Primary, of Lymphatic and Hematopoietic Tissue |
| 209 | Neuroendocrine Tumors |
| 210–229 | Benign Neoplasms |
| 230–234 | Carcinoma in Situ |
| 235–238 | Neoplasms of Uncertain Behavior |
| 239 | Neoplasms of Unspecified Nature |

In ICD-9-CM coding, neoplasms are classified according to three criteria:

1. Behavior of the neoplasm, such as malignant or benign
2. Anatomical site involved, such as lung, brain, or stomach
3. Morphology type, such as leukemia, melanoma, or adenocarcinoma

Common morphology types can be found in appendix E on the accompanying website.

## ICD-9-CM Coding Guidelines

The ICD-9-CM Official Guidelines for Coding and Reporting contain a chapter-specific set of rules concerning the coding of neoplasms. See Section I. C. Chapter-Specific Coding

Guidelines, Chapter 2, Neoplasms (140–239) for a complete review of the specific guidelines that address coding and sequencing of primary and secondary sites, complications, V10 codes for personal history, admissions for chemotherapy or radiation therapy, admissions to determine extent of malignancy, and sign and symptom codes. The guidelines also address encounters for prophylactic organ removal due to genetic susceptibility to cancer or a family history of cancer.

## Neoplasm Behavior

Definitions describing the behavior of seven specific neoplasms include:

- **Malignant:** Malignant neoplasms are collectively referred to as cancers. A malignant neoplasm can invade and destroy adjacent structures, as well as spread to distant sites to cause death.
- **Primary:** A primary neoplasm is the site where a neoplasm originated.
- **Secondary:** A secondary neoplasm is the site(s) to which the neoplasm has spread via:
  - Direct extension, in which the primary neoplasm infiltrates and invades adjacent structures
  - Metastasis to local lymph vessels by tumor cell infiltration
  - Invasion of local blood vessels
  - Implantation in which tumor cells shed into body cavities
- **In situ:** In an in situ neoplasm, the tumor cells undergo malignant changes but are still confined to the point of origin without invasion of surrounding normal tissue. The following terms also describe in situ malignancies: noninfiltrating, noninvasive, intraepithelial, or preinvasive carcinoma.
- **Benign:** In benign neoplasms, growth does not invade adjacent structures or spread to distant sites but may displace or exert pressure on adjacent structures.
- **Uncertain behavior:** Neoplasms of uncertain behavior are tumors that a pathologist cannot determine as being either benign or malignant because some features of each are present.
- **Unspecified nature:** Neoplasms of unspecified nature include tumors in which neither the behavior nor the histological type is specified in the diagnosis.

## ICD-9-CM Neoplasm Table

The Alphabetic Index to Diseases contains three tables. One of them is known as the neoplasm table. This table is indexed under the main term "Neoplasm."

The neoplasm table contains seven columns. The first column lists the anatomical sites in alphabetical order. The next six columns identify the behavior of the neoplasm. The first three of these six columns include codes for malignant neoplasms and are further classified as primary, secondary, and carcinoma (CA) in situ. The next column identifies codes for benign neoplasms. The last two columns include codes for neoplasms of uncertain behavior and of unspecified type.

**A point to remember:** When many sites are indented under a main term, the listing for that term may run several pages long. Remember to search through all of the subterms under the main heading.

## Exercise 5.1

Using only the neoplasm table, assign codes to the following:

1. Malignant neoplasm originating in the lingual tonsil

   ____________________

2. Neoplasm of pancreas (behavior unspecified)

   ____________________

3. Benign neoplasm of liver

   ____________________

4. Neoplasm of cerebrum, behavior uncertain

   ____________________

5. Carcinoma in situ of cervix

   ____________________

6. Secondary malignant neoplasm involving the lower lobe of lung

   ____________________

## Morphology Codes

Morphology codes explain the histology and behavior of a neoplasm. Morphology codes (M codes) consist of five digits: the first four digits identify the histological type of the neoplasm and the fifth digit indicates the behavior. The histology of a neoplasm identifies the minute structure of cells and tissue that comprise the tumor or new growth. The behavior of a neoplasm describes the type of tumor it is: malignant, benign, carcinoma-in-situ, or uncertain whether it is benign or malignant. Malignant tumors are composed of different types of cells but all have the capacity to metastasize or move to another location in the body. Benign tumors are also composed of different types of cells, but they do not metastasize; instead they can grow larger in their site of origin. A complete listing of morphology codes can be found in appendix A of ICD-9-CM, volume 1. The M codes are not used for billing purposes.

Morphology codes are four digits with a fifth digit separated by a forward slash. The fifth digit after the forward slash is called the behavior code. The behavior codes are as follows:

/0 Benign

/1 Uncertain whether benign or malignant
Borderline malignancy

/2 Carcinoma in situ
Intraepithelial
Noninfiltrating
Noninvasive

/3 Malignant, primary site

/6 Malignant, metastatic site
Secondary site

/9 Malignant, uncertain whether primary or metastatic site

Morphology codes appear next to each neoplastic term in the Alphabetic Index.

**EXAMPLE:** Adenocarcinoma (M8140/3)—*see also* Neoplasm, by site, malignant

In the preceding example, M8140 identifies the histological type as adenocarcinoma and the digit /3 indicates the malignant behavior as a primary site.

Although the behavior code listed in ICD-9-CM is appropriate to the histological type of neoplasm, the behavior type should be changed to fit the diagnostic statement.

**EXAMPLE:** Patient was admitted to the hospital with a diagnosis of adenocarcinoma of the lung with metastasis to the bone.

M8140/3 Adenocarcinoma (lung)
M8140/6 Metastatic adenocarcinoma (bone)

Occasionally, difficulty arises in assigning a morphologic number when a diagnosis contains two qualifying adjectives with different morphology codes. In such cases, the higher number should be selected.

**EXAMPLE:** Patient was admitted to the hospital with a diagnosis of papillary serous carcinoma of the ovary.

The following two morphology codes are available:

M8050/3 Papillary carcinoma (ovary)
M8460/3 Serous papillary carcinoma (ovary)

Because the higher number is M8460/3, this code is assigned.

## ICD-9-CM V Codes

V codes, which are discussed in greater detail in Chapter 23, provide a method for reporting encounters for chemotherapy, radiation therapy, and follow-up visits, as well as a way to indicate a history of primary malignancy or a family history of cancer.

### *Coding Guidelines for V Codes*

Following is a set of guidelines for using V codes:

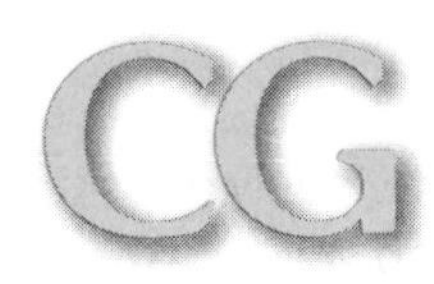


- If the treatment is directed at the malignancy, designate the malignancy as the principal diagnosis. The only exception to this guideline is if a patient admission or encounter is solely for the administration of chemotherapy, immunotherapy, or radiation therapy. When the purpose of the encounter or hospital admission is for radiation therapy or radiotherapy (V58.0), for antineoplastic chemotherapy (V58.11), or for antineoplastic immunotherapy (V58.12), use the V code as the principal diagnosis and sequence the malignancy as an additional diagnosis. Do not use V58.0, V58.11, or V58.12 as the only code reported. The need for the therapy should be explained with the use of an additional code from the 140–208 categories. Also, it is inappropriate to report

(*Continued*)

*(Continued)*

V58.0, V58.11, or V58.12 with a V10 category code as the only secondary code. V58.0, V58.11, or V58.12 can be used with the V10 category code when an additional code for a malignancy of a secondary site (for example, categories 196–198) is included. This indicates that the cancer treatment is being directed to the secondary site with the V10 category code indicating the primary site.

**EXAMPLE:** Female patient with right upper outer quadrant (UOQ) breast carcinoma was admitted for chemotherapy. The antineoplastic chemotherapy drug was administered intravenously.

The following codes are reported:

| | |
|---|---|
| V58.11 | Encounter for chemotherapy |
| 174.4 | Malignant neoplasm of upper outer quadrant of breast |
| 99.25 | Infusion of cancer chemotherapeutic substance (chemotherapy) |

- When a patient is admitted for the purpose of radiotherapy, immunotherapy or chemotherapy and develops a complication, such as uncontrolled nausea and vomiting or dehydration, the principal diagnosis is the admission for radiotherapy (V58.0) or the admission for the chemotherapy (V58.11), or encounter for antineoplastic immunotherapy (V58.12). Additional codes would include the cancer and the complication(s).

**EXAMPLE:** Patient was admitted for chemotherapy for acute lymphocytic leukemia. During the hospitalization, the patient developed severe nausea and vomiting treated with medications.

The following codes are reported:

| | |
|---|---|
| V58.11 | Encounter for chemotherapy |
| 204.00 | Acute lymphocytic leukemia, without mention of having achieved remission |
| 787.01 | Nausea with vomiting |
| 99.25 | Chemotherapy |

- When the primary malignancy has been previously excised or eradicated from its site, and there is no adjunct treatment directed to that site and no evidence of any remaining malignancy at the primary site, use the appropriate code from category V10 to indicate the former site of the primary malignancy. Any mention of extension, invasion, or metastasis to a nearby structure or organ or to a distant site is coded as a secondary malignant neoplasm to that site and may be the principal diagnosis in the absence of the primary site. The V10 category essentially describes the patient who is "cured" of the malignancy.

**A point to remember:** The instructional notes listed under each subcategory in category V10 refer to specific code ranges for primary malignancy categories (140–195 and 200–208) and carcinoma in situ categories (230–234). Therefore, history of secondary malignancies (196–198) is not reported with the V10 codes.

## Exercise 5.2

Use the Alphabetic Index to assign diagnosis and morphology codes (M codes) to questions 1–6. For questions 7 and 8, assign the appropriate disease, procedure, and morphology codes using the Tabular List to find the appropriate fifth digits.

1. Theca cell carcinoma

   ______________________________

2. Choriocarcinoma (male patient, age 31)

   ______________________________

3. Acute monocytic leukemia in relapse

   ______________________________

4. Multiple myeloma

   ______________________________

5. Wilms' tumor

   ______________________________

6. Patient was admitted with a diagnosis of bone metastasis originating from the right upper lobe (RUL) of the lung. Pathology was consistent with oat cell carcinoma. This admission was for chemotherapy that was administered.

   ______________________________

7. C cell carcinoma

   ______________________________

8. Female patient was admitted with a history of right breast carcinoma with mastectomy performed two years ago and no treatment currently given for breast carcinoma. Patient presents with complaints of vision disturbances. Workup revealed metastasis to the brain.

   ______________________________

## ICD-9-CM Alphabetic Index Instructions

The main terms and subentries in the Alphabetic Index to Diseases and Injuries assist the coder in locating the morphological type of neoplasms. When a specific code or site is not listed in the index, cross-references direct the coder to the neoplasm table. The following steps should be followed in coding neoplasms:

1. **Locate the morphology of the tumor in the Alphabetic Index.** ICD-9-CM classifies neoplasms by system, organ, or site. Exceptions to this rule include:

- Neoplasms of the lymphatic and hematopoietic system
- Malignant melanomas of the skin
- Lipomas
- Common tumors of the bone, uterus, and ovary

Because of these exceptions, the Alphabetic Index must first be checked to determine if a code has been assigned for that specific histology type.

**Leiomyoma** (M8890/0—*see also* . . .
uterus (cervix) (corpus) 218.9
interstitial 218.1
intramural 218.1
submucous 218.0
subperitoneal 218.2
subserous 218.2
vascular (M8894/0—*see* Neoplasm,
connective tissue, benign

As the preceding example shows, the Alphabetic Index offers direction to the neoplasm table for selection of codes, but occasionally the index itself will provide the codes more directly.

2. **Follow instructions under the main term in the Alphabetic Index.** Instructions in the Alphabetic Index should be followed when determining which column to use in the neoplasm table.

**Adenomyoma** (M8932/0—*see also*
Neoplasm, by site, benign
prostate 600.20

The subterms in the Alphabetic Index should be carefully reviewed if the documentation in the health record specifies a different behavior than normal for a particular type of neoplasm.

**EXAMPLE:** Malignant adenoma of colon
153.9 Malignant neoplasm of colon, unspecified

The Alphabetic Index says to "*see also* Neoplasm, by site, benign" next to the main term, Adenoma. However, the documentation clearly reflects that this adenoma is malignant. Under the main term, Adenoma, there is the subterm, malignant, which directs the coder to "*see* Neoplasm, by site, malignant. The coder should assign code 153.9, Malignant neoplasm of colon, unspecified, rather than code 211.3, Benign neoplasm of the colon.

When a diagnostic statement indicates which column of the neoplasm table to reference but does not identify the specific type of tumor, the neoplasm table should be consulted directly.

**EXAMPLE:** Carcinoma in situ of cervix
233.1 Carcinoma in situ of cervix uteri

After consulting the neoplasm table, code 233.1 from the in situ column is selected.

## ICD-9-CM Tabular List Instructions

Specific instructions for coding neoplasms appear in the Tabular List as well as in the Alphabetic Index. The following information applies to the coding of neoplasms:

1. **Code functional activity associated with a neoplasm.** Some categories in the neoplasm chapter in the Tabular List offer the instructional notation "Use additional code" as advice to also code any functional activity associated with a particular neoplasm, such as increased or decreased hormone production due to the presence of a tumor.

> **183 Malignant neoplasm of ovary and other uterine adnexa**
>
> *Excludes:* Douglas' cul-de-sac (158.8)
>
> **183.0 Ovary**
>
> Use additional code, if desired, to identify any functional activity

**EXAMPLE:** Patient was admitted to the hospital with carcinoma of the ovary and menometrorrhagia due to hyperestrogenism.

183.0 Malignant neoplasm of ovary
256.0 Hyperestrogenism
626.2 Excessive or frequent menstruation

2. **Note variations in categories 150 and 201.** Two categories in the malignant section depart from the usual principles of classification. In each case, the fourth-digit subdivisions are not mutually exclusive. The two categories are:

- Malignant neoplasms of the esophagus (150)
- Hodgkin's disease (201)

**EXAMPLE:**

150.0 Cervical esophagus
150.1 Thoracic esophagus
150.2 Abdominal esophagus
150.3 Upper third of esophagus
150.4 Middle third of esophagus
150.5 Lower third of esophagus

In the category 150 codes, the anatomy of the esophagus is classified in two ways because no uniform agreement exists on the use of these terms. Some physicians prefer the terms *upper, middle,* and *lower* to describe the site of the esophagus; others prefer *cervical, thoracic,* and *abdominal.* The code that correlates with documentation in the health record should be assigned.

**EXAMPLE:**

201.0x Hodgkin's paragranuloma
201.1x Hodgkin's granuloma
201.2x Hodgkin's sarcoma
201.4x Lymphocytic-histiocytic predominance
201.5x Nodular sclerosis
201.6x Mixed cellularity
201.7x Lymphocytic depletion
201.9x Hodgkin's disease, unspecified

In the preceding example, a dual axis reflects the different terminology used by pathologists when these codes were created.

### Exercise 5.3

Using volumes 1 and 2 of ICD-9-CM (referring to the Alphabetic Index to Diseases and the neoplasm table), assign codes to the following. Do not assign morphology codes.

1. Malignant melanoma of skin of scalp
2. Benign melanoma of skin of shoulder
3. Glioma of the parietal lobe of brain
4. Adenocarcinoma of prostate
5. Lipoma of face
6. Hypoglycemia due to islet cell adenoma of pancreas
7. Epidermoid carcinoma of the middle third of the esophagus
8. Galactorrhea due to pituitary adenoma
9. Adenoma of adrenal cortex with Conn's syndrome
10. Carcinoma in situ of vocal cord

## ICD-9-CM Coding of the Anatomical Site

ICD-9-CM provides guidelines for coding the anatomical site of a neoplasm to the highest degree of specificity. These guidelines are discussed in the following sections.

### *Classification of Malignant Neoplasms*

Malignant neoplasms are separated into primary sites (140–195) and secondary or metastatic sites (196–198), with further subdivisions by anatomic sites.

Neoplasms of the lymphatic and hematopoietic system are always coded to categories 200–208, regardless of whether the neoplasm is stated as primary or secondary. Neoplasms of the lymphatic and hematopoietic system, such as leukemias and lymphomas, are considered widespread and systemic in nature and, as such, do not metastasize. Therefore, they are not coded to category 196, Secondary and unspecified malignant neoplasms of lymph nodes, which includes codes identifying secondary or metastatic neoplasms of the lymphatic system.

Neuroendocrine tumors include both malignant (209.00–209.30) and benign tumors (209.40–209.69) that arise from endocrine or neuroendocrine cells scattered throughout the body. Neuroendocrine tumors are classified into two types: carcinoid tumors and pancreatic endocrine tumors. Many of these tumors are associated with the multiple endocrine neoplasia syndromes identified by ICD-9-CM subcategory codes 258.01–258.03. Different codes exist in category 209 for malignant and benign neuroendocrine tumors of various locations. There is a note under category 209 to code first any associated multiple endocrine neoplasia syndrome. There is also a note under category 209 to use additional code to identify associated endocrine syndrome such as carcinoid syndrome.

## Determination of the Primary Site

The primary site is defined as the origin of the tumor. Physicians usually identify the origin of the tumor in the diagnostic statement. In some cases, however, the physician cannot identify the primary site. For these situations, ICD-9-CM provides an entry in the neoplasm table titled "unknown site or unspecified" assigned to code 199.1. Code 199.1 can be assigned whether the site is primary or secondary (metastatic) in nature.

### Category 195

Category 195, Malignant neoplasms of other and ill-defined sites, is available for use only when a more specific site cannot be identified. This category includes malignant neoplasms of contiguous sites, not elsewhere classified, whose point of origin cannot be determined.

**EXAMPLE:** Carcinoma of the neck

195.0 Malignant neoplasm of head, face, and neck

## Definition of the Asterisk * in ICD-9-CM

At the beginning of the neoplasm table, a boxed note defines the use of the asterisk (*). When the asterisk follows a specific site in the neoplasm table, the following rules apply:

- When the neoplasm is identified as a squamous cell carcinoma or an epidermoid carcinoma, that condition should be classified as a malignant neoplasm of the skin.

  **EXAMPLE:** Squamous cell carcinoma of the ankle

  173.72 Squamous cell carcinoma of skin of lower limb, including hip

- The asterisk following the term *ankle* in the neoplasm table indicates that it would be incorrect in this case to assign code 195.5, Malignant neoplasm of lower limb, because the neoplasm is a squamous cell carcinoma. Instead, the malignant column for the entry "skin . . . ankle" in the neoplasm table should be referenced to assign the correct code.

  When the neoplasm is identified as a papilloma of any type, that condition should be classified as a benign neoplasm of the skin.

**EXAMPLE:** Papilloma of the arm

216.6 Benign neoplasm of skin of upper limb, including shoulder (arm)

- The asterisk following the term *arm* in the neoplasm table indicates that it would be incorrect to assign code 229.8, Benign neoplasm of other specified sites, if the neoplasm is a papilloma. The benign column for the entry "skin, . . . arm" in the neoplasm table should be referenced to assign the correct code.

The asterisk is not found in the ICD-10-CM Neoplasm Table. This only applies to ICD-9-CM.

### Coding of Contiguous Sites

In some cases, the origin of the tumor (primary site) may involve two adjacent, overlapping, or contiguous sites. Therefore, neoplasms with overlapping site boundaries are classified to the fourth-digit subcategory 8, titled "Other." These codes are provided to identify the circumstance when the physician cannot ascertain precisely where the neoplasm originated because, at the time the diagnosis was made, the tumor was overlapping into one or more anatomic sites.

**EXAMPLE:** A malignant lesion of the jejunum and ileum

152.8 Malignant neoplasm of other specified sites of small intestine

**152 Malignant neoplasm of small intestine, including duodenum**

**152.8 Other specified sites of small intestine**

Duodenojejunal junction

Malignant neoplasm of contiguous or overlapping sites of small intestine whose point of origin cannot be determined

Code 152.8 is obtained by referencing the entry "intestine . . . small . . . contiguous sites" in the neoplasm table.

## Exercise 5.4

Assign ICD-9-CM codes to the following. Do not assign the M codes for the morphology of the disease.

1. Subacute leukemia

2. Basal cell carcinoma of buttock

3. Adenocarcinoma of head of pancreas

4. Paget's disease with infiltrating duct carcinoma of right female breast involving central portion, nipple, and areola

5. Epidermoid carcinoma in situ of tongue, dorsal surface

6. Hemangioma of skin of lower right leg

7. Papilloma of back

8. Squamous cell carcinoma of leg

9. Hodgkin's granuloma of intra-abdominal lymph nodes and spleen

10. Acute myeloid leukemia in remission

## Classification of Primary Sites

As defined earlier in this chapter, a primary site refers to the site where the tumor originated. This subsection discusses some of the complexities involved in determining whether a neoplasm should be coded as a primary or a secondary site.

### Surgical Removal Followed by Adjunct Therapy

When surgical removal or eradication of a primary site malignancy is followed by adjunct chemotherapy or radiotherapy, the malignancy code (from Chapter 2 in the Tabular List) is assigned as long as chemotherapy or radiotherapy is actively administered. Even when the neoplasm has been removed surgically and the patient is still receiving therapy for that condition, the active code for the malignant neoplasm must be assigned, and not a V10 category code describing "history of malignant neoplasm."

### Surgical Removal Followed by Recurrence

If a primary malignant neoplasm previously removed by surgery or eradicated by radiotherapy or chemotherapy recurs, the primary malignant code for that site is assigned, unless the Alphabetic Index directs otherwise.

**EXAMPLE:** Recurrence of carcinoma of inner aspect of lower lip

140.4 Malignant neoplasm of lower lip, inner aspect

The Alphabetic Index refers to the neoplasm table, where code 140.4 is found for neoplasm of the inner aspect of the lower lip.

### "Metastatic from" in Diagnostic Statements

When cancer is described as "metastatic from" a specific site, it is interpreted as a primary neoplasm of that site.

**EXAMPLE:** Carcinoma in cervical lymph nodes metastatic from lower esophagus

150.5 Malignant neoplasm of lower third of esophagus
196.0 Secondary malignant neoplasm of lymph nodes of head, face, and neck

The lower esophagus is the primary site (150.5). The secondary site is the cervical lymph nodes (196.0).

### Malignant Neoplasm Associated with Transplanted Organ

A malignant neoplasm of a transplanted organ should be coded as a transplant complication. Assign first the appropriate code from subcategory 996.8, Complication of transplanted organ, followed by code 199.2, Malignant neoplasm associated with transplanted organ. Use an additional code for the specific malignancy.

**EXAMPLE:** Carcinoma in transplanted kidney

996.81 Complication of transplanted organ, kidney
199.2 Malignant neoplasm associated with transplanted organ
189.0 Malignant neoplasm, kidney

## Exercise 5.5

Assign ICD-9-CM codes to the following. Do not assign M codes to these exercises.

1. Recurrent choriocarcinoma in female patient

2. Cartilage Burkitt's lymphoma in multiple lymph nodes and spleen

3. Recurrence of papillary carcinoma of bladder dome, low-grade transitional cell

4. Carcinoma of cervical lymph nodes from epidermoid carcinoma of larynx

5. Carcinoma of the brain from the lower lobe of the lungs

## *Classification of Secondary Sites*

The patient's health record is the best source of information for differentiating between a primary and a secondary site. A secondary site may be referred to as a metastatic site in the record documentation. The following subsection describes some of the principal terms used in diagnostic statements that refer to secondary malignant neoplasms.

### "Metastatic To" and "Direct Extension To"

The terms "metastatic to" and "direct extension to" are both used in classifying secondary malignant neoplasms in ICD-9-CM. For example, cancer described as "metastatic to" a specific site is interpreted as a secondary neoplasm of that site.

**EXAMPLE:** Metastatic carcinoma of the colon to the lung

153.9 Malignant neoplasm of colon, unspecified
197.0 Secondary malignant neoplasm of lung

The colon (153.9) is the primary site, and the lung (197.0) is the secondary site.

### "Spread To" and "Extension To"

When expressed in terms of malignant neoplasm with "spread to" or "extension to," diagnoses should be coded as primary sites with metastases.

**EXAMPLE:** Adenocarcinoma of the stomach with spread to the peritoneum

151.9 Malignant neoplasm of stomach, unspecified
197.6 Secondary malignant neoplasm of retroperitoneum and peritoneum

The stomach (151.9) is the primary site, and the peritoneum (197.6) is the secondary site.

### Metastatic of One Site

If only one site is stated in the diagnostic statement and it is identified as metastatic, the coder determines whether the site should be coded as primary or secondary (assuming the health record does not provide additional information to assist in assigning a code).

**EXAMPLE:** Metastatic serous papillary ovarian carcinoma

In the preceding example, the diagnostic statement identifies the carcinoma as metastatic. Before the code can be assigned, however, the following six steps must be taken:

1. In the Alphabetic Index, locate the morphology type of the neoplasm as described in the diagnostic statement.

   **EXAMPLE:** In the preceding example, the morphology type is carcinoma with subterms "serous" and "papillary."

2. Review subterms for the specific site as identified in the diagnostic statement. If the specific site is identified, assign that code. If the specific site is not included as a subterm, assign the code for primary neoplasm of an unspecified site.

   **EXAMPLE:** In the preceding example, the specific site, ovary, is not identified; however, a code is provided for primary neoplasm of unspecified site.

   The following is displayed in the Alphabetic Index:

   **Carcinoma** (M8010/3) . . .
   serous (M8441/3)
   papillary (M8460/3)
   specified site—*see* Neoplasm, by site, malignant
   unspecified site 183.0

   Code 183.0, Malignant neoplasm of ovary, is assigned as the principal diagnosis to indicate the primary malignant site.

3. When the code obtained in step 2 is 199.0 or 199.1, the directions in step 5 must be followed.

4. Now that the primary site of the carcinoma has been identified, a code must be assigned to describe the metastatic or secondary site. A review of the diagnostic statement finds no other site identified. Therefore, the neoplasm table must be used to determine the metastatic code. Because the metastatic site is unspecified, review the neoplasm table for a subterm of "unknown site or unspecified." From the second column, "Malignant, Secondary," select the code 199.1.

5. When the morphology is not stated, or the code obtained in step 2 is 199.0 or 199.1, the site described as metastatic in the diagnostic statement should be coded as a primary malignant neoplasm, unless it is included in the following list of exceptions.

   The following sites are exceptions to this rule and must be coded as secondary neoplasms of that site:

   Bone
   Brain
   Diaphragm
   Heart
   Liver
   Lymph nodes
   Mediastinum
   Meninges
   Peritoneum
   Pleura
   Retroperitoneum
   Spinal cord
   Sites classifiable to 195.0–8

**EXAMPLE:** Metastatic carcinoma of the bronchus. The morphology is carcinoma. Upon indexing "Carcinoma," the first step is to look for a subterm of unspecified site. In reviewing the entries, no subterm is found for unspecified site. However, "*see also* Neoplasm, by site, malignant" appears after the main term "Carcinoma."

6. The next step is to turn to the neoplasm table and look for a subterm of unspecified site. A code is selected from the "Malignant, Primary" column—199.1. However, step 5 informs coders to assign the site listed in the diagnostic statement as the primary site if code 199.1 is identified. The next step is to review the exception list to determine if bronchus is included in the list. Because bronchus is not included in the list, it is assigned as the primary site and identified by code 162.9, Malignant neoplasm of bronchus and lung, unspecified. To assign a code for the secondary site, unknown in this example, use the "Malignant, Secondary" column of the neoplasm table to locate the subterm of "unknown site or unspecified"—199.1.

### Malignant Neoplasm of Lymphatic and Hematopoietic Tissue

Chapter 2 of ICD-9-CM includes the classification of malignant conditions of lymphatic and hematopoietic tissue. These conditions include lymphomas that arise out of lymph tissue, multiple myeloma that originates in bone marrow, and leukemia that forms in the blood with proliferation of abnormal leukocytes. These conditions are systemic and not isolated to a particular location, and the concept of metastatic coding discussed previously does not apply to these neoplasms. Lymphomas are classified according to their type and the specific lymph nodes involved when the diagnosis was made. Multiple myeloma is classified as to whether it is stated to be in remission or not. Leukemias are classified according to their type, such as lymphoid, myeloid, or monocytic, and their stage, such as acute or chronic. Fifth digits are added to the leukemia categories 204–208 to identify how the condition currently exists (without mention of having achieved remission, condition is in remission, or condition is in relapse). Remission occurs when the disease lessens in severity or the symptoms decrease and treatment may be discontinued. Relapse is the return of manifestations of the disease after an interval of improvement. Relapse may be considered a recurrence of the leukemia.

### Neoplasm-Related Pain

A patient with primary and/or secondary malignant neoplasms may seek medical care because of neoplasm-related pain. Code 338.3, neoplasm-related pain, is assigned to pain documented as being related, associated, or due to a primary or secondary malignant neoplasm. This code may be assigned for acute or chronic pain. The code may be assigned as a principal diagnosis or a first-listed diagnosis code when the stated reason for the admission or outpatient encounter is documented as pain control or pain management. The underlying neoplasm should also be reported as an additional diagnosis. When the reason for admission or outpatient care is the management of the neoplasm, and the pain associated with the malignancy is also documented, code 338.3 can be assigned as an additional diagnosis code.

### Other Conditions Described as Malignant

The medical term "malignant" has two meanings. In one context, it means resistant to treatment; occurring in severe form and frequently fatal; tending to become worse and leading to an ingravescent (increasing in severity) course. In reference to a neoplasm, malignant means having of the property of locally invasive and destructive growth and metastasis.

Effusion is the escape of fluid from blood vessels or lymphatics into the tissues or a cavity. This fluid can accumulate abnormally in the pleural cavity, pericardium, or the peritoneum. Pleural effusions due to tumors may or may not contain malignant cells. When the condition is symptomatic, thoracentesis or chest tube drainage is required. Symptomatic pericardial effusion is treated by creating a pericardial window. Fluid in the peritoneum or ascites is usually treated with repeated paracentesis of small volumes of fluid.

When ICD-9-CM was first developed, malignant ascites and malignant pleural effusion were classified to codes for secondary neoplasm of the peritoneum and secondary neoplasm of the pleura. It has been determined that this is not a valid default because the conditions, while due to a malignancy, are not all forms of a secondary neoplasm. Malignant pleural effusion is a physical sign that is important in the staging of lung cancer. Codes for malignant ascites (789.51) and malignant pleural effusion (511.81) are included in chapters other than ICD-9-CM Chapter 2, Neoplasms.

## Official Guidelines for Coding and Reporting Neoplasms

The ICD-9-CM Official Guidelines for Coding and Reporting include chapter-specific guidelines for coding and reporting neoplasms. Section 1, Part C, Chapter 2, Neoplasms (140–239) contains important rules for coding malignancies that all coders must be familiar with for accurate coding.

When treatment is directed at the malignancy, the malignancy is listed as the principal or first-listed diagnosis. The only exception to this guideline is in a case where a patient admission or encounter is solely for the administration of chemotherapy, immunotherapy, or radiation therapy. In this case, the appropriate V58.0, V58.11, or V58.12 code is listed first, and the malignancy for which the service is being provided is listed as a secondary code.

When a patient is admitted or treated for a primary malignancy with metastasis, and the treatment is directed toward the secondary site only, the secondary neoplasm is listed as the principal or first-listed diagnosis even though the primary malignancy is still present.

A patient with a neoplasm may suffer from complications associated with the malignancy or the therapy provided. For example, if the patient has anemia associated with the malignancy and is admitted or treated only for the anemia, the appropriate anemia code is listed first. An additional code is assigned for the malignancy (both primary and secondary sites if both exist). If the anemia is associated with the treatment of chemotherapy or immunotherapy and the only treatment is for the anemia, a code for the appropriate type of anemia is listed first, followed by code E933.1, Adverse effects of antineoplastic and immunosuppressive drugs. The appropriate neoplasm code is listed as an additional code. If the patient is admitted or treated for dehydration due to the malignancy—for example with intravenous hydration fluids—and the malignancy is not treated during this episode of care, the dehydration is coded and sequenced first, followed by the code(s) for the malignancy.

A patient may be referred to as having a "history" of cancer or be considered cancer-free. Instead of a primary malignancy (140–195) code, the assignment of a category V10, Personal history of malignant neoplasm, is appropriate when all of the following three situations exist:

- The primary malignancy has been previously excised or eradicated from its site
- There is no further treatment directed to that site
- There is no evidence of any existing primary malignancy

A patient may have a history of a primary site but later develop a secondary neoplasm or a metastatic site at another location. When this occurs, the treatment is likely to be directed to the secondary site. The secondary site code (196–199) is assigned first with a category V10 code used as an additional diagnosis code.

When the episode of care or hospital admission is for the purpose of surgically removing a primary- or secondary-site neoplasm, the neoplasm code should be listed first using codes in the 140–198 category or, when appropriate, codes in the 200–203 category. Even if, during this admission, the patient receives chemotherapy or radiation therapy before or after the surgical excision, the malignancy code is listed first. A "history of" neoplasm code would not be used during the episode of care when the surgery was performed.

If the patient's visit or admission is solely for the administration of chemotherapy, immunotherapy, or radiation therapy, the code for the therapy (V58.0, V58.11, or V58.12) is listed first, followed by additional code(s) for the primary and secondary neoplasms that exist. If the patient receives more than one of these therapies during the same visit or admission, more than one of these codes may be assigned, in any sequence. When the patient's visit or admission is for one of these therapies, and the patient develops a complication such as dehydration, nausea, or vomiting, the patient's first-listed diagnosis is still one of the V codes for the therapy. Even if the therapy was not performed or completed because of the complication, the V code for the therapy is still listed first. Additional codes are reported for the specific complication and the malignancy being treated.

A patient may be admitted to the hospital to study the extent of his or her disease or to "stage" the malignancy, or the patient may be admitted for a specific procedure intended to treat or evaluate the patient's condition. During this same admission, chemotherapy or radiation therapy may be performed. In this circumstance, the principal diagnosis is the primary malignancy or appropriate metastatic site, depending on the individual patient, even though the chemotherapy or radiation therapy was performed.

Symptoms, signs, and ill-defined conditions included in Chapter 16 of ICD-9-CM that are characteristic of or associated with an existing primary- or secondary-site malignancy cannot be used to replace the malignancy as the principal or first-listed diagnosis code.

Cancer patients may suffer from various types of pain caused by their malignancy. Code 338.3, Neoplasm related pain, is assigned to pain documented as being related to, associated with or due to cancer, primary or secondary malignancy, or tumor. This code is assigned for both acute and chronic types of pain. Code 338.3 can be assigned as the principal or first-listed code when the reason for the admission or visit is documented as being to provide pain management or pain control. The underlying neoplasm should be reported as an additional diagnosis code. When the reason for the admission or visit is to manage the neoplasm, and pain is noted to also exist and is treated, code 338.3 can be assigned as an additional diagnosis.

## Exercise 5.6

Assign ICD-9-CM codes to the following diagnoses. Do not assign M codes to these exercises.

1. Metastatic carcinoma of bone
   a. What is the morphology type of this neoplasm?
   b. What is the code for primary carcinoma of unspecified site?
   c. Is bone included in the exception list?
   d. What is the primary site?
   e. What is the secondary site?
2. Adenocarcinoma of sigmoid colon with extension to peritoneum
3. Adenocarcinoma of prostate with metastasis to pelvic bones
4. Metastatic carcinoma of bile duct to local lymph nodes
5. Metastatic carcinoma of mediastinum

## ICD-9-CM Review Exercises: Chapter 5

Assign the appropriate ICD-9-CM codes for the following diagnoses and procedures. For these exercises, the M code for the morphology of the disease can be assigned.

1. Ewing's sarcoma of the left femur with excision of lesion of bone

2. Lipoma of left kidney

3. Metastatic carcinoma to liver from rectum; chronic neoplasm-related pain

4. Hepatocellular carcinoma

5. Malignant carcinoid tumor of appendix with open appendectomy and open resection of cecum

6. Relapse of chronic leukemia

7. Hodgkin's disease (mixed cellularity), head and neck with cervical lymph node biopsy

8. Epidermoid carcinoma of the upper lip; wide resection of lesion; chemotherapy

9. Carcinoma in situ of cervix

10. Generalized carcinomatosis, primary site undetermined with abdominal paracentesis

11. Small cell carcinoma of the right lower lobe of the lung with metastasis to the mediastinum; partial right lower lobectomy

12. Poorly differentiated lymphocytic lymphoma of the brain; admission for photon radiation therapy; radiation administered without complications

13. Subacute monocytic leukemia in remission

14. Malignant melanoma of the lower left arm with radical excision

*(Continued on next page)*

## ICD-9-CM Review Exercises: Chapter 5 (Continued)

15. Admission for chemotherapy; 25-year-old man with inoperable giant cell glioblastoma; anemia due to antineoplastic chemotherapy; administration of intravenous chemotherapy

    ______________________________

16. Cavernous angioma of the trunk (skin) with excision of skin lesion

    ______________________________

17. Acute lymphocytic leukemia; admission for chemotherapy; chemotherapy

    ______________________________

18. Adenocarcinoma of the right breast, upper outer quadrant, with metastasis to the axillary lymph nodes; modified radical mastectomy

    ______________________________

19. Squamous cell carcinoma of the leg with excision of skin lesion

    ______________________________

20. Tumor of abdomen

    ______________________________

# ICD-10-CM Chapter 2, Neoplasms (C00–D49)

The neoplasm chapter has undergone some organizational changes, too. For example, in ICD-10-CM, the block of codes for *in situ neoplasms* is located before the block for *benign neoplasms*. An example of a classification improvement is the addition in ICD-10-CM of a separate fifth character for extranodal and solid organ sites for lymphomas and Hodgkin's. ICD-9-CM included these sites with the fifth digit for unspecified site in codes for Hodgkin's disease, non-Hodgkin's lymphoma, peripheral, and cutaneous T-cell lymphomas.

## Organization and Structure of ICD-10-CM Chapter 2

Chapter 2 of ICD-10-CM includes categories C00–D49 arranged in the following blocks:

- C00–C75 Malignant neoplasms stated or presumed to be primary (of specific sites) and certain specified histologies, except neuroendocrine, and of lymphoid, hematopoietic and related tissues
  - C00–C14 Malignant neoplasms of lip, oral cavity and pharynx
  - C15–C26 Malignant neoplasms of digestive organs
  - C30–C39 Malignant neoplasms of respiratory and intrathoracic organs
  - C40–C41 Malignant neoplasms of bone and articular cartilage
  - C43–C44 Melanoma and other malignant neoplasms of skin
  - C45–C49 Malignant neoplasms of mesothelial and soft tissue
  - C50 Malignant neoplasms of breast
  - C51–C58 Malignant neoplasms of female genital organs
  - C60–C63 Malignant neoplasms of male genital organs
  - C64–C68 Malignant neoplasms of urinary tract
  - C69–C72 Malignant neoplasms of eye, brain and other parts of central nervous system
  - C73–C75 Malignant neoplasms of thyroid and other endocrine glands
- C7A Malignant neuroendocrine tumors
- C7B Secondary neuroendocrine tumors
- C76–C80 Malignant neoplasms of ill-defined, other secondary and unspecified sites
- C81–C96 Malignant neoplasms of lymphoid, hematopoietic and related tissue
- D00–D09 In situ neoplasms
- D10–D36 Benign neoplasms except benign neuroendocrine tumors
- D3A Benign neuroendocrine tumors
- D37–D48 Neoplasms of uncertain behavior, polycythemia vera and myelodysplastic syndromes
- D49 Neoplasms of unspecified behavior

## Coding Guidelines and Instructional Notes for ICD-10-CM Chapter 2

It is essential to review the extensive chapter-specific guidelines for Chapter 2, Neoplasms, in the ICD-10-CM Official Guidelines for Coding and Reporting (CDC 2014). A sample of these guidelines include:

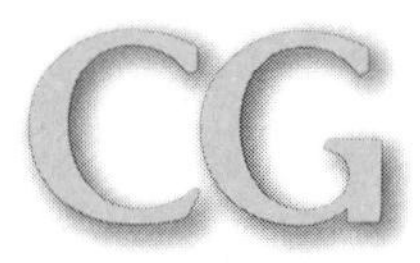

- Guidelines I.C.2. General neoplasm guidelines
  - The Neoplasm Table in the Alphabetic Index should be referenced first. However, if the histological term is documented, that term should be referenced first rather than going immediately to the Neoplasm Table in order to determine which column in the Neoplasm Table is appropriate.
- Guideline I.C.2.a. Treatment directed at the malignancy
  - "If the treatment is directed at the malignancy, designate the malignancy as the principal diagnosis. The only exception to this guideline is if a patient admission/encounter is solely for the administration of chemotherapy, immunotherapy or radiation therapy, assign the appropriate Z51 code as the first-listed or principal diagnosis and the diagnosis or problem for which the service is being performed as a secondary diagnosis."
- Guideline I.C.2.b. Treatment of secondary site
  - "When a patient is admitted because of a primary neoplasm with metastasis and treatment is directed toward the secondary site only, the secondary neoplasm is designated as the principal diagnosis even though the primary malignancy is still present."
- Guidelines I.C.2.c. Coding and sequencing of complications
  - Guidelines address the coding and sequencing of anemia associated with malignancy or as an adverse effect of chemotherapy, immunotherapy, and radiation therapy as well as the coding and sequencing of dehydration due to the malignancy and treatment of a complication resulting from a surgical procedure.
- Guideline I.C.2.d. Primary malignancy previously excised
  - "When a primary malignancy has been previously excised or eradicated from its site and there is no further treatment directed to that site and there is no

evidence of any existing primary malignancy, a code from category Z85, Personal history of malignant neoplasm, should be used to indicate the former site of the malignancy."

  - "Any mention of extension, invasion or metastasis to another site is coded as a secondary malignant neoplasm to that site. The secondary site may be the principal or first listed with the Z85 code used as a secondary code."

- Guidelines I.C.2.e. Admissions/encounters involving chemotherapy, immunotherapy and radiation therapy
  - Guidelines address the episode of care that involves the surgical removal of a neoplasm.
  - Patient admission/encounter solely for administration of chemotherapy, immunotherapy, and radiation therapy
  - Patient admitted for radiation therapy, chemotherapy, or immunotherapy and develops complications.
- Guidelines I.C.2.l. Sequencing of neoplasm codes
  - Specific guidelines exist to address the coding of an encounter for treatment of primary or secondary malignancy, malignant neoplasm in a pregnant patient, encounter for complications associated with a neoplasm; complications from surgical procedures for treatment of a neoplasm; and pathologic fracture due to a neoplasm.

The coding student should review all of the coding guidelines for Chapter 2 of ICD-10-CM, which appear in an ICD-10-CM code book at the website http://www.cdc.gov/nchs/icd/icd10cm.htm, or in appendix I of the accompanying website.

## ICD-10-CM Neoplasm Table

As in ICD-9-CM, the ICD-10-CM Neoplasm Table is organized into columns, with the left column listing the anatomic site and the next six columns providing codes for primary malignant, secondary malignant, CA [carcinoma] in situ, benign, uncertain, and unspecified behavior for each anatomic site. Malignant tumor codes start with the alphabetic character C in the range of C00–C96. Benign, in situ, and neoplasms of uncertain behavior and unspecified behavior are listed in the range of D00–D49.

A new feature in ICD-10-CM is the concept of laterality. Codes listed in the ICD-10-CM Neoplasm Table with a dash (-) following the code have a required fifth character for laterality. The Tabular List must be reviewed for the complete code. Neoplasm codes are specific as to whether the location is the right or left organ when a tumor is present in an organ that exists bilaterally. Examples of laterality would be a malignant neoplasm of the upper-outer quadrant of the right female breast (C50.411) and a benign neoplasm of the left kidney (D30.02). Codes also exist for an unspecified side of bilateral locations.

For each site, there are broad groupings for behavior—malignant, primary; malignant, secondary, CA in situ, benign, uncertain and unspecified behavior.

Definitions describing the behavior of seven specific neoplasms include:

- **Malignant:** Malignant neoplasms are collectively referred to as cancers. A malignant neoplasm can invade and destroy adjacent structures, as well as spread to distant sites to cause death.
- **Primary:** A primary neoplasm is the site where a neoplasm originated.
- **Secondary:** A secondary neoplasm is the site(s) to which the neoplasm has spread via:
    - Direct extension, in which the primary neoplasm infiltrates and invades adjacent structures
    - Metastasis to local lymph vessels by tumor cell infiltration
    - Invasion of local blood vessels
    - Implantation in which tumor cells shed into body cavities
- **In situ:** In an in situ neoplasm, the tumor cells undergo malignant changes but are still confined to the point of origin without invasion of surrounding normal tissue. The following terms also describe in situ malignancies: noninfiltrating, noninvasive, intraepithelial, or preinvasive carcinoma.
- **Benign:** In benign neoplasms, growth does not invade adjacent structures or spread to distant sites but may displace or exert pressure on adjacent structures.
- **Uncertain behavior:** Neoplasms of uncertain behavior are tumors that a pathologist cannot determine as being either benign or malignant because some features of each are present.
- **Unspecified nature:** Neoplasms of unspecified nature include tumors in which neither the behavior nor the histological type is specified in the diagnosis.

"Chapter 2 classifies neoplasms primarily by site (topography), with broad groupings for behavior (malignant, in situ, benign, and so on). The Neoplasm Table should be used to identify the correct topography code. In a few cases, such as for malignant melanoma and certain neuroendocrine tumors, the morphology (histologic type) is included in the category and codes." (CDC 2014)

## ICD-10-CM Chapter 2 Index Instructions

If the coder can identify the behavior and site of the neoplasm, the usual first step is to access the ICD-10-CM Neoplasm Table. However, the main terms and subterms in the ICD-10-CM Index to Diseases and Injuries assist the coder in locating the morphological type of neoplasms. When a specific code or site is not listed in the Index, cross-references direct the coder to the Neoplasm Table. The following instruction of classifying neoplasms should be followed:

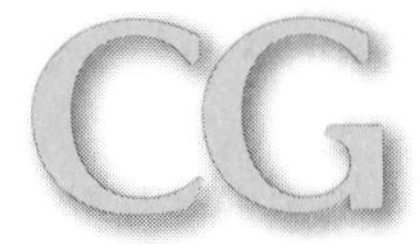

1. If the morphology is stated, the coder must locate the morphology of the tumor in the Index to Diseases and Injuries. For example, entries exist for lipoma, melanoma, sarcoma, etc. and specific codes for these types of these neoplasms are included in the Index and the coder does not need to reference the Neoplasm Table at all.
2. If the morphology is stated, the coder must locate the morphology of the tumor in the Index to Diseases and Injuries. However, not every entry in the Index will include codes. For example, if the doctor writes "subependymal glioma of the brain" as the diagnosis. The Index entry of glioma, subependymal, brain (specified site) is referenced and a cross reference directs the coder to see Neoplasm, uncertain behavior, by site (brain).
3. If the morphology is stated but the physician does not include an anatomic site, the coder should locate the morphology of the tumor in the Index to Diseases and Injuries. Certain types of morphology indicate the anatomic site as the only possible site where the tumor would develop. The physician would consider writing both the morphology and the site as redundant terminology. For example, the physician writes "serous papillary carcinoma" but the site is not stated. The Index entry of carcinoma, papillary, serous or carcinoma serous, papillary is referenced and the coder will find an entry for "unspecified" site with code C56.9. This is correct, code C56.9 is the code for malignant neoplasm of ovary, unspecified site. The coder can trust the entry because serous papillary carcinoma will only occur in an ovary.
4. If the coder is certain about the behavior of the neoplasm, for example, carcinoma is always a malignant primary tumor, the coder should reference the ICD-10-CM Neoplasm Table as the first step. The site of the neoplasm is located and the code is selected based on the behavior of the neoplasm.

## ICD-10-CM Chapter 2 Tabular List Instructions

In ICD-10-CM, instructional notes are found under many of the categories for malignant neoplasms. Instructional notes unique to ICD-10-CM direct coding professionals to use an additional code to identify such conditions as alcohol abuse and dependence, history of tobacco use, tobacco dependence, history of tobacco use, exposure to environmental tobacco smoke, and other facts.

All neoplasms are classified in this chapter, whether they are functionally active or not. An additional code from Chapter 4, Endocrine, Nutritional and Metabolic Diseases, may be used to identify functional activity associated with any neoplasm Functional activity, such as increased or decreased hormone production, which may occur when a neoplasm is present in a glandular organ. For example, when a patient has carcinoma of the ovary, she may also experience hyperestrogenism that produces excessive or frequent menstruation.

**EXAMPLE:** **C73** **Malignant neoplasm of thyroid gland**
Use additional code to identify any functional activity

An instructional note under category D3A, Benign neuroendocrine tumor and C7A, Malignant neuroendocrine tumors instructs the coding professional to code additional disorders.

**EXAMPLE:** **D3A** **Benign neuroendocrine tumors**
Code also any associated multiple endocrine neoplasia [MEN] syndromes (E31.2-)
Use additional code to identify any associated endocrine syndrome, such as: carcinoid syndrome (E34.0)

**EXAMPLE:** **C7A** **Malignant neuroendocrine tumors**
Code also any associated multiple endocrine neoplasia [MEN] syndromes (E31.2-)
Use additional code to identify any associated endocrine syndrome, such as: carcinoid syndrome (E34.0)

There have been other changes in the classification system regarding neoplasm coding. For example:

- Codes were moved from other chapters to Chapter 2 (for example, Waldenström's macroglobulinemia)
- Heading changes were made. For example, Malignant neoplasm of retroperitoneum and peritoneum moved from Malignant neoplasms of digestive organs and peritoneum to Malignant neoplasms of mesothelial and soft tissue
- Melanoma in situ has a unique category, D03 (previously included in ICD-9-CM category 172, Malignant melanoma of skin)

### *Primary Malignant Neoplasms Overlapping Site Boundaries*

A subcategory code of .8 is present in almost every category for primary malignant neoplasms in the range of C00–C69. Examples of these codes are C15.8, Malignant neoplasm of overlapping sites of esophagus or C50.811, Malignant neoplasm of overlapping sites of right female breast. A tumor may develop at one site in body and then overlaps into an area next to it. At the time the diagnosis is made it is often to determine exactly where the tumor originated, so it is described as a neoplasm of a contiguous or overlapping site. When there are multiple neoplasms of the same site that are not contiguous, such as tumors of different quadrants of the same breast, codes for each of the individual sites should be assigned.

## ICD-10-CM Review Exercises: Chapter 5

Assign the correct ICD-10-CM diagnosis codes to the following exercises.

1. Small cell carcinoma of the right lower lobe of the lung with metastasis to the intrathoracic lymph nodes, brain, and right rib

   ______________________________

2. Malignant mesothelioma of pleura

   ______________________________

3. Subacute monocytic leukemia in remission

   ______________________________

4. Melanoma of the left breast and left arm

   ______________________________

5. Benign carcinoid of the cecum

   ______________________________

6. Patient had left breast carcinoma four years ago and a left mastectomy was performed. She has been well since that time with no further treatment except for yearly checkups. The patient is now being seen with visual disturbances, dizziness, headaches, and blurred vision. Workup was completed which revealed metastasis to the brain, accounting for these symptoms. This was identified as being metastatic from the breast, not a new primary.

   ______________________________

7. The reason for the encounter is to receive chemotherapy following the recent diagnosis of carcinoma of the small intestines. The tumor was in the area where the duodenum and jejunum join. The cancer was resected two months ago and the patient has been receiving chemotherapy.

   ______________________________

8. Carcinoma of the head of the pancreas with metastasis to the right lung.

   ______________________________

9. Malignant carcinoid tumor of kidney

   ______________________________

10. Terminal carcinoma of the central portion of the right breast, metastatic to the liver and brain, was seen for dehydration and chronic intractable neoplasm-related pain. Patient was rehydrated with IVs and given IV pain medication with no treatment directed toward the cancer.

    ______________________________

# Chapter 6

# Endocrine, Nutritional and Metabolic Diseases, and Immunity Disorders

## Learning Objectives

At the conclusion of this chapter, you should be able to:

1. Describe the organization of the conditions and codes included in Chapter 3 of ICD-9-CM, Endocrine, Nutritional and Metabolic Diseases, and Immunity Disorders (240–279)
2. Describe the organization of the conditions and codes included in Chapter 4 of ICD-10-CM, Endocrine, Nutritional and Metabolic Diseases (E00–E89)
3. Define the term *diabetes mellitus*
4. Describe the different types of diabetes and how the type of diabetes impacts code selection in ICD-9-CM and in ICD-10-CM
5. Explain what the fourth and fifth digits indicate in ICD-9-CM when used to describe diabetes and diabetic conditions
6. Identify the codes included in Chapter 3 of ICD-9-CM that describe metabolic and immunity disorders such as gout, fluid and electrolyte imbalances, cystic fibrosis, and graft-versus-host disease
7. Assign ICD-9-CM diagnosis and procedure codes for endocrine, nutritional and metabolic diseases, and immunity disorders
8. Assign ICD-10-CM codes for endocrine, nutritional, and metabolic diseases

## ICD-9-CM, Chapter 3, Endocrine, Nutritional and Metabolic Diseases, and Immunity Disorders (240–279)

Chapter 3, Endocrine, Nutritional and Metabolic Diseases, and Immunity Disorders, in the Tabular List in volume 1 of ICD-9-CM includes conditions such as diabetes, cystic fibrosis, electrolyte imbalances, and disorders of the thyroid, parathyroid, and adrenal glands. In addition,

**Figure 6.1.** Endocrine system

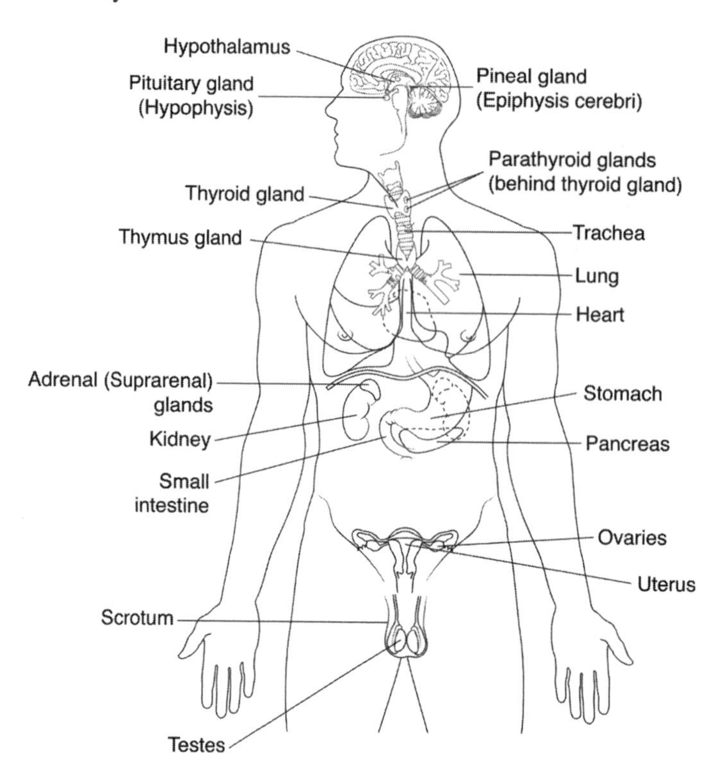




Chapter 3 provides codes for nutritional deficiencies, vitamin deficiencies, and other disorders of metabolism, as well as immune disorders. Figure 6.1 highlights the endocrine glands that cause or suffer from the diseases discussed in this chapter.

Chapter 3 is subdivided into the following categories and section titles:

| Categories | Section Titles |
|---|---|
| 240–246 | Disorders of Thyroid Gland |
| 249–259 | Diseases of Other Endocrine Glands |
| 260–269 | Nutritional Deficiencies |
| 270–279 | Other Metabolic and Immunity Disorders |

Chapter 6 in this book introduces coding instruction as it specifically relates to diabetes and to fluid, electrolyte, and acid-base imbalances.

## Diabetes Mellitus

Diabetes mellitus is a metabolic disease in which the pancreas does not produce insulin normally. The cause of diabetes mellitus can be attributed to both hereditary and nonhereditary factors, such as obesity, surgical removal of the pancreas, or the action of certain drugs. When the pancreas fails to produce insulin, glucose (sugar) is not broken down to be used and stored by the body's cells. As a result, too much sugar accumulates in the blood, causing hyperglycemia and resulting in spillover into the urine, causing glycosuria. Saturating the blood and urine with glucose draws water out of the body, causing dehydration and thirst. Other symptoms include excessive hunger, marked weakness, and weight loss.

Treatment may consist of insulin regulation by either insulin injection or oral antidiabetic agents, along with physical activity and a healthy diet.

## Category 250

Category 250, Diabetes mellitus, is subdivided into fourth-digit subcategories to identify the presence or absence of complications and/or manifestations.

**250 Diabetes Mellitus**
- **250.0 Diabetes mellitus, without mention of complication**
- **250.1 Diabetes with ketoacidosis**
- **250.2 Diabetes with hyperosmolarity**
- **250.3 Diabetes with other coma**
- **250.4 Diabetes with renal manifestations**
- **250.5 Diabetes with ophthalmic manifestations**
- **250.6 Diabetes with neurological manifestations**
- **250.7 Diabetes with peripheral circulatory disorders**
- **250.8 Diabetes with other specified manifestations**
- **250.9 Diabetes with unspecified complication**

### Fifth-Digit Subclassification

**Note:** *ICD-9-CM uses Roman numerals to describe the two types of diabetes (type I and type II); ICD-10-CM uses Arabic numerals (type 1 and type 2). In this text, we have moved to the more current treatment and will use "type 1 and type 2" in all narrative discussion of the disease. However, any examples using ICD-9-CM codes will use Roman numerals, as in the code set.*

Two types of diabetes are discussed here and impact the fifth digit subclassification of category 250 codes: type 1 and type 2. If the type of diabetes is not documented in the medical records, it is considered "unspecified" and the ICD-9-CM code assignment default is "type II or unspecified type." Type 1 and type 2 diabetes mellitus were previously known as insulin-dependent (IDDM) and noninsulin-dependent (NIDDM).

Type 1 diabetes was previously referred to as IDDM. Most patients with type 1 diabetes develop the condition as children or young adults, although it can develop at any age. Type 1 diabetes mellitus is also referred to as juvenile diabetes. Type 1 diabetes occurs when the pancreas produces little or no insulin.

Type 2 diabetes was previously referred to as NIDDM or adult-onset diabetes. Type 2 diabetes is the more common form of diabetes mellitus, affecting 90 to 95 percent of the diabetic population. It is common in older adults but also can occur in teenagers and young adults. Risk factors include obesity and heredity.

Type 1 diabetes mellitus refers to the absence of pancreatic beta cells. Type 2 diabetes mellitus occurs when the body is not able to use insulin effectively and insulin production decreases. The injection of insulin is not a determining factor in the type of diabetes present in a patient. Type 1 diabetic patients must use insulin. Type 2 diabetic patients may or may not use insulin depending on their diabetic condition and the other health conditions they may have. Pregnant women who develop gestational diabetes may also require insulin to maintain proper blood glucose levels during the pregnancy.

A diagnosis of "diabetic ketoacidosis" is coded to 250.13, Diabetes with ketoacidosis, type 1, uncontrolled, unless the physician specifically documents the type of diabetes in the patient to be type 2 By definition, diabetic ketoacidosis is uncontrolled diabetes. Type 1 diabetic patients are much more likely to develop ketoacidosis by the nature of their disease than patients with type 2 diabetes mellitus.

The following fifth digits with category 250 conform to the accepted terminology for diabetes mellitus. Also, an additional code to indicate the long-term (current) use of insulin is assigned with the fifth digits of 0 and 2. The use of insulin by patients with type 2 diabetes mellitus and women with gestational diabetes will be identified by the V58.67 code. The following fifth digits are available for use with category 250:

- 0 type 2 or unspecified type, not stated as uncontrolled

  Fifth digit 0 is for use for type 2 patients, even if the patient requires insulin.

  Use additional code, if applicable, for associated long-term (current) insulin use, V58.67

- 1 type 1 [juvenile type], not stated as uncontrolled
- 2 type 2 or unspecified type, uncontrolled

  Fifth digit 2 is used for type 2 patients, even if the patient requires insulin.

  Use additional code, if applicable, for associated long-term (current) insulin use, V58.67

- 3 type 1 [juvenile type], uncontrolled

When coding the case of a patient who receives insulin during a hospitalization, it should not be assumed that the patient is a type 1 diabetic. Type 2 diabetics often may require the administration of insulin to regulate blood glucose levels; however, this does not imply that the patient is now a type 1 diabetic.

If the documentation in a medical record does not indicate the type of diabetes but does indicate that the patient uses insulin, the appropriate fifth digit for type 2 must be used. For type 2 patients who routinely use insulin, code V58.67, Long-term (current) use of insulin, should also be assigned to indicate the patient uses insulin. Code V58.67 should not be assigned if insulin is given temporarily to bring a type 2 patient's blood sugar under control during an encounter. The use of insulin during an acute episode of care or hospitalization may be required to bring a type II diabetic condition under control during the encounter. This includes the temporary use of insulin during a patient's acute illness or after surgery.

Documentation in the health record must support assignment of type 1 diabetes. Furthermore, use of fifth digits 2 or 3 also must be confirmed by appropriate documentation. The physician must document the diabetes as "out of control" or "uncontrolled."

### Complications and Manifestations

Some patients with diabetes develop other conditions (for example, retinopathy, neuropathy, and others) that may or may not be due to diabetes mellitus. ICD-9-CM provides codes when a causal relationship exists between a condition and the diabetes:

**250.4 Diabetes with renal manifestations**
**250.5 Diabetes with ophthalmic manifestations**
**250.6 Diabetes with neurological manifestations**
**250.7 Diabetes with peripheral circulatory disorders**
**250.8 Diabetes with other specified manifestations**

To assign these codes, documentation in the health record must support this causal relationship. When a causal relationship exists, the principal diagnosis code assigned is a diabetic code from category 250, followed by the code for the manifestation or complication. The diabetes codes and the secondary codes that correspond to them are paired codes that follow the etiology/manifestation convention of the classification.

**EXAMPLE:** Proliferative diabetic retinopathy due to type I diabetes mellitus

250.51 Diabetes with ophthalmic manifestations, type I (juvenile type), not stated as uncontrolled
*362.02 Proliferative diabetic retinopathy*

The principal diagnosis is diabetes with ophthalmic manifestations (250.51), followed by proliferative diabetic retinopathy (362.02).

When a patient develops several complications due to diabetes, more than one code from category 250 may be assigned to describe the patient's condition completely. Assign as many codes from category 250 as needed to identify all of the associated conditions that the patient has.

**EXAMPLE:** Diabetic polyneuropathy and peripheral angiopathy due to type I diabetes mellitus

250.61 Diabetes with neurological manifestations, type I (juvenile type), not stated as uncontrolled
*357.2 Polyneuropathy in diabetes*
250.71 Diabetes with peripheral circulatory disorders, type I (juvenile type), not stated as uncontrolled
*443.81 Peripheral angiopathy in diseases classified elsewhere*

As in the preceding example of diabetic polyneuropathy, the Tabular List often displays a manifestation in italic type as a reminder that the underlying condition must be sequenced before the manifestation (for example, polyneuropathy).

Official coding guidelines exist for the coding of diabetes mellitus. See Section I. C. Chapter-Specific Guidelines, Chapter 3, Endocrine, Nutritional and Metabolic Diseases, and Immunity Disorders (240–279).

### Category 249

Category 249 codes describe secondary diabetes mellitus. Secondary diabetes mellitus is always caused by another disease, as indicated by the word "secondary." Secondary diabetes can occur in a patient with cystic fibrosis, Cushing's syndrome, a malignant neoplasm, and certain genetic disorders. Secondary diabetes can also be a late effect of poisoning.

The category 249, Secondary diabetes mellitus, has an Includes Note that describes the condition as diabetes (due to) (in) (secondary) (with): drug-induced or chemical-induced or infection. The Excludes Note refers the coders to other conditions classified elsewhere, such as gestational diabetes, hyperglycemia NOS, neonatal diabetes, nonclinical diabetes, type 1, and type 2 diabetes.

Category 249 codes parallel the diabetes codes in category 250 with the same manifestations and uncontrolled, not stated as uncontrolled, or unspecified status. Specific sequencing of category 249 codes will depend on the documentation in the health record, the circumstances of admission or encounter, and the official coding guidelines.

For patients routinely using insulin, code V58.67, Long-term (current) use of insulin should also be assigned. V58.67 should not be assigned if insulin is given temporarily to control a patient's blood sugar during a hospital stay or encounter.

When a patient has secondary diabetes mellitus with associated conditions as a result of the diabetes, the code(s) from category 249 must be listed first, followed by the codes for the associated conditions. The coder may assign as many codes from category 249 as needed to identify all the associated conditions. The corresponding codes for the associated conditions are listed under each of the secondary diabetes codes.

The sequencing of the secondary diabetes codes with the codes for the underlying condition or the cause of the secondary diabetes depends on the reason for the visit or admission, applicable ICD-9-CM sequencing conventions, and chapter-specific guidelines. If the patient is seen for treatment of the secondary diabetes or one of its associated conditions, a code from category 249 is listed first with the cause of the secondary diabetes, for example, cystic fibrosis, listed as an additional diagnosis. However, if the patient is seen for management of the condition causing the secondary diabetes, the code for the cause of the secondary diabetes should be listed first. An additional code (or codes) is reported for the type of secondary diabetes that is managed during the encounter as well.

A different form of diabetes occurs following a pancreatectomy (excision of the pancreas). This surgery produces hypoinsulinemia and/or hyperglycemia. Code 251.3, Postsurgical hypoinsulinemia, is assigned. Additionally, at least one code from subcategory 249, along with either code V88.11 or code V88.12, is assigned. The codes from subcategory V88.1 provide information as to whether the patient had a total or partial pancreatectomy. This post-surgical state may also have a diabetic manifestation, such as diabetic nephropathy, which would be coded with code 583.81, Nephritis and nephropathy in diseases classified elsewhere. For example, the ICD-9-CM codes for a patient who develops secondary diabetes mellitus with diabetic nephropathy due to a total pancreatectomy performed are 251.3, 249.20, 583.81, and V88.11.

## Metabolic and Immunity Disorders

Category 274 includes various conditions caused by gout such as arthropathy, nephropathy, and other manifestations. Gout is a disorder in which uric acid or urate crystals are deposited in joints and soft tissues with resulting inflammation and degenerative changes. The most common forms of gout affect the body's joints. Gout is associated with hyperuricemia or excessive uric acid in the blood. Acute gouty arthropathy is also known as acute gout, gout attack or flare. It is a symptomatic inflammation caused by urate crystals in one or more joints, with the large joint of the big toe being one of the most commonly affected joints. Acute gout is intermittent, unpredictable as to when it occurs, extremely painful and often debilitating. Chronic gouty arthropathy may occur with or without mention of tophus or tophi. Tophus is the deposit of urate crystals in and around the joints. This form of chronic arthritis is characterized by tender and swollen joints. Tophi usually appear after the patient has had gout for several years. Specific codes exist for gouty arthropathy:

**274.00 Gouty arthropathy, unspecified**
**274.01 Acute gouty arthropathy**
**274.02 Chronic gouty arthropathy without mention of tophus (tophi)**
**274.03 Chronic gouty arthropathy with tophus (tophi)**

Additionally, codes exist in category 274 for manifestations of gout and for gout, unspecified.

Category 276 includes the following conditions:

**276 Disorders of fluid, electrolyte and acid-base imbalance**
- **276.0 Hyperosmolality and/or hypernatremia**
- **276.1 Hyposmolality and/or hyponatremia**
- **276.2 Acidosis**
- **276.3 Alkalosis**
- **276.4 Mixed acid-base balance disorder**
- **276.5 Volume depletion**
- **276.6 Fluid overload**
- **276.7 Hyperpotassemia**
- **276.8 Hypopotassemia**
- **276.9 Electrolyte and fluid disorders, not elsewhere classified**

The preceding conditions are usually symptoms of a larger disease process and, as such, should be coded as additional diagnoses when documented in the health record. In some cases, however, the patient may be admitted for treatment of one of these symptoms, with the underlying condition not requiring much care. In such cases, the symptom or metabolic disorder may be assigned as the principal diagnosis.

"Volume depletion may refer to depletion of total body water (dehydration) or depletion of the blood volume (hypovolemia)." (*Coding Clinic for ICD-9-CM*, Fourth Quarter 2005, pp 54–55) Dehydration, a lack of adequate water in the body, can be a medical emergency. This condition is classified to 276.51 in ICD-9-CM. Common in infants and elderly people, severe dehydration can occur with vomiting, excessive heat and sweating, diarrhea, or lack of food or fluid intake. Blood volume may be maintained despite dehydration, with fluid being pulled from other tissues. Conversely, hypovolemia may occur without dehydration when "third-spacing" of fluids occurs, for example, with significant edema or ascites. Hypovolemia is an abnormally low circulating blood volume and is classified to 276.52 in ICD-9-CM. Blood loss may be due to internal bleeding from the intestine or stomach, external bleeding from an injury, or loss of blood volume and body fluid associated with diarrhea, vomiting, dehydration, or burns. If hypovolemia is severe, hypovolemic shock can occur with symptoms such as rapid or weak pulse, feeling faint, pale skin, cool or moist skin, rapid breathing, anxiety, overall weakness, and low blood pressure. Emergency medical attention must be sought. Given that the nature of these two conditions and their respective treatments are different, coding of hypovolemia is different from dehydration.

**EXAMPLE:** Patient admitted with severe dehydration and gastroenteritis. Treatment was directed toward resolving the dehydration.

276.51 Dehydration
558.9 Other and unspecified noninfectious gastroenteritis and colitis

In the preceding example, dehydration (276.51) is assigned as the principal diagnosis, followed by the underlying cause, gastroenteritis (558.9).

Cystic fibrosis is an inherited disease of the exocrine glands that affects the gastrointestinal and respiratory systems. Subcategory codes for cystic fibrosis (277.0) have fifth-digit codes to describe the different manifestations that often occur. Cystic fibrosis is characterized by chronic obstructive pulmonary disease, pancreatic insufficiency, and abnormally high sweat electrolytes. The degree of pulmonary involvement usually determines the course of the disease. The patient's demise is often the result of respiratory failure and cor pulmonale. The codes for cystic fibrosis describe the condition when it occurs with pulmonary manifestations, with complications of pancreatic enzyme replacement therapy, and with other manifestations.

Graft-versus-host disease (GVHD) can occur as a complication of bone marrow transplant. On occasion it can occur following blood transfusion or any organ transplant in which white blood cells are present in the organ that is transplanted. GVHD may be described as acute or chronic. Acute GVHD causes disorders in the skin, gastrointestinal tract, and liver and also causes increased susceptibility to infection. Chronic GVHD usually begins more than three months after transplant and may occur in patients who have had the acute form of the disease. Treatment of GVHD involves corticosteroids and other immune-suppressant drugs. Codes for GVHD identify whether the condition is considered acute form (279.51), chronic form (279.52), or acute-on-chronic form (279.53). The GVHD code is reported as an additional diagnosis after the code for complication of a transplanted organ (996.80–996.89) or complication of blood transfusion (999.89). Additional codes are used to describe the associated manifestations of GVHD.

## ICD-9-CM Review Exercises: Chapter 6

Assign ICD-9-CM codes to the following:

1. Type 2 diabetic with nephrosis due to the diabetes
2. Folic acid deficiency
3. Cushing's syndrome
4. Hypokalemia
5. Cystic fibrosis with pulmonary manifestations
6. Uncontrolled type 2 diabetes mellitus; mild malnutrition
7. Toxic diffuse goiter with thyrotoxic crisis
8. Sporadic hypogammaglobulinemia
9. Tyrosinemia
10. Panhypopituitarism
11. Lower extremity ulcer on skin of left heel secondary to brittle diabetes mellitus, type 1, uncontrolled
12. Diabetic proliferative retinopathy in a patient with controlled type 1 diabetes
13. Arteriosclerotic heart disease involving native arteries with familial hypercholesterolemia
14. Acute infantile rickets
15. Syndrome of inappropriate secretion of antidiuretic hormone (SIADH)
16. Marasmus secondary to AIDS

## ICD-9-CM Review Exercises: Chapter 6 (Continued)

17. Overweight adult with a body mass index (BMI) of 26.5

18. Hypoglycemia in type 1 diabetic

19. Hyperthyroidism with nodular goiter; partial thyroidectomy

20. Waldenström's hypergammaglobulinemia

21. Acute graft-versus-host disease, described as a complication of a recent bone marrow transplant

22. Hungry bone syndrome

23. Partial androgen insensitivity syndrome

24. Secondary diabetes mellitus with diabetic coma, uncontrolled

25. Acute gout

# ICD-10-CM, Chapter 4, Endocrine, Nutritional, and Metabolic Diseases (E00–E89)

Chapter 4 of ICD-10-CM, Endocrine, Nutritional, and Metabolic Diseases (E00–E89) contains many frequently coded conditions such as disorders of the thyroid gland, obesity, dehydration, and diabetes mellitus.

## Organization and Structure of ICD-10-CM Chapter 4

Chapter 4 of ICD-10-CM includes categories E00–E89 arranged in the following blocks:

| | |
|---|---|
| E00–E07 | Disorders of thyroid gland |
| E08–E13 | Diabetes mellitus |
| E15–E16 | Other disorders of glucose regulation and pancreatic internal secretion |
| E20–E35 | Disorders of other endocrine glands |

| | |
|---|---|
| E36 | Intraoperative complications of endocrine system |
| E40–E46 | Malnutrition |
| E50–E64 | Other nutritional deficiencies |
| E65–E68 | Overweight, obesity and other hyperalimentation |
| E70–E88 | Metabolic disorders |
| E89 | Postprocedural endocrine and metabolic complications and disorders, not elsewhere classified |

A number of new subchapters have been added to the chapter for endocrine, nutritional, and metabolic diseases. For example, diabetes mellitus and malnutrition have their own subchapter while these conditions were grouped with diseases of other endocrine glands and nutritional deficiencies respectively. Code titles have been revised in a number of places in Chapter 4. Code descriptors for goiter are now consistent with present terminology.

A significant change to ICD-10-CM is the classification of diabetes mellitus. There are five categories for diabetes mellitus in ICD-10-CM. Additionally, diabetes mellitus codes have been expanded to reflect manifestations and complications of the disease by using fourth or fifth characters rather than by using an additional code to identify the manifestation. ICD-10-CM does not classify inadequately controlled, out of control, and poorly controlled diabetes mellitus with fifth digit subclassification as is the case in ICD-9-CM. New to ICD-10-CM are codes to report diabetes mellitus, by type, with hyperglycemia.

**Note:** ICD-10-CM Five Categories for Diabetes Mellitus:

- E08, Diabetes mellitus due to underlying condition
- E09, Drug or chemical induced diabetes mellitus
- E10, Type 1 diabetes mellitus
- E11, Type 2 diabetes mellitus
- E13, Other specified diabetes mellitus

## Coding Guidelines and Instructional Notes for ICD-10-CM Chapter 4

Instructions for coding "late effects" or sequelae have been expanded in Chapter 4 of ICD-10-CM. For example, Excludes1 notes have been added to some categories between E50–E63 to indicate that the sequelae of the nutritional deficiency are assigned a code from category E64.

The National Center for Health Statistics (NCHS) has published chapter-specific guidelines for Chapter 4 of ICD-10-CM:

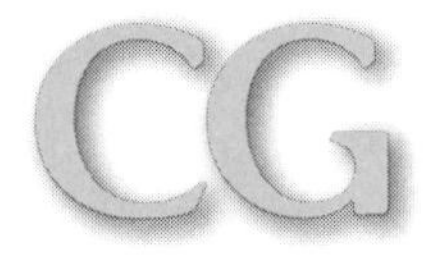

Guidelines I.C.4. Diabetes Mellitus. Some excerpts are included here:

- "The diabetes mellitus codes are combination codes that include the type of diabetes mellitus, the body system affected, and the complications affecting that body system. As many codes within a particular category as are necessary to describe all of the complications of the disease may be used. They should be sequenced based on the reason for a particular encounter. Assign as many codes from categories E08–E13 as needed to identify all of the associated conditions that the patient has."
- New guidelines that clarify code usage are also found under specific codes. "Codes under categories E08, Diabetes mellitus due to underlying condition, and E09, Drug or chemical induced diabetes mellitus, identify complications/manifestations associated with secondary diabetes mellitus. Secondary diabetes is always caused by another condition or event (for example, cystic fibrosis, malignant neoplasm of pancreas, pancreatectomy, adverse effect of drug, or poisoning)."

## Coding Overview for ICD-10-CM, Chapter 4

The coding of diabetes mellitus in ICD-10-CM is an example of the use of combination codes that have been expanded in the new classification system. In ICD-9-CM, when diabetes is present in a patient with complications and manifestations of the disease, at least two diagnosis codes are used: one for the diabetes code from category 249 or 250, followed by the code for the complication or manifestation, usually from another body system such as diseases of the eye or kidney.

In ICD-10-CM, the diabetes mellitus codes are combination codes that include the type of diabetes (type 1, type 2, due to underlying condition or due to drug or chemical), the body system affected, and the complications affecting that body system. For type 1 and type 2 diabetes, the diabetes code contains the details about the type of diabetes and most of the associated complications. A few of the diabetes codes require the use of an additional code, for example to identify the stage of the chronic kidney disease caused by the diabetes. For other types of diabetes, the underlying condition is listed first, followed by the diabetes code that includes any associated complication.

Each type of diabetes has a particular category of codes:

- E08, Diabetes mellitus due to underlying condition
  - Code first the underlying condition, such as Cushing's Syndrome
- E09, Drug or chemical induced diabetes mellitus

  - Code first poisoning due to drug or toxin if applicable (T36–T65). Use additional code for adverse effect, if applicable to identify drug (T36–T50)
- E10, Type 1 diabetes mellitus
- E11, Type 2 diabetes mellitus
  - Diabetes NOS or of an unspecified type defaults to Type 2
- E13, Other specified diabetes mellitus

Other forms of diabetes are coded elsewhere in ICD-10-CM:

- Gestational diabetes (O24.41)
- Neonatal diabetes mellitus (P70.2)

In addition to identifying the type of diabetes, the ICD-10-CM code includes one or more of the complications or manifestations that exists in a particular body system. For example:

- E08.21, Diabetes mellitus due to underlying condition with diabetic nephropathy
- E09.610, Drug or chemical induced diabetes mellitus with diabetic neuropathic arthropathy
- E10.321, Type 1 diabetes mellitus with mild nonproliferative diabetic retinopathy with macular edema
- E11.51, Type 2 diabetes mellitus with diabetic peripheral angiopathy without gangrene
- E13.620, Other specified diabetes mellitus with diabetic dermatitis

The coder may assign as many codes from categories E08–E13 as needed to identify all the associated conditions that a patient may have had treated. An additional code is available to indicate the use of insulin. Except for Type 1 diabetes, an additional code of Z79.4 is used to identify patients who routinely use insulin for the management of their type 2 or other forms of diabetes.

The coding guidelines state that "all neoplasms, whether functionally active or not, are classified in Chapter 2. Appropriate codes in Chapter 4 (namely, E05.8, E07.0, E16–E31, E34.-) may be used as additional codes to indicate either functional activity by neoplasms and ectopic endocrine tissue or hyperfunction and hypofunction of endocrine glands associated with neoplasms and other conditions classified elsewhere." (CMS 2014)

There is an Excludes1 note at the beginning of ICD-10-CM, Chapter 4 for transitory endocrine and metabolic disorders specific to the newborn (P70–P74).

## ICD-10-CM Review Exercises: Chapter 6

Assign the correct ICD-10-CM diagnosis codes to the following exercises.

1. Mild nonproliferative diabetic retinopathy, type 2 diabetes mellitus with macular edema, on daily insulin injections. Patient also has diabetic cataract in right eye.

2. Type 1 diabetic with diabetic chronic kidney disease, stage 3, being seen for regulation of insulin dosage. Patient also has an abscessed right molar.

3. Secondary diabetes mellitus due to acute idiopathic pancreatitis with diabetic hyperglycemia; long-term use of insulin.

4. Hyperthyroidism with multinodular goiter. The patient has the symptoms of nervousness, irritability, increased perspiration, shakiness and increased appetite with unexplained weight loss, increased heart rate, palpitations, and sleeping difficulties. The patient was started on oral anti-thyroid medication. Arrangements were also made for patient to see a cardiologist due to the fact that her palpitations were more pronounced than seen in other patients with hyperthyroidism.

5. Morbid obesity with a BMI of 42 in an adult.

6. Diagnosis: Dehydration. Salmonella gastroenteritis, abdominal cramping, nausea, vomiting, and diarrhea. The patient was seen with severe abdominal cramping, nausea and vomiting, and diarrhea. She ate turkey salad several hours before these symptoms developed 15 hours ago. Lab tests show dehydration. The patient was treated with IV therapy.

7. Bulimia with moderate protein–calorie malnutrition.

8. Patient has steroid-induced diabetes mellitus due to the prolonged use of corticosteroids, which have been discontinued. The patient's diabetes is managed with insulin.

9. A 25-year-old male patient with type 1 diabetes mellitus, taking insulin, is admitted because he is having symptoms of nausea, severe vomiting, increased frequency of urination, and polydipsia. The patient is also severely dehydrated. The patient was hydrated, and, as a result, his blood sugar decreased from more than 600 to normal levels. The patient was diagnosed with diabetic ketoacidosis, type 1.

10. Type 1 diabetes with a severe chronic diabetic left foot ulcer with diabetic peripheral angiopathy. Patient also has diabetic stage 2 chronic kidney disease. He is being evaluated to see if debridement is required for this ulcer with breakdown of the skin only.

# Chapter 7

# Diseases of the Blood and Blood-Forming Organs

## Learning Objectives

At the conclusion of this chapter, you should be able to:

1. Describe the organization of the conditions and codes included in Chapter 4 of ICD-9-CM, Diseases of the Blood and Blood-Forming Organs (280–289)
2. Describe the organization of the conditions and codes included in Chapter 3 of ICD-10-CM, Diseases of the blood and blood-forming organs and certain disorders involving the immune mechanism (D50–D89)
3. Define anemia and identify the causes of the specific types of anemia—deficiency, hemolytic, aplastic, and antineoplastic chemotherapy-induced
4. Define the term *coagulation defects,* give specific examples of these conditions, and briefly describe their treatment
5. Describe primary and secondary thrombocytopenia and briefly describe their treatments
6. Identify diseases of the white blood cells and give examples of these conditions
7. Assign ICD-9-CM diagnosis and procedure codes for blood and blood-forming organs
8. Assign ICD-10-CM codes for conditions categorized in ICD-10-CM Chapter 3

## ICD-9-CM Chapter 4, Diseases of the Blood and Blood-Forming Organs (280–289)

Chapter 4, Diseases of the Blood and Blood-Forming Organs, in the Tabular List in volume 1 of ICD-9-CM includes anemias, coagulation defects, purpura, and other hemorrhagic conditions and diseases of the white blood cells (WBCs).

## Anemias

Anemia is defined as a decrease in the number of erythrocytes (red blood cells), the quantity of hemoglobin, or the volume of packed red cells in the blood. Laboratory data reflect a decrease in red blood cells (RBCs), hemoglobin (Hgb), or hematocrit (Hct). Anemia is manifested by pallor of skin and mucous membranes, shortness of breath, palpitations of the heart, soft systolic murmurs, lethargy, and fatigability.

### Deficiency Anemias

Categories 280–281 include codes for deficiency anemias. The most common type of anemia, iron deficiency anemia (category 280), is caused by an inadequate absorption of or excessive loss of iron. Iron deficiency anemia due to chronic blood loss is reported with code 280.0. The underlying cause of the bleeding should be coded when documented in the health record. Without further specification, iron deficiency anemia is reported with code 280.9.

Acute posthemorrhagic anemia is anemia due to acute blood loss and is reported with code 285.1. It is defined as a normocytic, normochromic anemia developing as a result of rapid loss of large quantities of RBCs during bleeding. It may occur as a result of a massive hemorrhage that may be due to spontaneous or traumatic rupture of a large blood vessel, rupture of an aneurysm, arterial erosion from a peptic ulcer or neoplastic process, or complications of surgery from excessive blood loss. Coders should not assume that anemia following a procedure, or postoperative anemia, is acute blood loss anemia. When postoperative anemia is documented without specification of acute blood loss, code 285.9, Anemia, unspecified, is used.

Category 281 describes other deficiency anemias that may be referred to as megaloblastic anemias. The etiology of megaloblastic anemias includes a deficiency or defective utilization of vitamin $B_{12}$, or folic acid. The condition can also be caused by the presence of cytotoxic agents (usually antineoplastic or immunosuppressive drugs) that interfere with DNA synthesis. Megaloblastic anemias include:

**281.0** **Pernicious anemia**
**281.1** **Other vitamin $B_{12}$ deficiency anemia**
**281.2** **Folate deficiency anemia**
**281.3** **Other specific megaloblastic anemias, NEC**
**281.4** **Protein deficiency anemias**
**281.8** **Anemia associated with other specific nutritional deficiencies**
**281.9** **Unspecified deficiency anemia**

### Hemolytic Anemias

Hemolytic anemia refers to an abnormal reduction of RBCs caused by an increased rate of RBC destruction and the inability of the bone marrow to compensate. Hemolytic anemias may be hereditary (category 282) or acquired (category 283). Hereditary anemias are caused by intrinsic abnormalities involving structural defects of RBCs or defects of globin synthesis or structure. ICD-9-CM classifies hereditary hemolytic anemias to category 282, which includes the following common hematologic disorders:

**282.40–282.49** **Thalassemias**
**282.5** **Sickle cell trait**
**282.60–282.69** **Sickle cell disease**

Typically, acquired hemolytic anemias are caused by extrinsic factors such as trauma (surgery or burns), infection, systemic diseases (Hodgkin's lymphoma, leukemia, or systemic lupus erythematosus), drugs or toxins, liver or renal disease, or abnormal immune responses. ICD-9-CM classifies acquired hemolytic anemia to category 283, with the fourth and fifth digits (when applicable) describing the specific type or cause of disorder; for example:

**283.0** **Autoimmune hemolytic anemias**
**283.10–283.19** **Non-autoimmune hemolytic anemias**

### Aplastic Anemias

Aplastic anemias include a group of bone marrow disorders, most of which involve anemia as well as pancytopenia. Aplastic anemia is caused by an abnormal reduction of RBCs due to a lack of bone marrow blood production. Usually, this type of anemia is accompanied by agranulocytosis and thrombocytopenia, in which case it is called pancytopenia. Exposure to toxins such as radiation, chemotherapy, chloramphenicol, sulfonamides, and phenytoin can result in aplastic anemia. ICD-9-CM classifies aplastic anemias to category 284, with the fourth and fifth digits indicating the specific type. Constitutional RBC anemias (code 284.01), such as Blackfan-Diamond syndrome, are usually congenital or familial. Other constitutional anemias, such as Fanconi's anemia, code 284.09, also exist.

Pancytopenia is a decrease in all of the cellular elements in the blood, including red cells, white cells, and platelets. It may be caused by aplastic anemia as well as other conditions. The coder should refer to the excludes note that follows category 284.1, pancytopenia.

Acquired red cell aplasia is a form of aplastic anemia. Code 284.81, Red cell aplasia, may also be described as red cell aplasia with thymoma. Patients may acquire a form of aplastic anemia due to chronic systemic disease, due to drugs including chemotherapy, due to infection, and/or due to radiation, as well as other toxins. Code 284.89, Other specified aplastic anemias, is used to classify these forms of acquired aplastic anemias due to these specified substances.

### Other and Unspecified Anemias

Category 285 classifies other and unspecified anemias, including acute blood loss anemia (285.1) and sideroblastic anemia (285.0). Subcategory 285.2 allows three codes to be reported: 285.21, Anemia in chronic kidney disease; 285.22, Anemia in neoplastic disease; and 285.29, Anemia of other chronic disease.

Subcategory code 285.3, Antineoplastic chemotherapy-induced anemia is used to describe an anemia acquired from the administration of antineoplastic chemotherapy to treat a malignancy. Cancer drugs can inhibit the production of bone marrow and thereby reduce the number of RBCs produced. This produces an anemia that may be short term and does not reduce the bone marrow cellularity to a state of aplasia. Chemotherapy-induced anemia is one of the more common side effects of chemotherapy affecting 20 to 60 percent of all patients receiving chemotherapy as their cancer treatment. Patients with this type of anemia may suffer from significant fatigue and inability to perform normal activities of daily living. Drug treatment with erythropoiesis (red blood cell) stimulating proteins can restore the volume of RBCs and reduce the anemia. Commonly-used drugs to treat chemotherapy-induced anemia include epoetin alfa (Procrit) and darbepoetin alfa (Aranesp).

Code 285.9 is used to report anemia, unspecified. The diagnosis of "postoperative" anemia may be documented by the physician during a hospital stay without specification of acute blood loss. By following the ICD-9-CM Alphabetic Index, this statement would be coded as 285.9. However, if the physician stated postoperative anemia due to blood loss or stated acute posthemorrhagic anemia, code 285.1 should be reported—again, following the Alphabetic Index entries carefully.

## Coagulation Defects

Coagulation defects are disorders of the platelets that result in serious bleeding due to a deficiency of one or more clotting factors. ICD-9-CM classifies coagulation defects to category 286, with the fourth and fifth digits identifying the specific type of defect. Coagulation defects include:

1. Classic hemophilia (hemophilia A), which is the most common, occurs as a result of factor VIII deficiency. It is inherited as an X-linked recessive disorder affecting males and transmitted by females. ICD-9-CM classifies classic hemophilia to code 286.0.
2. Hemophilia B (Christmas disease) results from a deficiency of factor IX. As with hemophilia A, this type is transmitted as an X-linked recessive trait. ICD-9-CM classifies hemophilia B to code 286.1.
3. Hemophilia C is an autosomal recessive disease caused by a deficiency in factor XI. ICD-9-CM classifies this condition to code 286.2.

Other conditions are often confused with coagulation defects. For example, a patient being treated with Warfarin sodium (Coumadin), heparin, or another anticoagulant may develop bleeding or hemorrhage. Bleeding that occurs in a patient taking the drug Coumadin or heparin is an adverse effect of the anticoagulant therapy when the drug is taken as prescribed. When this occurs, a code for the condition and associated hemorrhage is assigned, with an additional code of E934.2 to indicate the drug documented by the physician and responsible for the bleeding. To locate the code for the drug responsible for the hemorrhage, the coder would access the Table of Drugs and Chemicals and locate the entry for "Coumadin" or "anticoagulants." Because Coumadin is a therapeutic agent, the adverse effect of the drug causing the hemorrhage would be coded with an External Cause code (E Code) of E934.2 to identify that the therapeutic use of this drug caused the problem. If a patient takes more anticoagulant than was prescribed and it results in bleeding, then the condition would be reported as an accidental poisoning rather than an adverse effect of a medication. Poisonings are in chapter 20 in this textbook.

A code from category 286.5, Hemorrhagic disorder due to intrinsic circulating anticoagulants, antibodies, or inhibitors, is not assigned for bleeding in a patient taking an anticoagulant drug, and doing so is a common coding error when identifying a hemorrhage caused by an anticoagulant drug that is taken by prescription.

Another condition confused with coagulation defects is prolonged prothrombin time or other abnormal coagulation profiles. This condition is not coded as a coagulation defect. Code 790.92 is assigned to report an abnormal laboratory finding. However, when a patient is receiving Coumadin therapy, it is expected that the patient will have a prolonged bleeding time, and in such a case, code 790.92 is not assigned for expected laboratory findings.

## Purpura and Other Hemorrhagic Conditions

Category 287 includes codes that describe purpura, thrombocytopenia, and other hemorrhagic disorders. Thrombocytopenia is diagnosed when the platelets fall below 150,000 cells per microliter (Melloni 2001). Two types of thrombocytopenia are recognized: primary or idiopathic and secondary. Idiopathic or immune thrombocytopenic purpura (ITP) is an autoimmune disorder with development of antibodies to one's own platelets. In children, the condition often resolves without treatment. In adults, medication such as corticosteroids or thrombopoietins are given. In severe cases, the spleen may be removed to eliminate the platelet destruction by phagocytosis. Primary thrombocytopenia may also be congenital or hereditary. Primary thrombocytopenia is classified in ICD-9-CM to 287.30–287.39 depending on the type.

Secondary thrombocytopenia is a complication of another disease. Causes may include viral or bacterial infections, systemic lupus erythematosus, chronic lymphocytic leukemia, sarcoidosis, or carcinoma of the ovary. Drugs such as chemotherapy, heparin, and rifampin can cause the condition. It is also a common, temporary complication of bone marrow transplant. The treatment of the secondary form of this condition centers on treating the underlying disease or changing medication. If bleeding is severe, a person is given transfusions of platelets to replace those destroyed. ICD-9-CM classifies secondary thrombocytopenia to codes 287.41 or 287.49. Posttransfusion purpura (PTP) is coded to 287.41. This condition is characterized by a sudden and severe thrombocytopenia (a platelet count of less than 10,000), usually occurring 5 to 10 days following transfusions of whole blood, plasma, platelets, or RBCs. PTP is a reaction associated with the presence of antibodies directed against the Human Platelet Antigen (HPA) system. Other forms of secondary thrombocytopenia are coded to 287.49 and may be due—among other causes—to drugs, extracorporeal circulation of blood during open heart or other procedures, or due to massive blood transfusions.

## Diseases of the White Blood Cells

Category 288 classifies diseases of the WBCs, with the fourth and fifth digits identifying the specific type of disorder. Two types of WBCs circulate in the body: granular and nongranular (agranular) leukocytes. Granular leukocytes include neutrophils, eosinophils, and basophils. Nongranular leukocytes include lymphocytes and monocytes. Agranulocytosis (now more commonly called neutropenia) is an acute condition characterized by the absence of neutrophils and an extremely low granulocyte count. The most common cause is drug toxicity or hypersensitivity caused by large doses of drugs and/or drugs taken over a long period of time. Neutropenia commonly occurs in patients receiving chemotherapy. ICD-9-CM classifies neutropenia to subcategory 288.0 with fifth digit codes for the various specific forms of neutropenia. Codes in the range of 288.50–288.59 describe decreased WBC counts. Codes in the range of 288.60–288.69 describe elevated WBC counts, including leukemoid reaction, monocytosis, basophilia, and bandemia.

Bandemia is defined as the presence of an excess number of immature WBCs or band cells, while the total WBC count is normal. Bandemia is frequently present in patients with bacterial infections. However, bandemia may be identified when a diagnosis of infection has not been established. Pediatricians frequently use this diagnosis in children when the source of an infection is unknown. ICD-9-CM specifically identifies bandemia with code 288.66.

## Other Blood and Blood-Forming Organ Diseases

The last category in Chapter 4 of ICD-9-CM (category 289) includes conditions not classified elsewhere, including familial and secondary polycythemia, chronic lymphadenitis, hypersplenism, chronic congestive splenomegaly, and methemoglobinemia. It also includes myelofibrosis, a chronic progressive disease in which fibrous tissue replaces normal bone marrow. A progressive anemia results even though the spleen attempts to replace the lost blood production and splenomegaly can occur. Myelofibrosis can be a primary hematologic disease or a secondary process. Code 238.76, Myelofibrosis with myeloid metaplasia is the primary form of the disease. Code 289.83 is used to code the unspecified form or the secondary form of myelofibrosis.

Secondary polycythemia occurs as a result of tissue hypoxia and is associated with chronic obstructive pulmonary disease, congenital heart disease, and prolonged exposures to high altitudes (higher than 10,000 feet). ICD-9-CM classifies secondary polycythemia to code 289.0.

Heparin-induced thrombocytopenia (HIT) is a life-threatening clinical event that can occur in 3 to 5 percent of all patients receiving unfractionated heparin for at least five days or in about 0.5 percent of patients receiving low molecular-weight heparin. HIT is a hypercoagulable state, not a hemorrhagic condition. The diagnosis is first suspected based on a fall in the platelet count by 50 percent or more occurring five to twelve days after beginning heparin therapy. Treatment involves the initiation of an alternative anticoagulant or direct thrombin inhibitor drugs.

## ICD-9-CM Review Exercises: Chapter 7

Assign ICD-9-CM codes to the following (morphology codes are not necessary):

1. Sickle cell (Hb-SS) disease with crisis

2. Iron deficiency anemia secondary to blood loss

3. Neutropenic fever

4. Fanconi's anemia

5. Congenital nonspherocytic hemolytic anemia

6. Idiopathic thrombocytopenic purpura

7. Toxic neutropenia

8. Von Willebrand's disease

9. Microangiopathic hemolytic anemia

10. Chemotherapy-induced anemia secondary to antineoplastic medication for breast cancer (currently being treated)

## ICD-9-CM Review Exercises: Chapter 7 (Continued)

11. Disseminated intravascular coagulation

12. Chronic congestive splenomegaly

13. Acquired hemolytic anemia due to AIDS

14. Chronic mesenteric lymphadenitis with biopsy of lymphatic structure

15. Cooley's anemia; splenectomy

16. Polycythemia secondary to living in a high-altitude region

17. Glucose-6-phosphate dehydrogenase (G-6-PD) anemia

18. Goat's milk anemia

19. Deficiency of factor I

20. Gross hematuria, identified as a result of the patient's Coumadin therapy, properly administered

21. Acute hemorrhaging duodenal ulcer with acute blood loss anemia

22. Sickle cell thalassemia with crisis

23. Pure red cell aplasia

24. Anemia in end-stage renal disease; ESRD

25. Heparin-induced thrombocytopenia

# ICD-10-CM Chapter 3, Diseases of the Blood and Blood-Forming Organs and Certain Disorders Involving the Immune Mechanism (D50–D89)

Coding professionals will find the organizational structure of ICD-10-CM's Chapter 3 an improvement over ICD-9-CM's Chapter 4, Diseases of the Blood and Blood-Forming Organs. Diseases and disorders have been grouped into subchapters or blocks making it easier to identify the type of conditions classified to ICD-10-CM Chapter 3. Modifications have also been made to specific categories that bring the terminology up to date with current medical practice. Other enhancements to Chapter 3 include classification changes that provide greater specificity than found in ICD-9-CM.

## Coding Overview for ICD-10-CM, Chapter 3

Chapter 3 of ICD-10-CM includes codes primarily from ICD-9-CM Chapter 4, Diseases of the Blood and Blood-Forming Organs, but also includes many codes from ICD-9-CM Chapter 3, Endocrine, Nutritional and Metabolic Diseases and Immunity Disorders. It also includes some codes from ICD-9-CM Chapter 1, Infectious and Parasitic Diseases (for example, sarcoidosis).

Similar to ICD-9-CM, ICD-10-CM contains codes for nutritional anemias, hemolytic anemias, and aplastic and other acquired anemias. Purpura, coagulation defects, and other disorders of blood and blood-forming organs are also included. Intraoperative and postprocedural complication codes are found within the body system chapters with codes specific to the organs and structures of that body system. However, Chapter 3 of ICD-10-CM also contains a new feature.

Category D78, Intraoperative and postprocedural complications of the spleen, includes codes for intraoperative hemorrhage and hematoma of the spleen, accidental puncture and laceration of the spleen, and postprocedural hemorrhage and hematoma of the spleen. These combination codes identify the specific complication and whether the complication occurred during a procedure on the spleen or the complication occurred during another surgical procedure. Two codes, D78.81 and D78.89, are available to identify another specified type of complication of the spleen beyond the codes in the range of D78.01–D78.22. An additional code is used to further identify what the complication was.

## Organization and Structure of ICD-10-CM Chapter 3

Chapter 3 of ICD-10-CM includes categories D50–D89 arranged in the following blocks:

| | |
|---|---|
| D50–D53 | Nutritional anemias |
| D55–D59 | Hemolytic anemias |
| D60–D64 | Aplastic and other anemias and other bone marrow failure syndromes |
| D65–D69 | Coagulation defects, purpura and other hemorrhagic conditions |
| D70–D77 | Other disorders of blood and blood-forming organs |
| D78 | Intraoperative and postprocedural complications of spleen |
| D80–D89 | Certain disorders involving the immune mechanism |

Codes in Chapter 7 have been expanded to allow the coding of specific forms of diseases of blood and blood-forming organs.

**EXAMPLE:** ICD-9-CM 281.2 Folate-deficiency anemia
In comparison in ICD-10-CM, there are four codes to describe different types of folate deficiency anemias.

ICD-10-CM D52 Folate deficiency anemia
D52.0, Dietary folate deficiency anemia
D52.1, Drug-induced folate deficiency anemia
Use additional code for adverse effect if applicable to identify the drug (T36-T50 with fifth or sixth character 5)
D52.8, Other folate deficiency anemias
D52.9, Folate deficiency anemia, unspecified

The last block in this chapter (D80–D89) groups disorders involving the immune mechanism. The immunodeficiency disorders have been reclassified from Chapter 4, Endocrine, Nutritional and Metabolic Diseases, and Immunity Disorders in ICD-9-CM to Chapter 3 in ICD-10-CM.

## Coding Guidelines and Instructional Notes for ICD-10-CM Chapter 3

At the time of this publication, there were no official ICD-10-CM official coding guidelines for Chapter 3, Diseases of the Blood and Blood-Forming Organs and Certain Disorders Involving the Immune Mechanism.

## Instructional Notes

In ICD-10-CM Chapter 3, there are several codes with a note that states to "use additional code" for adverse effects, if applicable, to identify drug (T36–T50) with fifth or sixth character 5.

**EXAMPLES:** **D52.1** **Drug-induced folate deficiency anemia**
Use additional code for adverse effect, if applicable, to identify drug (T36–T50 with fifth or sixth character 5)

**D59.0** **Drug-induced autoimmune hemolytic anemia**
Use additional code for adverse effect, if applicable, to identify drug (T36–T50 with fifth or sixth character 5)

**D61.1** **Drug-induced aplastic anemia**
Use additional code for adverse effect, if applicable, to identify drug (T36–T50 with fifth or sixth character 5)

Another instructional note found in this chapter is "Code first, if applicable, toxic effects of substances chiefly nonmedicinal as to source (T51–T59)."

**EXAMPLE:** **D61.2** **Aplastic anemia due to other external agents**
Code first, if applicable, toxic effects of substances chiefly nonmedicinal as to source (T51–T65)

Similarly, two instructional notes appears with a code as the type of anemia is produced by either a poisoning or an adverse effect of a drug. The following type of anemia is produced by either a poisoning or an adverse effect of a drug.

**EXAMPLE:** **D64.2** **Secondary sideroblastic anemia due to drugs and toxins**

Code first poisoning due to drug or toxin, if applicable (T36–T65 with fifth or sixth character 1–4, 6)
Use additional code for adverse effect, if applicable, to identify drug (T36-T50 with fifth or sixth character 5)

Other instructional notes apply to the entire category of codes or an individual code to use additional codes for associated conditions.

**EXAMPLES:** **D56.0** **Acute thalassemia**

Use additional code, if applicable, for hydrops fetalis due to alpha thalassemia (P56.99)

**D57** **Sickle-cell disorders**

Use additional code for any associated fever (R50.81)

**D59.3** **Hemolytic-uremic syndromes**

Use additional code to identify associated:
E. coli infection (B96.2-)
Pneumococcal pneumonia (J13)
Shigella dysenteriae (A03.9)

**D70** **Neutropenia**

Use additional code for any associated:
Fever (R50.81)
Mucositis (J34.81, K12.3-, K92.81, N76.81)

Instructions to "Code first" or "Code also" the underlying disease are also included in Chapter 3.

**EXAMPLE:** **D61.82** **Myelophthisis**

Code also the underlying disorder, such as:
Malignant neoplasm of breast (C50.-)
Tuberculosis (A15.-)

**EXAMPLE:** **D63.0** **Anemia in neoplastic disease**

Code first neoplasm (C00–D49)

**EXAMPLE:** **D63.1** **Anemia in chronic kidney disease**

Code first underlying chronic kidney disease (CKD) (N18.-)

Another instruction recognizes external causes can produce a blood disorder.

**EXAMPLE:** **D59.6** **Hemoglobinuria due to hemolysis from other external causes**

Use additional code (Chapter 20) to identify external cause

Certain blood disorders and disorders involving the immune mechanism are related to underlying diseases as well as influences of drugs and toxins. In addition, a blood disorder can produce other conditions or manifestations.

**EXAMPLE:** **D70.1 Agranulocytosis secondary to cancer chemotherapy**

Use additional code for adverse effect, if applicable, to identify drug (T45.1X5)
Code also underlying neoplasm

**D89.81 Graft-versus-host disease**

Code first underlying cause, such as:
Complications of transplanted organs and tissue (T86.-)
Complications of blood transfusion (T80.89)
Use additional codes to identify associated manifestations, such as:
Desquamative dermatitis (L30.8)
Diarrhea (R19.7)
Elevated bilirubin (R17)
Hair loss (L65.9)

At least one blood disorder in Chapter 3 of ICD-10-CM has at least three instructional codes, such as this example:

**EXAMPLE:** **D75.81 Myelofibrosis**

Code first the underlying disorder, such as L
Malignant neoplasm of breast (C50.-)
Use additional code, if applicable, for associated therapy-related myelodysplastic syndrome (D46.-)
Use additional code for adverse effect, if applicable, to identify drug (T45.1X5)

## Coding Guidelines

There are coding guidelines, I.C.2.c.1, in ICD-10-CM Chapter 2, Neoplasms for anemia associated with malignancy. When the admission or encounter is for management of an anemia associated with the malignancy, and the treatment is only for anemia, the appropriate code for the *malignancy* is sequenced as the principal or first listed diagnosis followed by the appropriate code for the anemia (such as code D63.0, Anemia in neoplastic disease).

There are directions provided in the guidelines for anemia associated with chemotherapy, immunotherapy, and radiation therapy. For example, when the patient is seen for management of anemia associated with an adverse effect of the administration of chemotherapy or immunotherapy and the only treatment is for the anemia, the following should be coded:

1. The type of anemia treated and sequenced first
2. The neoplasm being treated with chemo- or immunotherapy
3. The adverse effect (T45.1X5) of antineoplastic and immunosuppressive drugs

Another example is when the patient is seen for management of anemia associated with an adverse effect of radiation, the following should be coded:

1. The type of anemia treated and sequenced first
2. The neoplasm being treated with radiation therapy
3. Y84.2, Radiological procedure and radiotherapy as the cause of abnormal reaction of the patient, or of later complication, without mention of misadventure at the time of the procedure

## ICD-10-CM Review Exercises: Chapter 7

Assign the correct ICD-10-CM diagnosis codes to the following exercises

1. A patient receives a blood transfusion for severe anemia due to her left breast carcinoma

2. Sickle-cell crisis with acute chest syndrome

3. Congenital red cell aplastic anemia

4. Thalassemia, minor

5. Periodic neutropenia

6. Severe combined immunodeficiency [SCID] with low T- and B- cell numbers

7. Anemia due to chemotherapy for colon carcinoma

8. Acute hemorrhagic anemia

9. Leukocytosis

10. Idiopathic thrombocytopenic purpura

# Chapter 8

# Mental, Behavioral and Neurodevelopmental Disorders

## Learning Objectives

At the conclusion of this chapter, you should be able to:

1. Describe the organization of the conditions and codes included in Chapter 5 of ICD-9-CM, Mental, Behavioral and Neurodevelopmental Disorders (290–319)
2. Describe the organization of the conditions and codes included in Chapter 5 of ICD-10-CM, Mental, Behavioral and Neurodevelopmental Disorders (F01–F99)
3. Describe the *DSM-5* and explain its purposes
4. Describe the multiple coding rules related to the coding of mental disorders
5. Review the inclusion and exclusion notes for the classification of mental disorders
6. Define and differentiate between the terms *alcoholism, alcohol abuse,* and *alcohol use*
7. Define and differentiate between the terms *drug dependence, drug abuse,* and *drug use*
8. Describe the ICD-9-CM coding guidelines for the selection of principal diagnosis for patient admitted for alcohol or drug dependence treatment
9. Describe the ICD-10-CM coding guidelines for pain disorders and mental and behavioral disorders due to psychoactive substance use.
10. Define the terms *detoxification* and *rehabilitation* as related to alcohol and drug dependence treatment
11. Assign ICD-9-CM diagnosis and procedure codes for mental, behavioral, and neurodevelopmental disorders
12. Assign ICD-10-CM codes for mental and behavioral disorders

# ICD-9-CM Chapter 5, Mental, Behavioral and Neurodevelopmental Disorders (290–319)

Chapter 5, Mental, Behavioral and Neurodevelopmental Disorders, in the Tabular List in volume 1 of ICD-9-CM classifies mental disorders into the following categories and section titles:

| Categories | Section Titles |
|---|---|
| 290–299 | Psychoses |
| 300–316 | Neurotic Disorders, Personality Disorders, and Other Nonpsychotic Mental Disorders |
| 317–319 | Intellectual Disabilities |

The codes in Chapter 5 are compatible with those included in the *Diagnostic and Statistical Manual of Mental Disorders, Fifth Edition, (DSM-5),* published by the American Psychiatric Association (APA). The DMS-5 book contains dual codes for every psychiatric diagnosis to account for the currently used ICD-9-CM diagnosis codes as well as new ICD-10-CM codes. The ICD-9-CM and ICD-10-CM codes are included in parentheses within the diagnostic criteria box for each disorder. The inclusions of ICD codes in the DSM-5 code book allows the physician or practitioner to assign valid ICD-9-CM codes now and ICD-10-CM codes in the future for insurance purposes. DSM-5 codes are not usually submitted on billing claim forms unless required by a specific payer (APA 2013).

## Updating of Code Descriptions

Effective October 1, 2004, numerous substantial changes were made to the titles of category and subcategory codes within Chapter 5 of ICD-9-CM. Although the diagnostic codes used in the DSM-5 classification system have been taken from ICD-9-CM and ICD-10-CM, the diagnostic terminology has evolved over several revisions of the DSM-5 in order to keep up with current clinical usage. In contrast, the terminology used in ICD-9-CM has not changed much since the introduction of ICD-9-CM in the late 1970s. APA has worked closely with the National Center for Health Statistics (NCHS) over the years to ensure a seamless crosswalk between the two systems so that coders can easily determine the ICD-9-CM diagnosis codes that correspond to the DSM diagnoses. APA continually examines the relationship between the codes in DSM-5 and the ICD-9-CM and ICD-10-CM codes. A substantial number of changes and refinements to DSM-5 in 2014 were based on the ICD-10-CM edition to be implemented October 1, 2015. APA also continues to present diagnoses that are new to DSM-5 to the Cooperating Parties for review and inclusion in the ICD-10-CM system, most likely after the October 1, 2015 compliance date.

## Multiple Coding

When coding mental disorders, instructional notations to assign additional codes to fully describe the patient's condition are frequently encountered. Examples of three such instructional notations follow:

- Instructional note to assign an additional code to identify any associated neurological disorder.

**EXAMPLE:** **299.1 Childhood disintegrative disorder**
Heller's syndrome

Use additional code to identify any associated neurological disorder.

- Instructional note to assign an additional code to identify any associated mental disorder, as well as physical condition.

**EXAMPLE:** **301 Personality disorders**
Includes: character neurosis

Use additional code to identify any associated neurosis or psychosis, or physical condition.

- Instructional note to assign a specific code for the presence of another condition (for example, cerebral atherosclerosis).

**EXAMPLE:** **290.4 Vascular dementia**
Multi-infarct dementia or psychosis

Use additional code to identify cerebral atherosclerosis (437.0).

## Fifth-Digit Subclassification

The use of fifth digits occurs quite frequently in the chapter on mental disorders of ICD-9-CM. Although this specificity exists in the classification system, documentation in the health record often does not provide the information required to assign a specific fifth digit. The fifth digit for unspecified course of illness is assigned when further information is unavailable. Never assume the course of illness from general statements made in the health record.

### Exercise 8.1

Assign ICD-9-CM codes to the following:

1. Latent schizophrenia, chronic

2. Continuous cocaine dependence

3. Epileptic psychosis with generalized grand mal epilepsy

4. Acute senile dementia in Alzheimer's disease

5. Autistic disorder, active

## Inclusion and Exclusion Notes

Chapter 5 of ICD-9-CM contains many special inclusion notes, such as those in the following two examples:

**EXAMPLE:** **295 Schizophrenic disorders**

Includes: schizophrenia of the types described in 295.0–295.9 occurring in children

The preceding inclusion note says that codes 295.0–295.9 may be assigned in the pediatric population, if applicable.

**EXAMPLE:** **298 Other nonorganic psychoses**

Includes: psychotic conditions due to or provoked by:
emotional stress
environmental factors as major part of etiology

The preceding inclusion note serves to advise that psychotic conditions due to or provoked by emotional stress (for example, divorce) or environmental factors (for example, a forest fire) are assigned to category 298.

Exclusion notes also are used frequently in Chapter 5 to warn that specified forms of a condition are classified elsewhere, such as:

**290.0 Senile dementia, uncomplicated**
Senile dementia:
NOS
simple type

*Excludes:* *mild memory disturbances, not amounting to dementia, associated with senile brain disease (310.89)*
*senile dementia with:*
*delirium or confusion (290.3)*
*delusional [paranoid] features (290.20)*
*depressive features (290.21)*

The preceding exclusion note advises that mild memory disturbances associated with senile brain disease and senile dementia with specific features—such as confusion, paranoia, or depression—are classified elsewhere.

294.10 **Dementia in conditions classified elsewhere without behavioral disturbance**
Dementia in conditions classified elsewhere NOS
294.11 **Dementia in conditions classified elsewhere with behavioral disturbance**
Aggressive behavior
Combative behavior
Violent behavior

Use additional code, where applicable, to identify:
wandering in conditions classified elsewhere (V40.31)

Coders should pay special attention to inclusion and exclusion notes in the previous example regarding the treatment and long-term care of patients with dementia affected by the behavioral aspect of the dementia. Patients who are aggressive and combative pose a greater treatment dilemma. Subcategory code 294.1 was expanded to distinguish with and without behavioral disturbance. An inclusion note was added to 294.11 to list those conditions considered to be behavioral disturbances.

## Alcoholism and Alcohol Abuse

Alcoholism (alcohol dependence) is a chronic condition in which a patient has become dependent on alcohol with increased tolerance and is unable to stop using it, even while facing strong incentives such as impairment of health, deteriorated social interactions, and interference with job performance. Such patients often experience physical signs of withdrawal during any sudden cessation of drinking.

Alcoholism is classified to category 303, Alcohol dependence syndrome. The fourth digits identify a state of acute intoxication (303.0) or other and unspecified forms, including chronic forms (303.9). The fifth digits identify the stage of the alcoholism—unspecified, continuous, episodic, or in remission. An additional code should be assigned to identify any of the following associated conditions:

Alcoholic psychosis (291.0–291.9)
Drug dependence (304.0–304.9)
Physical complications of alcohol, such as:
  Cerebral degeneration (331.7)
  Alcoholic cirrhosis of the liver (571.2)
  Epilepsy or recurrent seizures (345.00–345.90)
  Alcoholic gastritis (535.30–535.31)
  Acute alcoholic hepatitis (571.1)
  Alcoholic liver damage (571.3)

Reported with code 305.0x, alcohol abuse is described as problem drinking and includes those patients who drink to excess but have not reached a stage of physical dependency. The fifth digit (shown as x in the previous sentence) again identifies the stage of the condition (unspecified, continuous, episodic, or in remission); for example: 305.01, Alcohol abuse, continuous.

**A point to remember:** The excludes note appearing below subcategory 305.0 indicates that a diagnosis of acute alcohol intoxication in a patient with alcoholism is reported with code 303.0x (*Coding Clinic* 2nd Quarter, 1991, 11). This note emphasizes the important fact that a patient who has alcoholism or alcohol dependence and can be identified with codes in the range of 303.00–303.03, which identifies the patient as also being acutely intoxicated at the particular time of the healthcare encounter. Specifically a code in the range of 305.00–305.03 and category 303 codes are never used together. The patient is either dependent on alcohol (category 303) or is not dependent on alcohol but uses it to excess or abuse (codes 305.00–305.03).

## Drug Dependence and Abuse

Drug dependence or drug addiction is a chronic mental and physical condition related to the patient's pattern of taking a drug or a combination of drugs. It is characterized by behavioral and physiological responses such as a compulsion to take the drug, to experience its psychic effects, or to avoid the discomfort of its absence. There is increased tolerance and an inability to stop the use of the drug, even with strong incentives.

Category 304 of ICD-9-CM classifies drug addiction. The fourth digit identifies the specific drug or class of drug involved. The fifth digit identifies the stage of the dependence—unspecified, continuous, episodic, or in remission. When several drugs are involved in the drug addiction, ICD-9-CM provides the following codes for use: 304.7x, Combination drugs including an opioid drug, and 304.8x, Combination drugs not including an opioid drug.

Nondependent drug abuse represents problem drug taking and includes those patients who take drugs to excess but have not yet reached a state of dependence. Included in category 305, Nondependent abuse of drugs, is the abuse of alcohol, tobacco, and other prescription and non-prescription, as well as illegal, drugs. Codes 305.00–305.03 describe "alcohol abuse" but not dependence. Also included in this category is the current use of tobacco (products) classified to code 305.1, tobacco use disorder. A patient with a history of smoking would be classified with code V15.82, history of tobacco use. ICD-9-CM classifies nondependent use of drugs, such as cannabis, hallucinogens, sedatives, opiates, cocaine, and others to codes 305.2x through 305.9x. The fourth digit identifies the specific class of drug, and the fifth digit indicates the stage of the abuse (*Coding Clinic* 1991).

## Fifth Digits for Alcohol/Drug Dependence and Abuse

The following information is provided to explain the intent of the appropriate fifth digit for categories 303, 304, and 305 (with the exception of 305.1). As always, the documentation in the health record should serve as the final determination for the code selected. The provider must specifically document the pattern of use.

| | | |
|---|---|---|
| 0 | Unspecified | Inadequate documentation in the health record |
| 1 | Continuous | Alcohol: Refers to daily intake of large amounts of alcohol or regular heavy drinking on weekends or days off from work<br>Drugs: Daily or almost daily use of drug(s) |
| 2 | Episodic | Alcohol: Refers to alcoholic binges lasting weeks or months, followed by long periods of sobriety<br>Drugs: Indicates short periods between drug use or use on the weekends |
| 3 | Remission | Refers to either a complete cessation of alcohol or drug intake or the period during which a decrease toward cessation is taking place (*Coding Clinic* 1991) |

## Principal Diagnosis Selection for Patients Admitted for Alcohol or Drug Dependence Treatment

The circumstances of admission for patients with alcohol and/or drug dependence and associated mental disorders govern the selection of the principal diagnosis. This is in keeping with the Uniform Hospital Discharge Data Set (UHDDS) definition of principal diagnosis as "the condition established after study to be chiefly responsible for occasioning the admission of the patient to the hospital for care." (UHDDS 1985, 31038–31040)

The following guidelines will help coders determine the appropriate principal diagnosis:

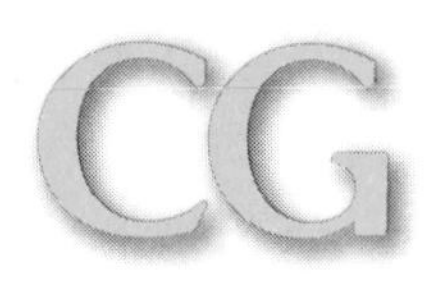


- If the patient is admitted in withdrawal or if withdrawal develops after admission, the withdrawal code is designated as the principal diagnosis. Categories 291 and 292 include codes that describe withdrawal symptoms. The code for the substance abuse/dependence is listed second; for example, 292.0, Drug withdrawal, and 304.01, Opioid-type dependence, continuous.
- If the patient is admitted with a diagnosis of a substance-related mental condition, such as alcoholic dementia, the principal diagnosis is the mental condition, followed by a code for alcohol/drug dependence or

abuse; for example, 291.2, Alcohol-induced persisting dementia, and 303.91, Chronic alcoholism, continuous.

- If the patient is admitted for detoxification or rehabilitation or both, and no related mental condition is documented, the principal diagnosis is the code describing the alcohol and/or drug abuse/dependence; for example, 304.22, Cocaine dependence, episodic.
- If the patient is admitted with an unrelated condition and has a diagnosis of alcohol and/or drug dependence/abuse, the unrelated condition is the principal diagnosis. The code for substance abuse/dependence is listed second; for example, 038.0, Streptococcal septicemia, and 303.90, Chronic alcoholism, unspecified.
- If the patient is admitted for treatment or evaluation of a physical complaint related to alcohol and/or drug abuse/dependence, the physical condition is the principal diagnosis, followed by the code for the alcohol and/or drug abuse/dependence (*Coding Clinic* 1991); for example, 535.30, Alcoholic gastritis, without mention of hemorrhage, and 303.91, Chronic alcoholism, continuous.

## Therapy for Alcohol or Drug Dependence

Therapies for patients with diagnoses of substance abuse or dependence consist of detoxification, rehabilitation, or both.

### Detoxification

Detoxification is the active management of withdrawal symptoms in a patient who is physically dependent on alcohol and/or drugs. Treatment includes evaluation, observation, and monitoring, as well as administration of thiamine and multivitamins for nutrition and other medications, such as methadone, clonidine, long-acting barbiturates, benzodiazepines, and carbamazepine.

### Rehabilitation

Rehabilitation is a structured program that results in controlling the alcohol or drug use and in replacing alcohol or drug dependence with activities that are nonchemical in nature. Modalities may include methadone maintenance (for opiate dependence), therapeutic communities (residential), and long-term outpatient drug- or alcohol-free treatments.

### Coding Therapies for Alcohol and Drug Dependence

The codes for therapies for alcohol and drug dependence are found in the Tabular List in volume 3 of ICD-9-CM.

Therapy for alcohol abuse and dependence is coded as follows:

**94.61 Alcohol rehabilitation**
**94.62 Alcohol detoxification**
**94.63 Alcohol rehabilitation and detoxification**

Therapy for drug abuse and dependence is coded as follows:

**94.64 Drug rehabilitation**
**94.65 Drug detoxification**
**94.66 Drug rehabilitation and detoxification**

Combined therapies for patients with both alcohol and drug dependence are coded as follows:

**94.67 Combined alcohol and drug rehabilitation**
**94.68 Combined alcohol and drug detoxification**
**94.69 Combined alcohol and drug rehabilitation and detoxification**

It may happen that a patient receives detoxification for either drug or alcohol dependence and rehabilitation for both alcohol and drug dependence. This would be coded as 94.62 for alcohol detoxification or 94.65 for drug detoxification, and 94.67 for combined alcohol and drug rehabilitation (*Coding Clinic,* 2nd Quarter 1991).

## ICD-9-CM Review Exercises: Chapter 8

Assign ICD-9-CM codes to the following:

1. Panic attacks

2. Acute exacerbation of chronic undifferentiated schizophrenia

3. Reactive depressive psychosis due to death of child

4. Dissociative fugue

5. Drug withdrawal; diazepam dependence, continuous; patient underwent detoxification services

6. Alcoholic gastritis due to chronic alcoholism, episodic

7. Disruptive behavior disorder

## ICD-9-CM Review Exercises: Chapter 8 (Continued)

8. Senile dementia with acute confusional state

9. Hypochondriac with continuous laxative habit

10. Anxiety reaction manifested by fainting

11. Attention deficit disorder with hyperactivity (ADDH)

12. Alcohol dependence syndrome in remission, resulting in cirrhosis of liver

13. Cerebral arteriosclerotic vascular dementia

14. Bipolar II disease

15. Psychogenic mucous colitis

16. Acute alcoholic intoxication in a patient with chronic alcoholism

17. Addiction to crack cocaine, continuous form

18. Excessive drinking (15-year-old teen)

19. Alzheimer's dementia with behavioral disturbances

20. Anxiety in an acute stress reaction

# ICD-10-CM Chapter 5, Mental, Behavioral and Neurodevelopmental Disorders (F01–F99)

## Organization and Structure of ICD-10-CM Chapter 5

Chapter 5 contains more subchapters, categories, subcategories, and codes than ICD-9-CM. Rather than grouping by psychotic, nonpsychotic disorders, or intellectual disabilities as in ICD-9-CM, ICD-10-CM organizes mental and behavioral disorders in the following blocks:

| | |
|---|---|
| F01–F09 | Mental disorders due to known physiological conditions |
| F10–F19 | Mental and behavioral disorders due to psychoactive substance use |
| F20–F29 | Schizophrenia, schizotypal and delusional, and other non-mood psychotic disorders |
| F30–F39 | Mood [affective] disorders |
| F40–F48 | Anxiety, dissociative, stress-related, somatoform and other nonpsychotic mental disorders |
| F50–F59 | Behavioral syndromes associated with physiological disturbances and physical factors |
| F60–F69 | Disorders of adult personality and behavior |
| F70–F79 | Mental retardation |
| F80–F89 | Pervasive and specific developmental disorders |
| F90–F98 | Behavioral and emotional disorders with onset usually occurring in childhood and adolescence |
| F99 | Unspecified mental disorder |

Changes were necessary in many parts of Chapter 5 because of outdated terminology. For example, given what has been discovered in the past 20 years about the effects of nicotine, ICD-10-CM contains a separate category F17 for nicotine dependence with subcategories to identify the specific tobacco product and nicotine-induced disorders. ICD-9-CM has a single code, 305.1, for tobacco use disorder or tobacco dependence.

### *DSM-5*

The codes in Chapter 5 of ICD-10-CM parallel the codes in *The Diagnostic and Statistical Manual of Mental Disorders, Fifth Edition, (DSM-5.)* Because the DSM-5 diagnostic codes are limited to codes in the ICD system, new DSM-5 disorders are assigned to the best available ICD codes. The names connected with the ICD codes sometimes do not match the DSM-5 name. APA continues to work with the NCHS and the Centers for Medicare and Medicaid Services to include the new DSM-5 terms in ICD-10-CM. The APA website provides resources for the reader interested in learning more about the DSM-5 classification for mental disorders (www.psych.org and www.dsm5.org).

*DSM-5* provides clear descriptions of diagnostic categories that allow clinicians and investigators to diagnose, communicate about, study, and treat people with various mental disorders. Definitions of mental disorders classified in Chapter 5 of ICD-9-CM and Chapter 5 of ICD-10-CM can be found in the DSM-5. Keep in mind that coders must assign diagnosis codes based on medical record documentation by a provider who is legally qualified to render a medical diagnosis. DSM-5 uses the codes within ICD-9-CM and ICD-10-CM for all mental disorders, including personality disorders and intellectual disabilities, but the ICD system does not contain the detailed descriptions of how to diagnose these conditions as used by the psychiatrists and mental health practitioners. The DMS-5 book contains dual codes for every psychiatric diagnosis to account for the currently used ICD-9-CM diagnosis codes as well as new ICD-10-CM codes. The ICD-9-CM and ICD-10-CM codes are included in parentheses within the diagnostic criteria box for each disorder. The inclusion of ICD codes in the DSM-5 code book allows the physician or practitioner to assign valid ICD-9-CM codes now and ICD-10-CM codes in the future for insurance purposes. DSM-5 codes are not usually submitted on billing claim forms unless required by a specific payer (American Psychiatric Association 2013).

## Coding Guidelines and Instructional Notes for Chapter 5

There are changes to a number of instructional notes in ICD-10-CM Chapter 5. There is a change in sequencing involving the intellectual disabilities codes (F70–F79). In ICD-9-CM, an additional code for any associated psychiatric or physical condition(s) should be sequenced after the intellectual disabilities code. In ICD-10-CM, any associated physical or developmental disorder should be coded first. In ICD-10-CM, beneath code F54, there is a note that states to "code first" the associated physical disorder.

The NCHS has published chapter-specific guidelines for Chapter 5 in the *ICD-10-CM Official Guidelines for Coding and Reporting* (contained in Appendix I of the website accompanying this text):

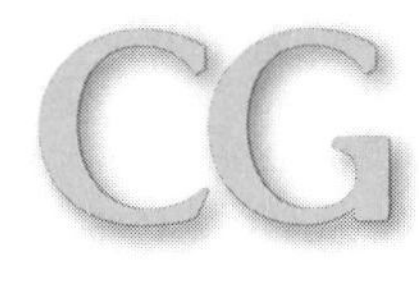

- Guideline I.C.5.a. Pain disorders related to psychological factors
    - There are two codes for pain disorders related to psychological factors. Assign code F45.41 for pain disorders exclusively psychological. There is an Excludes1 note under category G89, Pain, not elsewhere classified that indicates a code from G89 is not to be used with code F45.41. Another code is F45.42, pain disorder with related psychological factors. This code should be used following the appropriate code from category G89 for acute or chronic pain if there is documentation of a psychological component for a patient with acute or chronic pain.
- Guidelines I.C.5.b. Mental and behavioral disorders due to psychoactive substance use
    - The coding of conditions described as "in remission" is done only when documented by the responsible physician or practitioner. There are codes for "in remission" that appear in categories F10–F19, mental and behavioral disorders due to psychoactive substance use (categories F10–F19 with -.21).
    - The coding of these disorders is based on the provider documentation. Unfortunately multiple practitioners treating the patient may use the terminology of use,

(*Continued*)

(*Continued*)

abuse and dependence interchangeably in the record of the patient. When the attending physician or provider refers to the use, abuse and dependence of the same substance (that is, alcohol, opioid, cannabis, and such), only one code should be assigned to identify the pattern of use based on the following hierarchy:

- If both use and abuse of the psychoactive substance are documented, the coder should assign only the code for **abuse**.
- If both abuse and dependence are documented, the coder should assign only the code for **dependence**.
- If use, abuse, and dependence are all documented, the coder should assign only the code for **dependence**.
- If both use and dependence are documented, assign only the code for **dependence**.

- Psychoactive Substance Use
    - As is true for coding all other diagnoses, the codes for psychoactive substance use (F10.9-, F11.9-, F12.9-, F13.9-, F14.9-, F15.9-, F16.9-) should only be assigned based on provider documentation. The codes should only be used when they meet the definition of a reportable diagnosis (see Section III, Reporting Additional Diagnoses.) In addition, the coding guidelines state the codes are to be used only when the psychoactive substance use is associated with a mental or behavioral disorder, and such a relationship is documented by the provider.

## Coding Overview for ICD-10-CM Chapter 5

Chapter 5 of ICD-10-CM, Mental, Behavioral and Neurodevelopmental Disorders (F01–F99), allows for more specific coding of these conditions consistent with the language of behavioral health and substance abuse services as documented in health and client records today. For example, mental and behavioral disorders due to psychoactive substance use (F10–F19) include an extensive number of codes that link the substance involved (alcohol or specific drug) with the specific disorder caused by it. For instance, code F14.280 identifies cocaine dependence with cocaine-induced anxiety disorder. The Alphabetic Index provides access to these codes under the main term "dependence," with the substance and subterms beneath it to identify the behavioral disturbance associated with the substance.

Other categories in this chapter, including schizophrenia, mood disorders, anxiety, dissociative, or other nonpsychotic disorders, allow for more specific reporting of the current episode of illness. Chapter 5 also includes, with updated terminology and specificity, codes for eating disorders, sleep disorders not due to a substance or known physiological condition, impulse disorders, gender identity disorders, as well as specific developmental disorders.

The codes in this chapter include disorders of psychological development, but exclude symptoms, signs, and abnormal clinical laboratory findings (R00–R99). The arrangement of the codes within the various sections of ICD-10-CM is significantly different.

A number of changes to category and subcategory titles have been made. For example, ICD-9-CM subcategory 296.0 is titled "Bipolar I disorder, single manic episode," but the ICD-10-CM counterpart, category F30, is titled "Manic episode."

There are unique codes for alcohol and drug use (not specified as abuse or dependence), and abuse and dependence, so careful review of the documentation is required. And there are changes to the codes for drug and alcohol abuse and dependence as they no longer identify continuous or episodic use. A history of drug or alcohol dependence is coded as "in remission" but the diagnosis of history or in remission requires the provider's clinical judgment and must be specifically documented in the patient's record. Further, there are combination codes for drug and alcohol use and associated conditions, such as withdrawal, sleep disorders, or psychosis. Under the category F10, there is a "use additional code" note for blood alcohol level (Y90.-), if applicable. Blood alcohol level can be indexed in the External Cause of Injuries index.

## ICD-10-CM Review Exercises: Chapter 8

Assign the correct ICD-10-CM diagnosis codes to the following exercises.

1. Alcohol abuse with intoxication

2. Alcohol dependence. The doctor stated the patient also has a history of cocaine dependence but has received drug treatment, and is no longer using cocaine.

3. Patient requesting counseling for dependence on chewing tobacco

4. Patient was brought to the ER and then admitted because of acute alcohol inebriation. Blood alcohol level shows 22 mg/100 ml. The discharge diagnosis is acute and chronic alcoholic, continuous.

5. Borderline personality disorder, specifically described as "cluster B personality disorder." The patient is also a recovering alcoholic, which the provider describes as being "in remission."

6. Dependence on amphetamines

7. Bipolar disorder with current episode of severe depression

8. Anxiety reaction

9. Restricting type anorexia nervosa

10. Postpartum depression

# Chapter 9

# Diseases of the Nervous System and Sense Organs

## Learning Objectives

At the conclusion of this chapter, you should be able to:

1. Describe the organization of the conditions and codes included in Chapter 6 of ICD-9-CM, Diseases of the Nervous System and Sense Organs (320–389)
2. Describe the organization of the conditions and codes included in Chapter 6 of ICD-10-CM, Diseases of the Nervous System (G00–G99)
3. Describe the organization of the conditions and codes included in Chapter 7 of ICD-10-CM, Diseases of the Eye and Adnexa (H00–H59)
4. Describe the organization of the conditions and codes included in Chapter 8 of ICD-10-CM, Diseases of the Ear and Mastoid Process (H60–H95)
5. Describe meningitis, including the circumstances in which two ICD-9-CM codes are required to classify the condition
6. Describe the types of codes ICD-9-CM includes for pain
7. Define the terms *hemiplegia* and *hemiparesis*
8. Define and differentiate between *epilepsy, seizures,* and *convulsions*
9. Describe the different ICD-9-CM codes used to identify epilepsy, seizures, and convulsions
10. Describe different types of headaches, including intractable and chronic headaches, and differentiate among these terms
11. Identify and describe the various types of eye disorders, including retinopathy, glaucoma, and cataract
12. Identify and describe the various types of ear infections, including otitis externa and otitis media
13. Identify and describe the various types of hearing loss
14. Assign ICD-9-CM diagnosis and procedure codes for diseases of the nervous system and sense organs
15. Assign ICD-10-CM codes for diseases of the nervous system and sense organs

# ICD-9-CM Chapter 6, Diseases of the Nervous System and Sense Organs (320–389)

Chapter 6, Diseases of the Nervous System and Sense Organs, in the Tabular List in volume 1 of ICD-9-CM classifies conditions affecting the brain and spinal cord, as well as the peripheral nervous system. In addition, it classifies a variety of eye and adnexal disorders, and diseases of the ear and mastoid process.

Chapter 6 is subdivided into the following categories and section titles:

| Categories | Section Titles |
|---|---|
| 320–326 | Inflammatory Diseases of the Central Nervous System |
| 327 | Organic Sleep Disorders |
| 330–337 | Hereditary and Degenerative Diseases of the Central Nervous System |
| 338 | Pain |
| 339 | Other Headache Syndromes |
| 340–349 | Other Disorders of the Central Nervous System |
| 350–359 | Disorders of the Peripheral Nervous System |
| 360–379 | Disorders of the Eye and Adnexa |
| 380–389 | Diseases of the Ear and Mastoid Process |

## Inflammatory Diseases of the Nervous System (320–326)

This subsection describes how to code for meningitis and the late effects of conditions within the description of inflammatory diseases of the nervous system.

### *Meningitis*

Meningitis is the inflammation of the meninges, which cover the brain and the spinal cord. A variety of microorganisms or viruses can cause meningitis, which is classified in ICD-9-CM in Chapter 6, Diseases of the Nervous System and Sense Organs, and Chapter 1, Infectious and Parasitic Diseases. Because of this particular classification, the instructions provided in the Alphabetic Index to Diseases must be followed to ensure accurate code assignment.

**Meningitis** . . . 322.9
  abacterial NEC *(see also* Meningitis, aseptic) 047.9
  actinomycotic 039.8 *[320.7]*
  adenoviral 049.1
  Aerobacter aerogenes 320.82
    anaerobes (cocci) (gram-negative)
      (gram-positive) (mixed) (NEC) 320.81
  arbovirus NEC 066.9 *[321.2]*
    specified type NEC 066.8 *[321.2]*

Note that in the preceding example two codes are required in some cases, and in other cases, one code is sufficient. However, accurate sequencing of the two codes is essential. The second code listed is in brackets and set in italic type, meaning that this code must always follow the code describing the underlying cause.

### *Category 326, Late Effects of Intracranial Abscess or Pyogenic Infection*

Category 326 is used to identify late effects of conditions classified in categories 320–325. The note under category 326 must be reviewed carefully because some codes in categories 320–325 are excluded. Instructions to "Use additional code to identify condition," such as hydrocephalus or paralysis, also must be reviewed.

**EXAMPLE:** Residual hemiplegia due to late effect of encephalitis

342.90 Hemiplegia, unspecified, affecting unspecified side
326 Late effects of intracranial abscess or pyogenic infection

## Organic Sleep Disorders (327)

The category 327, Organic sleep disorders, includes fourth and fifth digit codes to classify various types of insomnia, hypersomnia, and sleep apnea. Several of the subclassification codes contain the direction "Code first underlying condition." Additional codes for other forms of sleep disturbances (780.50–780.59) are included in Chapter 16, Symptoms, Signs, and Ill-Defined Conditions.

## Hereditary and Degenerative Diseases of the Central Nervous System (330–337)

Categories 330–337 describe hereditary and degenerative diseases of the central nervous system that range in severity from mild to severe.

### *Category 331 Other Cerebral Degeneration*

Acute and chronic forms of cerebral degenerative disease are included in this category, such as Alzheimer's disease, 331.0; Pick's disease, 331.11; Idiopathic normal pressure hydrocephalus, 331.5; Cerebral degeneration in diseases classified elsewhere, 331.7; Reye's syndrome, 331.81; and Dementia with Lewy bodies, 331.82.

Code 331.83 identifies the condition described by physicians as "mild cognitive impairment." This disease entity is defined as an impairment in memory (or any other cognitive domain) that is beyond what is normal for the aging process, with relatively intact function in the other cognitive domains. The patient will first have a memory complaint that is corroborated by other individuals and, for this reason, seek medical evaluation. The diagnosis is used by physicians as the reason for diagnostic testing services.

## Pain, Not Elsewhere Classified (338)

Pain, Not Elsewhere Classified (338) was added to ICD-9-CM to create unique codes for encounters for pain management. A "use additional code" note appears at the top of this category to direct the coder to assign a code for pain associated with psychological factors, as documented by the physician. Excludes notes under this category state that generalized pain is coded to the ICD-9-CM symptoms chapter (780.96), and localized pain should be coded to pain by the site identified. The excludes note also states that a pain disorder exclusively attributed to psychological factors should not be coded with category 338, but instead with code 307.80.

Code 338.0, central pain syndrome, describes the condition that can be caused by damage to the central nervous system by trauma or brain-related disease (for example, cardiovascular accident [CVA], multiple sclerosis, tumors, epilepsy, or Parkinson's disease). The condition may also be described as "thalamic pain syndrome."

Other codes exist for acute pain (338.11–338.19) and chronic pain (338.21–338.29) due to trauma or surgery. There is no timeframe defining when pain becomes chronic. The physician's documentation should be used to guide the use of chronic pain codes.

Neoplasm-related pain may be described with code 338.3 for pain due to the primary or secondary malignancy or tumor. This code is assigned regardless of whether the pain is described as acute or chronic. Code 338.3 can be used as a principal diagnosis or first-listed diagnosis if the reason for the admission or outpatient visit is for pain control or pain management. The underlying neoplasm should be reported as an additional diagnosis code. The neoplasm-related pain code can be reported as an additional diagnosis when the reason for the admission or outpatient visit is management of the neoplasm, and the pain associated with the neoplasm is also documented.

Finally, a single code, 338.4, is provided for the diagnostic statement "chronic pain syndrome," often stated as the reason for ongoing pain management services. The code for chronic pain syndrome should only be used when the physician has specifically documented this condition.

Category 338 codes are acceptable as the principal or first-listed diagnosis codes. Codes from category 338 can be reported with codes that identify the site of the pain, including symptom codes from ICD-9-CM, Chapter 16, if the category 338 code provides additional information. For example, if a code from Chapter 16 identifies the site of the pain but does not describe the pain as acute or chronic, both codes should be assigned.

If the encounter is for pain control or pain management, the code from category 338 is sequenced first, followed by the code for the specific site of the pain or the underlying cause of the pain, if known. For example, a patient with known displacement of lumbar intervertebral disc is seen in the Pain Clinic for management of his acute low back pain secondary to displacement of the lumbar intervertebral disc. For this encounter the acute pain, 338.19, would be listed first with an additional code 722.10 for the underlying condition of the displacement of the lumbar intervertebral disc.

The sequencing of category 338 codes with site-specific pain codes depends on the circumstances of the admission or outpatient visit. When an admission or encounter is for a procedure aimed at treating the underlying condition, a code for the underlying condition should be assigned as the principal or first-listed diagnosis. No code from category 338 should be assigned. For example, a patient with known displacement of lumbar intervertebral disc and chronic back pain due to the displaced disc is admitted for a laminectomy with excision of the herniated intervertebral disc. This patient's principal diagnosis is the displacement of the intervertebral disc, 722.10. The procedure performed is coded as 80.51 from ICD-9-CM, Volume 3. No additional diagnosis code for the chronic back pain is assigned.

When an admission or encounter is for any other reason except pain control or pain management, and a related definitive diagnosis has not been established or confirmed by the provider, the coder should assign the code for the specific site of pain first, followed by the appropriate code from category 338. For example, a patient comes to the physician's office complaining of hip pain that has been present for several months. The physician orders x-rays to be performed and concludes the patient has chronic hip pain of unknown etiology. For this encounter the code for the hip pain, 719.45, is listed as the first code with an additional code for the chronic pain, 338.29.

Codes for postoperative or post-thoracotomy pain are classified to the subcategories of 338.1 or 338.2 depending on whether the pain is acute or chronic. If the postoperative pain is not specified as acute or chronic, the default code is the code for the acute form. Postoperative pain may be a principal or first-listed diagnosis when the reason for the admission or outpatient visit is documented as postoperative pain control or management. Postoperative pain can be reported as a secondary diagnosis code when a patient has outpatient surgery and develops an unusual amount of postoperative pain. Routine or expected postoperative pain immediately after surgery is not coded.

## Other Disorders of the Nervous System (340–349)

The following subsections discuss the categories of other disorders of the nervous system, including paralytic conditions and epilepsy.

### *Categories 342–344, Paralytic Conditions*

Categories 342–344 classify paralytic conditions such as hemiplegia, infantile cerebral palsy, and quadriplegia.

#### Category 342, Hemiplegia and Hemiparesis

The terms *hemiplegia* and *hemiparesis* both refer to the paralysis of one side of the body. Category 342 has fourth-digit subcategories that differentiate between flaccid and spastic hemiplegia. Flaccid refers to the loss of muscle tone in the paralyzed parts with the absence of tendon reflexes, whereas spastic refers to the spasticity of the paralyzed parts with increased tendon reflexes. The 342 codes often are assigned when the health record provides no further information, when the cause of the hemiplegia and hemiparesis is unknown, or as an additional code when the condition results from a specified cause. For example, if a patient has a cerebral infarction and is also treated for hemiplegia resulting from the infarction, a diagnosis code from the 342 category is used in addition to the principal diagnosis code for the cerebral infarction, such as 434.91.

A fifth-digit subclassification is included in category 342 to identify whether the dominant or nondominant side of the body is affected. This type of specificity may not be available in the health record; if not, assign the fifth digit 0.

#### Category 343, Infantile Cerebral Palsy

Infantile cerebral palsy is a nonprogressive, brain-damaging disturbance that originates during the prenatal and perinatal period. It is characterized by persistent, qualitative motor dysfunction, paralysis, and, in severe cases, intellectual disabilities. Fourth-digit subcategories identify the different forms of infantile cerebral palsy.

#### Category 344, Other Paralytic Syndromes

Category 344 includes conditions such as quadriplegia, paraplegia, diplegia, and monoplegia. Also classified in this section are codes for cauda equina syndrome, with or without neurogenic bladder.

### *Category 345, Epilepsy and Recurrent Seizures*

The term *epilepsy* denotes any disorder characterized by recurrent seizures. A seizure is a transient disturbance of cerebral function caused by an abnormal paroxysmal neuronal discharge in the brain.

Physicians often document "recurrent seizure" or "seizure disorder" as well as epilepsy in a health record. Recurrent seizures or seizure disorders are classified in the same category as epilepsy because the terminology is synonymous in medicine. Localization-related epilepsy is the terminology used today for an older term, partial epilepsy.

Other terms used to describe convulsions are not classified to category 345. Such phrases as convulsion or convulsive disorder, convulsive seizures, fits, or recurrent convulsions are not accepted as equivalent to epilepsy or recurrent seizures. Instead the codes for the convulsive conditions are included in code 780.39 within the ICD-9-CM Chapter 16 for symptoms. The term *seizure* and the plural term *seizures* are also coded to the symptom code 780.39 by following the Alphabetic Index carefully. Coders must not use the terms *seizures* and *convulsions* interchangeably. By using the physician's description of the patient's condition and following the Alphabetic Index precisely, different terminology will produce different ICD-9-CM diagnosis codes. Seizures, repetitive seizures, convulsions, recurrent convulsions, repetitive convulsions, epileptiform convulsions, and convulsive disorder are assigned to code 780.39, Other convulsions. Recurrent seizures, epileptic convulsions, and seizure disorder are assigned to category 345, Epilepsy and recurrent seizures.

ICD-9-CM identifies several types of epilepsy, including grand mal and petit mal status. Again, documentation in the health record provides direction as to what code to select. If the health record does not identify a particular form of epilepsy, assign code 345.90, Epilepsy, unspecified, without mention of intractable epilepsy.

Fifth digits are used with category 345 to identify the mention of intractable epilepsy as follows:

**EXAMPLE:** The following fifth-digit subclassification is for use with categories 345.0, 345.1, and 345.4–.9:

**0 without mention of intractable epilepsy**
**1 with intractable epilepsy**

**A point to remember:** The physician must state intractable epilepsy or describe the condition as pharmacoresistant, poorly controlled, refractory or treatment resistent in the health record before the fifth digit 1 can be assigned. Never assume that the epilepsy is intractable based on generalities in the health record.

## Category 339 and Category 346—Headaches

ICD-9-CM provides codes for various types of headaches. Chapter 6, Diseases of the Nervous Systems and Sense Organs, includes codes for migraine, post-procedural, and other forms of headaches. Headaches without a known cause are included in Chapter 16, Signs, Symptoms and Ill-Defined Conditions. The ICD-9-CM chapter for mental disorders includes codes for tension and psychogenic headaches.

Various headache syndromes and tension-type headaches are classified to category 339, Other headache syndromes. Contained within category 339 are cluster headaches and other trigeminal autonomic cephalgias (339.00–339.09), tension-type headaches (339.10–339.12), post-traumatic headaches (339.20–339.22), drug induced headaches, not elsewhere classified (339.3), complicated headache syndromes (339.41–339.44), and other headache syndromes (339.81–339.89).

The classification of migraine headaches has long been reported with category codes 346, Migraine. Many types of migraine headaches can be identified with specific codes in subcategories for migraine with aura, migraine without aura, hemiplegic migraine, menstrual migraine, persistent migraine aura with and without cerebral infarction, chronic migraine, and other forms of migraine. Category 346 requires the use of the following fifth digit subclassification:

0 without mention of intractable migraine without mention of status migrainosus
without mention of refractory migraine without mention of status migrainosus
1 with intractable migraine, so stated, without mention of status migrainosus
with refractory migraine, so stated, without mention of status migrainosus
2 without mention of intractable migraine with status migrainosus
without mention of refractory migraine with status migrainosus
3 with intractable migraine, so stated, with status migrainosus
with refractory migraine, so stated, with status migrainosus

Intractable migraine is usually defined as headaches with duration greater than 72 hours. Status migrainous is debilitating and incapacitating, with symptoms that typically leave the patient restricted to bed. The coding of these conditions must be based on provider documentation and not the timing of the headaches as may be recorded in the record.

An additional code to identify the cerebral infarction (codes from 433 and 434 with fifth digit 1) are required to be used with subcategory codes from 346.6, Persistent migraine aura with cerebral infarction. The definition of "chronic" in primary episodic headache disorders is a headache that occurs on more days than not for more than three months. For trigeminal autonomic cephalgias, "chronic" is not used until the headache is unremitting for more than a year.

## Disorders of the Peripheral Nervous System (350–359)

The peripheral nervous system consists of the nerves outside of the brain and the spinal cord. These are 31 pairs of spinal nerves that branch off the spinal cord and extend to all parts of the body including the internal organs, trunk and extremities. The nerves coming off the cervical region of the spinal cord supply sensation to the head, neck, shoulders, arms, hands, and diaphragm. Off the thoracic region, the nerves extend to the chest and parts of the abdomen. From the lumbar region, the nerves provide communication to the lower back, and upper legs. Finally, nerve pairs coming off the sacral area innervate the buttocks, legs, feet, and genital regions of the body. The peripheral nervous system is divided into the somatic and autonomic nervous systems. The somatic nerve system are sensory neurons that bring information from organs and muscles back to the central nervous system, the brain, and spinal cord. The autonomic nervous system are motor nerves that bring information from the brain and spinal cord to the muscles and all parts of the body (NLM 2014).

### *Category 357, Inflammatory and Toxic Neuropathy*

Category 357 contains different forms of polyneuritis and polyneuropathy, some of which are the result of other diseases, such as diabetes, malignancy, and collagen vascular diseases. Subcategories 357.1, 357.2, 357.3, and 357.4 include a direction to "code first underlying disease." Other forms of polyneuropathy included in this category can be coded as a first code or a single code, such as Guillain-Barré syndrome or acute infective polyneuritis, 357.0.

Diabetic polyneuropathy or peripheral neuropathy is a serious and progressive complication of diabetes associated with significant morbidity, loss of quality of life, and increase in healthcare costs. Although there are different stages of diabetic peripheral neuropathy, a single code (357.2) is used to represent the entire spectrum. This italicized code contains a direction to "code first underlying disease (249.6, 250.6)."

### *Critical Illness Neuropathy and Myopathy (357.82 and 359.81)*

Critical illness neuropathy has two components: critical illness polyneuropathy (CIP) and critical illness myopathy (CIM). CIP is a major cause of prolonged morbidity associated with sepsis and multiple organ failure, which produces severe weakness and causes difficulty in weaning from mechanical ventilation. CIM also causes difficulty in weaning from mechanical ventilation and prolongs recovery time after illness. CIM has also been described in asthma and organ transplant patients receiving both neuromuscular blocking agents and corticosteroids. Codes exist to describe these conditions: 357.82, Critical illness polyneuropathy, and 359.81, Critical illness myopathy.

## Disorders of the Eye and Adnexa (360–379)

The "Disorders of the Eye and Adnexa" section in Chapter 6 classifies conditions such as cataracts, retinal disorders, glaucoma, corneal ulcers, conjunctivitis, and disorders of the eyelids, orbits, and optic nerve.

### *Category 362, Other Retinal Disorders*

Within category 362, various stages and severity of diabetic retinopathy are classified as 362.01–362.06. Diabetic retinopathy is a complication of diabetes that is caused by changes in the blood vessels of the eye. It is the leading cause of legal blindness among working-age Americans. Diabetic retinopathy in its earliest stages is called nonproliferative diabetic retinopathy (NPDR). As the disease advances, moderate or severe NPDR is diagnosed. The more advanced stage is known as proliferative diabetic retinopathy (PDR). In addition, a code exists for diabetic macular or retinal edema (362.07), which cannot be reported without a code for diabetic retinopathy. Diabetic macular edema (DME) is swelling of the retina in patients with diabetes mellitus, caused by leaking of fluid from the blood vessels within the macula. DME cannot occur in the absence of diabetic retinopathy. Subcategory 362.0, Diabetic retinopathy, is an italicized code that indicates that the etiology, diabetes with ophthalmic complications (249.5x or 250.5x), must be listed first.

Retinopathy of prematurity (ROP) is a serious vasoproliferative disorder involving the developing retina in premature infants. ROP is the disease name used to describe the acute retinal changes seen in premature infants. Mild forms usually cause little or no vision loss. Severe forms lead to vision loss due to retinal scarring and damage. Even with optimal treatment, many preterm infants will develop some level of ROP, especially the smallest and most premature infants. Retrolental fibroplasia is an older medical term used to describe the condition in which the retina is actually scarred. Codes 362.20–362.27 identify the specific stages of ROP as well as retrolental fibroplasia.

### *Category 365, Glaucoma*

Glaucoma is a group of eye diseases characterized by an increase in intraocular pressure that causes pathological changes in the optic disk and typical visual field defects. Category 365 is subdivided to identify the various types of glaucoma. For example, patients developing glaucoma as a result of corticosteroid therapy are classified to subcategory 365.3. Glaucoma associated with a congenital anomaly, dystrophy, or systemic syndrome is classified to subcategory 365.4. Code 365.44 is set in italic type, with an instruction to first code the associated disease or disorder, such as neurofibromatosis. Subcategory 365.8 includes code 365.83, Aqueous misdirection, formerly known as malignant glaucoma. Aqueous misdirection usually requires surgical treatment. It is neither angle-closure nor open-angle glaucoma. In this form of glaucoma, the aqueous flows into the vitreous instead of flowing into the anterior chamber. Finally, if documentation in the health record states glaucoma only, code 365.9, Unspecified glaucoma, should be assigned. Many of the codes in the category 365, glaucoma, direct the coder to use an additional code to identify the glaucoma stage. Codes in subcategory 365.7 are always used as additional codes to reflect the stage of the glaucoma disease: mild stage glaucoma (365.71), moderate stage glaucoma (365.72), severe stage or advanced stage glaucoma (365.73), and indeterminate stage glaucoma (365.74.) There is also a code 365.70 for glaucoma stage, unspecified. There are specific coding guidelines in section I. C. 6. b, Glaucoma, that provide direction on how to code unilateral and bilateral glaucoma in patients with the same or different stage in each eye.

### Category 366, Cataract

A cataract is the opacity of the crystalline lens of the eye, or its capsule, which results in a loss of vision. ICD-9-CM identifies many types of cataracts. However, the exclusion note under category 366 directs coders to codes 743.30–743.34 for congenital cataracts.

The first two subcategories of cataracts, 366.0 and 366.1, classify cataracts according to their onset in life. Subcategory 366.3 describes cataracts that are secondary to ocular disorders. Subcategory 366.4 describes cataracts associated with other disorders.

Codes 366.41–366.44 are set in italic type and, as such, are not used for primary coding. The underlying disease—such as calcinosis or craniofacial dysostosis—is coded first. If documentation in the health record states only cataract, assign code 366.9, Unspecified cataract.

## Diseases of the Ear and Mastoid Process (380–389)

The Diseases of the Ear and Mastoid Process section in Chapter 6 includes conditions such as otitis externa, otitis media (OM), Meniere's disease, cholesteatoma, hearing loss, and tinnitus.

### Otitis Externa

Otitis externa (external otitis, swimmer's ear) is an infection of the external auditory canal that may be classified as acute or chronic. Acute otitis externa is characterized by moderate to severe pain, fever, regional cellulitis, and partial hearing loss. Instead of pain, chronic otitis externa is characterized by pruritus, which leads to scaling and a thickening of the skin.

ICD-9-CM classifies otitis externa to subcategories 380.1, Infective otitis externa, and 380.2, Other otitis externa. When otitis externa is not further specified, the following codes may be reported: 380.10, Infective otitis externa, unspecified, and 380.23, Chronic otitis externa.

### Otitis Media

Otitis Media is an inflammation of the middle ear that may be further specified as suppurative or secretory, and acute or chronic. These variations and their symptoms follow:

- Acute suppurative OM is characterized by severe, deep, throbbing pain; sneezing and coughing; mild to high fever; hearing loss; dizziness; nausea; and vomiting.
- Acute secretory OM results in severe conductive hearing loss and, in some cases, a sensation of fullness in the ear with popping, crackling, or clicking sounds on swallowing or with jaw movement.
- Chronic OM has its origin in the childhood years but usually persists into adulthood. Cumulative effects of chronic OM include thickening and scarring of the tympanic membrane, decreased or absent tympanic mobility, cholesteatoma, and painless purulent discharge.

ICD-9-CM classifies OM to categories 381, Nonsuppurative otitis media and Eustachian tube disorders, and 382, Suppurative and unspecified otitis media. Both of these categories are subdivided to identify acute and chronic forms of OM and other specific types of OM. The following codes identify common forms of OM:

**381.00 Acute nonsuppurative otitis media, unspecified**
**381.01 Acute serous otitis media**
**381.10 Chronic serous otitis media, simple or unspecified**
**381.3 Other and unspecified chronic nonsuppurative otitis media**
**381.4 Nonsuppurative otitis media, not specified as acute or chronic**
**382.00 Acute suppurative otitis media, without spontaneous rupture of ear drum**
**382.2 Chronic atticoantral suppurative otitis media**
**382.4 Unspecified suppurative otitis media**
**382.9 Unspecified otitis media**
Otitis media:
NOS
Acute otitis media NOS
Chronic otitis media NOS

### Hearing Loss

ICD-9-CM category code 389, hearing loss, contains several subcategory codes that describe various forms of hearing loss or deafness. Conductive hearing loss is the decreased ability to hear sounds because of a defect of the sound-conducting apparatus of the ear. Conductive hearing loss in one ear (unilateral) is classified with code 389.05 whereas bilateral conductive hearing loss is classified with code 389.06. Sensorineural hearing loss is the decreased ability to hear sounds due to a defect in the sensory mechanisms within the ear or the nerves within the ear. Sensorineural hearing loss may be described as sensory, neural, or central hearing loss. Specific codes exist for unilateral mixed conductive and sensorineural with conductive hearing loss (389.21) and bilateral mixed hearing loss (389.22), as well as code 389.20 for use when the condition is not specified as unilateral or bilateral. The condition described as "deaf nonspeaking" is also classified to this category with code 389.7 to identify the condition when a patient has the absence of both hearing and the faculties of speech.

## ICD-9-CM Review Exercises: Chapter 9

Assign ICD-9-CM codes to the following (no need to assign morphology codes):

1. Aerobacter aerogenes meningitis

2. Plateau iris syndrome

3. Fungal meningitis

4. Postvaccinal encephalitis

## ICD-9-CM Review Exercises: Chapter 9 (Continued)

5. Conjunctivochalasis; excision of redundant conjunctival tissue

6. Intracranial abscess

7. Partial retinal detachment with single retinal defect

8. Congenital diplegic cerebral palsy

9. Tic douloureux

10. Tay-Sachs disease with profound mental retardation

11. Carpal tunnel syndrome; surgical release of carpal tunnel syndrome

12. Tonic-clonic epilepsy

13. Acute chemical conjunctivitis

14. Infantile spastic quadriplegia

15. Senile mature cataract; phacoemulsification extraction of cataract and aspiration of cataract

16. Chronic serous otitis media; bilateral myringotomy and placement of tubes

17. Cerebellar ataxia in alcoholism

18. Communicating hydrocephalus; insertion of ventriculoperitoneal shunt

19. Cholesteatoma of middle ear; excision of cholesteatoma

20. Type I diabetes mellitus with polyneuropathy

*(Continued on next page)*

## ICD-9-CM Review Exercises: Chapter 9 (Continued)

21. Episodic cluster headache

22. Migraine with aura

23. Retinopathy of prematurity, stage 3

24. Hemiplegic migraine with intractable migraine

25. Carotid sinus syndrome

# ICD-10-CM Chapter 6, Diseases of the Nervous System (G00–G99)

## Organization and Structure of ICD-10-CM Chapter 6

Chapter 6 of ICD-10-CM includes categories G00–G99 arranged in the following blocks:

| | |
|---|---|
| G00–G09 | Inflammatory diseases of the central nervous system |
| G10–G14 | Systemic atrophies primarily affecting the central nervous system |
| G20–G26 | Extrapyramidal and movement disorders |
| G30–G32 | Other degenerative diseases of the nervous system |
| G35–G37 | Demyelinating diseases of the central nervous system |
| G40–G47 | Episodic and paroxysmal disorders |
| G50–G59 | Nerve, nerve root and plexus disorders |
| G60–G65 | Polyneuropathies and other disorders of the peripheral nervous system |
| G70–G73 | Diseases of myoneural junction and muscle |
| G80–G83 | Cerebral palsy and other paralytic syndromes |
| G89–G99 | Other disorders of the nervous system |

In ICD-9-CM, Chapter 6 includes diseases of the nervous system and sense organs, such as disorders of the eye, ear, and mastoid process. ICD-10-CM has three separate chapters (Chapters 6, 7, and 8) for these same conditions. Sense organs have been separated from nervous system disorders, creating two new chapters for diseases of eye and adnexa (Chapter 7) and diseases of the ear and mastoid process (Chapter 8).

The organization of Chapter 6 in ICD-10-CM is comparable to that in ICD-9-CM. One change to note is that only diseases of the nervous system are contained in Chapter 6 of ICD-10-CM. Diseases of the sense organs, namely eye/adnexa and ear/mastoid processes, each have their own chapter in ICD-10-CM, while they are combined into a single chapter in

ICD-9-CM. A few categories in Chapter 6 have rephrased titles and in some cases encompass a combination of conditions. Additionally, a number of codes for diseases of the nervous system have been expanded in ICD-10-CM.

Category for Alzheimer's disease (G30) has been expanded to reflect onset (early versus late). ICD-10-CM has two codes for phantom limb syndrome, differentiating whether pain is present or not.

Classification of organic sleep disorders have undergone a significant change in ICD-10-CM. First, these disorders are now included in Chapter 6 rather than the signs and symptoms chapter where ICD-9-CM had classified them. Second, sleep apnea has its own subcategory with fifth character specificity identifying the type.

## Coding Guidelines and Instructional Notes for ICD-10-CM Chapter 6

No instructional note is found at the start of Chapter 6 in ICD-9-CM. However, this is not the case in ICD-10-CM. A series of excluded conditions are listed that are applicable to all conditions classifiable to Chapter 6. Additional modifications were made to specific codes.

In ICD-10-CM beneath category G89, Pain, not elsewhere classified, there is a note that states "Code also related psychological factors associated with pain (F45.42)."

By contrast to the above note, below ICD-9-CM category 338, Pain, not elsewhere classified, the note instructs coding professionals to "use additional code to identify pain associated with psychological factors (307.89)."

The National Center for Health Statistics (NCHS) has published chapter-specific guidelines for Chapter 6 in the *ICD-10-CM Official Guidelines for Coding and Reporting*:

- Guideline I.C.6.a. Dominant/nondominant side
  - Codes from category G81, hemiplegia and hemiparesis, and subcategories G83.1–G83.3, Monoplegia of lower limb, upper limb or unspecified, identify whether the dominant or non-dominant side is affected. Should the affected side be documented, but not specified as dominant or non-dominant, and the classification does not indicate a default, code selection is as follows:
    - For ambidextrous patients, the default should be dominant
    - If the left side is affected, the default is non-dominant
    - If the right side is affected, the default is dominant
- Guidelines I.C.6.b. Pain—Category G89. Guidelines address general instructions for the coding of pain. Guidelines on the pain codes are very similar to ICD-9-CM's guidelines for pain codes.
  - When category G89 codes are used as principal or first-listed diagnoses
  - The use of category G89 codes in conjunction with site specific pain codes
- Guidelines 1.C.6.2. Pain due to devices, implants, and grafts
- Guideline 1.C.6.3 Postoperative Pain
- Guideline 1.C.6.4 Chronic Pain
- Guideline 1.C.6.5 Neoplasm Related Pain
- Guideline 1.C.6.6 Chronic Pain Syndrome

## Coding Overview for ICD-10-CM Chapter 6

ICD-10-CM's Chapter 6, Diseases of the Nervous System (G00–G99), includes diseases of the central and peripheral nervous systems as well as epilepsy, migraine, and other headache syndromes. Laterality is included in the nerve root and plexus disorders to identify whether the mononeuropathy occurs on the right or left side. Codes from category G81, Hemiplegia and hemiparesis, and subcategories G83.1–G83.2–G83.3, Monoplegias, identify whether the right or left dominant or nondominant side is affected. Also in this chapter are the intraoperative and postprocedural complication codes. For example, cerebrospinal fluid leak from spinal puncture is coded here with G97.0. Other codes identify intraoperative hemorrhage or hematoma, accidental puncture of dura or other nervous system organ or postprocedural hemorrhage, or hematoma that occurred during a nervous system procedure or affecting a nervous system organ during another procedure.

The following conditions have been moved from ICD-9-CM Chapter 7, Diseases of the Circulatory System, to ICD-10-CM Chapter 6, Diseases of the Nervous System: basilar and carotid artery syndromes, transient global amnesia, and transient cerebral ischemic attack.

A note at categories G81 (Hemiplegia and hemiparesis), G82 (Paraplegia and quadriplegia) and G83 (Other paralytic syndromes) provides this information: This category is to be used only when the listed conditions are reported without further specification, or are stated to be old or longstanding but of unspecified cause. The category is also for use in multiple coding to identify these conditions resulting from any cause. Paralytic sequelae of cerebral infarct/stroke are in Chapter 9, Diseases of the Circulatory System.

The terminology for epilepsy has been updated, with terms to classify the disorder such as: Localization-related idiopathic epilepsy, generalized idiopathic epilepsy, and special epileptic syndromes. Within those various categories, more specificity is possible, such as identifying seizures of localized onset, complex partial seizures, intractable, and status epilepticus. A note with Category G40, Epilepsy and recurrent seizures and G43, Migraine provides the following terms to be considered equivalent to intractable: pharmacoresistent (pharmacologically resistant), treatment resistant, refractory (medically), and poorly controlled.

## ICD-10-CM Review Exercises: Chapter 6 of ICD-10-CM, Diseases of the Nervous System

Assign the correct ICD-10-CM diagnosis codes to the following exercises.

1. A patient had been noted to have dementia and forgetfulness. He has been leaving his home and forgetting where he is or where he is going. The diagnosis of dementia due to early-onset Alzheimer's was established.

________________

2. Juvenile myoclonic epilepsy with intractable seizures

________________

3. Left-sided hemiplegia

________________

4. The patient was admitted with high fever, stiff neck, chest pain, and nausea. A lumbar puncture was performed and results were positive for meningitis. Chest x-ray revealed pneumonia. Sputum cultures grew pneumococcus. Patient was treated with IV antibiotics. The established diagnoses were pneumococcal meningitis and pneumococcal pneumonia. Code only the diagnoses for this case.

________________

## ICD-10-CM Review Exercises: Chapter 6 of ICD-10-CM, Diseases of the Nervous System (Continued)

5. Diagnosis: Secondary Parkinsonism due to Haloperidol. This patient has been taking Haloperidol as prescribed for paranoid schizophrenia and developed a change in facial expressions and stiffness in the arms and legs. The drug will be discontinued.

   ______________________________

6. Female patient has breast cancer of the right breast with multiple metastases to the liver. She is seen to control the severe acute pain of the liver metastases.

   ______________________________

7. The patient, a type 2 diabetic with neuropathy, developed weakness of the left arm and leg. The patient was brought to the emergency room where he could speak but was unable to use his left arm and leg. Patient was able to ambulate with no neurological deficits within 24 hours. Due to the complete recovery, it was determined that the patient had experienced a TIA. During this encounter the patient also was treated for an intractable classical migraine.

   ______________________________

# ICD-10-CM Chapter 7, Diseases of Eye and Adnexa (H00–H59)

## Organization and Structure of ICD-10-CM Chapter 7

Chapter 7 of ICD-10-CM includes categories H00–H59 arranged in the following blocks:

| | |
|---|---|
| H00–H05 | Disorders of eyelid, lacrimal system and orbit |
| H10–H11 | Disorders of conjunctiva |
| H15–H22 | Disorders of sclera, cornea, iris and ciliary body |
| H25–H28 | Disorders of lens |
| H30–H36 | Disorders of choroid and retina |
| H40–H42 | Glaucoma |
| H43–H44 | Disorders of vitreous body and globe |
| H46–H47 | Disorders of optic nerve and visual pathways |
| H49–H52 | Disorders of ocular muscles, binocular movement, accommodation and refraction |
| H53–H54 | Visual disturbances and blindness |
| H55–H57 | Other disorders of eye and adnexa |
| H59 | Intraoperative and postprocedural complications and disorders of eye and adnexa, not elsewhere classified |

Chapter 7 is an entirely new chapter in ICD-10-CM. A diagram of the eye is shown in figure 9.1. In ICD-9-CM, the conditions classified in this chapter are located in Chapter 6, Diseases of the Nervous System and Sense Organs. Chapter 7 in ICD-10-CM also has a

**Figure 9.1.** Diagram of the Eye

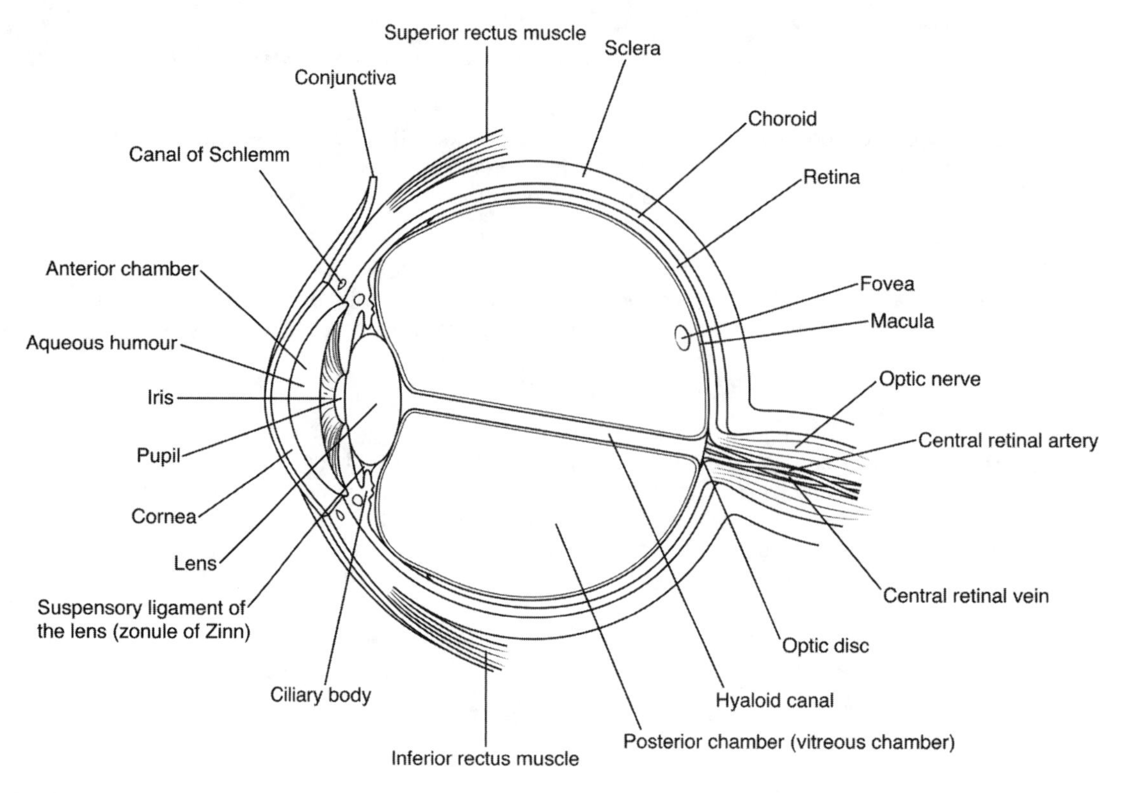




different organization than what is found in ICD-9-CM. While the structure is still by "site" for diseases of the eye and adnexa, the order differs.

Some categories in Chapter 7 have undergone title changes to reflect the terminology used today. For example, ICD-9-CM uses *senile cataract,* while ICD-10-CM utilizes the descriptor *age-related cataract.* Many of the classification changes in Chapter 7 have to do with the expansion of characters to provide for laterality. ICD-10-CM contains codes for right side, left side, and in some instances bilateral sides for diseases of the eye and adnexa.

**EXAMPLE:** **H16.01** **Central corneal ulcer**
H16.011, Central corneal ulcer, right eye
H16.012, Central corneal ulcer, left eye
H16.013, Central corneal ulcer, bilateral
H16.019, Central corneal ulcer, unspecified eye

## Coding Guidelines and Instructional Notes for ICD-10-CM Chapter 7

With the formation of a new chapter for Diseases of the eye and adnexa come new instructions on which conditions are excluded from Chapter 7 of ICD-10-CM. Since the placement of the note is at the beginning of Chapter 7, none of the listed conditions would be coded here.

Included in this chapter are a number of notes for code usage that are code specific.

Under ICD-10-CM subcategory H47.5, Disorders of other visual pathways, is a note to code also the underlying condition. This differs from ICD-9-CM in that a single code is used to identify the visual pathway disorder and the associated condition.

Under ICD-10-CM subcategory H54, Blindness and low vision, is a note to code first any associated underlying cause of the blindness. No such note appears under ICD-9-CM category 369, Blindness and low vision.

The ICD-10-CM Draft Official Coding Guidelines for Coding and Reporting contain directions for the coding of the different types of glaucoma with seventh characters used to identify the different stages of glaucoma in the patient.

## Coding Overview for ICD-10-CM Chapter 7

Chapter 7 is a new chapter in ICD-10-CM, and these conditions were previously included with Diseases of the Nervous System and Sense Organs.

Chapter 7, Diseases of the Eye and Adnexa (H00–H59), includes very specific codes, with the laterality of the condition identified as right eye or left eye as well as right or left upper eyelid or lower eyelid. Codes also exist to describe whether the condition occurs bilaterally or in both eyes. There are unspecified codes to use if the physician or provider does not specify the right or left side for the condition. The term "senile" is not used in ICD-10-CM to describe a type of cataract; the term "age-related" is used instead.

In addition to the intraoperative or postprocedural hemorrhages or accidental puncture or laceration for conditions of the eye, specific complications of the eye due to a procedure are included. For example, keratopathy (bullous aphakia) following cataract surgery (H59.011–H59.019) and cataract (lens) fragments in eye following cataract surgery (H59.021–H59.029) are included in this chapter.

### ICD-10-CM Review Exercises: Chapter 7 of ICD-10-CM, Diseases of the Eye and Adnexa

1. Nonulcerative bilateral blepharitis of the upper eyelids

2. Recurrent pterygium, bilateral

3. Age-related nuclear cataract, left eye only

4. Primary open-angle glaucoma of the left eye, moderate stage

5. Bullous keratopathy, left eye, due to cataract surgery

6. Right eye age-related cortical cataract with cataract extraction surgery performed at an ambulatory surgery. After the procedure was completed, the patient suffered an immediate postoperative hemorrhage of the eye, while still in the operating room, which was addressed by the surgeon. Assign the diagnosis codes only.

# ICD-10-CM Chapter 8, Diseases of the Ear and Mastoid Process (H60–H95)

## Organization and Structure of ICD-10-CM Chapter 8

Chapter 8 of ICD-10-CM includes categories H60-H95 arranged in the following blocks:

| | |
|---|---|
| H60–H62 | Diseases of external ear |
| H65–H75 | Diseases of middle ear and mastoid |
| H80–H83 | Diseases of inner ear |
| H90–H94 | Other disorders of ear |
| H95 | Intraoperative and postprocedural complications and disorders of ear and mastoid process, not elsewhere classified |

Chapter 8 is an entirely new chapter in ICD-10-CM. A diagram of the external, middle and inner ear is shown in figure 9.2. In ICD-9-CM, the conditions classified in this chapter are located in Chapter 6, Diseases of the Nervous System and Sense Organs. Diseases of the ear and mastoid process have been arranged into blocks making it easier to identify the types of conditions that would occur in the external ear (block 1), middle ear and mastoid (block 2), and inner ear (block 3). Block 4 is used for other disorders of the ear. Block 5 contains the codes for intraoperative and postprocedural complications. The intraoperative and postprocedural complications are grouped at the end of the chapter rather than scattered throughout different categories. Category and subcategory titles have been revised in a number of locations in Chapter 8.

| | | |
|---|---|---|
| **EXAMPLES:** | ICD-9-CM: | 381, Nonsuppurative otitis media and Eustachian tube disorders |
| | ICD-10-CM: | H65, Nonsuppurative otitis media |
| | ICD-9-CM: | 380.10, Infective otitis externa, unspecified |
| | ICD-10-CM: | H60.0, Abscess of external ear |
| | ICD-9-CM: | 386, Vertiginous syndromes and other disorders of vestibular system |
| | ICD-10-CM: | H81, Disorders of vestibular function |

Although Chapter 8 in ICD-10-CM basically parallels the corresponding section in Chapter 6 of ICD-9-CM, there are quite a few changes. These changes include greater specificity added at the fourth-, fifth-, and sixth-character levels; the delineation of laterality and the addition of many more "code first underlying disease" notes.

One last noted classification change in this chapter is that the ICD-9-CM category 381, Nonsuppurative otitis media and Eustachian tube disorders, has been split into two categories in ICD-10-CM; H65, Nonsuppurative otitis media and H68, Eustachian salpingitis and obstruction.

## Coding Guidelines and Instructional Notes for ICD-10-CM Chapter 8

Instructions on the use of codes may change from one revision to the next. For example, ICD-9-CM contains a note excluding otitis media with perforation of tympanic membrane from subcategory 384.2. In ICD-10-CM, the note directly under H72, Perforation of tympanic membrane, states "code first any associated otitis media."

**Figure 9.2.** Diagram of the ear

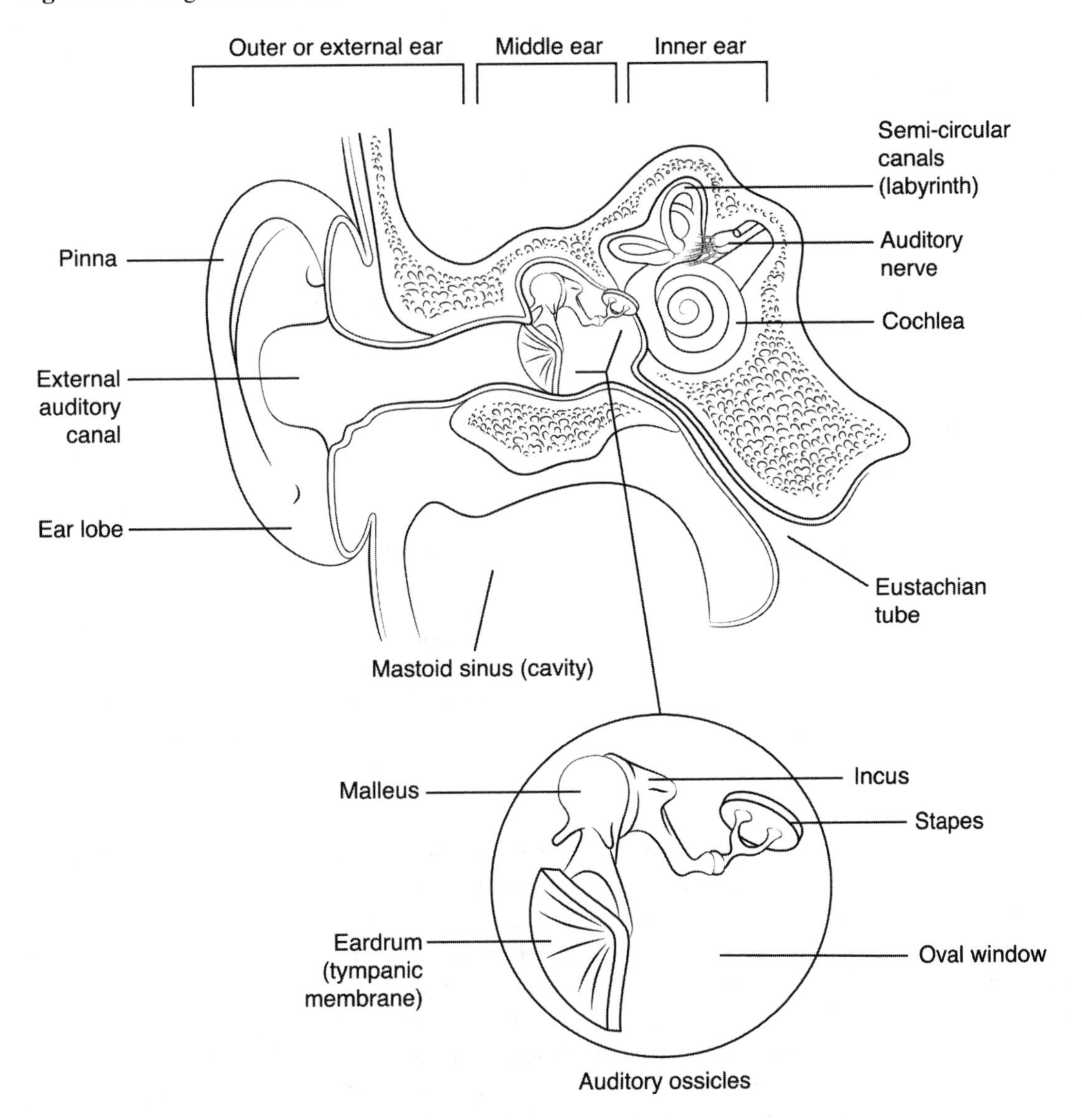




**EXAMPLE:** ICD-9-CM: **384.2, Perforation of Tympanic Membrane**
Excludes: otitis media with perforation of tympanic membrane (382.00–382.9)

ICD-10-CM: **H72, Perforation of tympanic membrane**
Code first any associated otitis media (H65.-, H66.1-, H66.2-, H66.3-, H66.4-, H66.9-,H67.-)

Excludes1: acute suppurative otitis media with rupture of the tympanic membrane (H66.01-)
traumatic rupture of ear drum (S09.2-)

At the beginning of Chapter 8, there is a note to the coder to use an external cause code following the code for the ear condition, if applicable, to identify the cause of the ear condition. There is an instructional note in categories H65, H66.1–H66.9, and H67 to use an additional code for any associated perforated tympanic membrane (H72.-).

At this time, there are no chapter-specific guidelines related to Chapter 8, Diseases of the Ears and Mastoid Process.

## Coding Overview for ICD-10-CM Chapter 8

Chapter 8 is also a new chapter in ICD-10-CM, and includes conditions previously found in the Nervous System and Sense Organs chapter.

Codes have also been expanded to increase anatomic specificity and add the concept of laterality.

A number of new instructional notes have been added. The note at the beginning of the chapter states to use an external cause code following the code for the ear condition, if applicable, to identify the cause of the ear condition.

The following note addresses otitis media categories H65 and some of the codes in H66:

> Use additional code for any associated perforated tympanic membrane (H72.-)
> Use additional code to identify:
> exposure to environmental tobacco smoke (Z77.22)
> exposure to tobacco smoke in the perinatal period (P96.81)
> history of tobacco use (Z87.891)
> occupational exposure to environmental tobacco smoke (Z57.31)
> tobacco dependence (F17.-)
> tobacco use (Z72.0)

Notes indicating that the underlying disease should be coded first have been added, for example, there is a note under the ICD-10-CM category for perforation of tympanic membrane indicating that any associated OM should be coded first.

Hearing loss, ear pain, tinnitus, as well as other acoustic disorders are included in the chapter with left, right, or bilateral distinctions where applicable.

Specific ear complications that occur following a mastoidectomy as well as the intraoperative hemorrhage, hematoma, accidental puncture or laceration, and postprocedural hemorrhage or hematoma following ear or mastoid procedures or other procedures are found at the end of the chapter in the range of codes from H95.00–H95.89.

## ICD-10-CM Review Exercises: Chapter 8 of ICD-10-CM, Diseases of the Ear and Mastoid Process

1. Left acute serous otitis media with a total perforated tympanic membrane of the left ear.

_______________

2. Ménière's vertigo of left ear.

_______________

3. Bilateral conductive hearing loss due to nonobliterative otosclerosis of the stapes at the oval window. She is unable to hear with hearing aids and has decided to undergo left stapedectomy. During the surgery an inadvertent laceration was made to the tympanic meatal flap, which was repaired. Assign the diagnosis codes only.

_______________

4. Subperiosteal mastoid abscess, left year

_______________

5. Tinnitus, right ear

_______________

6. Conductive hearing loss, left ear, with normal hearing in right ear

_______________

7. Cholesteatoma, right external ear

_______________

# Chapter 10

# Diseases of the Circulatory System

## Learning Objectives

At the conclusion of this chapter, you should be able to:

1. Describe the organization of the conditions and codes included in Chapter 7 of ICD-9-CM, Diseases of the Circulatory System (390–459)
2. Describe the organization of the conditions and codes included in Chapter 9 of ICD-10-CM, Diseases of the Circulatory System (I00–I99)
3. Define *rheumatic fever and chronic rheumatic heart disease* and identify the Alphabetic Index entries for the types of heart valve diseases associated with them
4. Describe the format of the hypertension table in the ICD-9-CM Alphabetic Index
5. Describe the coding guidelines for the use of the combination codes for hypertensive heart disease and hypertensive kidney disease and the codes to describe hypertension with other illnesses.
6. Apply the correct fourth- and fifth-digit subclassification ICD-9-CM codes for acute myocardial infarction
7. Apply the ICD-10-CM coding guidelines for the correct coding of current and subsequent acute myocardial infarctions
8. Describe the ICD-9-CM coding sequencing rule of angina and coronary disease
9. Explain the differences between the ICD-9-CM codes 414.00–414.07 used to describe chronic ischemic heart disease
10. Identify the ICD-9-CM codes that describe various types of cardiac arrhythmias and conduction disorders
11. Describe the circumstances in which the ICD-9-CM code 427.5 for cardiac arrest is assigned for a patient
12. Identify the ICD-9-CM code for acute cerebrovascular accident (CVA) and describe the circumstances in which additional codes are used with the CVA code to identify associated conditions

13. Describe the circumstances in which the ICD-9-CM category code 438 is used to describe the late effect of cerebrovascular disease and contrast them with those in which code V12.54 is used
14. Briefly describe the ICD-9-CM procedure coding for cardiac catheterization, coronary angiography, and percutaneous transluminal coronary angioplasty
15. Briefly describe the ICD-9-CM procedure coding for cardiac pacemakers and automatic implantable cardioverter-defibrillator devices
16. Assign ICD-9-CM diagnosis and procedure codes for Chapter 7 of ICD-9-CM, Diseases of the Circulatory System
17. Assign ICD-10-CM codes for ICD-10-CM Chapter 9, Diseases of the circulatory system

## Chapter 7, Diseases of the Circulatory System (390–459)

Chapter 7, Diseases of the Circulatory System, in the Tabular List in volume 1 of ICD-9-CM is subdivided into the following categories and section titles:

| Categories | Section Titles |
|---|---|
| 390–392 | Acute Rheumatic Fever |
| 393–398 | Chronic Rheumatic Heart Disease |
| 401–405 | Hypertensive Disease |
| 410–414 | Ischemic Heart Disease |
| 415–417 | Diseases of Pulmonary Circulation |
| 420–429 | Other Forms of Heart Disease |
| 430–438 | Cerebrovascular Disease |
| 440–449 | Diseases of Arteries, Arterioles, and Capillaries |
| 451–459 | Diseases of Veins and Lymphatics, and Other Diseases of Circulatory System |

Circulatory diagnoses are often difficult to code because a variety of nonspecific terminology is used to describe these conditions. All inclusion and exclusion notes within ICD-9-CM Chapter 7 should be carefully reviewed prior to selecting a code.

In this chapter, the following conditions and procedures are highlighted: acute rheumatic fever and rheumatic heart disease, hypertension, myocardial infarction, angina, atherosclerosis, congestive heart failure, and cerebrovascular disease.

### Acute Rheumatic Fever and Rheumatic Heart Disease

Acute and chronic diseases of rheumatic origin are classified in categories 390–398. This section also covers diseases of mitral and aortic valves, because when the ICD classification system was set up, clinicians believed that mitral stenosis was caused by rheumatic heart disease. Rheumatic heart disease continues to be the most common cause for mitral stenosis, and rarely do other factors cause the condition. Rheumatic fever does not occur as often in recent years due to the effective treatment of streptococcal infections with appropriate antibiotics. For this reason, the number of patients with mitral stenosis is decreasing (PubMed Health 2012).

### Categories 390–392, Acute Rheumatic Fever

Rheumatic fever occurs after a streptococcal sore throat (Group A streptococcus hemolyticus). The acute phase of the illness is marked by fever, malaise, sweating, palpitations, and polyarthritis, which varies from vague discomfort to severe pain felt chiefly in the large joints. Most patients have elevated titers of antistreptolysin antibodies and increased sedimentation rates.

The importance of rheumatic fever derives entirely from its capacity to cause severe heart damage. Salicylates markedly reduce fever, relieve joint pain, and may reduce joint swelling, if present. Because rheumatic fever often recurs, prophylaxis with penicillin is recommended and has markedly reduced the incidence of rheumatic heart disease in the general population.

### Categories 393–398, Chronic Rheumatic Heart Disease

Rheumatic heart disease develops with an initial attack of rheumatic fever in about 30 percent of cases (Merck 2014). The cardiac involvement may affect all three layers of the heart muscle, causing pericarditis, scarring and weakening of the myocardium, and endocardial involvement of heart valves. The latter condition occurs more often in children who have had rheumatic fever and, to a lesser extent, in adults with rheumatic fever. A murmur heard over the heart is symptomatic of a valvular lesion. Rheumatic fever causes inflammation of the valves, thus damaging the valve cusps so that the opening may become permanently narrowed (stenosis). The mitral valve is involved in the great majority of such cases; the aortic valve is involved to a lesser extent; and the tricuspid and pulmonary valves, in a small percentage of the patients. In about 10 percent of patients, two of these valves are involved (Merck 2014).

When stenosis affects the mitral valve, blood flow decreases from the left atrium into the left ventricle. As a result, blood is held back in the lungs, then in the right side of the heart, and, finally, in the veins of the body. Incompetence of a valve may also occur because the cusps will not retract. If the mitral valve cannot close, blood escapes from the mitral valve back into the left atrium. In the case of the aortic valve, blood escapes from the aorta into the left ventricle. In such cases, plastic and metal replacement valves that function as well as normal valves may be surgically inserted.

In coding diseases of the mitral valve and diseases affecting both the mitral and aortic valves, the Alphabetic Index to Diseases offers direction to codes from categories 393–398. Remember to always trust the Alphabetic Index to Diseases and assign the code it indicates.

**Insufficiency, insufficient** . . .
  mitral (valve) 424.0
    with
      aortic (valve) disease 396.3
        insufficiency, incompetence, or regurgitation 396.3
        stenosis or obstruction 396.2
      obstruction or stenosis 394.2
        with aortic valve disease 396.8
    congenital 746.6
    rheumatic 394.1
      with

aortic (valve) disease 396.3
insufficiency, incompetence, or regurgitation 396.3
stenosis or obstruction 396.2
obstruction or stenosis 394.2
with aortic valve disease 396.8
active or acute 391.1
with chorea, rheumatic (Sydenham's) 392.0

The inclusion note under category 396 states that category 396 includes involvement of both mitral and aortic valves, whether specified as rheumatic or not.

## Exercise 10.1

Assign ICD-9-CM codes to the following:

1. Congestive rheumatic heart failure
2. Mitral valve stenosis with aortic valve insufficiency
3. Acute rheumatic heart disease
4. Mitral valve stenosis with regurgitation
5. Chronic rheumatic endocarditis

## Hypertensive Disease

The Alphabetic Index to Diseases uses a table to display hypertensive diseases. This table provides a complete listing of all conditions due to, or associated with, hypertension. Part of the table for hypertensive diseases follows:

**Alphabetic Index to Diseases: Hypertension**

| | Malignant | Benign | Unspecified |
|---|---|---|---|
| **Hypertension, hypertensive** (arterial) (arteriolar) (crisis) (degeneration) (disease) (essential) (fluctuating) (idiopathic) (intermittent) (labile) (low renin) (orthostatic) (paroxysmal) (primary) (systemic) (uncontrolled) (vascular) | 401.0 | 401.1 | 401.9 |
| with | | | |

| | | | |
|---|---|---|---|
| chronic kidney disease | | | |
| stage I through stage IV, or unspecified | 403.00 | 403.10 | 403.90 |
| stage V or end stage renal disease | 403.01 | 403.11 | 403.91 |
| heart involvement (conditions classifiable to 429.0–429.3, 429.8, 429.9 due to hypertension) (*see also* Hypertension, heart) | 402.00 | 402.10 | 402.90 |
| with kidney involvement—*see* Hypertension, cardiorenal | | | |
| renal (kidney) involvement (*only* conditions classifiable to 585, 587) *(excludes conditions classifiable to 584)* (*see also* Hypertension, kidney) | 403.00 | 403.10 | 403.90 |
| with heart involvement—*see* Hypertension, cardiorenal | | | |
| failure (and sclerosis) (*see also* Hypertension, kidney) | 403.01 | 403.11 | 403.91 |
| sclerosis without failure (*see also* Hypertension, kidney) | 403.00 | 403.10 | 403.90 |
| accelerated (*see also* Hypertension, by type, malignant) | 401.0 | — | — |
| antepartum—*see* Hypertension, complicating pregnancy, childbirth, or the puerperium | | | |
| borderline | | | 796.2 |
| cardiorenal (disease) | 404.00 | 404.10 | 404.90 |

The first column in the table identifies the hypertensive condition, such as accelerated, antepartum, cardiovascular disease, cardiorenal, and cerebrovascular disease. The remaining three columns are titled "Malignant," "Benign," and "Unspecified," and they constitute the subcategories of hypertensive disease. The documentation in the patient's health record often will not specify a hypertensive condition as malignant or benign; therefore, the unspecified code to describe that hypertensive condition must be assigned.

## Definition of Hypertension

A threshold of blood pressure that an individual could overshoot and then be considered hypertensive has not been defined. However, the standard commonly applied is that a sustained diastolic pressure above 90 mm Hg and a sustained systolic pressure above 140 mm Hg constitutes hypertension. The prevalence of hypertension increases with age. About 90 percent of hypertension is primary (essential hypertension), and its cause is unknown. The remaining 10 percent is due to other diseases, often secondary to renal disease (Madhur 2014). Both essential and secondary hypertension can be either benign or malignant. Complications of hypertension include left ventricular failure, arteriosclerotic heart disease, retinal hemorrhages, cerebrovascular insufficiency, and renal failure.

### Benign Hypertension

In most cases, benign hypertension remains fairly stable over many years and is compatible with a long life. If untreated, however, it becomes an important risk factor in coronary heart disease and cerebrovascular disease. Benign hypertension is also asymptomatic until complications develop. Effective antihypertensive drug therapy is the treatment of choice.

### Malignant Hypertension

Malignant hypertension is far less common, occurring in only a small percent of patients with elevated blood pressure. Physicians may also refer to malignant hypertension as "accelerating" or "necrotizing" hypertension and this terminology is included in the hypertension table in the Alphabetic Index leading to the same code as malignant hypertension. The malignant form is frequently of abrupt onset. It often ends with renal failure or cerebral hemorrhage. Usually a person with malignant hypertension will complain of headaches and difficulties with vision. Blood pressures of 200/140 are common, and an abnormal protrusion of the optic nerve (papilledema) occurs with microscopic hemorrhages and exudates seen in the retina. The initial event appears to be some form of vascular damage to the kidneys. This may result from long-standing benign hypertension with damage of the arteriolar walls, or it may derive from arteritis of some form. The chances for long-term survival depend on early treatment before significant renal insufficiency has developed.

### Hypertensive Heart Disease

Hypertensive heart disease refers to the secondary effects on the heart of prolonged sustained systemic hypertension. The heart has to work against greatly increased resistance in the form of high blood pressure. The primary effect is thickening of the left ventricle, finally resulting in heart failure. The symptoms are similar to those of heart failure from other causes. Many persons with controlled hypertension do not develop heart failure. However, when a patient has heart failure due to hypertension, additional codes are required to be used with category 402 codes to specify the type of heart failure that exists, such as 428.0, 428.20–428.23, 428.30–428.33, or 428.40–428.43, if known.

### ICD-9-CM Official Coding Guidelines

The following guidelines are applicable in coding hypertensive diseases:

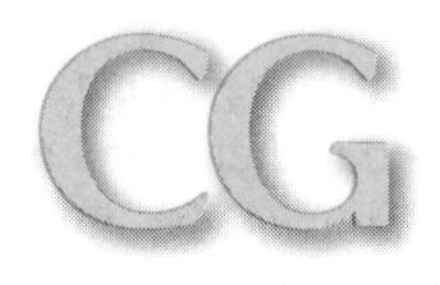


1. **Hypertension, essential or NOS:** Assign hypertension (arterial) (essential) (primary) (systemic) (NOS) to category 401, with the appropriate fourth digit to indicate malignant (.0), benign (.1), or unspecified (.9). Do not use either .0 (malignant) or .1 (benign) unless the documentation in the health record supports such a designation.
2. **Hypertension with heart disease:** When hypertension and heart disease are present at the same time, they are coded differently depending on whether the heart disease is caused by the hypertension or not.
   a. When heart disease is caused by hypertension or the heart disease is described as hypertensive, a combination code from category 402 is used to describe it.

   Heart conditions (425.8, 429.0–429.3, 429.8, 429.9) are assigned to a code from category 402 when a causal relationship is stated (due to hypertension) or implied (hypertensive). Use an additional code from category 428 to identify the type of heart failure in those patients with heart failure. More than one code from category 428 may be assigned if the patient has systolic or diastolic failure and congestive heart failure.

In ICD-9-CM, a stated causal relationship is usually documented using the term due to (for example, congestive heart failure due to hypertension). An implied causal relationship is documented using the term hypertensive. In ICD-9-CM, hypertensive is interpreted to mean "due to."

**EXAMPLE:** Hypertensive cardiomegaly (or cardiomegaly due to hypertension)

402.90 Hypertensive cardiomegaly

In category 402, Hypertensive heart disease, the fourth-digit subcategory describes whether the hypertensive condition is malignant, benign, or unspecified. The fifth-digit subclassification states the absence or presence of heart failure.

b. When heart disease and hypertension coexist in a patient, but the heart disease is not due to the hypertension, the two conditions are coded separately.

The same heart conditions (425.8, 429.0–429.3, 429.8, 429.9) with hypertension, but without a stated causal relationship, are coded separately and sequenced according to the circumstances of the admission or encounter.

**EXAMPLE:** Cardiomegaly and hypertension

429.3 Cardiomegaly
401.9 Essential hypertension, unspecified

c. Do not assume heart disease is caused by hypertension.

Although hypertension is frequently the cause of various forms of heart and vascular disease, ICD-9-CM does not presume a cause-and-effect relationship. The mention of "heart disease with hypertension only" should not be interpreted as a "due to" condition. Use of the terms *and* and *with* in the diagnostic statement does not imply cause and effect.

3. **Hypertensive chronic kidney disease:** Assign codes from category 403, Hypertensive chronic kidney disease, when conditions classified to categories 585 or 587 are present with hypertension. Unlike hypertension with heart disease, ICD-9-CM presumes a cause-and-effect relationship and classifies chronic kidney disease with hypertension as hypertensive chronic kidney disease. chronic kidney disease.

(*Continued*)

*(Continued)*

Fifth digits for category 403 should be assigned as follows:

0—with CKD stage I through stage IV, or unspecified

1—with CDK stage V or end stage renal disease

The appropriate code from category 585, Chronic kidney disease, should be used as a secondary code with a code from category 403 to identify the stage of chronic kidney disease.

As with hypertensive heart disease, the fourth-digit subcategory describes whether the hypertensive condition is malignant, benign, or unspecified. The fifth-digit subclassification specifies the stage of chronic kidney disease present, from stage I through stage V, and end-stage renal disease or the unspecified type of chronic kidney disease. Under the codes within category 403 is the direction to "use additional code to identify the stage of chronic kidney disease (585.1–585.6, 585.9)."

**EXAMPLE:** Hypertension and chronic kidney disease, stage I

403.90 Hypertensive renal disease, unspecified with chronic kidney disease, stage I, with code 585.1

4. **Hypertensive heart and chronic kidney disease:** Assign codes from category 404, Hypertensive heart and kidney disease, when both hypertensive kidney disease and hypertensive heart disease are stated in the diagnosis. Assume a causal relationship between the hypertension and the chronic kidney disease, whether or not the condition is designated that way. (Remember, the fourth-digit subcategory describes whether the hypertensive condition is malignant, benign, or unspecified. The fifth-digit subclassification identifies the presence, absence, or combination of heart failure with chronic kidney disease.) An additional code from category 428 is required to identify the type of heart failure. More than one code from category 428 may be assigned if the patient has systolic or diastolic failure and congestive heart failure. An additional code from 585.1–585.6, 585.9 is required to identify the stage of chronic kidney disease.

   Fifth digits for category 404 should be assigned as follows:

   0—without heart failure and with chronic kidney disease (CKD) stage I through stage IV or unspecified

   1—with heart failure and with CKD stage I through stage IV, or unspecified

   2—without heart failure and with CKD stage V or end stage renal disease

3—with heart failure and with CKD stage V or end stage renal disease

The appropriate code from category 585, Chronic kidney disease, should be used as a secondary code with a code from category 404 to identify the stage of chronic kidney disease

**EXAMPLE:** Hypertensive cardiomegaly and hypertensive kidney disease, stage III

404.90 Hypertensive heart and kidney disease, unspecified with chronic kidney disease, stage III, with code 585.3

In this example, the fifth digit 0 reflects the presence of chronic kidney disease alone, and at stage III. A second code indicates the stage of chronic kidney disease.

5. **Hypertensive cerebrovascular disease:** Two codes are required to fully describe a hypertensive cerebrovascular condition. The first code assigned describes the cerebrovascular disease (430–438), followed by the appropriate code describing the hypertension (401–405).

**EXAMPLE:** Cerebrovascular accident and benign hypertension

434.91 Cerebral artery occlusion, unspecified, with cerebral infarction

401.1 Benign essential hypertension

6. Hypertensive retinopathy: Two codes are required to identify the hypertensive retinopathy condition. First, assign code 362.11, Hypertensive retinopathy, followed by the appropriate code from categories 401 through 405 describing the hypertension (for example, 401.1, Benign essential hypertension).

7. Hypertension, secondary: Two codes are required: one to identify the underlying etiology and one from category 405 to identify the hypertension. Sequencing of codes is determined by the reason for admission/encounter.

When a physician documents that the hypertension is due to another disease (secondary hypertension), two codes are required to completely describe the condition. One code describes the underlying condition, and the other code is selected from category 405, Secondary hypertension. Sequencing of codes is determined by the reason for the admission or encounter. If the patient is admitted for or the focus of the visit is on the treatment of the secondary hypertension, the secondary hypertension code is listed first with an additional code for the condition

(*Continued*)

*(Continued)*

causing the hypertension. If the patient is admitted for or the focus of the visit is on the underlying disease that is producing the secondary hypertension, the underlying disease code is listed first with an additional code for the secondary hypertension.

Category 405 is subdivided at the fourth-digit level to describe whether the hypertensive condition is malignant, benign, or unspecified. The fifth-digit subclassification identifies the underlying condition of renovascular origin or of another origin.

Renovascular origin can include renal artery aneurysm, anomaly, embolism, fibromuscular hyperplasia, occlusion, stenosis, or thrombosis. Other types of diseases causing secondary hypertension can include a calculus of the ureter or kidney, a brain tumor, polycystic kidneys, or polycythemia.

**EXAMPLE:** Uncontrolled hypertension due to a malignant neoplasm of the brain (admitted primarily to treat the hypertension)

405.99 Other unspecified secondary hypertension
191.9 Malignant neoplasm of brain, unspecified

8. **Hypertension, transient:** Assign code 796.2, Elevated blood pressure reading without diagnosis of hypertension, unless patient has an established diagnosis of hypertension. Assign code 642.3x for transient hypertension of pregnancy.
9. **Controlled hypertension:** Assign the appropriate code from categories 401 through 405 to describe a diagnostic statement of controlled hypertension. This type of statement usually refers to an existing state of hypertension under control by therapy.
10. Uncontrolled hypertension: Uncontrolled hypertension may refer to untreated hypertension or to hypertension not responding to current therapeutic regimen. In either case, assign the appropriate code from categories 401 through 405 to designate the stage and type of hypertension, with the appropriate fourth and fifth digits.
11. **Elevated blood pressure:** For a statement of elevated blood pressure without further specificity, assign code 796.2, Elevated blood pressure reading without diagnosis of hypertension, rather than a code from category 401.

**EXAMPLE:** After the patient was told at an employer's health screening program that his blood pressure was high, the patient made an appointment with the physician. In the office, the patient's blood pressure readings ranged from 150/90 to 144/95 measured repeatedly in both arms. The patient was counseled about changes in his diet and exercise regime that could impact his elevated blood pressure readings. The patient was advised to return to the office in two weeks. At this time the doctor did not document the diagnosis of hypertension in the record. The correct code for this encounter would be:

796.2, Elevated blood pressure reading without diagnosis of hypertension.

## Exercise 10.2

Assign ICD-9-CM codes to the following:

1. Hypertensive cardiovascular disease, malignant
2. Congestive heart failure; benign hypertension
3. Secondary benign hypertension; stenosis of renal artery
4. Congestive heart failure and chronic kidney disease due to accelerated hypertension with end-stage renal disease (ESRD)
5. Acute renal failure; essential hypertension
6. Congestive heart failure due to hypertensive heart disease
7. Malignant hypertensive nephropathy with chronic kidney disease, stage V
8. Hypertensive cardiorenal disease with congestive heart failure and chronic kidney disease, stage II
9. Uncontrolled hypertension due to Cushing's disease (focus of care is hypertension)
10. Hypertension with chronic kidney disease, stage I

## Categories 410–414, Ischemic Heart Disease

Ischemic heart disease includes arteriosclerotic heart disease, coronary ischemia, and coronary artery disease. It is the generic name for three forms of heart disease: myocardial infarction, angina pectoris, and chronic ischemic heart disease. All three diseases result from an imbalance between the need of the myocardium for oxygen and the oxygen supply. Usually, the imbalance results from insufficient blood flow due to arteriosclerotic narrowing of the coronary arteries.

At the beginning of the ischemic heart disease section, the inclusion note states that this section includes ischemic heart conditions with mention of hypertension. The statement "Use additional code to identify presence of hypertension" also appears at the beginning of this section as an instruction to assign an additional code to describe hypertension, if present. An illustration of the coronary arteries of the heart are shown in figure 10.1.

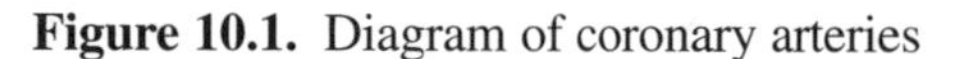

**Figure 10.1.** Diagram of coronary arteries

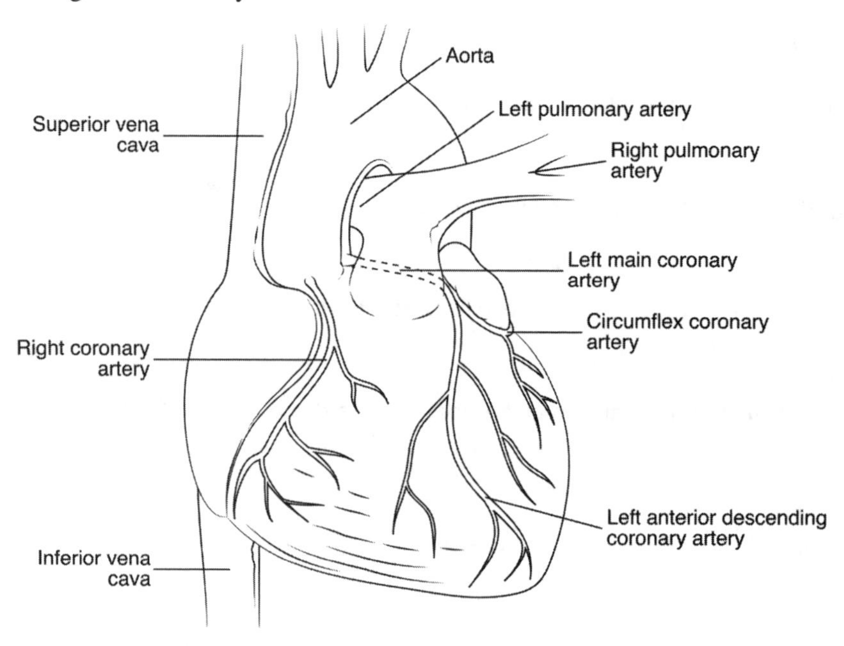




### Acute Myocardial Infarction

Acute myocardial infarction (AMI) usually occurs as a result of a sudden inadequacy of coronary flow. The first symptom of AMI is the development of deep substernal pain described as aching or pressure, often with radiation to the back or left arm. The patient is pale, diaphoretic (sweaty), and in severe pain. Peripheral or carotid cyanosis may be present, as well as arrhythmias. Treatment is designed to relieve the patient's distress, reduce cardiac work, and prevent and treat complications. Major complications include tachycardia, frequent ventricular premature beats, Mobitz II heart block, and ventricular fibrillation. Heart failure often occurs.

When the physician describes a condition as "aborted myocardial infarction," the code 411.1, Intermediate coronary syndrome, should be assigned. This condition usually means the patient did not have any myocardial damage and an acute myocardial infarction has not occurred.

Included under category 410, Acute myocardial infarction, is the terminology of "ST elevation (STEMI) and non-ST elevation (NSTEMI) myocardial infarction" that coders may see documented by physicians in the records of patients with AMI. Other terminology used by physicians for cardiac emergencies is "acute coronary syndrome," which ranges from STEMI to NSTEMI to unstable angina. A thorough review of the documentation in the record is required to clarify which condition is present prior to coding.

### Diagnostic Tools

The diagnosis of AMI depends on the patient's clinical history, the physical examination, interpretation of electrocardiogram (EKG), chest radiograph, and measurement of serum levels of cardiac enzymes, such as troponins or the MB isoenzyme of creatine kinase (CK-MB).

Diagnostic uncertainty frequently arises because of various factors. Many patients with acute AMI have atypical symptoms. Other people with typical physical symptoms do not have AMI. EKGs may also be nondiagnostic. Laboratory tests known as biochemical or serum markers of cardiac injury are commonly relied upon to diagnose or exclude an AMI.

Creatine kinase and lactate dehydrogenase have been the "gold standard" for the diagnosis of AMI for many years. However, single values of these tests have limited sensitivity and specificity. Serum markers currently in use are troponin T and I, myoglobin, and CK-MB. These markers are used instead of, or along with, the standard markers.

EKGs also prove useful in diagnosing myocardial infarctions. The initial EKG may be diagnostic in acute transmural myocardial infarction, but serial EKGs may be necessary to confirm the diagnosis for other myocardial infarction sites.

A patient diagnosed with an acute myocardial infarction or an acute ischemic stroke may be given intravenous tissue plasminogen activator (tPA), which is a thrombolytic agent also known as a "clot-busting drug." In order to be effective, tPA must be given within the first three hours after the onset of symptoms. The fact that a patient has received tPA is important information. A patient may be seen in hospital #1 and receive tPA intravenously and then be transferred to hospital #2 for further management of the acute myocardial infarction. If the patient has received tPA within the 24 hours prior to admission to the current facility then the coder at hospital #2 should code V45.88, Status post administration of tPA (rtPA) in a different facility within the last 24 hours prior to admission to the current facility. The condition requiring the tPA administration is coded first, such as acute MI or acute cerebral infarction. Hospital #1 does not use diagnosis code V45.88.

### Fourth-Digit Subcategories and Fifth-Digit Subclassifications

ICD-9-CM classifies myocardial infarction to category 410, with the following fourth-digit subcategories describing the specific site involved:

**410.0 Of anterolateral wall**
**ST elevation myocardial infarction of anterolateral wall**

**410.1 Of other anterior wall**
**ST elevation myocardial infarction of other anterior wall**

**410.2 Of inferolateral wall**
**ST elevation myocardial infarction of inferolateral wall**

**410.3 Of inferoposterior wall**
**ST elevation myocardial infarction of inferoposterior wall**

**410.4 Of other inferior wall**
**ST elevation myocardial infarction of other inferior wall**

**410.5 Of other lateral wall**
**ST elevation myocardial infarction of other lateral wall**

**410.6 True posterior wall infarction**
**ST elevation of true posterior wall myocardial infarction**

**410.7 Subendocardial infarction**
**Non-ST elevation myocardial infarction**

**410.8 Of other specified sites**
**ST elevation myocardial infarction of other specified sites**

**410.9 Unspecified site**
**Myocardial infarction NOS**

The following fifth-digit subclassifications to category 410, Acute myocardial infarction, are used to indicate the episode of care:

**0 episode of care unspecified**

Use fifth digit 0 when the source document does not contain sufficient information for the assignment of fifth digit 1 or 2.

**1 initial episode of care**

Use fifth digit 1 to designate the first episode of care (regardless of facility site) for a newly diagnosed myocardial infarction. The fifth digit 1 is assigned regardless of the number of times a patient may be transferred during the initial episode of care.

The fifth digit 1 is used to describe all care provided to a newly diagnosed myocardial infarction until the patient has been discharged from acute care. Acute care treatment includes any transfers to and from other acute care facilities prior to the patient's discharge that occurs within the 8-week time period. This includes transfers between acute care hospitals. It also includes transfers from acute care hospitals to long-term acute-care hospitals (LTACH), provided that the patient has not been discharged from medical care for the myocardial infarction, and the transfer to the LTACH is within the 8-week time period. The code for the acute myocardial infarction treated in the LTACH is the fifth digit 1.

**2 subsequent episode of care**

Use fifth digit 2 to designate episode of care following the initial episode when the patient is admitted for further observation, evaluation, or treatment for a myocardial infarction that has received initial treatment but is still less than eight weeks old.

If the patient is transferred to a nonacute care facility, such as a skilled nursing facility (SNF), intermediate care facility (ICF), home care, rehabilitation facility, or hospice, the fifth digit 2 is assigned when the acute myocardial infarction is treated in a nonacute care facility, and the care is provided within the 8-week time period. The fifth digit 2 is assigned if the patient is readmitted to an acute care facility from a nonacute setting or home within the 8-week time period.

**EXAMPLE:** A male patient was admitted to Hospital A with the diagnosis of acute anterolateral wall myocardial infarction. The patient was transferred to Hospital B four days later. The patient was discharged from Hospital B after undergoing cardiac catheterization.

Principal diagnosis code for Hospital A: 410.01

Principal diagnosis code for Hospital B: 410.01

**EXAMPLE:** A female patient was admitted to University Hospital for aortocoronary bypass six weeks after experiencing a myocardial infarction that was treated at a community hospital.

MI diagnosis code for University Hospital: 410.92

**EXAMPLE:** An 80-year-old woman was admitted to the SNF after a total hip replacement to treat a fractured hip. Seven weeks ago, the patient was treated for an acute inferolateral wall myocardial infarction.

MI diagnosis code for the SNF: 410.22

**EXAMPLE:** A 65-year-old man was admitted to Community Medical Center and treated for an anterior wall myocardial infarction. Subsequent coronary angiography demonstrated four-vessel coronary artery disease. The patient was discharged home to contemplate future coronary artery bypass surgery. Four weeks later, the patient was readmitted to Community Medical Center for the coronary artery bypass surgery.

MI diagnosis for first hospital stay: 410.11

MI diagnosis for second hospital stay: 410.12

#### Old Myocardial Infarction

Code 412, Old myocardial infarction, is assigned when the diagnostic statement mentions the presence of a healed MI presenting no symptoms during the current episode of care.

### *Angina*

There are two types of angina: unstable angina and angina pectoris.

#### Category 411.1, Unstable Angina

Unstable angina, also known as crescendo and preinfarction angina, is defined as the development of prolonged episodes of anginal discomfort, usually occurring at rest and requiring hospitalization to rule out a myocardial infarction.

ICD-9-CM classifies unstable angina under code 411.1, Intermediate coronary syndrome, which includes the types of angina just discussed, as well as impending or aborted myocardial infarction. Code 411.1 is assigned when a patient is admitted to the hospital and treated for unstable angina without documentation of infarction, occlusion, or thrombosis.

#### Category 413, Angina Pectoris

Angina pectoris refers to chest pain due to ischemia (loss of blood supply to a part) of the heart. The blood flow, with its supply of oxygen, is reduced because of atherosclerosis (hardening of arteries). Immediate causes of angina pectoris are exertion, stress, cold weather, or digestion of a large meal. Pain is most commonly felt beneath the sternum, and a vague or a sharp pain sometimes radiates down the left arm. Blood pressure and heart rate are increased during an attack; however, angina lasts only a few minutes and is relieved by rest and/or sublingual nitroglycerin. Angina pectoris is a warning of more severe heart disease, such as myocardial infarction or congestive heart failure.

ICD-9-CM classifies angina pectoris to category 413. The fourth-digit subcategories identify specific types of angina pectoris, such as angina decubitus and Prinzmetal angina. Other terminology includes vasospastic coronary disease, coronary vasospasm, or focal coronary artery, which is consistent with the definition of Prinzmetal or variant angina: chest pain at rest secondary to myocardial ischemia.

### Sequencing of Angina and Coronary Disease

Keep in mind the definition of principal diagnosis: "The condition established after study to be chiefly responsible for occasioning the admission of the patient to the hospital for care." (UHDDS 1985, 31038–31040).
This definition must be used when a patient suffers from angina.

**EXAMPLE:** A patient was admitted with angina. Diagnostic cardiac catheterizations determined that the angina was due to coronary atherosclerosis of the native vessels. The patient was discharged on antianginal medications.

The coronary atherosclerosis, 414.01, is listed as the principal diagnosis. Angina, 413.9, is listed as an additional diagnosis.

**EXAMPLE:** A patient was admitted with symptomatic angina that evolved into an AMI.

The AMI is sequenced as the principal diagnosis, 410.91, and no additional code is assigned for angina as it is an inherent part of the condition.

**EXAMPLE:** A patient with unstable angina was admitted to the hospital for left heart cardiac catheterization. He was found to have significant four-vessel coronary atherosclerosis. He had four-native-vessel coronary artery bypass surgery performed during the same admission.

The principal diagnosis is the coronary atherosclerosis, 414.01. The diagnosis of unstable angina, 411.1, may be listed as an additional diagnosis.

**EXAMPLE:** A patient who experienced an AMI 5 weeks ago was admitted with unstable angina. The angina was treated and no further infarction occurred.

The principal diagnosis is the unstable angina, 411.1. An additional diagnosis of the AMI, subsequent episode of care, 410.92, is also used.

Further examples of coding and sequencing of angina and coronary heart disease can be found in *Coding Clinic* 1993, 10:5, 17–24.

### Category 414, Chronic Ischemic Heart Disease

ICD-9-CM classifies chronic ischemic heart disease to category 414. Chronic ischemic heart disease (arteriosclerotic heart disease) refers to those cases in which ischemia has induced general myocardial atrophy and scattered areas of interstitial scarring. Generally, chronic ischemic heart disease results from slow, progressive narrowing of the coronary arteries. This course, however, may be altered by episodes of sudden severe coronary insufficiency. The patient with chronic ischemic heart disease may develop angina or an AMI.

### Atherosclerosis

Atherosclerosis is the formation of lesions on the inside of arterial walls from the accumulation of fat cells and platelets. The gradual enlargement of the lesion eventually weakens the arterial wall and narrows the lumen, or channel of the blood vessel, decreasing the volume of blood flow. The large arteries—the aorta and its main branches—are primarily affected, but smaller arteries such as the coronary and cerebral arteries can also be affected. In such a case, the patient experiences chest pain, shortness of breath, and sweating. Blood pressure is high; pulse is rapid and weak. An x-ray reveals cardiomegaly and narrowing, or occlusion, of the affected vessel wall. Blood tests may show hypercholesterolemia.

Atherosclerosis is the major cause of ischemia of the heart, brain, and extremities. Its complications include stroke, congestive heart failure, angina pectoris, myocardial infarction, and kidney failure. Treatment is directed toward the specific manifestation.

### Subcategories of 414, Other Forms of Chronic Ischemic Heart Disease

ICD-9-CM classifies chronic ischemic heart disease to category 414, Other forms of chronic ischemic heart disease. The fourth-digit subcategories describe specific types of ischemic heart diseases, such as coronary atherosclerosis (414.0) and aneurysm of the heart (414.1).

Subcategory code 414.0 is further expanded to fifth-digit subclassifications to identify whether the atherosclerosis is present in a native artery, in a bypass graft, or in a coronary artery of a transplanted heart. These fifth-digit codes are vessel specific and should be assigned when the physician's documentation states that atherosclerosis has been found in that specific vessel. A fifth-digit code should not be assigned based solely on the fact that a patient has atherosclerosis and a history of bypass surgery. An explanation of these fifth-digit codes follows:

1. Code 414.00 is assigned when there is no information in the health record as to whether the disease is present in a native vessel or a graft.
2. Code 414.01 is assigned to show coronary artery disease in a native coronary artery. This code is used when a patient has coronary artery disease and no history of coronary artery bypass graft (CABG) surgery. This code may be used if a patient, who in the past had a percutaneous transluminal coronary angioplasty (PTCA), has vessels that have reoccluded as demonstrated by a recent cardiac catheterization (AHA 1995, 17).
3. Code 414.02 is assigned to show coronary artery disease in an autologous vein bypass graft. Vein bypass grafts have been the most commonly performed CABG in the past. Patients who had a CABG procedure several years ago probably had saphenous veins used for graft material. Often these patients are readmitted for a "redo" CABG procedure.
4. Code 414.03 is assigned to show coronary artery disease in a nonautologous biological bypass graft.
5. Code 414.04 is assigned if the physician documents the diagnosis of coronary atherosclerosis in an artery used for a bypass graft.

6. Code 414.05 is assigned if the physician documents the diagnosis of coronary atherosclerosis in a bypass graft and the patient has a history of CABG surgery. This code is used when there is no further documentation of the type of bypass graft used.
7. Code 414.06 is assigned when atherosclerosis develops in the native coronary artery of a transplanted heart. It is presumed that the development of atherosclerosis is a natural process and not a complication of the transplant.
8. Code 414.07 is assigned when coronary atherosclerosis is present in the artery or vein bypass graft(s) of the transplanted heart.

Subcategory code 414.1 differentiates between aneurysms and dissections of the heart. Code 414.12 is included for dissection of the coronary artery. An arterial dissection is characterized by blood coursing within the layers of the arterial wall and is not an aneurysm. The term *dissecting aneurysm* has been removed from code 441.0, Dissection of aorta. Arterial dissections are a common complication of interventional radiology procedures. Although the aorta is the most common site for dissections, they can occur in other arteries in the body. Subcategory, 443.2, Other arterial dissection, contains fifth-digit subclassifications to describe dissections of the carotid, iliac, renal, vertebral, and other arteries.

Subcategory 414.2, Chronic total occlusion of coronary artery, is used as an additional code when a patient with coronary atherosclerosis (414.00–414.07) also has the complete blockage of a coronary artery. There is an increased risk of myocardial infarction or death for individuals with chronic total occlusion of a coronary artery. Chronic total occlusion of a coronary artery may be treated with angioplasty or stent placement, which is technically more difficult to perform than an angioplasty or stent placement in a patient with less than total occlusion of a coronary artery.

Subcategory 414.3, Coronary atherosclerosis due to lipid rich plaque, identifies the type of plaque within a coronary artery. This diagnostic information is important to the cardiologist in determining the most appropriate type of stent (drug-eluting or bare metal) to place in the vessel depending on the location and amount of lipid-rich plaque present. Code 414.3 is used in addition to a code for the location and type of coronary artherosclerosis (414.00–414.07) that exists in the patient.

Subcategory code 414.8, Other specified forms of chronic ischemic heart disease, includes an important note:

**414.8 Other specified forms of chronic ischemic heart disease**

Chronic coronary insufficiency
Ischemia, myocardial (chronic)
Any condition classifiable to 410 specified as chronic, or
presenting with symptoms after 8 weeks from date of infarction

*Excludes:* *coronary insufficiency (acute) (411.89)*

The preceding note advises that code 414.8 should be assigned if a diagnosis states chronic myocardial infarction with symptoms presenting eight weeks after the date of the infarction.

## Exercise 10.3

Assign ICD-9-CM codes to the following:

1. AMI of inferolateral wall, initial episode of care

2. Old myocardial infarction

3. Arteriosclerotic heart disease (native coronary artery) with angina pectoris

4. Coronary arteriosclerosis involving an autologous vein bypass graft

5. Preinfarction syndrome

## Category 428, Heart Failure

Heart failure is the heart's inability to contract with enough force to properly pump blood. This condition may be caused by coronary artery disease (usually in a patient with a previous myocardial infarction), cardiomyopathy, hypertension, or heart valve disease. Sometimes the exact cause of heart failure is not found. Heart failure may develop gradually or occur acutely.

Heart failure has the following three effects:

- **Pressure in the lungs is increased.** Fluid collects in the lung tissue, inhibiting $O_2$ and $CO_2$ exchange.
- **Kidney function is hampered.** Blood does not filter well, and body sodium and water retention increase, resulting in edema.
- **Blood is not properly circulated throughout the body.** Fluid collects in tissues, resulting in edema of the feet and legs.

Symptoms of heart failure include:

- Sudden weight gain, such as three or more pounds a day or five or more pounds a week
- Shortness of breath or difficulty breathing, especially while at rest or when lying flat in bed
- Waking up breathless at night, trouble sleeping, using more pillows
- Frequent dry, hacking cough, especially when lying down
- Increased fatigue and weakness, feeling tired all the time
- Dizziness or fainting

- Swollen feet, ankles, and legs
- Nausea with abdominal swelling, pain, and tenderness (HHS 1994)

The symptoms are caused by the inability of the heart to pump with adequate strength. Heart failure can involve the heart's left side, right side or both sides. However, it usually affects the left side first. An illustration of the blood flow within the heart and lungs is shown in figure 10.2.

**Figure 10.2.** Blood flow within the heart and lungs

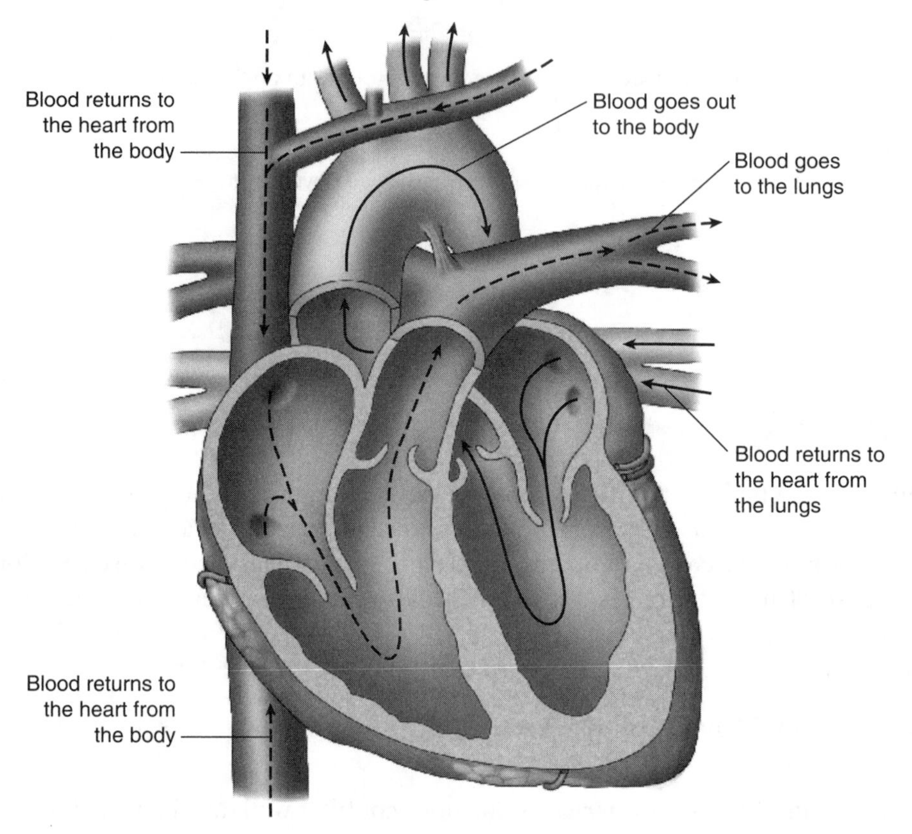




### Left-sided Heart Failure

The heart's pumping action moves oxygen-rich blood from the lungs to the left atrium and then on to the left ventricle, which pumps it to the rest of the body. The left ventricle supplies most of the heart's pumping power, so it is larger than the other chambers and essential for normal function. In left-sided or left ventricular (LV) heart failure, the left side of the heart must work harder to pump the same amount of blood.

There are two types of left-sided heart failure. Drug treatments are different for the two types.

- Systolic failure: The left ventricle loses its ability to contract normally. The heart cannot pump with sufficient force to push enough blood into circulation.
- Diastolic failure: The left ventricle loses its ability to relax normally (because the muscle has become stiff). The heart cannot properly fill with blood during the resting period between each beat.

### Right-sided Heart Failure

The heart's pumping action also moves deoxygenated blood, which returns through the veins to the heart, through the right atrium, and into the right ventricle. The right ventricle then pumps the blood back out of the heart into the lungs to be replenished with oxygen.

Right-sided or right ventricular (RV) heart failure usually occurs as a result of left-sided failure. When the left ventricle fails, increased fluid pressure is, in effect, transferred back through the lungs, ultimately damaging the heart's right side. When the right side loses pumping power, blood backs up in the body's veins. This usually causes swelling in the legs and ankles.

### Congestive Heart Failure

Congestive heart failure is another type of heart failure (sometimes the terms "congestive heart failure" and "heart failure" are used interchangeably) that requires seeking timely medical attention.

As bloodflow out of the heart slows, blood returning to the heart through the veins backs up, causing congestion in the body's tissues. Most often there is swelling in the legs and ankles, but it can occur in other parts of the body, too.

Sometimes fluid collects in the lungs and interferes with breathing, causing shortness of breath, especially when a person is lying down. This condition is called pulmonary edema and, if left untreated, can cause respiratory distress.

Heart failure also affects the kidneys' ability to dispose of sodium and water. This retained water also increases swelling in the body's tissues.

ICD-9-CM category 428 includes codes that distinguish between congestive heart failure (428.0), systolic heart failure (428.2), diastolic heart failure (428.3), and combined systolic and diastolic heart failure (428.4.) With the exception of 428.0, the subcategories require a fifth digit to describe the acute, chronic, acute on chronic, and unspecified forms of heart failure that can exist.

### Diagnostic Tests

Several diagnostic tests are important in diagnosing heart failure in a patient. Typical remarks on a chest x-ray indicating heart failure include hilar congestion, "butterfly" or "batwing" appearance of vascular markings, bronchial edema, Kerley B lines signifying chronic elevation of left atrial pressure, and heart enlargement. An echocardiograph measures the amount of blood pumped from the heart with each beat. This measurement is known as the ejection fraction. A normal heart pumps one half (50 percent) or more of the blood in the left ventricle with each heartbeat. With heart failure, the weakened heart may pump 40 percent or less, and less blood is pumped with less force to all parts of the body.

Urinalysis results show slight albuminuria, increased concentration with specific gravity of 1.020, and urine sodium decreased. Laboratory findings may include blood urea nitrogen (BUN) 60 mg/100 ml; acidosis –pH 7.35 due to increased $CO_2$ in blood from pulmonary insufficiency; blood volume increased with decrease in chloride, albumin, and total protein.

For most patients, heart failure is a chronic condition, which means it can be treated and managed, but not cured. Usually the patient's management plan consists of medications, such as angiotensin-converting enzyme (ACE) inhibitors; diuretics and digitalis; low sodium diet; possibly some modifications in daily activities; regular exercise such as walking and swimming; and other changes in lifestyle and health habits such as reducing alcohol consumption and quitting smoking.

## Cardiac Arrhythmias and Conduction Disorders

Cardiac arrhythmias identify disturbances or impairments of the normal electrical activity of heart muscle excitation. ICD-9-CM classifies cardiac arrhythmias to several categories depending on the specific type. Without further specification as to the type of cardiac arrhythmia, code 427.9 may be reported. A discussion of common arrhythmias follows:

**Atrial fibrillation (427.31)** is commonly associated with organic heart diseases, such as coronary artery disease, hypertension and rheumatic mitral valve disease, thyrotoxicosis, pericarditis, and pulmonary embolism. Treatment includes pharmacologic therapy (verapamil, digoxin, or propranolol) and cardioversion.

**Atrial flutter (427.32)** is associated with organic heart diseases, such as coronary artery disease, hypertension, and rheumatic mitral valve disease. Treatment is similar to that for atrial fibrillation.

**Ventricular fibrillation (427.41)** involves no cardiac output and is associated with cardiac arrest. Treatment is consistent with that for cardiac arrest.

**Paroxysmal supraventricular tachycardia (427.0)** is associated with congenital accessory atrial conduction pathway, physical or psychological stress, hypoxia, hypokalemia, caffeine and marijuana use, stimulants, and digitalis toxicity. Treatment includes pharmacologic therapy (quinidine, propranolol, or verapamil) and cardioversion.

**Sick sinus syndrome (SSS) (427.81)** is an imprecise diagnosis with various characteristics. SSS may be diagnosed when a patient presents with sinus arrest, sinoatrial exit block, or persistent sinus bradycardia. This syndrome is often the result of drug therapy, such as digitalis, calcium channel blockers, beta-blockers, sympatholytic agents, or antiarrhythmics. Another presentation includes recurrent supraventricular tachycardias associated with bradyarrhythmias. Prolonged ambulatory monitoring may be indicated to establish a diagnosis of SSS. Treatment includes insertion of a permanent cardiac pacemaker.

**Various forms of conduction disorders** may be classified in ICD-9-CM. Conduction disorders are disruptions or disturbances in the electrical impulses that regulate the heartbeats.

**Wolff-Parkinson-White (WPW) syndrome (426.7)** is caused by conduction from the sinoatrial node to the ventricle through an accessory pathway that bypasses the atrioventricular node. Patients with WPW syndrome present with tachyarrhythmias, including supraventricular tachycardia, atrial fibrillation, or atrial flutter. Treatment includes catheter ablation following electrophysiologic evaluation.

**Atrioventricular (AV) heart blocks** are classified as first, second, or third degree.

- **First-degree AV block** is associated with atrial septal defects or valvular disease. ICD-9-CM classifies first-degree AV block to code 426.11.
- **Second-degree AV block** is further classified as follows:
  - **Mobitz type I (Wenckebach)** is associated with acute inferior wall myocardial infarction or with digitalis toxicity. Treatment includes discontinuation of digitalis and administration of atropine. ICD-9-CM classifies Mobitz type I AV block to code 426.13.
  - **Mobitz type II** is associated with anterior wall or anteroseptal myocardial infarction and digitalis toxicity. Treatment includes temporary pacing and, in some cases, permanent pacemaker insertion, as well as discontinuation of digitalis and administration of atropine. ICD-9-CM classifies Mobitz type II AV block to code 426.12.

- **Third-degree heart block,** also referred to as complete heart block, is associated with ischemic heart disease or infarction, postsurgical complication of mitral valve replacement, digitalis toxicity, and Stokes-Adams syndrome. Treatment includes permanent cardiac pacemaker insertion. ICD-9-CM classifies third-degree heart block to code 426.0. When this type of heart block is congenital in nature, code 746.86 is reported rather than 426.0.
- Without further specification, AV block is reported with code 426.10.

**Sinus tachycardia** is a heart rate over 90 beats per minute triggered by the sinoatrial node, usually in response to exogenous factors, such as fever, exercise, anxiety, stress, pain, thyroid hormone, hypoxia, and dehydration. It may also accompany shock, left ventricular failure, cardiac tamponade, anemia, hyperthyroidism, hypovolemia, pulmonary embolism, and anterior myocardial infarction. Tachycardia is also a response to stimulants such as caffeine, cocaine, or amphetamines. Treatment is geared toward correcting the underlying cause. ICD-9-CM classifies sinus tachycardia, as well as supraventricular tachycardia, to code 427.89.

## Cardiac Arrest

Cardiac arrest, code 427.5 (excluding cardiac arrest that occurs with pregnancy, anesthesia overdose or wrong substance given, and postoperative complications), may be assigned as a principal diagnosis under the following circumstance:

- The patient arrives in the hospital in a state of cardiac arrest and cannot be resuscitated or is only briefly resuscitated, and is pronounced dead with the underlying cause of the cardiac arrest not established or unknown. This applies whether the patient is only seen in the emergency department or is admitted to the hospital and the underlying cause is not determined prior to death.

Cardiac arrest may be used as a secondary diagnosis in the following situations:

- The patient arrives at the hospital's emergency department in a state of cardiac arrest and is resuscitated and admitted with the condition prompting the cardiac arrest known, such as trauma or ventricular tachycardia. The condition causing the cardiac arrest is sequenced first with the cardiac arrest code listed as a secondary code.
- When cardiac arrest occurs during the course of the hospital stay and the condition prompting the cardiac arrest is known, the condition causing the arrest is sequenced first, followed by code 427.5, when it meets the definition of a reportable additional diagnosis, regardless of whether the patient is resuscitated or not.
- When cardiac arrest occurs during or following surgery, assign two codes, 997.1, Complications affecting specified body systems, not elsewhere classified, cardiac complications and 427.5, Cardiac arrest, as additional diagnosis, when cardiac arrest is documented as occurring during or following surgery, regardless of outcome (successfully resuscitated or not resuscitated).

When the physician documents cardiac arrest to describe an inpatient death, code 427.5 should not be assigned when the underlying cause or contributing cause of death is known. The patient's discharge disposition as expired will be collected as a data element required under the Uniform Hospital Discharge Data Set (UHDDS).

## Exercise 10.4

Assign ICD-9-CM codes to the following:

1. Benign hypertensive cardiomegaly

2. Pulmonary hypertension

3. Alcoholic cardiomyopathy

4. Atrial fibrillation

5. Acute endocarditis due to *Streptococcus* infection

6. Atrioventricular block, Mobitz type II

7. Chronic cor pulmonale

8. Sick sinus syndrome

9. Acute pulmonary edema with left ventricular failure

10. Cardiac arrest, etiology unknown

## Cerebrovascular Disease (430–438)

Cerebrovascular disease is an insufficient blood supply to a part of the brain and is usually secondary to atherosclerotic disease, hypertension, or a combination of both.

At the beginning of the Cerebrovascular Disease section, the inclusion note states that this section includes cerebrovascular diseases with mention of hypertension. The statement "Use additional code to identify presence of hypertension" also appears at the beginning of this section as an instruction to assign an additional code to describe hypertension, if present.

ICD-9-CM classifies cerebrovascular disease according to the following types of conditions:

**430 Subarachnoid hemorrhage**
**431 Intracerebral hemorrhage**
**432 Other and unspecified intracranial hemorrhage**
**433 Occlusion and stenosis of precerebral arteries**

**434 Occlusion of cerebral arteries**
**435 Transient cerebral ischemia**
**436 Acute, but ill-defined cerebrovascular disease**
**437 Other and ill-defined cerebrovascular disease**
**438 Late effects of cerebrovascular disease**

Categories 433 and 434 provide a fifth-digit subclassification that identifies the presence or absence of cerebral infarction.

### *Carotid Artery Stenosis*

Occlusion and stenosis of precerebral arteries include the carotid artery. The condition may be unilateral or bilateral. Code 433.10, Occlusion and stenosis of precerebral arteries, carotid artery, without mention of cerebral infarction, is assigned for carotid artery stenosis. Code 433.30, Occlusion and stenosis of precerebral arteries, multiple and bilateral, is assigned when any of the precerebral arteries occur bilaterally, or if multiple vessels are involved. If the physician documents the specific vessel that is occluded or stenotic and the condition exists bilaterally, it is acceptable to assign two codes. For example, if the patient has bilateral carotid artery stenosis, codes 433.10 and 433.30 may be assigned. Assigning both codes will describe both the specific artery involved and the laterality as bilateral.

### *Code 434.91, Default Code for Acute Cerebrovascular Accident*

Code 434.91, Cerebral artery occlusion, unspecified, with cerebral infarction, is assigned when the diagnosis states stroke, cerebral, or cerebrovascular accident (CVA) without further specification. The health record should be reviewed to make sure nothing more specific is available.

Conditions resulting from an acute cerebrovascular disease, such as aphasia or hemiplegia, should be coded as well, even when the deficit has been resolved at the time of discharge from the hospital.

**EXAMPLE:** Patient was admitted with aphasia and hemiplegia due to an acute CVA. The CVA and the resulting conditions were treated. On discharge, the aphasia had cleared; however, the hemiplegia is still present and will require outpatient physical therapy. Codes include 434.91, default code for acute cerebrovascular accident (CVA); 342.90, Hemiplegia and hemiparesis, unspecified; and 784.3, aphasia.

### *Category 438, Late Effects of Cerebrovascular Disease*

Category 438 codes identify late effects of cerebrovascular disease. Category 438 is used to indicate conditions classifiable to categories 430–437 as the causes of late effects (neurologic deficits), themselves classified elsewhere. These late effects include neurologic deficits that persist after initial onset of conditions classifiable to 430–437. The neurologic deficits caused by cerebrovascular disease may be present from the onset or may arise at any time after the onset of the condition classifiable to 430–437.

**EXAMPLE:** Patient was admitted for physical therapy for monoplegia of the leg affecting the nondominant side due to an old CVA. Codes include V57.1, Other physical therapy; 438.42, Late effect of cerebrovascular disease, monoplegia of lower limb affecting nondominant side.

The documentation in the health record may state the late effect in any of the following ways:

- 438.11, Aphasia, late effect of a CVA
- 438.21, Hemiplegia of the dominant side following a CVA one year ago
- 438.82, Dysphagia, sequelae of old CVA

When the health record documentation indicates previous CVA with no neurologic deficits, assign code V12.54, Personal history of transient ischemic attack (TIA), and cerebral infarction without residual deficits. In this circumstance, it is incorrect to assign a code from category 438.

The code V12.54 is located in the Alphabetic Index under "History (personal), stroke without residual deficits, V12.54" and "History (personal), infarction, cerebral, without residual deficits V12.54."

Codes from category 438 may be assigned on a healthcare record with codes from 430–437, if the patient has a current CVA and deficits from an old CVA.

**EXAMPLE:** Patient was admitted with occlusion of cerebral arteries resulting in infarction. Patient has a history of previous CVA 1 year ago with residual hemiplegia affecting the dominant side. Codes include 434.91, Cerebral artery occlusion, unspecified, with cerebral infarction; 438.21, Late effect of cerebrovascular disease, hemiplegia affecting dominant side.

## Venous Embolism and Thrombosis

Venous embolism and thrombosis, also referred to as venous thromboembolism (VTE), is an occlusion within the venous system. The terms deep vein thrombosis (DVT) and VTE are commonly documented in health records. Venous embolism and thrombosis may occur in deep and superficial veins. These conditions may occur in the thorax, neck, and upper and lower extremities. The patient with a new or acute venous embolism and thrombosis conditions requires the initiation of anticoagulant therapy. The patient with the diagnosis of chronic or old venous embolism and thrombosis continues to receive anticoagulant therapy over a period of time but is no longer in the acute phase of the illness.

Category code 453, Other venous embolism and thrombosis, contains three and four digit codes that distinguish between the location of the VTE and the acute versus chronic status of the condition. Excluded from this category is the personal history of venous thrombosis and embolism, V12.51, which describes the VTE condition that has resolved or no longer exists. A "use additional code" note appears under the subcategory codes for chronic VTEs to use code V58.61 for associated long-term (current) use of anticoagulants, if applicable.

Deep veins in the lower extremity include the femoral, iliac, popliteal, peroneal, and tibial vessels in the thigh and calf. Superficial veins in the lower extremity include the greater and lesser saphenous vein. Deep veins in the upper extremity include the brachial, radial, and ulnar veins. Superficial veins in the upper extremity include the antecubital, basilica, and cephalic veins.

Specific diagnosis codes for VTEs are:

Lower extremity occurring in the:
Deep veins with acute status, 453.40–453.42
Deep veins with chronic status, 453.50–453.52
Superficial veins, 453.6

Upper extremity occurring in the:
  Deep, superficial and unspecified veins with acute status, 453.81–453.82–453.83
  Deep, superficial and unspecified veins with chronic status, 453.71–453.72–453.73

Thorax and neck vessels such as the axillary, subclavian, internal jugular and other thoracic veins as:
  Acute, 453.84–453.85–453.86–453.87
  Chronic, 453.74–453.75–453.76–453.77

Other specified veins described as:
  Acute, 453.89
  Chronic 453.79

## Exercise 10.5

Assign ICD-9-CM codes to the following:

1. Bilateral thrombosis of carotid artery; bilateral endarterectomy

2. Hypertension due to kidney stone; percutaneous kidney stone removal

3. Insufficiency of precerebral arteries

4. Acute DVT of the iliac vein

5. Generalized cerebral ischemia

6. Thrombotic infarction of brain; no residual effects

7. Nontraumatic subdural hematoma

8. Atherosclerosis of lower extremity with intermittent claudication and gangrene; right femoro-popliteal artery bypass graft

9. Varicose veins of lower extremities with stasis dermatitis

10. Bleeding esophageal varices in patient with portal hypertension

11. Ruptured berry aneurysm

*(Continued on next page)*

## Exercise 10.5 (Continued)

12. Acute nontransmural myocardial infarction, initial episode; ventricular fibrillation

13. Congestive heart failure with severe pleural effusion; diabetes mellitus, type I; thoracentesis

14. Congestive heart failure; malignant hypertension

15. Mitral valve insufficiency, nonrheumatic

16. Chronic kidney disease, stage II with benign hypertension

17. Endocarditis in patient due to disseminated lupus erythematosus

18. Thrombophlebitis of deep femoral vein; chronic pulmonary emboli on anticoagulant drug therapy

19. Internal hemorrhoids with bleeding and prolapse; hemorrhoidectomy by ligation

20. Wolff-Parkinson-White syndrome

# Cardiovascular Procedures

This section highlights several cardiovascular procedures commonly performed, including diagnostic catheterization studies, coronary angioplasty, coronary bypass surgery, and insertion of pacemakers and defibrillators.

## Cardiac Catheterization (37.21–37.23)

Cardiac catheterization is a common diagnostic test used to identify, measure, and verify almost every type of intracardiac condition. The technique includes the passage of a flexible catheter through the arteries or veins into the heart chambers and vessels. Cardiac catheterizations can determine the size and location of a coronary lesion, evaluate left and right ventricular function, and measure heart pressures.

In addition to serving as a diagnostic tool, cardiac catheterizations may be therapeutic in nature. For example, both PTCAs and intracoronary streptokinase injections can be performed via cardiac catheterization.

Cardiac catheterization is most commonly performed on the left side of the heart, using the antecubital and femoral vessels. In a right heart catheterization, a catheter is inserted through the femoral or antecubital vein, advanced first into the superior or inferior vena cava, then into the right atrium, the right ventricle, and, finally, into the pulmonary artery.

In a left heart catheterization, a catheter enters the body through either the brachial artery or the femoral artery. The catheter is advanced into the aorta, through the aortic valve, and then into the left ventricle.

ICD-9-CM provides the following codes to describe cardiac catheterizations:

**37.21 Right heart catheterization**
**37.22 Left heart catheterization**
**37.23 Combined right and left heart catheterization**

## Percutaneous Transluminal Coronary Angioplasty

Percutaneous transluminal coronary angioplasty (PTCA) is used to relieve obstruction of coronary arteries. PTCA is performed to widen a narrowed area of a coronary artery by employing a balloon-tipped catheter. The catheter is passed to the obstructed area, and the balloon is inflated one or more times to exert pressure on the narrowed area. A thrombolytic agent may be infused into the heart.

A PTCA procedure may also include the insertion of one or more coronary stents. It is possible to insert stents in several different vessels during the same operative episode. It is also possible to insert multiple adjoining or overlapping stents.

Under the category heading, 36, Operations on vessels of heart, three "code also" notes are included:

- Code also any injection or infusion of platelet inhibitor (99.20)
- Code also any injection or infusion of thrombolytic agent (99.10)
- Code also cardiopulmonary bypass, if performed [extracorporeal circulation] [heart-lung machine] (39.61)

The PTCA or coronary angioplasty is identified with procedure code 00.66. It may also be referred to as a "balloon angioplasty" of a coronary artery. Another related procedure is tranluminal coronary atherectomy, identified with procedure code 17.55.

Beneath procedure codes 00.66 and 17.55 are directional notes to "code also:"

- Injection or infusion of thrombolytic agent (99.10)
- Insertion of coronary artery stent(s) (36.06–36.07)
- Intracoronary artery thrombolytic infusion (36.04)
- Number of vascular stents inserted (00.45–00.48)
- Number of vessels treated (00.40–00.43)
- Procedure on vessel bifurcation (00.44)
- SuperSaturated oxygen therapy (00.49)
- Transluminal coronary angioplasty (00.66) or atherectomy (17.55)

Code 36.06 is used for the insertion of nondrug-eluting coronary artery stent(s), which may also be referred to as bare or bare-metal stents, bonded stents, or drug-coated stents. Code 36.07 is used for the insertion of drug-eluting coronary artery stent(s).

Beneath procedure codes 36.06 and 36.07 are directional notes to "code also:"

- Number of vascular stents inserted (00.45–00.48)
- Number of vessels treated (00.40–00.43)
- Open chest coronary angioplasty (36.03)
- Percutaneous transluminal coronary angioplasty (PTCA) (00.66)
- Procedure on vessel bifurcation (00.40)
- Transluminal coronary atherectomy (17.55)

**EXAMPLE:** PTCA of left anterior descending artery with insertion of single drug-eluting stent: 00.66, 36.07, 00.40, 00.45

**EXAMPLE:** PTCA of left anterior descending artery and circumflex vessels with insertion of three non-drug-eluting stents: 00.66, 36.06, 00.41, 00.47

**A point to remember:** PTCA may also be performed on other arteries, such as carotid, renal, femoral, femoropopliteal, and vertebral.

Code 39.50, Angioplasty or atherectomy of noncoronary vessel, is available for classifying an angioplasty of the vessels of the lower extremity, mesenteric artery, renal artery, or upper extremity vessels.

Codes 00.61–00.62 describe percutaneous angioplasty or atherectomy of the precerebral (extracranial-carotid, basilar, vertebral) vessels or of the intracranial vessels.

Insertion of stents into peripheral, precerebral, and intracranial vessels is reported with the following codes:

39.90 Insertion of non-drug-eluting peripheral vessel stent(s),
00.55 Insertion of drug-eluting stent(s) of other peripheral vessel stent(s),
00.60 Insertion of drug-eluting stent(s) of superficial femoral artery
00.63 Percutaneous insertion of carotid artery stent(s),
00.64 Percutaneous insertion of other extracranial artery stent(s)
00.65 Percutaneous insertion of intracranial vascular stent(s)

In addition, the number of vascular stents inserted (00.45–00.48) and the number of vessels treated (00.40–00.43) is also coded.

## Coronary Artery Bypass Graft

Category 36.1, Bypass anastomosis for heart revascularization, includes codes for the CABG procedure. An illustration of the coronary arteries of the heart are shown in figure 10.1.

The coronary circulation consists of two main arteries, the right and the left, that are further subdivided into several branches:

- Right coronary artery
  - Right marginal
  - Right posterior descending
- Left main coronary artery
  - Left anterior descending branch
    - Diagonal
    - Septal
  - Left circumflex
    - Obtuse marginal
    - Posterior descending
    - Posterolateral

The following three surgical approaches are used in CABG procedures:

- Aortocoronary bypass uses the aorta to bypass the occluded coronary artery.
- Internal mammary-coronary artery bypass uses the internal mammary artery to bypass the occluded coronary artery.
- Abdominal-coronary artery bypass uses an abdominal artery.

### Aortocoronary Bypass or Coronary Artery Bypass Graft (CABG)

Aortocoronary bypass brings blood from the aorta into the obstructed coronary artery using a segment of the saphenous vein, radial vein, or a segment of the internal mammary artery for the graft. The procedure is commonly referred to as coronary artery bypass graft(s) or by the abbreviation CABG, pronounced "cabbage." ICD-9-CM provides the following codes to classify aortocoronary bypass, depending on the number of coronary arteries involved:

**36.10 (Aorto)coronary bypass for heart revascularization, not otherwise specified**
**36.11 (Aorto)coronary bypass of one coronary artery**
**36.12 (Aorto)coronary bypass of two coronary arteries**
**36.13 (Aorto)coronary bypass of three coronary arteries**
**36.14 (Aorto)coronary bypass of four or more coronary arteries**

### Internal Mammary-Coronary Artery Bypass

Internal mammary-coronary artery bypass is accomplished by loosening the internal mammary artery from its normal position and using the internal mammary artery to bring blood from the subclavian artery to the occluded coronary artery. Codes are selected based on whether one or both internal mammary arteries are used, regardless of the number of coronary arteries involved. ICD-9-CM provides the following two codes to classify internal mammary-coronary artery bypass:

**36.15 Single internal mammary-coronary artery bypass**
**36.16 Double internal mammary-coronary artery bypass**

### Abdominal-Coronary Artery Bypass

This type of procedure involves creating an anastomosis between an abdominal artery, commonly the gastro-epiploic, and a coronary artery beyond the occluded portion, for example, 36.17, Abdominal-coronary artery bypass (*Coding Clinic* First Quarter 1991, 7 and Coding Clinic Fourth Quarter, 1996, 64).

## Cardiac Pacemakers

A cardiac pacemaker has the following three basic components:

- The pulse generator is the pacing system that contains the pacemaker battery (power source) and the electronic circuitry.
- The pacing lead carries the stimulating electricity from the pulse generator to the stimulating electrode.
- The electrode is the metal portion of the lead that comes in contact with the heart.

There are different types of pacemakers:

- Single-chamber pacemakers use a single lead that is placed in the right atrium or the right ventricle.

- Dual-chamber pacemakers use leads that are inserted into both the atrium and the ventricle.
- Rate-responsive pacemakers have a pacing rate modality that is determined by physiological variables other than the atrial rate.
- Cardiac resynchronization pacemakers without a defibrillator (CRT-P), also are known as biventricular pacing without internal cardiac defibrillator.

### ICD-9-CM Coding Format for Pacemakers

ICD-9-CM classifies cardiac pacemakers to subcategory 37.8, Insertion, replacement, removal, and revision of pacemaker device. The note at the beginning of this subcategory states: Code also any lead insertion, lead replacement, lead removal, and/or lead revision (37.70–37.77). Therefore, a second code must be assigned to describe the insertion, replacement, removal, or revision of a lead by using codes 37.70–37.77. For example:

- In coding initial insertion of a permanent cardiac pacemaker, two codes are required: one for the pacemaker (37.80–37.83) and one for the lead (37.70–37.74).
- When a pacemaker is replaced with another pacemaker, only the replaced pacemaker is coded (37.85–37.87). Removal of the old pacemaker is included in the code for the replacement.
- Removal of a pacemaker is assigned code 37.89, Revision or removal of pacemaker device.

Also note the exclusion note in subcategory 37.8, which states that these codes exclude implantation of cardiac resynchronization pacemaker (00.50) and implantation or replacement of cardiac resynchronization pacemaker pulse generator only (00.53). Replacement of cardiac resynchronization devices or the component parts are classified with codes 00.52, 00.53, or 00.54. A simple illustration of a pacemaker is shown in figure 10.3.

**Figure 10.3.** Cardiac pacemaker

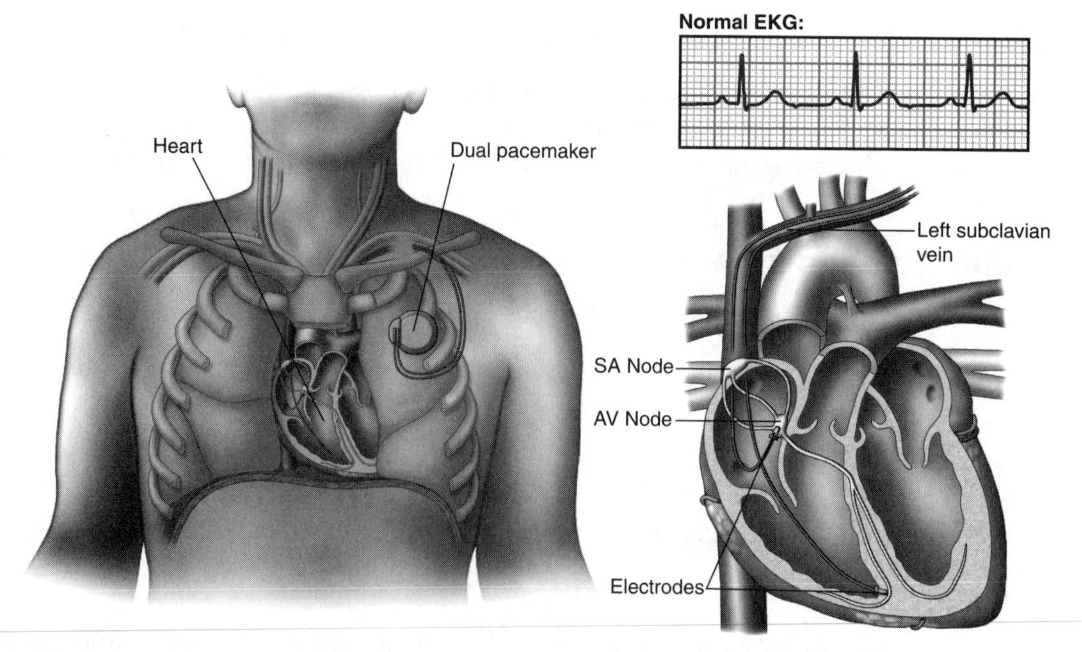

### Reprogramming of Cardiac Pacemakers

Patients admitted for reprogramming of a cardiac pacemaker are assigned diagnostic code V53.31, Fitting and adjustment of cardiac pacemaker. No procedure code in ICD-9-CM exists to describe reprogramming.

## Automatic Implantable Cardioverter-Defibrillators

The automatic implantable cardioverter-defibrillator (AICD) is a special type of pacemaker that proves effective for patients with recurring, life-threatening dysrhythmias, such as ventricular tachycardia or fibrillation.

The AICD is an electronic device consisting of a pulse generator and three leads. The pulse generator is implanted under the patient's skin, usually in the shoulder area. The first lead senses heart rate at the right ventricle; the second lead, sensing morphology and rhythm, defibrillates at the right atrium; the third lead defibrillates at the apical pericardium. The AICD can be programmed to suit each patient's needs, and it uses far less energy than an external defibrillator.

ICD-9-CM classifies the AICD to code 37.9, Other operations on heart and pericardium, and to 00.5, Other cardiovascular procedures, with the following codes available:

**37.94** **Implantation or replacement of automatic cardioverter/defibrillator, total system (AICD)**—Assign this code when a total system AICD is inserted. Total system refers to the implantation of the defibrillator with leads, formation of pocket, and any transvenous lead.

**37.95** **Implantation of automatic cardioverter/defibrillator lead(s) only**

**37.96** **Implantation of automatic cardioverter/defibrillator pulse generator only**

**37.97** **Replacement of automatic cardioverter/defibrillator lead(s) only**

**37.98** **Replacement of automatic cardioverter/defibrillator pulse generator only**

**37.99** **Other (Operations on heart and pericardium)**

**00.51** **Implantation of cardiac resynchronization defibrillator, total system (CRT-D)**

**00.54** **Implantation or replacement of cardiac resynchronization defibrillator, pulse generator device only (CRT-D)**

## Diagnostic Procedures

The following procedures are often performed during a cardiac catheterization:

- Cardiac angiography
- Coronary arteriography
- Ventriculography

### Cardiac Angiography

Cardiac angiography can be performed on the right or left side of the heart, or in a combined process including both the right and left sides of the heart. Right-side cardiac angiography is useful in detecting pericarditis and congenital lesions, such as Ebstein's malformation of the tricuspid valve. Left-side cardiac angiography reveals congenital and acquired lesions affecting the mitral valve, including mitral stenosis and mitral regurgitation.

In ICD-9-CM, cardiac or coronary angiograms are assigned to the following codes:

**88.52 Angiocardiography of right heart structures**
**88.53 Angiocardiography of left heart structures**
**88.54 Combined right and left heart angiocardiography**

### Coronary Arteriography

Coronary arteriography serves as a diagnostic tool in detecting obstruction within the coronary arteries. The following two techniques are used in performing a coronary arteriography:

- Sones technique uses a single catheter inserted via a brachial arteriotomy.
- Judkins technique uses two catheters inserted percutaneously through the femoral artery.

ICD-9-CM provides the following codes to describe coronary arteriograms:

**88.55 Coronary arteriography using a single catheter (Sones technique)**
**88.56 Coronary arteriography using two catheters (Judkins technique)**
**88.57 Other and unspecified coronary arteriography**

### Ventriculography

Ventriculograms measure stroke volume and ejection fraction. The ejection fraction is the amount of blood ejected from the left ventricle per beat; it is presented as a percentage of the total ventricular volume. The normal ejection fraction is usually between 55 and 70 percent. A fraction below 40 percent is usually a sign of heart failure A fraction between 40 and 55 percent indicates heart damage, perhaps from a previous acute myocardial infarction (American Heart Association 2014).

The Alphabetic Index in volume 3 of ICD-9-CM offers directions for coding ventriculograms. Use codes 88.52–88.54 for cardiac angiograms.

## Exercise 10.6

Assign ICD-9-CM procedure codes to the following:

1. Insertion of dual-chamber cardiac pacemaker and atrial and ventricular leads

   ______________________

2. Percutaneous transluminal angioplasty of single coronary artery with thrombolytic agent

   ______________________

3. Insertion of total system automatic implantable cardioverter-defibrillator

   ______________________

4. Right and left cardiac catheterization with Judkins coronary arteriogram and right and left ventriculogram

   ______________________

5. Coronary artery bypass graft of four vessels with cardiopulmonary bypass

   ______________________

## ICD-9-CM Review Exercises: Chapter 10

Assign the appropriate ICD-9-CM codes to the following diagnoses and procedures:

1. Venous thrombosis, greater saphenous vein, right leg

2. Acute pericardial effusion; pericardiocentesis

3. Atrial fibrillation; insertion of single-chamber, rate-responsive cardiac pacemaker with ventricular lead

4. Arteriosclerotic heart disease of autologous vein bypass graft; left cardiac catheterization, left ventriculogram, Sones arteriogram

5. Arteriosclerosis of the right lower extremity (native arteries) with rest pain, right popliteal-tibial bypass

6. Thoracic aortic aneurysm; Endovascular repair of aneurysm (EVAR) in the thoracic aorta with stent graft and with insertion of intra-aneurysm sac pressure monitoring device intra-operatively

7. Mitral valve insufficiency with prosthetic mitral valve replacement; cardiopulmonary bypass

8. AMI of the posterolateral wall, initial episode; triple coronary artery bypass using saphenous vein graft to diagonal branch and circumflex, and left internal mammary artery to left anterior descending; cardiopulmonary bypass

9. Subacute bacterial endocarditis secondary to *Staphylococcus aureus*; ventricular tachycardia

10. Acute myocardial infarction, anterior wall (initial episode); PTCA of two vessels with infusion of thrombolytic agent

11. Raynaud's disease with gangrene

12. End-stage renal disease (ESRD) with hypertension; venous catheterization for dialysis; renal dialysis

*(Continued on next page)*

## ICD-9-CM Review Exercises: Chapter 10 (Continued)

13. Infected varicose veins of the lower extremity with development of ulcer

    ______________________________

14. Occlusive disease of iliac artery; percutaneous angioplasty of iliac artery with drug-eluting stent insertion

    ______________________________

# ICD-10-CM Chapter 9, Diseases of the Circulatory System (I00–I99)

## Organization and Structure of ICD-10-CM Chapter 9

Chapter 9 of ICD-10-CM includes categories I00–I99 arranged in the following blocks:

| | |
|---|---|
| I00–I02 | Acute rheumatic fever |
| I05–I09 | Chronic rheumatic heart diseases |
| I10–I15 | Hypertensive diseases |
| I20–I25 | Ischemic heart diseases |
| I26–I28 | Pulmonary heart disease and diseases of pulmonary circulation |
| I30–I52 | Other forms of heart disease |
| I60–I69 | Cerebrovascular diseases |
| I70–I79 | Diseases of arteries, arterioles and capillaries |
| I80–I89 | Diseases of veins, lymphatic vessels and lymph nodes, not elsewhere classified |
| I95–I99 | Other and unspecified disorders of the circulatory system |

The organization of Chapter 9 in ICD-10-CM is comparable to Chapter 7 in ICD-9-CM. One change to note is the order of conditions within the block for ischemic heart disease.

In ICD-9-CM, the first condition is acute myocardial infarction. However, in ICD-10-CM angina pectoris begins the block for ischemic heart disease.

The terminology used to describe several cardiovascular conditions has been revised to reflect more current medical practice.

**EXAMPLES:**

| | | |
|---|---|---|
| **EXAMPLES:** | ICD-9-CM | 410, Acute myocardial infarction |
| | ICD-10-CM | I21, ST, elevation (STEMI) and non-ST elevation (NSTEMI) myocardial infarction |
| | ICD-9-CM | 411.1, Intermediate coronary syndrome |
| | ICD-10-CM | I20.0, Unstable angina |
| | ICD-9-CM | 411.81, Acute coronary occlusion without myocardial infarction |
| | ICD-10-CM | I24.0, Acute coronary thrombosis not resulting in myocardial infarction |

In ICD-9-CM, the code for gangrene (785.4) is classified in Chapter 16, Symptoms, Signs and Ill-Defined Conditions, whereas in ICD-10-CM this condition is classified in Chapter 9 and is coded as I96, Gangrene, NEC. Additionally, Binswanger's Disease has been reclassified from Chapter 5, Mental Disorders in ICD-9-CM to Chapter 9 in ICD-10-CM and is coded as I67.3.

The classification of hypertension has changed. In ICD-9-CM, hypertension codes classify the type of hypertension (benign, malignant, unspecified). In ICD-10-CM, hypertension codes no longer classify the type.

## Coding Guidelines and Instructional Notes for ICD-10-CM Chapter 9

The NCHS has published chapter-specific guidelines for Chapter 9 in *ICD-10-CM Official Guidelines for Coding and Reporting*:

*To gain an understanding of these rules, access the 2014 guidelines from NCHS website (http://www.cdc.gov/nchs/icd/icd10cm.htm) and read Chapter 9, Diseases of the Circulatory System guidelines I.C.9.a through I.C.9.e on starting on page 41.*

There are changes to a number of codes in this chapter. For example, in ICD-10-CM beneath categories I21, I22, and I23 for acute myocardial infarction are notes that state how the specific category must be used within four weeks (28 days) or less from onset. However, below category 410 in ICD-9-CM, the note refers to an 8-week or less time period.

The instructional notes and guidelines are very important for these three categories to indicate correct code usage. A code from category I22, Subsequent acute myocardial infarction, must be used in conjunction with a code from category I21, ST elevation myocardial infarction (STEMI) and non-ST elevation myocardial infarction (NSTEMI). A code from category I23, Certain current complications following ST elevation (STEMI) and non-ST elevation (NSTEMI) myocardial infarction must be used in conjunction with a code from category I21 or I22.

Instructional notes that clarify code usage are also found under specific codes. Under code I05, rheumatic mitral valve diseases, is a note that states this category includes conditions classifiable to both I05.0 and I05.2–I05.9, whether specified as rheumatic or not.

Examples of the coding guidelines for the circulatory system are:

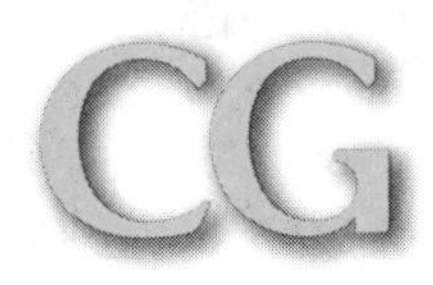


**Coding Guideline I.C.9.a.3. Hypertensive Heart and Chronic Kidney Disease**

Assign codes from combination category I13, Hypertensive heart and chronic kidney disease, when both hypertensive kidney disease and hypertensive heart disease are stated in the diagnosis. Assume a relationship between the hypertension and the chronic kidney disease, whether or not the condition is so designated. If heart failure is present, assign an additional code from category I50 to identify the type of heart failure.

**Coding Guideline I.C.9.b. Atherosclerotic Coronary Artery Disease and Angina**

ICD-10-CM has combination codes for atherosclerotic heart disease with angina pectoris. The subcategories for these codes are I25.11, Atherosclerotic heart disease

(*Continued*)

(*Continued*)

of native coronary artery with angina pectoris, and I25.7, Atherosclerosis of coronary artery bypass graft(s) and coronary artery of transplanted heart with angina pectoris.

When using one of these combination codes, it is not necessary to use an additional code for angina pectoris. A causal relationship can be assumed in a patient with both atherosclerosis and angina pectoris, unless the documentation indicates the angina is due to something other than the atherosclerosis.

**Coding Guideline I.C.9.d.1. Category I69, Sequelae of Cerebrovascular Disease**

Category I69 is used to indicate conditions classifiable to categories I60–I67 as the causes of late effect (neurologic deficits), themselves classified elsewhere. These "late effects" include neurologic deficits that persist after the initial onset of conditions classifiable to categories I60–I67. The neurologic deficits caused by cerebrovascular disease may be present from the onset or may arise at any time after the onset of the condition classifiable to categories I60–I67.

**Coding Guideline I.C.9.e.1. ST Elevation Myocardial Infarction (STEMI) and Non-ST Elevation Myocardial Infarction (NSTEMI)**

If NSTEMI evolves to STEMI, assign the STEMI code. If STEMI converts to NSTEMI due to thrombolytic therapy, it is still coded as a STEMI.

**Coding Guideline I.C.9.e.3. AMI Documented as Nontransmural or Subendocardial but Site Provided.**

If an AMI is documented as nontransmural or subendocardial but the site is provided, it is still coded as subendocardial AMI.

**Coding Guideline I.C.9.e.4. Subsequent Myocardial Infarction**

A code from category I22, Subsequent ST elevation (STEMI) and non-ST elevation (NSTEMI) myocardial infarction is to be used when a patient who has suffered an AMI has a new AMI within the 4-week time frame of the initial AMI. A code from category I22 must be used in conjunction with a code from category I21.

The sequencing of I22 and I21 codes depends on the circumstances of the encounter. Should a patient who is in the hospital due to an AMI have a subsequent AMI while still in the hospital, code I21 would be sequenced first as the reason for admission, with code I22 sequenced as a secondary code. Should a patient have a subsequent AMI after discharge for care of an initial AMI, and the reason for admission is the subsequent AMI, the I22 code should be sequenced first followed by the I21. An I21 code must accompany an I22 code to identify the site of the initial AMI, and to indicate that the patient is still within the 4-week time frame of healing from the initial AMI.

## Coding Overview for ICD-10-CM Chapter 9

ICD-10-CM's Chapter 9, Diseases of the Circulatory System (I00–I99), contains an expanded number of very specific codes that describe coronary, cerebral, and vascular diseases. "Use additional code to identify" notes appear throughout the chapter to direct the coder to identify exposure to, history of current use, and dependence of tobacco. Codes also specify the laterality of vessels to identify the specific location of disease, for example, left middle cerebral artery.

### Hypertensive Disease

The hypertension table was eliminated in ICD-10-CM and replaced with regular Alphabetic Index entries. The codes follow the same pattern as ICD-9-CM, with combination codes for hypertensive heart and hypertensive kidney disease and additional codes for coding heart failure and chronic kidney disease as applicable for each patient. The type of hypertension (benign, malignant, unspecified) is not used as an axis for the ICD-10-CM hypertension codes. There is only one code for essential hypertension (I10).

### Ischemic Heart Disease

Combination codes in ICD-10-CM include atherosclerotic heart disease with angina and appear in category I25, Chronic ischemic heart disease. This placement eliminates the need to use an additional code for angina pectoris or unstable angina. The I25 category codes in ICD-10-CM contain details about the location of the coronary artery disease, such as native vessel or bypass graft, and the type of angina, such as unstable, with documented spasm, as well as other forms of angina pectoris.

### Cerebrovascular Disease

ICD-10-CM contains very specific codes to identify various forms of cerebral vascular accidents (CVAs). The codes specify whether the condition is a cerebral hemorrhage or infarction due to a thrombosis, embolism, or unspecified occlusion or stenosis in the cerebral vessel. The cerebral infarction codes identify the specific cerebral artery involved and laterality (right or left). Category I69, Sequelae of cerebrovascular disease, contains many codes for very specific conditions that remain after the acute CVA is treated.

The category for late effects of cerebrovascular disease has been retitled "Sequelae of cerebrovascular disease," and it has been restructured by expanding all subcategory codes. This expansion involves specifying laterality, changing subcategory titles, making terminology changes, adding sixth characters, and providing greater specificity in general. Sequelae of cerebrovascular disease are differentiated by type of stroke (hemorrhage, infarction).

### Venous Embolism, Thrombosis, and Thrombophlebitis

Very specific codes exist in ICD-10-CM to describe acute and chronic deep and superficial vein thrombosis. The codes identify the specific vessel involved and the right or left side of the body. This same type of detail is also included in the thrombophlebitis and varicose vein codes.

### Intraoperative and Postprocedural Circulatory Complications

Intraoperative and postprocedural circulatory complications can be identified with greater specificity in ICD-10-CM than in ICD-9-CM. For example, different codes exist for:

- Intraoperative versus postprocedural cardiac arrest
- Postprocedural hypertension
- Postprocedural heart failure
- Intraoperative and postprocedural cerebral infarction
- Accidental puncture or laceration during a circulatory system procedure
- Accidental puncture or laceration of a circulatory system organ during another body system procedure

## Acute Myocardial Infarction (AMI)

The coding of AMI is quite different in ICD-10-CM than in ICD-9-CM. The AMI codes—ICD-10-CM categories I21 and I22—do not use a fifth digit to describe the episode of care as was the case in ICD-9-CM. Instead, codes are described as STEMI and NSTEMI conditions involving different parts of the heart wall and arteries.

Certain current complications following STEMI and NSTEMI myocardial infarctions are reported with category I23 codes when the condition occurs within 28 days after the infarction. This is a different time period than the eight weeks identified by the subsequent MI codes in ICD-9-CM.

Specific ICD-10-CM coding guidelines exist for the coding of current and subsequent AMIs with AMI complication codes and likely will challenge new ICD-10-CM coders as they begin to use the classification system.

In the acute myocardial infarction codes, STEMI and NSTEMI are in the ICD-10-CM code titles instead of just being inclusion terms.

Chapter 9 contains codes for initial AMIs (I21) and subsequent AMIs (I22). A code from category I22, Subsequent STEMI and NSTEMI myocardial infarction is to be used when a patient who has suffered an AMI has a new AMI within the 4-week time frame of the initial AMI. A code from category I22 must be used in conjunction with a code from category I21, STEMI and NSTEMI myocardial infarction. Category I22 is never used alone. The sequencing of the I22 and I21 codes depends on the circumstances of the encounter.

An important note to remember is that a code from category I22 must be used in conjunction with a code from category I21. The I22 code should be sequenced first, if it is the reason for encounter, or, it should be sequenced after the I21 code if the subsequent MI occurs during the encounter for the initial MI. Also watch for notes to use additional codes to identify body mass index (BMI), if known, and tobacco use or exposure.

## ICD-10-CM Review Exercises: Chapter 10

Assign the correct ICD-10-CM diagnosis codes to the following.

1. Benign hypertension

2. Stage 3 chronic kidney disease with congestive heart failure (CHF) due to hypertension

3. Acute non-ST anterior wall myocardial infarction. Atrial fibrillation.

4. Acute on chronic diastolic congestive heart failure

5. Postinfarction angina. Patient was discharged two days ago after treatment for an anterior wall ST elevation myocardial infarction

6. Coronary artery disease (CAD) with angina. This patient has no previous history of CABG.

7. Unstable angina. History of 2-vessel coronary artery bypass approximately 18 months ago. A recent cardiac catheterization shows continued evidence of coronary arteriosclerosis but both of the bypass grafts are patent. Also, this patient suffered a cerebrovascular infarction three years ago which resulted in right-side (dominant) hemiparesis.

8. Progressive episodes of chest pain determined to be crescendo angina. The patient has no previous history of CABG. He had myocardial infarction five years ago and was diagnosed with coronary artery disease and progressively has been having more frequent episodes of chest pain.

9. Acute cerebral infarction, thrombosis of the left anterior cerebral artery with residual right-sided hemiplegia

10. Cerebrovascular infarction six months ago with remaining aphasia and left-sided hemiparesis on his nondominant side

11. Acute cerebrovascular infarction—embolism of the left cerebellar artery with dysphagia and right hemiplegia.

12. Continuing unstable angina found to be due to atherosclerosis of his bypass using autologous artery. Hypertensive congestive heart failure.

13. Current inferolateral ST elevation myocardial infarction complicated by the development a hemopericardium as a result of the infarction.

*(Continued on next page)*

## ICD-10-CM Review Exercises: Chapter 10 (Continued)

14. The same patient from exercise #3 presented to the emergency department two weeks later and was diagnosed with an acute inferior wall myocardial infarction. She is still being monitored following her initial heart attack three weeks earlier and continues to have atrial fibrillation.

 ______________________________

15. Postprocedural hematoma right groin vessel following/due to a cardiac catheterization procedure.

 ______________________________

# Chapter 11

# Diseases of the Respiratory System

## Learning Objectives

At the conclusion of this chapter, you should be able to:

1. Describe the organization of the conditions and codes included in Chapter 8 of ICD-9-CM, Diseases of the Respiratory System (460–519)
2. Describe the organization of the conditions and codes included in Chapter 10 of ICD-10-CM, Diseases of the Respiratory System (J00–J99)
3. Define *bronchitis* and identify the different ICD-9-CM and ICD-10-CM codes used to describe it
4. Understand how ICD-9-CM and ICD-10-CM organizes the codes for various types of pneumonia
5. Define *asthma* and identify the different ICD-9-CM and ICD-10-CM codes used to describe it
6. Define *chronic obstructive pulmonary disease* (COPD) and identify the various conditions that may be described as forms of COPD
7. Define *respiratory failure* and understand the ICD-9-CM and ICD-10-CM coding and sequencing rules for assigning respiratory failure codes
8. Briefly describe the ICD-9-CM procedure coding of mechanical ventilation and the procedures associated with it
9. Assign ICD-9-CM diagnosis and procedure codes for diseases of the respiratory system
10. Assign ICD-10-CM codes for disease of the respiratory system

# ICD-9-CM Chapter 8, Diseases of the Respiratory System (460–519)

Chapter 8, Diseases of the Respiratory System, in the Tabular List in volume 1 of ICD-9-CM is subdivided into the following categories and section titles:

| Categories | Section Titles |
|---|---|
| 460–466 | Acute Respiratory Infections |
| 470–478 | Other Diseases of the Upper Respiratory Tract |
| 480–488 | Pneumonia and Influenza |
| 490–496 | Chronic Obstructive Pulmonary Disease and Allied Conditions |
| 500–508 | Pneumoconioses and Other Lung Diseases Due to External Agents |
| 510–519 | Other Diseases of the Respiratory System |

This chapter highlights coding instructions for specific respiratory conditions. A diagram of the respiratory track including the trachea, bronchi and lungs is shown in figure 11.1.

**Figure 11.1.** Diagram of the respiratory track

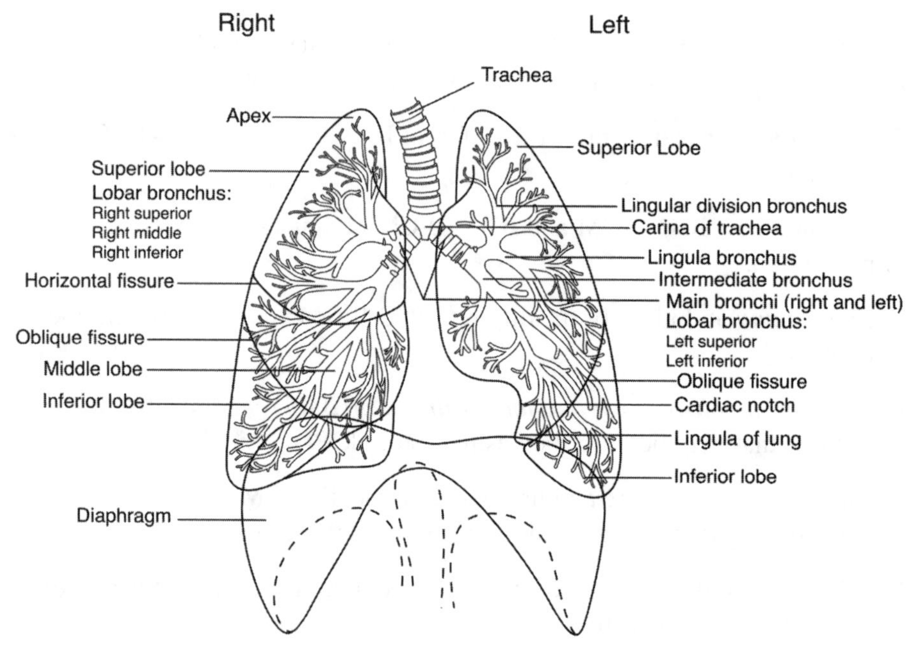




## Bronchitis

Bronchitis is an inflammation of the bronchi and can be acute or chronic in nature. Acute bronchitis is an inflammation of the tracheobronchial tree with a short and more or less severe course. It is often due to exposure to cold, inhalation of irritant substances, or acute infections. Chronic bronchitis is a condition associated with prolonged exposure to nonspecific bronchial irritants and is accompanied by mucus hypersecretion and certain structural changes in the bronchi. Usually associated with cigarette smoking, one form of bronchitis is characterized clinically by a chronic productive cough.

ICD-9-CM provides separate codes to describe acute and chronic bronchitis. The following acute conditions of bronchitis are classified to code 466.0:

**466.0 Acute bronchitis**
Bronchitis, acute or subacute:
fibrinous
membranous
pneumococcal
purulent
septic
viral
with tracheitis
Croupous bronchitis
Tracheobronchitis, acute

Code 490, Bronchitis, not specified as acute or chronic, is assigned when the specific type of bronchitis is not documented in the health record. Chronic bronchitis is included in the section titled "Chronic Obstructive Pulmonary Disease and Allied Conditions." Category 491, Chronic bronchitis, is subdivided to describe the types of chronic bronchitis, such as simple, mucopurulent, and obstructive.

**A point to remember:** When chronic bronchitis is described as obstructive or is associated with COPD, a code from subcategory 491.2 should be reported.

## Pneumonia

The third and fifth sections of Chapter 8 include codes for pneumonias, with the following separate categories identifying the underlying organism or site:

| | |
|---|---|
| **480** | **Viral pneumonia** |
| **481** | **Pneumococcal pneumonia [Streptococcus pneumoniae pneumonia]** |
| **482** | **Other bacterial pneumonia** |
| **483** | **Pneumonia due to other specified organism** |
| **484** | **Pneumonia in infectious diseases classified elsewhere** |
| **485** | **Bronchopneumonia, organism unspecified** |
| **486** | **Pneumonia, organism unspecified** |
| **487.0** | **Influenza with pneumonia** |
| **488.01 and 488.11** | **Influenza due to certain identified influenza viruses with pneumonia** |
| **488.81** | **Influenza due to identified novel influenza A virus with pneumonia** |
| **507** | **Pneumonitis due to solids and liquids** |
| **516.3** | **Idiopathic interstitial pneumonia** |
| **516.8** | **Other specified alveolar and parietoalveolar pneumonopathy** |

### *Category 480, Viral Pneumonia*

Category 480, Viral pneumonia, is subdivided to fourth-digit subcategories that identify the specific virus. Viral pneumonia is a highly contagious disease affecting both the trachea and the bronchi of the lungs. Inflammation destroys the action of the cilia and causes hemorrhage. Isolation of the virus is difficult, and x-rays do not reveal any pulmonary changes.

### Category 481, Pneumococcal Pneumonia

Category 481, Pneumococcal pneumonia [Streptococcus pneumoniae pneumonia], describes pneumonia caused by the pneumococcal bacteria. The bacteria lodge in the alveoli and cause an inflammation. If the pleura are involved, the irritated surfaces rub together and cause painful breathing. On examination, pleural friction can be heard. A chest x-ray demonstrates a consolidation of the lungs that results from pus forming in the alveoli and replacing the air. Lobar pneumonia is a type of acute bacterial pneumonia usually limited to one lobe of the lung and the most common type is pneumococcal pneumonia (Dorland 2012).

### Category 482, Other Bacterial Pneumonia

Category 482, Other bacterial pneumonia, is subdivided to fourth-digit subcategories that identify specific bacteria, such as *Klebsiella pneumoniae* (482.0), *Pseudomonas* (482.1), *Hemophilus influenzae* (482.2), *Streptococcus* (482.3x), and *Staphylococcus* (482.4x). Bacteria are the most common cause of pneumonia in adults. Gram staining is a rapid and cost-effective method for diagnosing bacterial pneumonia, if a good sputum sample is available.

### Category 483, Pneumonia Due to Other Specified Organism

Category 483 includes codes for pneumonia due to other specified organisms, including *Mycoplasma pneumoniae* (483.0). The fourth digit identifies the specific organism.

### Category 484, Pneumonia in Infectious Diseases Classified Elsewhere

Category 484, Pneumonia in infectious diseases classified elsewhere, is subdivided to fourth-digit subcategories that identify the specific infectious disease. These codes are set in italic type and thus are not meant for primary tabulation. In addition, instructional notations in this category direct coders to code first the underlying disease.

### Category 485, Bronchopneumonia, Organism Unspecified

Category 485, Bronchopneumonia, organism unspecified, is a three-digit code that describes the site of the pneumonia. Bronchopneumonia usually begins in the terminal bronchioles of the lung and causes the air space to become filled with exudates.

### Category 486, Pneumonia, Organism Unspecified

Category 486, Pneumonia, organism unspecified, is a three-digit code that should be assigned only when the physician does not identify the causative organism.

### Category 487, Influenza

Influenza with respiratory manifestations is classified to 487.0–487.8. A "use additional code" note is included under code 487.0, Influenza with pneumonia, to identify the type of pneumonia (480.0–480.9, 481, 482.0–482.9, 483.0–483.8, 485). Code 486, Pneumonia, organism unspecified, would be inappropriate to use with code 487.0 because the connection has been made between the influenza and the resulting pneumonia. An excludes note appears under code 487.8, Influenza with other manifestations. Intestinal flu [viral gastroenteritis] would not be coded here, but instead to code 008.8. Influenzal conditions classified to category 487 are viral respiratory conditions other than those caused by avian influenza, identified 2009 H1N1 influenza, or novel influenza A virus.

### Category 488, Influenza Due to Certain Identified Influenza Viruses

Avian influenza virus and novel H1N1 influenza virus can cause respiratory illnesses such as pneumonia. Avian influenza (H5N1) and avian influenza A (H7N9) viruses have not been reported in the United States, but outbreaks of identified 2009 H1N1 influenza virus with the accompanying complications were widely reported in 2009 (AHA Coding Clinic, 4th quarter 2009, 92 and 4th quarter 2007, 87). According to Reuters Health Information published on Medscape, there have been 38 cases worldwide of H5N1, avian influenza, primarily occurring in China. A Canadian man died of H5N1 in 2014 after returning from a trip to China. H5N1 is normally spread by contact with infected birds and kills about 60 percent of those infected (Reuters 2014). There are no reported cases in the United States according to the CDC (CDC 2014).

Subcategory 488.0, Influenza due to identified avian influenza virus, is further subdivided to report:

**488.01 Influenza due to identified avian influenza virus with pneumonia**

**488.02 Influenza due to identified avian influenza virus with other respiratory manifestations, such as laryngitis, pharyngitis, or upper respiratory tract infection**

**488.09 Influenza due to identified avian influenza virus with other manifestation, such as involvement of the gastrointestinal tract or encephalopathy**

Subcategory 488.1, Influenza due to identified 2009 H1N1 influenza virus is further subdivided to report:

**488.11 Influenza due to identified 2009 H1N1 influenza virus with pneumonia**

**488.12 Influenza due to identified 2009 H1N1 influenza virus with other respiratory manifestations, such as laryngitis, pharyngitis, or upper respiratory tract infection**

**488.19 Influenza due to identified 2009 H1N1 influenza virus with other manifestations, such as involvement of the gastrointestinal tract or encephalopathy**

Subcategory 488.8, Influenza due to novel influenza A is further subdivided to report:

**488.81 Influenza due to identified novel Influenza A virus with pneumonia**

**488.82 Influenza due to identified novel influenza A virus with other respiratory manifestations**

**488.89 Influenza due to identified novel influenza A virus with other manifestations**

### Category 507, Pneumonitis Due to Solids and Liquids

Category 507, Pneumonitis due to solids and liquids, is subdivided to fourth-digit subcategories that describe the causative agent. This category also is referred to as aspiration pneumonia. If the causative agent is unspecified, the Alphabetic Index to Diseases offers direction to code 507.0.

**A point to remember:** When the patient develops both aspiration pneumonia and bacterial pneumonia, codes for both types of pneumonia should be assigned.

**EXAMPLE:** Patient was admitted with aspiration pneumonia, as well as *Klebsiella pneumoniae*: 507.0, Pneumonitis due to inhalation of food or vomitus; 482.0, Pneumonia due to *Klebsiella pneumoniae*

## Exercise 11.1

Assign ICD-9-CM codes to the following:

1. Allergic pneumonitis

______________________________

2. Streptococcal group B pneumonia

______________________________

3. Staphylococcal bronchopneumonia

______________________________

4. Aspiration pneumonia due to regurgitated food

______________________________

5. Pneumonia in cytomegalic inclusion disease

______________________________

## Category 493, Asthma

Asthma is a condition marked by recurrent attacks of paroxysmal dyspnea, with wheezing due to spasmodic contraction of the bronchi. In some cases, it is an allergic manifestation in sensitized persons. The term *reactive airway disease* is considered synonymous with asthma.

### Fourth-Digit Subcategories

ICD-9-CM classifies asthma to category 493, with the following subcategories that describe the specific types of asthma:

**493.0** **Extrinsic asthma** (an asthmatic condition caused by environmental allergen factors)

**493.1** **Intrinsic asthma** (a form of asthma caused by the body's own immunological response)

**493.2** **Chronic obstructive asthma** (a chronic form of asthma coexisting with chronic obstructive pulmonary disease [COPD] that includes chronic asthmatic bronchitis)

**493.81** **Exercise-induced bronchospasm**

**493.82** **Cough variant asthma**

**493.9** **Asthma, unspecified** (the subcategory used when the documentation does not specify one of the types listed above)

### Fifth-Digit Subclassification

The fifth-digit subclassifications of category 493 apply to subcategory codes 493.0, 493.1, 493.2, and 493.9 only. The fifth-digit subclassifications describe whether the patient was in status asthmaticus or suffered what may be described as an exacerbation or acute exacerbation of the asthma. Status asthmaticus (fifth digit 1) is an acute asthmatic attack in which the degree of bronchial obstruction is not relieved by usual treatments such as epinephrine or aminophylline. A patient in status asthmaticus fails to respond to therapy administered during an asthmatic attack. This is a life-threatening complication that requires emergency care and, most likely, inpatient hospitalization. An acute exacerbation or with exacerbation (fifth digit 2) is an increase in the severity of the disease or any of its signs or symptoms, such as wheezing or shortness of breath. Chronic obstructive asthma is another form of the disease. A physician may document that the patient has COPD and asthma. Following the Alphabetic Index entries, these two conditions combine into one code, 493.2, Chronic obstructive asthma, which requires a fifth digit. An acute exacerbation of this type of asthma is a worsening or a decompensation of a chronic condition.

A fifth digit of 0, 1, or 2 must be added as applicable to subcategories 493.0, 493.1, 493.2, and 493.9 only. Fifth digit 0, unspecified, indicates that there is no mention of status asthmaticus or exacerbation. Fifth digit 1 indicates that status asthmaticus is mentioned. Fifth digit 2 describes the asthma as having an acute exacerbation or with exacerbation (the term "acute" does not need to be stated).

**0 unspecified**
**1 with status asthmaticus**
**2 with (acute) exacerbation**

Keep in mind that documentation in the health record must support the use of the fifth digits 1 and 2. In a patient in whom the physician describes the condition as both acute exacerbation and status asthmaticus, only the fifth digit 1, with status asthmaticus, should be assigned.

**Note:** Bronchospasm or the spasmodic contraction of the smooth muscle of the bronchi may occur in several respiratory conditions. For example, when bronchospasm occurs with acute bronchitis, both conditions are included in the code 466.0. Bronchospasm is frequently a feature of asthma and, as part of the disease, is included in the codes for asthma in category 493 or is identified with a single code 493.81 when the bronchospasm is identified as "exercise induced." However, there are other patients, usually children, who experience bronchospasm but have not been diagnosed with asthma or bronchitis. A unique code for this form of bronchospasm, code 519.11, allows for the chronicity or recurrence of the condition to be better identified and tracked.

## Category 494, Bronchiectasis

Bronchiectasis is a chronic, congenital, or acquired disease characterized by irreversible dilation of the bronchi with secondary infection. The incidence of bronchiectasis has decreased with the widespread use of antibiotics and immunizations in pediatrics. In adults, the condition may develop following a necrotizing pneumonia or lung abscess. Category 494 was expanded to describe bronchiectasis without acute exacerbation (494.0) and bronchiectasis with acute exacerbation or acute bronchitis with bronchiectasis (494.1).

## Chronic Obstructive Pulmonary Disease

Chronic obstructive pulmonary disease (COPD) is a diffuse obstruction of the smaller bronchi and bronchioles that results in coughing, wheezing, shortness of breath, and disturbances of gas exchange. Exacerbations of COPD, such as episodes of increased shortness of breath and cough, often are treated on an outpatient basis. More severe exacerbations, such as an infection, usually result in admission to the hospital. When acute bronchitis is documented with COPD, code 491.22, Obstructive chronic bronchitis with acute bronchitis, should be assigned. It is not appropriate to assign code 466.0 with 491.22. Code 491.22 supersedes code 491.21, Chronic obstructive bronchitis with (acute) exacerbation. Code 491.21 is used when the medical record includes documentation of COPD with acute exacerbation, without mention of acute bronchitis.

Code 496, Chronic airway obstruction, not elsewhere classified, should not be used with any code from categories 491–493. Code 496 is an unspecified form of COPD. Categories 491 and 493 identify specified forms of COPD. The patient cannot have both an unspecified form and a specified form of the same disease. The diagnosis of COPD does not identify what type of COPD the patient has. Sometimes physicians use COPD as a short-cut diagnosis, and other times the diagnosis of COPD is used because the patient has several forms of COPD, such as chronic bronchitis, obstructive asthma or emphysema. Code 496 is an unspecified form of COPD and should not be used if the documentation from the provider is more specific as to what type of COPD is present in the patient.

ICD-9-CM classifies COPD to the following codes:

**491.2x** **COPD with chronic bronchitis**

**491.20** **Obstructive chronic bronchitis without exacerbation**
**Emphysema with chronic bronchitis**

**491.21** **Chronic obstructive bronchitis with (acute) exacerbation**

**491.22** **Obstructive chronic bronchitis with acute bronchitis**

**492.8** **COPD with emphysema**

**493.2x** **COPD with asthma**

**496** **COPD without further specification**

## Respiratory Failure

Respiratory failure is the inability of the respiratory system to supply adequate oxygen to maintain proper metabolism and/or to eliminate carbon dioxide ($CO_2$). ICD-9-CM classifies different forms of respiratory failure to the following codes in category 518, Other diseases of lung:

**518.51** **Acute respiratory failure following trauma and surgery**

**518.53** **Acute and chronic respiratory failure following trauma and surgery**

**518.81** **Acute respiratory failure**
**Respiratory failure, not otherwise specified**

**518.83** **Chronic respiratory failure**

**518.84** **Acute and chronic respiratory failure**

Respiratory failure is assigned when documentation in the health record supports its use. It may be due to, or associated with, other respiratory conditions such as pneumonia, chronic bronchitis, or COPD. Respiratory failure also may be due to, or associated with, nonrespiratory conditions such as myasthenia gravis, congestive heart failure, myocardial infarction, or CVA.

Arterial blood gases may be useful in diagnosing respiratory failure; however, normal values may vary from person to person depending on individual health status. Coders should not assume the condition of respiratory failure exists based solely on laboratory and radiology test findings.

### *Coding and Sequencing of Acute Respiratory Failure*

The coding and sequencing of acute respiratory failure presents many challenges to both the new and the experienced clinical coder. Various coding rules and guidelines must be considered.

Acute respiratory failure, code 518.81, may be assigned as a principal or secondary diagnosis depending on the circumstances of the inpatient admission. Chapter-specific coding guidelines (obstetrics, poisoning, HIV, newborn) provide specific sequencing direction. Respiratory failure may be listed as a secondary diagnosis. In addition, if respiratory failure occurs after admission, it may be listed as a secondary diagnosis.

When a patient is admitted in acute respiratory failure with another acute condition, the principal diagnosis will not be the same in every situation. There is not one respiratory failure coding rule. This is true whether or not the other acute condition is a respiratory or nonrespiratory condition. Selection of the principal diagnosis will depend on the circumstances of the admission. If both the respiratory failure and the other acute condition are equally responsible for the patient's admission to the hospital, and there are no chapter-specific sequencing rules, the guideline regarding two or more diagnoses that equally meet the definition for principal diagnosis (Section II, C) may be applied. If the documentation is not clear as to whether the acute respiratory failure and another condition are equally responsible for occasioning the admission, the physician must be asked for clarification.

Respiratory failure is a life-threatening condition that is always caused by an underlying condition. It may be caused by diseases of the circulatory system, respiratory system, central nervous system, peripheral nervous system, respiratory muscles, and chest wall muscles. The primary goal of the treatment of acute respiratory failure is to assess the severity of underlying disease and to correct the inadequate oxygen delivery and tissue hypoxia.

The following are examples of the appropriate coding and sequencing of acute respiratory failure in association with the underlying disease.

**EXAMPLE 1:** A patient with chronic myasthenia gravis suffers an acute exacerbation and develops acute respiratory failure. The patient is admitted to the hospital to treat the respiratory failure.

Principal diagnosis: 518.81, Acute respiratory failure
Secondary diagnosis: 358.01, Myasthenia gravis with (acute) exacerbation

**EXAMPLE 2:** A patient with emphysema develops acute respiratory failure. The patient is admitted to the hospital for treatment of the respiratory failure.

Principal diagnosis: 518.81, Acute respiratory failure
Secondary diagnosis: 492.8, Emphysema

**EXAMPLE 3:** A patient with congestive heart failure is brought to the emergency department in acute respiratory failure. The patient is intubated and admitted to the hospital. The physician documents that acute respiratory failure is the reason for the admission.

Principal diagnosis: 518.81, Acute respiratory failure
Secondary diagnosis: 428.0, Congestive heart failure

In the above example, the physician has stated that the reason for the admission is to treat the respiratory failure. If the documentation is not clear regarding whether the congestive heart failure or the acute respiratory failure was the reason for admission, the coder should ask the physician for clarification.

**EXAMPLE 4:** A patient with asthma in status asthmaticus develops acute respiratory failure and is admitted to the hospital for treatment of the acute respiratory failure.

| | |
|---|---|
| Principal diagnosis: | 518.81, Acute respiratory failure |
| Secondary diagnosis: | 493.91, Asthma, unspecified, with status asthmaticus |

**EXAMPLE 5:** A patient is admitted to the hospital during the postpartum period as a result of developing pulmonary embolism leading to respiratory failure.

| | |
|---|---|
| Principal diagnosis: | 673.24, Obstetrical blood clot embolism, postpartum condition or complication |
| Secondary diagnosis: | 518.81, Acute respiratory failure |

The above example is one of a chapter-specific guideline. The obstetric code is sequenced first because Chapter 11 (obstetric) codes have sequencing priority over codes from other ICD-9-CM chapters (Guideline Section I. C. 11. a. 1).

**EXAMPLE 6:** A patient who is diagnosed as having overdosed on crack cocaine is admitted to the hospital with respiratory failure.

| | |
|---|---|
| Principal diagnosis: | 970.81, Poisoning by cocaine |
| Secondary diagnosis: | 518.81, Acute respiratory failure |

This is another example of a chapter-specific guideline. The poisoning code is sequenced first because a chapter-specific guideline (Section I. C. 17. e. 2. d) provides sequencing directions specifying that the poisoning code is listed first, followed by a code for the manifestation of the poisoning. In example 6, the respiratory failure is a manifestation of the poisoning or overdose.

**EXAMPLE 7:** A patient is admitted with respiratory failure due to *Pneumocystis carinii* pneumonia, which is associated with AIDS.

| | |
|---|---|
| Principal diagnosis: | 042, Human immunodeficiency virus (HIV) disease |
| Secondary diagnosis: | 518.81, Acute respiratory failure; 136.3, Pneumocystosis |

In example 7, the AIDS code (042) is listed as the principal diagnosis with the respiratory failure and pneumonia listed as secondary diagnoses according to the chapter-specific guidelines regarding HIV-related conditions. In this case, the pneumocystosis is the HIV-related condition that caused the respiratory failure. The guidelines in Section I. C. 1. a. 2. a. state that if a patient is admitted for an HIV-related condition, the principal diagnosis should be 042, AIDS, followed by additional diagnosis codes for all reported HIV-related conditions.

**EXAMPLE 8:** A patient is admitted to the hospital with severe *Staphylococcus aureus* sepsis and acute respiratory failure.

| | |
|---|---|
| Principal diagnosis: | 038.11, *Methicillin Susceptible Staphylococcus aureus* septicemia |
| Secondary diagnosis: | 995.92, Severe sepsis; 518.81, Acute respiratory failure |

In this example, the *Staphylococcus aureus* sepsis is sequenced first because there is an instructional note under subcategory 995.92 indicating to "code first" the underlying systemic infection. In addition, code 995.92 has a "use additional code" note to specify organ dysfunction and lists acute respiratory failure (518.81). This instruction would indicate that the respiratory failure would be a secondary diagnosis. This is an example of code selection based on using both the Alphabetic Index and the Tabular List directions.

## Exercise 11.2

Assign ICD-9-CM codes to the following:

1. Respiratory failure due to myasthenia gravis with exacerbation (patient admitted to the hospital to treat the respiratory failure)

2. Obstructive chronic bronchitis

3. COPD with emphysema

4. Acute bronchiolitis due to respiratory syncytial virus

5. Acute respiratory failure due to emphysema (patient admitted to the hospital to treat the respiratory failure)

6. Pneumococcal pneumonia due to HIV infection/AIDS

7. Intrinsic asthma in status asthmaticus

8. Pansinusitis with hypertrophy of nasal turbinates

9. Pneumonia with whooping cough

10. Emphysema with acute exacerbation of chronic obstructive bronchitis

# Respiratory Procedures

This section describes the ICD-9-CM coding of two respiratory procedures: closed endoscopic biopsy and other endoscopic procedures.

## Closed Endoscopic Biopsy

When coding closed endoscopic biopsies, take special note of the existence of combination codes that describe both the endoscopy and the biopsy. For example:

**31.43 Closed [endoscopic] biopsy of larynx**
**31.44 Closed [endoscopic] biopsy of trachea**

**33.20 Thoracoscopic lung biopsy**
**33.24 Closed [endoscopic] biopsy of bronchus**
**33.27 Closed [endoscopic] biopsy of lung**
**34.20 Thoracoscopic pleural biopsy**

## Endoscopic Procedures in the Respiratory System

Because many lesions in the respiratory tract can be removed by endoscopic means that do not require opening the chest, ICD-9-CM provides codes for this type of procedure. For example:

**32.01 Endoscopic excision or destruction of lesion or tissue of bronchus**
**32.28 Endoscopic excision or destruction of lesion or tissue of lung**
**32.41 Thoracoscopic lobectomy of lung**
**34.06 Thoracoscopic drainage of pleural cavity**
**34.52 Thoracoscopic decortication of lung**

In the above cases, it would be inaccurate to assign two separate codes to identify the endoscopy and the surgical procedures because one code describes both procedures.

## Invasive and Noninvasive Mechanical Ventilation

Mechanical ventilation is clinically indicated for patients with apnea, acute respiratory failure, and impending acute respiratory failure. Invasive mechanical ventilation pumps air into the patient's lungs even when there is no attempt by the patient to breathe on his or her own. Subcategory 96.7 is used to classify other continuous invasive mechanical ventilation. Code 96.7 is subdivided to classify the number of hours a patient is on continuous mechanical ventilation. A note at the beginning of this subcategory describes how to calculate the number of hours a patient was on continuous mechanical ventilation.

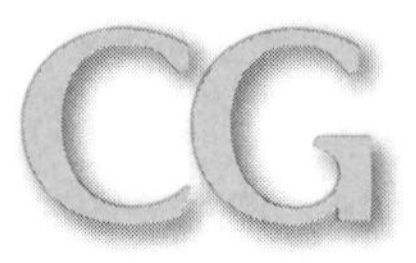


To calculate the number of hours (duration) of continuous mechanical ventilation during a hospitalization, begin the count from the start of the (endotracheal) intubation. The duration ends with (endotracheal) extubation.

If a patient is intubated prior to admission, begin counting the duration from the time of the admission. If a patient is transferred (discharged) while intubated, the duration would end at the time of transfer (discharge).

For patients who begin on (endotracheal) intubation and subsequently have a tracheostomy performed for mechanical ventilation, the duration begins with (endotracheal) intubation and ends when the mechanical ventilation is turned off (after the weaning period).

For patients with a tracheostomy, the second note states:

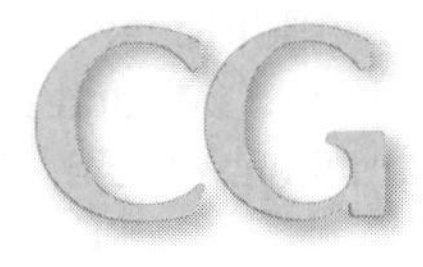

To calculate the number of hours of continuous mechanical ventilation during a hospitalization, begin counting the duration when mechanical ventilation is started. The duration ends when the mechanical ventilator is turned off (after the weaning period).

If a patient has received a tracheostomy prior to admission and is on mechanical ventilation at the time of admission, begin counting the duration from the time of admission. If the patient is transferred (discharged) while still on mechanical ventilation via tracheostomy, the duration would end at the time of the transfer (discharge).

Weaning the patient from the ventilation, that is, getting the patient to breathe on their own without the support of the mechanical ventilator, may occur over several days. The weaning period often consists of increasing the number of hours over several days when the patient is receiving less support from the ventilator and is called a weaning trial. The weaning trial is a period of time when the support from the ventilator is reduced and the patient starts the work of breathing on their own. This process may occur over minutes or hours in one day for a healthier patient, however, the sicker patient may need a gradual process of re-breathing on their own over several days. During this time the patient begins breathing on their own for increasing number of hours in a day but the mechanical ventilator is still turned on with varying degrees of volume or pressure support available to the patient. The hours for mechanical ventilation are calculated for the entire weaning period until the mechanical ventilator is finally turned off. A patient may also have intermittent ventilation, for example, overnight called nocturnal ventilation and then weaned off of all ventilation. Again, the hours for mechanical ventilation are calculated for the entire weaning period until the mechanical ventilator is turned off.

During the continuous mechanical ventilation period a patient may extubate himself by removing the endotracheal tube from the throat. Some patients may be able to breathe on their own immediately and the mechanical ventilation is turned off. However other patients are likely to still require ventilatory support and are reintubated. Although the patient may self-extubate one or more times during a hospital stay, the amount of time the patient is on mechanical ventilation continues to be counted. If the patient is placed back on the ventilator each time, the hours of mechanical ventilation continues to be counted. Discontinuation of mechanical ventilation depends on a physician's order and clinical indicators and not on the fact that the patient removed the breathing tube.

There is a "Code any associate" procedure note under the subcategory heading for 96.7, Other continuous invasive mechanical ventilation. Coders should review this note. Additional codes should be assigned, when applicable, to describe endotracheal tube insertion (96.04) and tracheostomy (31.1–31.29). The use of an invasive interface such as an endotracheal tube or the tracheostomy is required to deliver invasive mechanical ventilation.

Mechanical ventilation is considered noninvasive when it is delivered by a face mask, nasal mask, nasal pillow, oral mouthpiece or oronasal mask, or without an endotracheal tube or tracheostomy. Types of respiratory assistance considered noninvasive include continuous positive airway pressure (CPAP), bilevel positive airway pressure (BiPAP), noninvasive positive pressure ventilation (NIPPV), and nonpositive pressure ventilation (NPPV.) With CPAP and BiPAP, the patient is breathing on their own by initiating their own inspirations and exhalations. These methods of respiratory assistance augment the patient's breathing by providing continuous positive airway pressure as the patient breathes on a spontaneous basis.

Code 93.90, Non-invasive mechanical ventilation is assigned for the use of any of these noninvasive respiratory assistance procedures. However, if CPAP or BiPAP is delivered via a tracheostomy or through an endotracheal tube, this form of respiratory assistance is considered invasive and should be coded as invasive mechanical ventilation with codes from subcategory 96.7.

When a patient receives both invasive and noninvasive mechanical ventilation during the same episode of care but on different days in the hospital or in another health care facility, both types of mechanical ventilation are coded. For example, the patient may be admitted requiring noninvasive CPAP but later require invasive mechanical ventilation on a continuous basis.

## ICD-9-CM Review Exercises: Chapter 11

Assign ICD-9-CM diagnosis and procedure codes to the following:

1. Respiratory failure following surgery

2. Hypertrophy of tonsils and adenoids; tonsillectomy and adenoidectomy

3. Postoperative pneumothorax

4. Vocal cord paralysis, complete; diagnostic laryngoscopy

5. Acute respiratory failure; COPD; continuous mechanical ventilation for 20 hours; endotracheal intubation (patient admitted to the hospital to treat the acute respiratory failure)

6. Hay fever due to pollen

7. Tension pneumothorax with thoracentesis

8. Carcinoma of left upper lobe of the lung with endoscopic excision of lesion in left upper lobe

## ICD-9-CM Review Exercises: Chapter 11

9. Chronic simple bronchitis; closed biopsy of the bronchus

10. Chronic laryngotracheitis; endoscopic biopsy of larynx

11. Gram-negative bacterial pneumonia

12. Frontal sinus polyp with excision of polyp

13. Viral pneumonia due to severe acute respiratory syndrome (SARS)-associated coronavirus

14. Black lung disease; CPAP delivered via oronasal mask

15. Pneumonia due to *Haemophilus influenzae*

# ICD-10-CM Chapter 10, Diseases of the Respiratory System (J00–J99)

## Organization and Structure of ICD-10 Chapter 10

Chapter 10 of ICD-10-CM includes categories J00–J99 arranged in the following blocks:

| | |
|---|---|
| J00–J06 | Acute upper respiratory infections |
| J09–J18 | Influenza and pneumonia |
| J20–J22 | Other acute lower respiratory infections |
| J30–J39 | Other diseases of upper respiratory tract |
| J40–J47 | Chronic lower respiratory diseases |
| J60–J70 | Lung diseases due to external agents |
| J80–J84 | Other respiratory diseases principally affecting the interstitium |
| J85–J86 | Suppurative and necrotic conditions of the lower respiratory tract |
| J90–J94 | Other diseases of the pleura |
| J95 | Intraoperative and postprocedural complications and disorders of respiratory system, not elsewhere classified |
| J96–J99 | Other diseases of the respiratory system |

While overall Chapter 10 of ICD-10-CM is organized similarly to ICD-9-CM, diseases have been grouped into more blocks of codes to recognize upper and lower respiratory tract infections, diseases of the pleura and intraoperative, and postprocedural complications and disorders of the respiratory system.

Modifications have also been made to specific categories that bring the terminology up-to-date with current medical practice. For example, ICD-10-CM category J43, Emphysema, contains codes with panlobular emphysema and centrilobular emphysema in the titles. ICD-10-CM category J45, Asthma, classifies asthma as mild intermittent, mild persistent, moderate persistent, and severe persistent.

Other enhancements to Chapter 10 include classification changes that provide greater specificity than found in ICD-9-CM. ICD-10-CM has individual codes for acute recurrent sinusitis for each sinus. Subcategory J10.8, Influenza due to other identified influenza virus with other manifestations has been expanded to reflect the manifestations of the influenza. Category J20, Acute bronchitis, has been expanded to reflect the causes of the acute bronchitis.

## Coding Guidelines and Instructional Notes for ICD-10-CM Chapter 10

At the beginning of Chapter 10 of ICD-10-CM, the following instructional guideline appears: "When a respiratory condition is described as occurring in more than one site and is not specifically indexed, it should be classified to the lower anatomic site." For example, Tracheobronchitis is classified to bronchitis in J40, Bronchitis, not specified as acute or chronic.

An additional instructional note also appears at the beginning of Chapter 10 which instructs the coding professional to use an additional code, where applicable to identify: exposure to environmental tobacco smoke (Z77.22), exposure to tobacco smoke in the perinatal period (P96.81), history of tobacco use (Z87.891), occupational exposure to environmental tobacco smoke (Z57.31), tobacco dependence (F17.-), or tobacco use (Z72.0). Since these instructional notes appear at the beginning of the chapter, they should be followed when assigning any code from this chapter.

In the Tabular, there is a note under category J44 to code also type of asthma, if applicable (J45.-). There is also an Excludes2 note under category J45 for asthma with COPD.

By definition, when an Excludes2 note appears under a code, it is acceptable to use both the code and the excluded code together if the patient has both conditions at the same time.

The NCHS has published chapter-specific guidelines for Chapter 10 in the *ICD-10-CM Official Guidelines for Coding and Reporting*:

- Guideline I.C.10.a. Chronic obstructive pulmonary disease and asthma
- Guidelines I.C.10.b. Acute respiratory failure
- Guideline I.C.10.c. Influenza due to certain identified influenza viruses
- Guidelines I.C.10.d. Ventilator-associated pneumonia

To gain an understanding of these rules, access the 2014 guidelines from NCHS website (http://www.cdc.gov/nchs/icd/icd10cm.htm) and read Chapter 10, Diseases of the Respiratory System guidelines I.C.10.a through I.C.10.d on pages 46–48.

## Coding Overview for ICD-10-CM Chapter 10

Throughout Chapter 10 of ICD-10-CM, Diseases of the Respiratory System (J00–J99), use additional code where applicable notes appear to direct the coder to assign an additional code for exposure to environmental tobacco smoke (Z77.22), exposure to tobacco smoke in the perinatal period (P96.81), history of tobacco use (Z87.891), occupational exposure to environmental tobacco smoke (Z57.31), tobacco dependence (F17.-), and tobacco use (Z72.0).

Procedural complication codes are included in the category J95 to identify specific respiratory complications such as tracheostomy complications, acute pulmonary insufficiency following thoracic surgery and nonthoracic surgery, ventilator-associated pneumonia, as well as the other postprocedural complications seen in other chapters for hemorrhage, hematoma, and accidental puncture or laceration. Again, the complication can be identified as occurring during a respiratory system procedure or as complicating another body system procedure.

Certain codes have moved to Chapter 10 from other locations; for example, streptococcal sore throat moved from Chapter 1, Infectious and Parasitic Diseases in ICD-9-CM to the respiratory chapter in ICD-10-CM.

Lobar pneumonia has a unique code in a category for pneumonia, unspecified organism. Other codes are available if the lobar pneumonia is further specified as to type. In ICD-9-CM the condition was classified to the code for pneumococcal pneumonia.

The terminology used to describe asthma has been updated to reflect the current clinical classification of asthma. The following terms have been added to describe asthma: mild intermittent and three degrees of persistent—mild persistent, moderate persistent, and severe persistent. Intrinsic asthma (nonallergic) and extrinsic (allergic) are both classified to J45.909, Unspecified asthma, uncomplicated, if not further specified.

The physicians with the World Allergy Organization classify allergic asthma into four clinical phases, based upon symptoms and pulmonary function testing. This classification system allows physicians to communicate more uniformly regarding asthma severity and facilitates the creation of general guidelines for treatment (Li and Kaliner 2006). The four categories currently employed are:

| Asthma Severity | Frequency of Daytime Symptoms | Types of Symptoms and Pulmonary Function Studies |
|---|---|---|
| Intermittent | Less than or equal to 2 times per week | The patient is otherwise asymptomatic. Pulmonary function studies are normal except during periods of disease and exacerbations are brief and easily treated. |
| Mild Persistent | More than 2 times per week | The symptoms are severe enough to interfere with daily activities and may interrupt sleep up to twice a month. Pulmonary function studies are normal or show mild airflow obstruction which is reversible with the inhalation of a bronchodilator. |
| Moderate Persistent | Daily. May restrict physical activity | Patients are constantly aware of their disease, require medications on a daily basis, have their sleep interrupted at least weekly, and have to accommodate their lifestyle to the disease. Pulmonary function is moderately abnormal, with the FEV1 being 60–80% of the predicted value. |
| Severe Persistent | Throughout the day. Frequent severe attacks limiting ability to breathe. | Severe persistent asthma is defined as continuous symptoms despite the correct use of medications. The severity of the disease limits physical activities and is associated with frequent exacerbations and sleep interruption. Treatment requires combinations of medications on a constant basis. Pulmonary function tests are severely affected with the FEV1 being <60% of predicted. |

Source: Li and Kaliner 2006

According to the World Allergy Organization, a patient may fit into one category upon initial visit and another after treatment or during an exacerbation. For example, a patient with mild persistent disease can be exposed to allergens or develop a respiratory infection and have a severe exacerbation of asthma, changing the disease classification from mild to severe, until the exacerbation is resolved. Conversely, a patient with severe persistent symptoms can be treated effectively with resolution of symptoms and be reclassified to a mild category while on treatment (Li and Kaliner 2006).

A note at the beginning of the chapter states that when a respiratory condition is described as occurring in more than one site and is not specifically indexed, it should be classified to the lower anatomic site (for example, tracheobronchitis to bronchitis in J40).

Some of the codes in Chapter 10 have been expanded to include notes indicating that an additional code should be assigned or an associated condition should be sequenced first. The following are examples of the notations:

- Use additional code to identify the infectious agent
- Use additional code to identify the virus
- Code first any associated lung abscess
- Code first the underlying disease
- Use additional code to identify other conditions such as tobacco use or exposure

## ICD-10-CM Review Exercises: Chapter 11

Assign the correct ICD-10-CM diagnosis codes to the following

1. The patient has aspiration pneumonia because of his difficulty in swallowing (neurogenic) due to a previous cerebral infarction. The patient also has stage 1 decubitus ulcers on both his left and right hip.

2. Acute respiratory insufficiency due to acute exacerbation of COPD and tobacco dependence

3. Patient with a high fever, cough, and chest pain. Gram stain of the sputum showed numerous small gram-negative coccobacilli. Diagnosis: H. influenzae pneumonia.

4. Acute respiratory failure, acute bronchitis with acute exacerbation of COPD. The patient was admitted to treat the acute respiratory failure and treated with mechanical ventilation after intubation in the ER.

5. Severe persistent asthma with acute exacerbation

6. Novel H1N1 influenza with upper respiratory tract infection

7. Moderate persistent asthma with status asthmaticus. Acute exacerbation of chronic obstructive pulmonary disease.

8. Aspiration pneumonia treated with respiratory therapy and antibiotics. Patient has severe gastroesophageal reflux causing him to aspirate food.

9. Chronic mucopurulent chronic bronchitis

10. Acute pulmonary insufficiency following thoracic surgery (confirmed by the physician as being a postoperative complication)

# Chapter 12
# Diseases of the Digestive System

## Learning Objectives

At the conclusion of this chapter, you should be able to:

1. Describe the organization of the conditions and codes included in Chapter 9 of ICD-9-CM, Diseases of the Digestive System (520–579)
2. Describe the organization of the conditions and codes included in Chapter 11 of ICD-10-CM, Diseases of the Digestive System (K00–K95)
3. Identify the ICD-9-CM and ICD-10-CM codes for the various ulcers of the gastrointestinal tract
4. Identify the definitions of various types of hernia conditions that can be classified with ICD-9-CM and ICD-10-CM
5. Identify various types of noninfectious enteritis and colitis conditions that can be classified with ICD-9-CM and ICD-10-CM
6. Identify the ICD-9-CM and ICD-10-CM codes for the various types of gallbladder disease and calculus, including the required fourth and fifth digits
7. Understand the use of ICD-9-CM category 578, Gastrointestinal hemorrhage, and its relationship with other digestive conditions and ICD-10-CM category K92, Other diseases of digestive system
8. Briefly describe the methods of repairing various digestive system hernias
9. Describe the types of procedures that can be performed endoscopically within the digestive system
10. Define the terms *gastrostomy, colostomy, ileostomy,* and *enterostomy* and explain the coding of these procedures
11. Identify the types of procedures performed for intestinal resection and anastomosis
12. Assign ICD-9-CM diagnosis and procedure codes for diseases of the digestive system
13. Assign ICD-10-CM codes for diseases of the digestive system

# ICD-9-CM Chapter 9, Diseases of the Digestive System (520–579)

Chapter 9, Diseases of the Digestive System, in the Tabular List in volume 1 of ICD-9-CM contains the following categories and section titles:

| Categories | Section Titles |
|---|---|
| 520–529 | Diseases of Oral Cavity, Salivary Glands, and Jaws |
| 530–539 | Diseases of Esophagus, Stomach, and Duodenum |
| 540–543 | Appendicitis |
| 550–553 | Hernia of Abdominal Cavity |
| 555–558 | Noninfectious Enteritis and Colitis |
| 560–569 | Other Diseases of Intestine and Peritoneum |
| 570–579 | Other Diseases of Digestive System |

The organs of the gastrointestinal tract are featured in the diagram in figure 12.1.

**Figure 12.1.** Diagram of the gastrointestinal tract

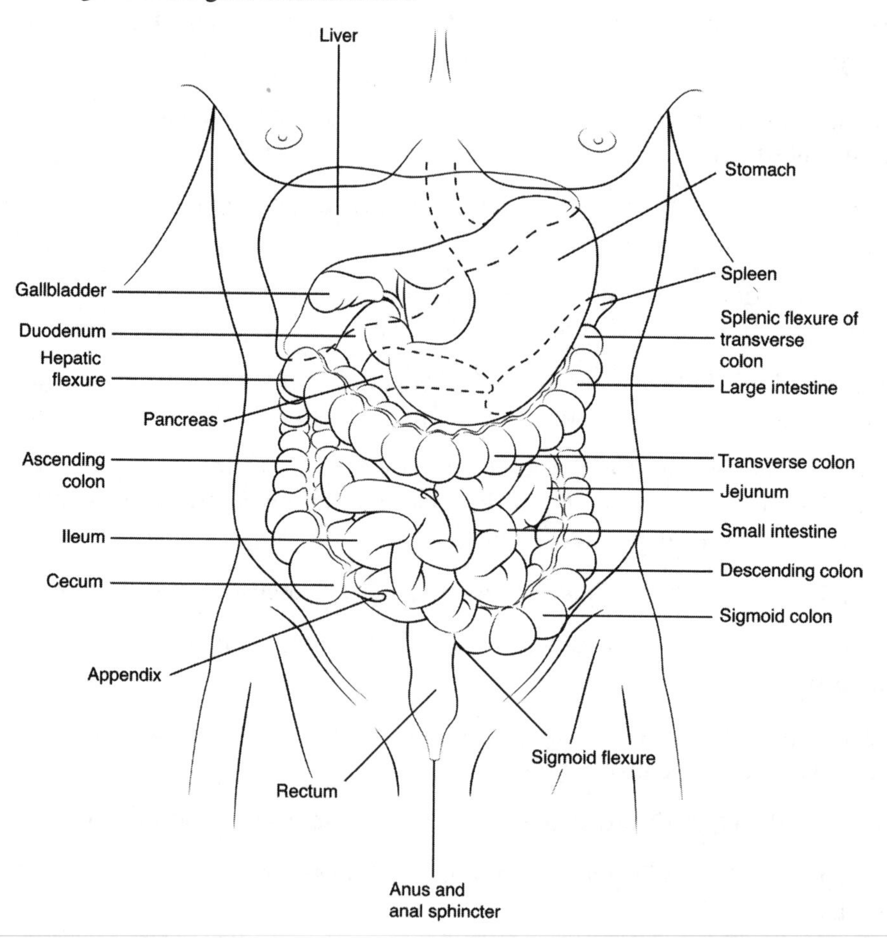

## Diseases of Oral Cavity, Salivary Glands, and Jaws

In the past, diagnosis coding was not widely used in dentistry. However, the need for dental diagnosis codes has become urgent with the advent of electronic health records and the desire of dentists to track patient conditions with their outcomes. The use of codes also support educational and research needs of dentistry. Codes describe types of dental caries, abrasions and erosions, gingival and periodontal disease, dentofacial anomalies, diseases of supporting structures, and diseases of oral soft tissues.

Mucositis can occur as an adverse effect of antineoplastic treatment and other medications. There is redness and/or ulcerative sores in the soft tissue of the mucosal surfaces throughout the body, resulting in severe pain as well as difficulty in eating, drinking, and taking oral medications. The most common location for mucosal toxicity is the oral cavity. Unique codes for stomatitis and mucositis due to antineoplastic therapy and other drugs are included in the digestive system chapter of ICD-9-CM with codes 528.01 and 528.02.

Mucositis can occur in other parts of the digestive system as well as in the respiratory and female genital organs as a result of cancer treatment.

## Gastrointestinal Ulcers

Ulcers of the gastrointestinal (GI) tract can be found in the following categories:

**531 Gastric ulcer**
**532 Duodenal ulcer**
**533 Peptic ulcer, site unspecified**
**534 Gastrojejunal ulcer**

The preceding categories are subdivided to fourth-digit subcategories that describe acute and chronic conditions and the presence of hemorrhage or perforation. The bleeding ulcer or hemorrhage does not have to be actively bleeding at the time of the examination procedure, such as an endoscopy, to use the code for ulcer with hemorrhage. A statement by the physician that bleeding has occurred and it is attributed to the ulcer is sufficient. The fifth-digit subclassification identifies the presence or absence of obstructions.

## Category 535, Gastritis and Duodenitis

ICD-9-CM classifies gastritis and duodenitis to category 535, which is subdivided to fourth-digit subcategories that describe types of gastritis and duodenitis. The fifth-digit subclassification identifies the presence or absence of hemorrhage. Active bleeding during the current examination or procedure does not have to be present to use the fifth digit to describe the hemorrhage. It may be diagnosed clinically by the physician based on the patient's history and/or physical examination.

## Categories 550–553, Hernias

Hernias of the abdominal cavity are classified to categories 550–553. A fifth digit is used to describe whether the hernia is unilateral, bilateral, or unspecified as to one- or two-sided and whether it is recurrent.

A hernia is the protrusion of a loop or knuckle of an organ or tissue through an abdominal opening. Many different types of hernias exist, including the following:

- An inguinal hernia is a hernia of an intestinal loop into the inguinal canal. An inguinal hernia may be referred to as "direct" or "indirect," which describes the anatomical location more precisely but cannot be coded as specifically with ICD-9-CM diagnosis codes. However, ICD-9-CM procedure codes do allow for differentiation of the repair of a direct or indirect inguinal hernia.
- A femoral hernia is a hernia of a loop of intestine into the femoral canal.
- A hiatal hernia is the displacement of the upper part of the stomach into the thorax through the esophageal opening (hiatus) of the diaphragm.
- A diaphragmatic hernia is the protrusion of an abdominal organ into the chest cavity through a defect in the diaphragm.
- A ventral hernia, or abdominal hernia, is a herniation of the intestine or some other internal body structure through the abdominal wall.
- An incisional hernia is an abdominal hernia at the site of a previously made incision.
- An umbilical hernia is a type of abdominal hernia in which part of the intestine protrudes at the umbilicus and is covered by skin and subcutaneous tissue. This type may also be described as an omphalocele.
- A hernia may be described as "reducible." This means the physician can manipulate the displaced structure(s) back into position.

ICD-9-CM uses the term *obstruction* to indicate that incarceration, irreducibility, or strangulation is present with the hernia.

- An "irreducible" hernia is also known as an "incarcerated" hernia. An incarcerated hernia is a hernia of intestine that cannot be returned or reduced by manipulation; it may or may not be strangulated.
- A strangulated hernia is an incarcerated hernia that is so tightly constricted as to restrict the blood supply to the contents of the hernial sac and possibly cause gangrene of the contents, such as the intestine. This represents a medical emergency requiring surgical correction.

Codes for different type of hernias of the abdominal cavity are included in the following categories:

**550 Inguinal hernia**
**551 Other hernia of abdominal cavity, with gangrene**
**552 Other hernia of abdominal cavity, with obstruction, but without mention of gangrene**
**553 Other hernia of abdominal cavity without mention of obstruction or gangrene**

## Categories 555–558, Noninfectious Enteritis and Colitis

ICD-9-CM classifies noninfectious enteritis and colitis to categories 555–558 in Chapter 9. Infectious enteritis and colitis are classified in Chapter 1, Infectious and Parasitic Diseases.

## Regional Enteritis (555)

Regional enteritis, also known as Crohn's disease and granulomatous enteritis, is defined as a chronic inflammatory disease commonly affecting the distal ileum and colon. Regional enteritis is characterized by chronic diarrhea, abdominal pain, fever, anorexia, weight loss, right lower quadrant mass or fullness, and lymphadenitis of the mesenteric nodes.

ICD-9-CM classifies regional enteritis to category 555, with the fourth digit identifying the specific site affected, such as the large intestine. Without further specification as to site, assign code 555.9.

## Gastroenteritis

Gastroenteritis is characterized by diarrhea, nausea and vomiting, and abdominal cramps. It can be caused by bacteria, amoebae, parasites, viruses, ingestion of toxins, reaction to drugs, or enzyme deficiencies. Allergic reactions as a response to food allergens may manifest as GI reactions, the most common of which are nausea, vomiting, diarrhea, and abdominal cramping. Codes exist to describe allergic and dietetic gastroenteritis and colitis.

Gastroenteritis is classified by cause in Chapters 1 and 9 in the Tabular List in volume 1 of ICD-9-CM.

**003.0 Salmonella gastroenteritis**
**005.9 Gastroenteritis due to food poisoning, unspecified**
**008.8 Viral gastroenteritis, NEC**
**009.0 Infectious gastroenteritis**
**556.9 Ulcerative gastroenteritis**
**558.3 Allergic gastroenteritis and colitis**
**558.9 Other and unspecified noninfectious gastroenteritis and colitis**
Colitis, enteritis, gastroenteritis, ileitis, jejunitis, and sigmoiditis, NOS, dietetic or noninfectious

## Categories 567 and 568, Peritonitis and Retroperitoneal Infections and Other Disorders of Peritoneum

Peritonitis is inflammation of the peritoneum, usually accompanied by abdominal pain and tenderness, constipation, vomiting, and moderate fever. It may be caused by a bacteria, such as *Staphylococcus, Pseudomonas,* or *Mycobacterium*; it may be fungal, most commonly *Candida* peritonitis, or caused by other factors, such as trauma or childbirth.

ICD-9-CM codes distinguish between generalized (acute) peritonitis, code 567.21, and peritoneal abscess of a specific location, such as mesenteric or subphrenic, code 567.22. Similarly, a retroperitoneal abscess (567.38) is coded differently than other forms of retroperitoneal infections (such as 567.39). Unique codes exist for spontaneous bacterial peritonitis as well as other acute bacterial forms of the disease. Choleperitonitis, code 567.81, occurs as the result of bile in the peritoneal cavity. Sclerosing mesenteritis, code 567.82, refers to a number of inflammatory processes involving the mesenteric fat, including fat necrosis and fibrosis. Each condition requires specific treatment.

## Cholecystitis and Cholelithiasis

Two categories are available to classify cholecystitis and cholelithiasis:

**574 Cholelithiasis**
**575 Other disorders of gallbladder**

Cholelithiasis is the presence of one or more calculi (gallstones) in the gallbladder. Gallstones tend to be asymptomatic. The most common symptom is biliary colic. More serious complications include cholecystitis, biliary tract obstruction (from stones in the bile ducts or choledocholithiasis), bile duct infection (cholangitis), and gallstone pancreatitis. A diagnosis is usually made by ultrasonography. If cholelithiasis causes symptoms or complications, a cholecystectomy may be necessary.

Choledocholithiasis is the presence of stones in the bile ducts. The stones can form in the gallbladder or in the bile ducts. The stones cause biliary colic, biliary obstruction, gallstone pancreatitis, or cholangitis. Cholangitis can lead to stricture, stasis, and choledocholithiasis. The diagnosis is usually made by magnetic resonance cholangiopancreatography (MRCP) or endoscopic retrograde cholangiopancreatography (ERCP).

Category 574 is divided into the following four-digit subcategories to describe the existence of calculus or stones in the gallbladder or in the bile ducts or both locations with acute or chronic cholecystitis:

**574.0 Calculus of gallbladder with acute cholecystitis**
**574.1 Calculus of gallbladder with other cholecystitis**
**574.2 Calculus of gallbladder without mention of cholecystitis**
**574.3 Calculus of bile duct with acute cholecystitis**
**574.4 Calculus of bile duct with other cholecystitis**
**574.5 Calculus of bile duct without mention of cholecystitis**
**574.6 Calculus of gallbladder and bile duct with acute cholecystitis**
**574.7 Calculus of gallbladder and bile duct with other cholecystitis**
**574.8 Calculus of gallbladder and bile duct with acute and chronic cholecystitis**
**574.9 Calculus of gallbladder and bile duct without cholecystitis**

In category 574, the fifth-digit subclassification describes the presence or absence of obstructions.

The coder must be careful in following the Alphabetic Index directions when coding gallbladder disease. For example, if a patient had acute and chronic cholecystitis with cholelithiasis, the coder may access the Index using the diagnosis "cholecystitis." There is a connecting term "with" beneath the main term cholecystitis that is very important to read. The coder must follow the direction when reviewing "Cholecystitis" with "calculus, stones in gallbladder—see Cholelithiasis." The coder must then go to the main term "cholelithiasis" and see the connecting term "with" and find codes following "cholecystitis, acute" and "cholecystitis, chronic." Two codes are required to code acute and chronic cholecystitis with cholelithiasis (without mention of obstruction): 574.00 and 574.10.

Category 575 contains the following two codes relating to cholecystitis without mention of calculus or stones in the gallbladder or bile duct:

**575.0 Acute cholecystitis**
**575.1 Other cholecystitis**

In subcategory 575.1, the fifth-digit subclassification indicates severity.

**575.10 Cholecystitis, unspecified**
**575.11 Chronic cholecystitis**
**575.12 Acute and chronic cholecystitis**

## Category 578, Gastrointestinal Hemorrhage

Category 578 includes subcategories for hematemesis (578.0), blood in stool or melena (578.1), and unspecified gastrointestinal hemorrhage (578.9).

The use of category 578 is limited to cases where a GI bleed is documented, but no bleeding site or cause is identified. A hemorrhage in the GI tract may produce either dark black, tarry, clotted stools (also referred to as melena) or bright red blood in the stool or vomitus. This is not the same as "occult blood," which is invisible and only detected by microscopic examination or by a guaiac test. Occult blood is a small amount of blood coming from the GI tract. Occult blood or guaiac-positive stool is reported with ICD-9-CM diagnosis code 792.1, Nonspecific abnormal findings in other body substances, stool contents.

Note the lengthy excludes note under the category 578. This note identifies a number of GI conditions that can be coded based on the presence of hemorrhage or bleeding. The use of the 578 category code is not appropriate when one of the conditions listed under the excludes note is present.

Even though ICD-9-CM includes the combination codes describing a GI hemorrhage with a GI condition (angiodysplasia, diverticulitis, gastritis, duodenitis, and ulcer), these codes should not be assigned unless the physician identifies a causal relationship. The coder should not assume a causal relationship between GI bleeding and a single finding such as a gastric ulcer, gastritis, diverticulitis, and so on. The physician must identify the source of the bleeding and link the clinical findings from the colonoscopy or upper endoscopy because these findings may be unrelated to the bleeding. Active bleeding does not have to be occurring at the time of the examination or procedure, but it does have to be identified in the patient's history. Two codes should be assigned when the physician states that the GI hemorrhage is unrelated to a coexisting GI condition: one for the GI hemorrhage, and one for the GI condition without hemorrhage.

## Exercise 12.1

Assign ICD-9-CM diagnosis and procedure codes to the following:

1. Small bowel obstruction with peritoneal adhesions; lysis of peritoneal adhesions

2. Unilateral femoral hernia with gangrene; repair of hernia with graft

3. Cholesterolosis of gallbladder

4. Regional enteritis of large intestine

5. Mesio-occlusion dentofacial anomaly, Angle's class III

6. Melena; esophagogastroduodenoscopy with biopsy

7. Acute perforated peptic ulcer

*(Continued on next page)*

## Exercise 12.1 (Continued)

8. Acute hemorrhagic gastritis with acute blood loss anemia

9. Acute appendicitis with perforation and peritoneal abscess; open appendectomy

10. Allergic diarrhea

11. Temporomandibular joint disorder with clicking sounds when moving the jaw

12. Diverticulosis and diverticulitis of colon; flexible fiberoptic colonoscopy

13. Esophageal reflux with esophagitis

14. Infection of colostomy

15. Acute cholecystitis with cholelithiasis; laparoscopic cholecystectomy

# Gastrointestinal Procedures

This section highlights coding for GI procedures such as:

- Laparoscopic and open repair of hernia
- Closed endoscopic biopsies
- Endoscopic excisions of lesions
- GI ostomies

## Laparoscopic and Open Repair of Hernia

Surgery is the only treatment and cure for most hernias. Hernia repair is one of the most commonly performed surgeries in the United States. While the majority of the procedures are performed via the "open" or incisional technique, the procedures can be performed laparoscopically. Open hernia repairs are performed through an incision with sutured tissue repair. Using synthetic mesh materials to repair the hernia has become fairly standard technique. Laparoscopic hernia repair is a less invasive procedure, with a small incision made to allow a thin, lighted instrument called a laparoscope to be inserted through the incision. The instruments used to repair the hernia are inserted through other small incisions. Laparoscopic procedures also use mesh that is fixated to the fascia with tacks or sutures to repair the hernia. Laparoscopic hernia repair is often preferred because it causes less postoperative pain, and the patients are able to return to their normal activities more quickly than after an open or incisional procedure.

Using ICD-9-CM volume 3, Procedures, laparoscopic and open hernia repairs are coded with different procedure codes. Laparoscopic (unilateral) repair of direct, indirect, or unspecified inguinal hernia with graft or prosthesis is coded with the procedure codes 17.11–17.13. The same procedures performed bilaterally are coded with the procedure codes 17.21–17.24. The repair of direct, indirect, or unspecified inguinal hernia using an incisional, open, or other technique is reported with ICD-9-CM procedure codes 53.01–53.05. If a bilateral direct, indirect, or unspecified hernia is repaired by the open or other techniques, ICD-9-CM procedure codes 53.10–53.17 are assigned.

A direct inguinal hernia requires the repair of the herniation that passes through the inguinal triangle in the groin and enters the inguinal canal. The repair involves the abdominal wall between the deep epigastric artery and the edge of the rectus muscle. An indirect inguinal hernia occurs when the hernial sac enters the inguinal canal through the deep inguinal ring and may descend farther and emerge from the canal through the superficial inguinal ring. An indirect inguinal hernia repair involves the internal inguinal ring and passes into the inguinal canal.

Other hernias can be repaired laparoscopically or by the open technique. Umbilical hernias can be repaired by laparoscopic repair with graft or prosthesis (53.42), by other laparoscopic umbilical herniorrhaphy (53.43), or by other open umbilical herniorrhaphy (53.49). Incisional hernias can be repaired by laparoscopic repair with graft or prosthesis (53.62) or by other laparoscopic repair of other hernia of anterior abdominal wall with graft or prosthesis (53.63). The same incisional or other anterior abdominal wall hernias can be repaired by an open technique (53.61 or 53.69).

A diaphragmatic hernia can be repaired via an abdominal approach either laparoscopically (53.71) or by an open or other approach (53.72), or an unspecified code may be used to describe the abdominal approach repair (53.75). The same type of hernia can be repaired via a thoracic approach either laparoscopically (53.83) or by an open or other approach (53.84), or an unspecified code may be used to describe the thoracic approach repair (53.80).

## Closed Endoscopic Biopsies

In coding closed endoscopic biopsies, note the following combination codes that describe both the endoscopy and the biopsy:

**42.24 Closed [endoscopic] biopsy of esophagus**
**44.14 Closed [endoscopic] biopsy of stomach**
**45.14 Closed [endoscopic] biopsy of small intestine**
**45.16 Esophagogastroduodenoscopy [EGD] with closed biopsy**
**45.25 Closed [endoscopic] biopsy of large intestine**
**48.24 Closed [endoscopic] biopsy of rectum**
**51.14 Other closed [endoscopic] biopsy of biliary duct or sphincter of Oddi**
**52.14 Closed [endoscopic] biopsy of pancreatic duct**

## Endoscopic Excision of Lesions

Many lesions in the digestive tract can be removed using endoscopic methods so that opening the abdomen is not required. ICD-9-CM provides the following codes for this type of procedure:

**42.33 Endoscopic excision or destruction of lesion or tissue of esophagus**
**43.41 Endoscopic excision or destruction of lesion or tissue of stomach**
**45.30 Endoscopic excision or destruction of lesion of duodenum**
**45.42 Endoscopic polypectomy of large intestine**
**45.43 Endoscopic destruction of other lesion or tissue of large intestine**
**49.31 Endoscopic excision or destruction of lesion or tissue of anus**
**51.64 Endoscopic excision or destruction of lesion of biliary ducts or sphincter of Oddi**
**52.21 Endoscopic excision or destruction of lesion or tissue of pancreatic duct**

## Gastrointestinal Ostomies

Notations must be reviewed carefully when coding GI ostomies because additional codes are required to describe the performance of any synchronous resection.

### Gastrostomy

A gastrostomy involves making an incision into the stomach to permit insertion of a synthetic feeding tube. This surgery is performed on patients who are unable to ingest food normally because of stricture or lesion of the esophagus. ICD-9-CM classifies gastrostomy to code 43.19, Other gastrostomy. Code 43.11 describes percutaneous [endoscopic] gastrostomy [PEG].

### Colostomy

A colostomy is the creation of an artificial opening of the colon through the abdominal wall. ICD-9-CM classifies all types of colostomies to subcategory 46.1. However, loop colostomy is assigned to code 46.03, and a colostomy performed with synchronous anterior rectal resection is assigned to code 48.62.

Code 46.03, Exteriorization of large intestine (a loop colostomy), involves bringing a loop of the large intestine out through a small abdominal incision, suturing it to the skin, and opening it. This resulting colostomy provides a temporary channel for the emptying of feces. This procedure is performed to give the bowel a rest following a colon resection. When the bowel is able to return to normal functioning, the loop colostomy is closed.

### Ileostomy

An ileostomy is the creation of an opening of the ileum through the abdominal wall. ICD-9-CM classifies ileostomy to subcategory 46.2; however, loop ileostomy is assigned to code 46.01, Exteriorization of small intestine. A loop ileostomy involves transposing a segment of the small intestine to the exterior of the body.

### Other Enterostomies

Other enterostomies are classified to subcategory 46.3. This subcategory includes percutaneous (endoscopic) jejunostomy, duodenostomy, and feeding enterostomy.

### Revision and Closure of Intestinal Stoma

Subcategory 46.4, Revision of intestinal stoma, includes codes for the revision of both the small and large intestinal stoma. Subcategory 46.5, Closure of intestinal stoma, includes codes for the closure of both the small and large intestinal stoma.

## Intestinal Resection and Anastomosis

Colorectal surgery is often the treatment of colon cancer or other diseases of the colon, such as ulcerative colitis or Crohn's disease. Colectomy procedures remove portions of the large intestine to treat the disease. The procedures can be performed through an incision (open procedure) or done with a laparoscope. Open surgeries can require six- to ten-inch incisions and are highly invasive procedures that require long recovery periods. Open and other partial excisions of the large intestine are reported with the ICD-9-CM procedure codes in the range of 45.71–45.79. Specific procedures—such as right and left hemicolectomy, sigmoidectomy, resection of the transverse colon, and multiple segmental resections of the large intestine—are included in these codes.

Laparoscopic or minimally-invasive surgery involves making a series of small incisions in the abdomen, inserting a video camera or "scope" through one incision, and placing surgical instruments in other incisions via portals called trocars; this procedure allows the surgeon to work inside the body and remove the diseased portion of the colon. Laparoscopic surgery allows the patient to have a short hospital stay and quicker recovery period. Laparoscopic partial excision of the large intestine is described by specific ICD-9-CM procedure codes in the range of 17.31–17.39. Specific procedures such as right and left hemicolectomy, sigmoidectomy, resection of the transverse colon, and multiple segmental resections of the large intestine are included in these codes.

Diseases of the colon and rectum are treated with other surgical procedures. A total intra-abdominal colectomy may be performed laparoscopically (45.81), by an open total technique (45.82), or as an other or unspecified procedure (45.83). A pull-through resection of the rectum can be performed via an open or other technique (48.40, 48.41, 48.43, and 48.49). The same procedure can be performed laparoscopically as well (48.42). An abdominoperineal (AP) resection of the rectum can be performed laparoscopically (48.51) or through an open or other approach (48.50, 48.52, and 48.59).

When coding excision of the small and large intestine, note the following instructions:

**45.5 Isolation of intestinal segment**
Code also any synchronous:
anastomosis other than end-to-end (45.90–45.94)
enterostomy (46.10–46.39)

**45.6 Other excision of small intestine**
Code also any synchronous:
anastomosis other than end-to-end (45.90–45.93, 45.95)
colostomy (46.10–46.13)
enterostomy (46.10–46.39)

**45.7 Open and other partial excision of large intestine**
Code also any synchronous:
anastomosis other than end-to-end (45.92–45.94)
enterostomy (46.10–46.39)

**48.4 Pull-through resection of rectum**
Code also any synchronous anastomosis other than end-to-end (45.90, 45.92–45.95)

**48.5 Abdominoperineal resection of rectum**
Includes: With synchronous colostomy
Code also any synchronous anastomosis other than end-to-end (45.90, 45.92–45.95)

The codes for anastomosis other than end-to-end or colostomy are appropriate to code when the procedures were performed in addition to the bowel resection.

## Laparotomy

Laparotomy is an incision into the abdominal wall. ICD-9-CM classifies laparotomy to subcategory 54.1, which is further subdivided to describe exploratory laparotomy, reopening of a recent laparotomy, and drainage of intraperitoneal abscess or hematoma.

**A point to remember:** Take special note of the exclusion note in code 54.11, Exploratory laparotomy: "exploration incidental to intra-abdominal surgery—omit code." In such a case, the laparotomy is the surgical approach and, as such, should not be coded.

## Application of Adhesion Barrier

In many categories of codes in this section, a note instructs that an additional code is to be assigned for any application or administration of an adhesion barrier substance (99.77).

The adhesion barrier is a temporary bioresorbable membrane used during the primary surgical procedure to assist in the prevention of postoperative adhesions following abdominopelvic procedures.

## ICD-9-CM Review Exercises: Chapter 12

Assign ICD-9-CM diagnosis and procedure codes to the following:

1. Chronic gastric ulcer with proximal gastrectomy
2. Postsurgical malabsorption syndrome
3. Right inguinal hernia, recurrent; open repair of direct inguinal hernia
4. Chronic ulcerative enterocolitis; colonoscopy with biopsy
5. Chronic duodenal ulcer with hemorrhage; esophagogastroduodenoscopy
6. Hepatitis due to infectious mononucleosis
7. Adenocarcinoma of the sigmoid colon; open resection of the sigmoid colon with end-to-end anastomosis
8. Acute cholecystitis with choledocholithiasis; percutaneous removal of common bile duct calculi

## ICD-9-CM Review Exercises: Chapter 12 (Continued)

9. Irritable bowel syndrome (IBS)

10. Rectal ulcer; colonoscopy with biopsy of the rectum

11. Severe dysphagia secondary to old cerebrovascular accident; percutaneous endoscopic gastrostomy (PEG)

12. Polyp of the distal colon; endoscopic polypectomy

13. Acute and chronic pancreatitis with atrophic gastritis

14. Incarcerated incisional hernia; repair of hernia

15. Chronic active hepatitis

# ICD-10-CM Chapter 11, Diseases of the Digestive System (K00–K94)

## Organization and Structure of ICD-10-CM Chapter 11

Chapter 11 of ICD-10-CM includes categories K00–K95 arranged in the following blocks:

| | |
|---|---|
| K00–K14 | Diseases of oral cavity and salivary glands |
| K20–K31 | Diseases of esophagus, stomach and duodenum |
| K35–K38 | Diseases of appendix |
| K40–K46 | Hernia |
| K50–K52 | Noninfective enteritis and colitis |
| K55–K64 | Other diseases of intestines |
| K65–K68 | Diseases of peritoneum and retroperitoneum |
| K70–K77 | Diseases of liver |
| K80–K87 | Disorders of gallbladder, biliary tract and pancreas |
| K90–K95 | Other diseases of digestive system |

A number of new subchapters have been added to the chapter. For instance, in ICD-10-CM, diseases of the liver have their own subchapter or block while these conditions were grouped with other diseases of the digestive system in ICD-9-CM. Some terminology changes and revisions to the classification of specific digestive conditions have occurred in ICD-10-CM as well. For example, the term "hemorrhage" is used when referring to ulcers. The term "bleeding" is used when classifying gastritis, duodenitis, diverticulosis, and diverticulitis:

- K25.0, Acute gastric ulcer with hemorrhage
- K29.01, Acute gastritis with bleeding
- K57.31, Diverticulosis of large intestine without perforation or abscess with bleeding

ICD-10-CM category K50, Crohn's disease, has been expanded to the fourth, fifth, and sixth character in contrast to ICD-9-CM category 555, Regional enteritis. The expansion at the fourth character level specifies the site of the Crohn's disease, the fifth character indicates whether a complication was present and the sixth character further classifies the specific complication. When classifying ulcers, in ICD-9-CM, the presence or absence of obstruction is used as an axis for classifying ulcers. In ICD-10-CM a fairly substantial classification change was made and the identification of obstruction is no longer a part of the ICD-10-CM ulcer code structure.

## Coding Guidelines and Instructional Notes for ICD-10-CM Chapter 11

Modifications were made to specific codes in this chapter. For example, in ICD-9-CM ulcerative colitis does not have any instructions for code usage listed below category 556. In contrast, guidelines for category K51, Ulcerative colitis, state to use an additional code to identify manifestations.

No instructional note is found at the start of the subchapter for hernias in ICD-9-CM. However, this is not the case in ICD-10-CM. The note "hernia with both gangrene and obstruction is classified to hernia with gangrene" applies to all conditions coded to categories K40–K46.

Instructional notes indicating that an additional code should be assigned for associated conditions and external causes or that an underlying condition should be coded first have been expanded.

At this time, there are no chapter-specific guidelines related to Chapter 11, Diseases of the Digestive System.

## Coding Overview for ICD-10-CM Chapter 11

Chapter 11 in ICD-10-CM, Diseases of the digestive system (K00–K95), contains many of the same conditions that appear in ICD-9-CM for the digestive diseases, with some combination codes that previously required a second code or the use of a fifth digit.

For example, in ICD-10-CM, the codes for gastric, duodenal, peptic, and gastrojejunal ulcers do not include the classification of obstruction but maintain the acute and chronic types of ulcers with and without hemorrhage and perforation.

The new codes for hernias of the abdominal cavity are differentiated as bilateral or unilateral, with or without obstruction and gangrene.

The ulcerative colitis and regional enteritis codes include the accompanying complication—such as rectal bleeding, intestinal obstruction, fistula, or abscess—within each code.

Complications of artificial openings of the digestive system, including colostomy, enterostomy, and gastrostomy infections and malfunctions, are included in this chapter. As in other chapters of ICD-10-CM, codes for intraoperative and postprocedural complications have been incorporated into the applicable chapters. In the digestive system, intraoperative and postprocedural complications such as postprocedural intestinal obstruction, as well as those for hemorrhage, hematoma, and accidental puncture and laceration, are found in category K91.

Some of the disease categories in Chapter 11 have been restructured to bring together those groups that are in some way related. For example, Chapter 11 contains two new sections: Diseases of liver (K70–K77) and Disorders of gallbladder, biliary tract, and pancreas (K80–K87). And in some cases, headings of subcategories have been changed, for example, angiodysplasia of intestine is in a subcategory for "other specified disorders of intestine" in ICD-9-CM, whereas it is in a subcategory for "vascular disorders of intestine" in ICD-10-CM.

## ICD-10-CM Review Exercises: Chapter 12

Assign the correct ICD-10-CM diagnosis codes to the following exercises.

1. This patient has extensive cellulitis of the abdominal wall due to an infection of the existing gastrostomy site. A feeding tube was inserted four months ago because of the patient's carcinoma of the middle esophagus. The physician confirmed that the responsible organism for the infection is Staph aureus.

2. Acute gastric ulcer with hemorrhage

3. Recurrent right inguinal hernia with gangrene and obstruction

4. Crohn's disease of the small intestine with a small bowel obstruction as the result of an exacerbation of the Crohn's disease

5. Choledocholithiasis with acute cholangitis and obstruction

6. A 68-year-old man was admitted to the hospital for bilateral inguinal hernia repair. The patient also had evaluation and treatment of COPD, chronic low back pain, and hypertension while in the hospital. After being prepared for surgery, the patient complained of precordial chest pain. The surgery was cancelled. Cardiac studies failed to find a reason for the chest pain which resolved later that day.

7. The patient came to the emergency room with the symptoms of vomiting blood and having very dark stools that appeared to be bloody. The patient is also being treated for congestive heart failure and atrial fibrillation. After study, it was determined the patient had a chronic gastric ulcer with bleeding.

8. Generalized chronic periodontitis

9. Diverticulitis of large intestine with perforation and peritonitis

10. Alcoholic cirrhosis of liver with ascites

# Chapter 13

# Diseases of the Genitourinary System

## Learning Objectives

At the conclusion of this chapter, you should be able to:

1. Describe the organization of the conditions and codes included in Chapter 10 of ICD-9-CM, Diseases of the Genitourinary System (580–629)
2. Describe the organization of the conditions and codes included in Chapter 14 of ICD-10-CM, Diseases of the Genitourinary System (N00–N99)
3. Identify the types of conditions considered to be chronic kidney disease
4. Define the term *cystitis* and describe the various codes that are available to classify these conditions
5. Define the term *benign prostatic hypertrophy (BPH)* and identify the associated urinary conditions that can be coded
6. Review the types of female genital tract disorders that can be classified using codes
7. Define the abbreviations of CIN I, CIN II, CIN III, and VIN I, VIN II, VIN III
8. Describe the circumstances in which subcategory codes 795.0 are used in place of codes described in ICD-9-CM Chapter 10, Diseases of the Genitourinary System
9. Identify the options for coding various types of menopause states
10. Assign ICD-9-CM diagnosis and procedure codes for diseases of the genitourinary system
11. Assign ICD-10-CM codes for diseases of the genitourinary system

# ICD-9-CM Chapter 10, Diseases of the Genitourinary System (580–629)

Chapter 10, Diseases of the Genitourinary System, in the Tabular List in volume 1 of ICD-9-CM contains the following categories and section titles:

| Categories | Section Titles |
|---|---|
| 580–589 | Nephritis, Nephrotic Syndrome, and Nephrosis |
| 590–599 | Other Diseases of Urinary System |
| 600–608 | Diseases of Male Genital Organs |
| 610–612 | Disorders of Breast |
| 614–616 | Inflammatory Disease of Female Pelvic Organs |
| 617–629 | Other Disorders of Female Genital Tract |

## Nephritis, Nephrotic Syndrome, and Nephrosis (580–589)

The exclusion note at the beginning of the section "Nephritis, Nephrotic Syndrome, and Nephrosis" reads "hypertensive chronic kidney disease (403.00–403.91), (404.00–404.93)." As discussed in chapter 10 of this book, "Diseases of the Circulatory System," when hypertension and chronic kidney disease exist in a patient, a causal relationship is presumed unless documentation in the health record states that the hypertension is secondary. A cross section diagram of the kidney is shown in figure 13.1.

**Figure 13.1.** Diagram of the kidney

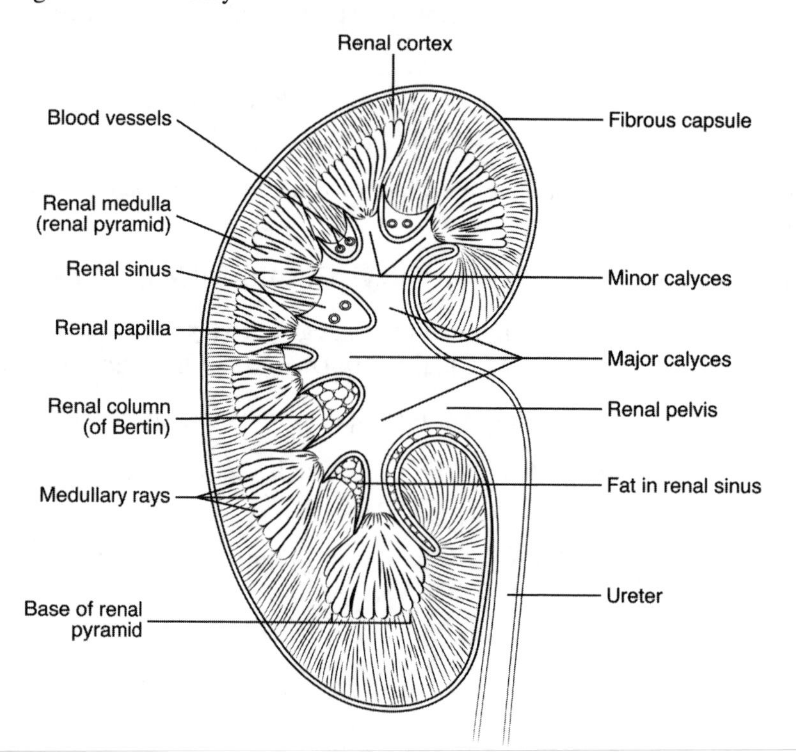

Renal failure and renal insufficiency represent a range of disease processes that occur when the kidneys have problems eliminating metabolic products from the blood. These problems can be caused by various underlying conditions such as hypertension and diabetes, or they may affect patients with a single kidney or those with a family history of kidney disease. There are both acute and chronic renal failure and acute and chronic renal insufficiency, which are identified as separate conditions with different codes in ICD-9-CM.

Proper terminology, as used in ICD-9-CM, is chronic kidney disease (CKD), rather than the vague terms of chronic renal failure and chronic renal insufficiency. CKD has five stages based on the glomerular filtration rate (GFR.) Care of patients with stage IV and V is intensive and complicated. For any patient, the goal is to slow the progression of CKD or better prepare the patient for renal replacement therapy. The determination of GFR is based on a well-established formula. Only patients in need of dialysis or receiving kidney transplants may be considered as having end-stage renal disease (ESRD). Code 585.6, End stage renal disease (ESRD), is assigned when the provider has documented end-stage renal disease. It is not up to the coder to render the diagnosis of ESRD but rather to code the diagnosis based on documentation by the provider.

Chronic renal insufficiency is a form of CKD classified with code 585.9, Chronic kidney disease, unspecified. Also included in this unspecified code are the vague diagnoses of CKD and chronic renal failure. A specific form of CKD and chronic renal insufficiency should not be coded in the same record. Acute renal insufficiency, a vague but different condition from CKD, is classified to code 593.9, Unspecified disorder of kidney and ureter, with other vague descriptions such as acute renal disease or renal disease unspecified. These forms of chronic kidney disease develop gradually in the patient over time, often associated with hypertension or diabetes. The condition may be controlled but generally are irreversible.

Acute renal failure (ARF) is assigned to category 584, with the fourth-digit subcategories identifying the location of the lesion. ARF occurs suddenly, usually as the result of physical trauma, infection, inflammation, or toxicity. Symptoms include oliguria or anuria with hyperkalemia and pulmonary edema. Physicians may identify ARF with more specificity by referring to it as prerenal, intrarenal, or postrenal, which more specifically identifies underlying causes such as congestive heart failure (prerenal), acute nephritis or nephrotoxicity (intrarenal), or obstruction of urine flow out of the kidneys (postrenal). ARF is treated differently from CKD and is classified to category 584, Acute renal failure. Acute renal failure typically develops over a short period of time as part of another illness and is generally reversible and is corrected as the underlying disease is treated or controlled.

## Other Diseases of Urinary System (590–599)

The section "Other Diseases of Urinary System" classifies many genitourinary infections, such as pyelonephritis, urinary tract infection, and cystitis, as well as other disorders of the bladder, ureter, and urethra. It is important to read all the notes at the beginning of the categories and subcategories in Chapter 10 because many conditions in this chapter require assignment of an additional code to identify the organism involved. The organs and vascular structures of the urinary system are shown in figure 13.2.

**EXAMPLE:** Chronic pyelitis due to *E. coli*: 590.00, Chronic pyelonephritis without lesion of renal medullary necrosis; 041.49, *Escherichia [E. coli]* infection in conditions classified elsewhere and of unspecified site

**Figure 13.2.** Diagram of the urinary system

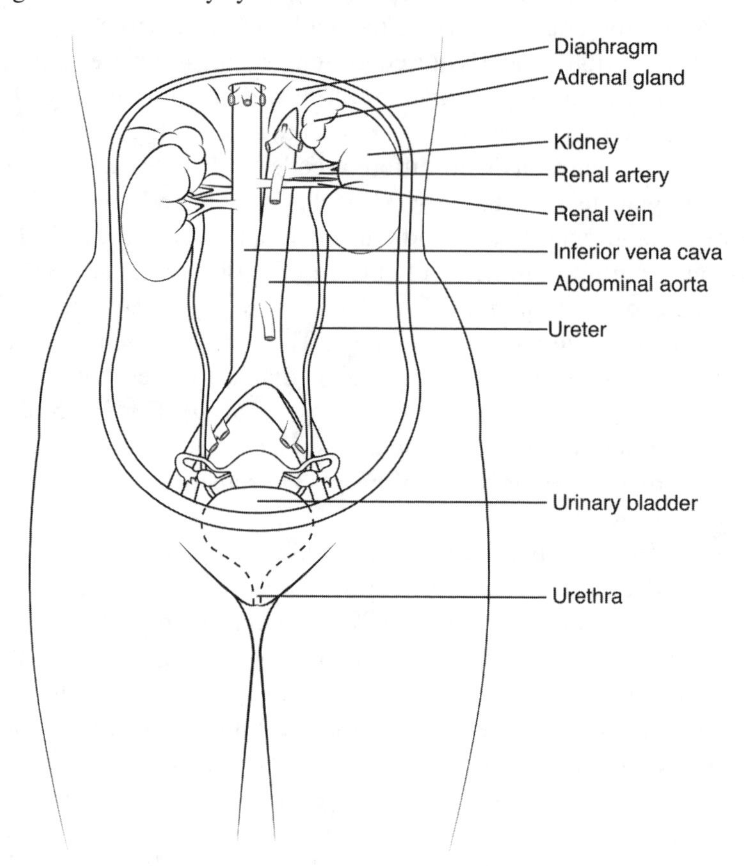




### Cystitis

Cystitis is a bacterial infection of the urinary bladder. Most common in women, this condition is often recurrent. Most cases are due to a vaginal infection that extends through the urethra to the bladder. Cystitis in men is due to urethral or prostatic infections or catheterizations. Symptoms include burning or painful urination, urinary urgency and frequency, nocturia, suprapubic pain, and lower back pain. A cross section diagram of the bladder is shown in figure 13.3.

A diagnosis of cystitis is made by obtaining a urine specimen from the bladder by either catheterization or a clean-catch midstream sample. A bacterial colony count of > (more than) 1,000 colonies/mL in a catheterized specimen indicates cystitis, as does a bacterial count of > (more than) 100,000/mL in a midstream sample. Urine also may be positive for pyuria and hematuria. Therapy with antibiotics is prescribed for uncomplicated infections.

**Note:** The coder should not arbitrarily record an additional diagnosis on the basis of an abnormal laboratory finding alone. If the specific diagnosis is not clearly stated in the health record, the physician should always be queried (CDC 2014).

ICD-9-CM classifies cystitis to category 595, with the fourth-digit subcategories describing type, severity, and location. An instruction at the beginning of this category advises that an additional code from Chapter 1, Infectious and Parasitic Diseases, should be assigned to identify the organism involved.

**Figure 13.3.** Diagram of the urinary bladder

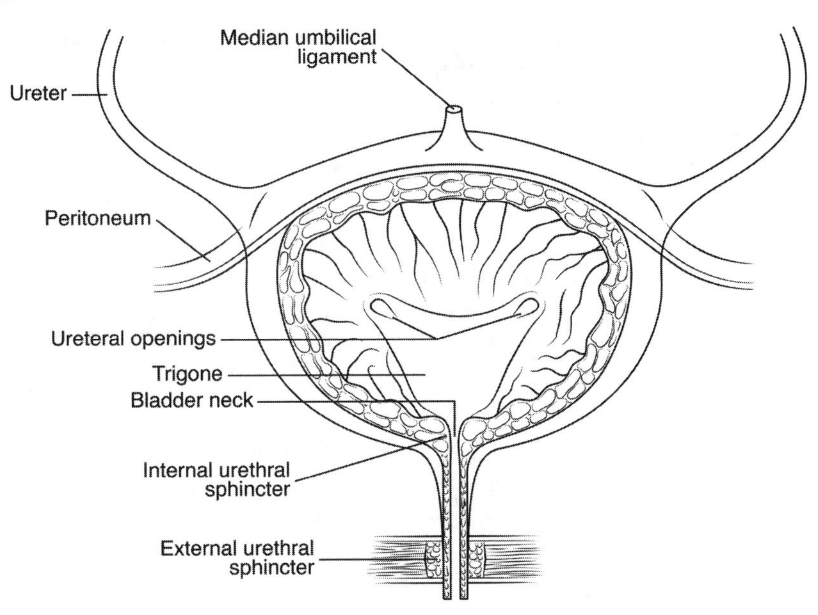




**595.0** **Acute cystitis**
**595.1** **Chronic interstitial cystitis**
**595.2** **Other chronic cystitis**
**595.3** **Trigonitis**
**595.4** **Cystitis in diseases classified elsewhere**
**595.8x** **Other specified types of cystitis**
**595.9** **Cystitis, unspecified**

### Hematuria

Hematuria (599.70) is the presence of blood or red blood cells in the urine. Gross hematuria (599.71) is the presence of blood in the urine in sufficient quantity to be visible to the naked eye. Microscopic hematuria (599.72) is the presence of blood cells in the urine visible only under the microscope. Hematuria can be caused by a number of underlying urinary conditions, including urinary tract infections, benign prostatic hypertrophy, and kidney and ureteral calculi. In patients with certain risk factors, hematuria is a cardinal sign of bladder cancer. These patients require more intensive workup than the primary hematuria patients. Patients presenting with hematuria who are at high risk for bladder cancer have other distinct risk factors: currently smoking or history of tobacco use, voiding dysfunction, personal history of urinary tract infections, and personal history of irradiation. Bladder cancer is generally associated with environmental or occupational factors and less often familial or inherited.

## Diseases of Male Genital Organs (600–608)

The section "Diseases of Male Genital Organs" also has notes requiring the use of an additional code to identify the organism involved.

**EXAMPLE:** Infected hydrocele; organism involved, *Staphylococcus:* 603.1, Infected hydrocele; 041.10, Unspecified *Staphylococcus* infection in conditions classified elsewhere and of unspecified site

### Benign Prostatic Hypertrophy

Benign prostatic hypertrophy, as well as benign prostatic hyperplasia, (both abbreviated BPH) is a condition commonly occurring in men by the age of 60 years, as part of the normal aging process. The prostate gland, which encircles the urethra at the base of the bladder, becomes enlarged and presses on the urethra, obstructing the flow of urine from the bladder. This is known as benign bladder neck obstruction or BNO. Symptoms of BPH, BNO, or what may also be referred to as lower urinary tract symptoms (LUTS) include urinary frequency, urgency, nocturia, incontinence, and hesitancy; decreased size and force of stream; and/or complete urinary retention. Straining to void may rupture veins of the prostate, causing hematuria. The code for benign prostatic hypertrophy is 600.00, whereas the code for benign prostatic hyperplasia is 600.90. These terms are not synonymous and use different codes in ICD-9-CM. However, in ICD-10-CM, these two conditions are reported using the same code.

A diagnosis of BPH is made by a rectal examination that finds the prostate enlarged and with a rubbery texture. Urinalysis shows WBC, RBC, albumin, bacteria, and blood. Cystoscopy reveals the extent of enlargement. A postvoiding cystogram shows the amount of residual urine in the bladder.

ICD-9-CM classifies the forms of hyperplasia and hypertrophy of the prostate to category 600. Some forms of hyperplasia may be indicative of the need for further testing due to the increased risk for prostatic cancer. Hyperplasia of the prostate often produces the symptom of urinary obstruction or the inability to urinate. The urinary obstruction is the problem that typically brings the patient to the physician or to the hospital emergency department.

Category 600 is expanded to the fifth-digit subclassification level to describe the type of hyperplasia of prostate and whether or not urinary obstruction or urinary retention is present. The term "enlarged prostate" is also included in this category. For example:

**600.00** **Hypertrophy (benign) of prostate without urinary obstruction and other urinary tract symptoms (LUTS)**

**600.01** **Hypertrophy (benign) of prostate with urinary obstruction and other lower urinary tract symptoms (LUTS)**

Some of the BPH codes (600.01, hypertrophy [benign] of prostate, 600.21, benign localized hyperplasia of prostate, and 600.91, hyperplasia of prostate, unspecified) include the fact that the patient also has urinary obstruction or urinary retention. In addition, the patient may exhibit other lower urinary tract symptoms. Under each of the BPH with obstruction codes, a directional note states "Use additional code to identify symptoms." Additional codes are used when the patient with prostatic hypertrophy or hyperplasia also has incomplete bladder emptying (788.21), nocturia (788.43), straining on urination (788.65), urinary frequency (788.41), hesitancy (788.64), incontinence (788.30–788.39), obstruction (599.69), retention (788.20), urgency (788.63), or weak urinary stream (788.62).

## Disorders of Breast (610–611)

Disorders such as gynecomastia, fibroadenosis, inflammatory disease, and solitary cyst of the breast are included in this section. Fibrocystic disease of the breast is classified to code 610.1, Diffuse cystic mastopathy. An image of the structures of the breast is shown in figure 13.4.

**Figure 13.4.** Structures within the breast

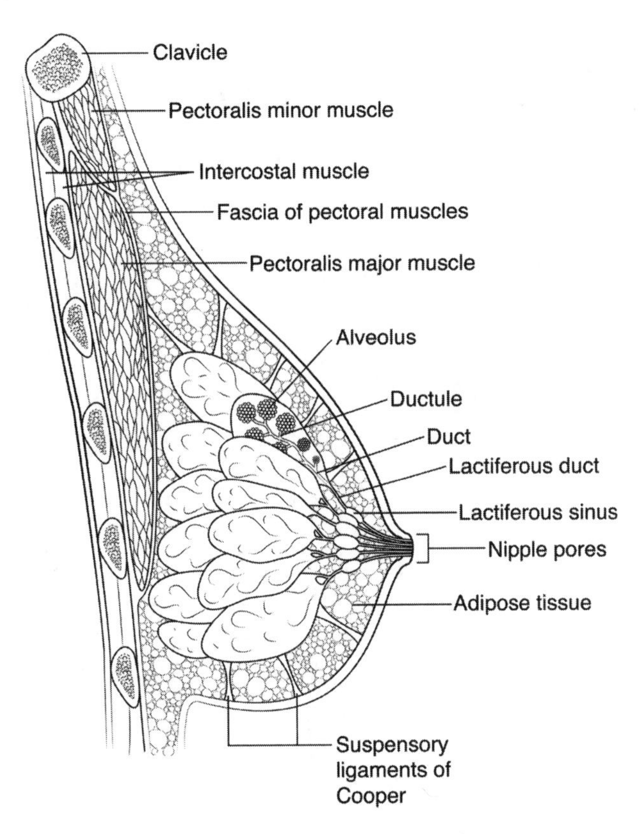




Certain signs and symptoms of breast disease, such as mastodynia, breast lump, and nipple discharge, are included in category 611, rather than in Chapter 16, with other symptoms, signs, and ill-defined conditions. Neoplasms of the breast are classified in Chapter 2, Neoplasms, in ICD-9-CM.

Specific codes describe conditions of the breast related to staged breast reconstruction following full or partial mastectomy due to breast disease or trauma. Codes identify the various stages for which a breast reconstruction encounter may occur or distinguish between the disorders of reconstructed breasts and native breasts. Specific conditions requiring reconstruction may be described with codes in the range of 611.81–611.89 for ptosis, hypoplasia, capsular contracture, and other specified disorders of breast. Deformity or disproportion of reconstructed breast is identified with ICD-9-CM codes 612.0–612.1.

## Inflammatory Disease of Female Pelvic Organs (614–616)

This section includes infections of the female pelvic organs. The note at the beginning of the section indicates "Use additional code to identify organism, such as *Staphylococcus* or *Streptococcus*."

**EXAMPLE:** Acute salpingitis; organism involved—*Streptococcus:* 614.0, Acute salpingitis and oophoritis; 041.00, Unspecified *Streptococcus* infection in conditions classified elsewhere and of unspecified site

An illustration of the various cavities of the female body is shown in figure 13.5 including the pelvic cavity where many of the female disorders discussed in this chapter are located.

**Figure 13.5.** Diagram of the body cavities in the female body

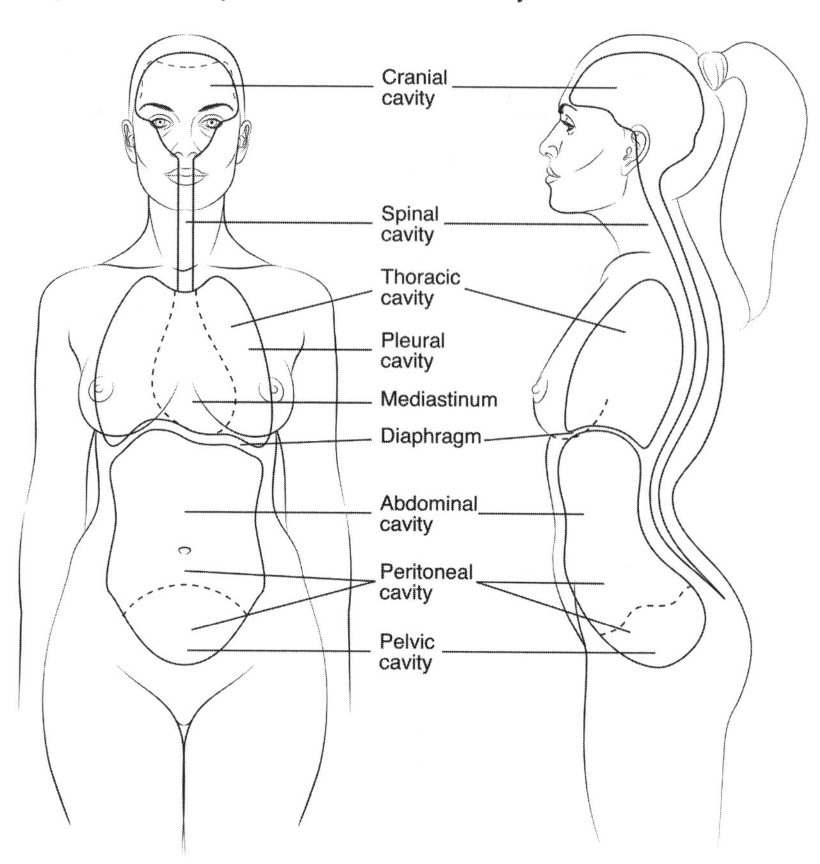




## Disorders of Female Genital Tract (617–629)

The "Other Disorders of Female Genital Tract" section includes conditions such as the following:

- Endometriosis, which occurs when endometrial glands or stroma are present outside the uterine cavity; for example, in the ovaries, uterine ligaments, rectovaginal septum, and pelvic peritoneum. Many women in the United States suffer from endometriosis, and it is one of the common causes of infertility in women (Puscheck 2013).
- Genital prolapse, or prolapse of the vaginal walls with and without uterine prolapse, can be described with ICD-9-CM codes to identify precise forms of these conditions.
- Ovarian cysts of a variety of types are the most common pelvic masses diagnosed in women.

Other gynecological conditions described in this chapter of ICD-9-CM include:

- Noninflammatory disorders of the female genital organs, including dysplasia of the cervix and vulva
- Disorders of menstruation
- Menopausal and postmenopausal disorders
- Infertility

### *Abnormal Pap Smear Findings*

The classification of abnormal cervical Papanicolaou (Pap) smears has become more sophisticated over time. More than 90 percent of the laboratories in the United States use the Bethesda system for reporting the results of Pap smears. The ICD-9-CM classification system is consistent with the Bethesda terminology. The descriptive diagnoses included in the Bethesda system include benign cellular changes, reactive cellular changes, and epithelial cell abnormalities. These abnormalities include:

- Nonneoplastic findings such as reactive cellular changes
- Epithelial cell abnormalities such as atypical squamous cells, low-grade and high-grade squamous intraepithelial lesions including mild to severe cervical dysplasia, and squamous cell carcinoma
- Glandular cell abnormalities that include endocervical adenocarcinoma in situ and other adenocarcinomas

ICD-9-CM codes 622.10–622.12 describe mild dysplasia of the cervix or cervical intraepithelial neoplasia I (CIN I), moderate dysplasia of cervix (CIN II), and unspecified dysplasia of cervix. However, if the condition is described as carcinoma in situ of the cervix, severe cervical dysplasia, or cervical intraepithelial neoplasia III (CIN III), it is classified in subcategory 233.1. ICD-9-CM codes 624.01–624.02 describe vulvar intraepithelial neoplasia I and II, which may be documented as VIN I and VIN II. These conditions are also known as mild dysplasia of vulva (624.01), moderate dysplasia of vulva (624.02), and other dystrophy, kraurosis, or leukoplakia of vulva (624.09). If the condition is described as carcinoma in situ of the vulva, severe dysplasia of vulva, or vulvar intraepithelial neoplasia III (VIN III), ICD-9-CM code 233.32 is used to classify the disease. The Alphabetic Index entry used to locate the codes for these conditions is the term "dysplasia, cervix" or "dysplasia, vulva."

Codes under subcategory 795.0 are used to describe the results of other abnormal Pap smears of the cervix. The Alphabetic Index entries to locate codes to describe these conditions are "Findings, abnormal, Papanicolaou" or "Papanicolaou smear." The following codes describe various ways to explain why results were not available and why a Pap smear must be repeated:

- Abnormal glandular Pap smear of cervix (795.00)
- Squamous cell abnormalities (795.01–795.04)
- Cervical high-risk human papillomavirus (HPV) DNA test positive (795.05)
- Pap smear of cervix with cytologic evidence of malignancy (795.06)
- Unsatisfactory smear or inadequate sample (795.08)

Subcategory 795.0 is used to describe nonspecific abnormal Pap smear of the cervix. Diagnoses such as atypical squamous cells of undetermined significance, as well as low-grade squamous intraepithelial lesion (LGSIL) or high-grade squamous intraepithelial lesion (HGSIL), are included here. Terminology that may also be noted in health records includes "ASCUS favor benign" (for atypical squamous cells of undetermined significance, once coded to 795.01) and "ASCUS favor dysplasia" (for atypical squamous cells, high grade, once coded to 795.02). These same conditions currently are described as ASC-US and ASC-H. Also within this subcategory, codes exist to describe a Pap smear of cervix with high-risk HPV DNA test positive (795.05) and Pap smear of cervix with low-risk HPV DNA test positive. Finally, a code exists to describe an unsatisfactory smear or inadequate sample (795.08) to explain why results were not available and why a Pap smear must be repeated.

Codes under subcategory 795.1 are used to describe abnormal Pap smears of vagina and vulva. Pap smears of the vagina and vulva are performed in women who do not have a uterus or cervix as the result of surgery. Cancer cells can occur in the vaginal walls and the vulva and require the same cancer prevention and screening procedures. Coders should use an additional code with codes in subcategory 795.1 to identify the acquired absence of the uterus and cervix, if applicable (V88.01–V88.03). Various types of abnormal results of Pap smears of the vagina and vulva are reported with codes 795.10–795.14. High-risk and low-risk human papilloma-virus (HPV) DNA tests positive of the vagina or vulva are reported with code 795.15 or 795.19. Other codes exist in this subcategory to describe Pap smear of vagina and vulva with cytologic evidence of malignancy, as well as an unsatisfactory vaginal or vulvar smear that produces an inadequate sample for testing.

## Menopause

The diagnosis of menopause or menopausal syndrome often needs to be more specific. ICD-9-CM includes several options for coding. Codes exist for both symptomatic menopausal syndrome and asymptomatic menopausal status. A crucial factor is whether the menopause is the result of the natural aging process or whether surgical intervention or other treatment such as radiation has created artificially induced menopause. The patient who has a menopausal disorder or symptom associated with artificial or postsurgical menopause may be coded with:

**256.2 Postablative ovarian failure**
**627.4 Symptomatic states associated with artificial menopause**

The patient who is menopausal as a result of having her ovaries removed surgically but who is asymptomatic may be coded with either:

**256.2 Postablative ovarian failure**
**V45.77 Acquired absence of genital organ (ovary)**

The patient who has a menopausal disorder or symptoms associated with age-related or naturally-occurring menopause may be coded with:

**256.39 Other ovarian failure**
**627.2 Symptomatic menopausal or female climacteric states**

Other codes in the 627 category may also be used to describe menopausal-related disorders such as bleeding, atrophic vaginitis, and so forth. Other symptoms may be classified with codes from other chapters.

The patient who is postmenopausal as a result of the natural or age-related process and is asymptomatic is coded with:

**V49.81 Postmenopausal status (age-related) (natural)**

## ICD-9-CM Review Exercises: Chapter 13

Assign ICD-9-CM diagnosis and procedure codes to the following:

1. Vesicoureteral reflux with bilateral reflux nephropathy

2. Acute glomerulonephritis with necrotizing glomerulitis

3. High risk human papillomavirus DNA test positive, vagina

4. Subserosal uterine leiomyoma, cervical polyp, and endometriosis of uterus; total abdominal hysterectomy with bilateral salpingo-oophorectomy

5. Moderate dysplasia of the cervix (CIN II); biopsy of cervix

6. Absence of menstruation

7. Symptomatic menopausal symptoms associated with ovarian failure as the result of age-related menopause

8. Actinomycotic cystitis

9. Benign prostatic hypertrophy with urinary obstruction and incomplete bladder emptying; transurethral resection of prostate

10. Unilateral gynecomastia in male patient with reduction mammoplasty

11. Wilms' tumor; right radical/total nephrectomy

12. Left ureteral stone; ureteral stent insertion

13. Fibrocystic disease of the breast; needle biopsy of the breast

14. Diabetic nephrotic syndrome, type I

*(Continued on next page)*

## ICD-9-CM Review Exercises: Chapter 13 (Continued)

15. Hyperplasia of prostate with lower urinary tract symptoms including urinary obstruction; transurethral microwave thermotherapy (TUMT) of prostate

16. Female midline cystocele, rectocele with pelvic muscle wasting; repair of cystocele and rectocele

17. Female infertility secondary to Stein-Leventhal syndrome

18. Infected hydrocele with hydrocelectomy (spermatic cord)

19. Acquired multiple cysts of the kidney

20. Acute pyelonephritis due to *Pseudomonas*

21. Microscopic hematuria. Personal contact and exposure to benzene (chemicals)

22. Disproportion (breast asymmetry) of reconstructed breast

23. Acute abscess of breast with incision and drainage of abscess

24. Postmenopausal uterine bleeding; Diagnostic D & C

25. Anal intraepithelial neoplasia I (AIN I) histologically confirmed

# ICD-10-CM Chapter 14, Diseases of the Genitourinary System (N00–N99)

## Organization and Structure of ICD-10-CM Chapter 14

Chapter 14 of ICD-10-CM includes categories N00–N99 arranged in the following blocks:

| | |
|---|---|
| N00–N08 | Glomerular diseases |
| N10–N16 | Renal tubulo-interstitial diseases |
| N17–N19 | Acute kidney failure and chronic kidney disease |
| N20–N23 | Urolithiasis |
| N25–N29 | Other disorders of kidney and ureter |
| N30–N39 | Other diseases of the urinary system |
| N40–N53 | Diseases of male genital organs |
| N60–N65 | Disorders of breast |
| N70–N77 | Inflammatory diseases of female pelvic organs |
| N80–N98 | Noninflammatory disorders of female genital tract |
| N99 | Intraoperative and postprocedural complications and disorders of genitourinary system, not elsewhere classified |

Genitourinary disorders in diseases classified elsewhere have been placed in their own category at the end of each block of Chapter 14. This differs from ICD-9-CM in that these conditions were classified within different subcategories. For example, one category, N08, Glomerular disorders in diseases classified elsewhere, is used to identify glomerulonephritis, nephritis, and nephropathy in diseases classified elsewhere.

Changes were necessary in some sections of Chapter 14 because of outdated terminology. For example, given what has advanced in terms of the diagnostic workup, surgery, treatments, and medications available to treat erectile dysfunction (ED) since the last revision of ICD, a new category N52, male erectile dysfunction has been added to ICD-10-CM in comparison to one code in ICD-9-CM, 607.84 (Kim 2014). ICD-10-CM includes category N52 for this condition with subcategories to identify the different causes of the dysfunction. ICD-9-CM has a single code, 607.84, for impotence of organic origin.

To code to the highest level of specificity for posttraumatic urethral stricture, coding professionals will need to identify the patient's gender. This is not necessary for ICD-9-CM code selection for this disorder.

## Coding Guidelines and Instructional Notes for ICD-10-CM Chapter 14

Throughout Chapter 14 are new includes notes that help to clarify the types of disorders that are classified to the various categories.

**EXAMPLE:** **N00 Acute nephritis syndrome**

Includes: acute glomerular disease
acute glomerulonephritis
acute nephritis

**N71 Inflammatory disease of uterus, except cervix**

Endo (myo) metritis
Metritis
Myometritis
Pyometra
Uterine abscess

A similar change has occurred to the instruction for menopausal and other perimenopausal disorders. In ICD-9-CM, there is no note under category 627 to help coding professionals in their selection of a code for these disorders other than an excludes note. However, ICD-10-CM includes a note stating menopausal and other perimenopausal disorders due to naturally occurring (age-related) menopause and perimenopause are classified to category N95.

Coding guidelines state that patients who have undergone kidney transplant may still have some form of CKD because the kidney transplant may not fully restore kidney function. Therefore, the presence of CKD alone does not constitute a transplant complication. Assign the appropriate N18 code for the patient's stage of CKD and code Z94.0, Kidney transplant status. If a transplant complication such as failure or rejection or other transplant complication is documented, see section I.C.19.g for information on coding complications of a kidney transplant. If the documentation is unclear as to whether the patient has a complication of the transplant, query the physician.

To gain an understanding of the genitourinary system coding guidelines, access the 2014 guidelines from NCHS website (http://www.cdc.gov/nchs/icd/icd10cm.htm) and read Chapter 14, Diseases of the Genitourinary System guidelines I.C.14.a.1–I.C.14.a.3. The guidelines are also available in Appendix I of the website accompanying this text.

## Coding Overview for ICD-10-CM Chapter 14

Chapter 14 of ICD-10-CM, Diseases of the Genitourinary System (N00–N99), includes many of the same conditions found in ICD-9-CM. Chronic kidney disease (N18) is divided into stage 1, 2, 3, 4, and 5, as well as end-stage renal disease. Combination codes exist to identify the presence of an infection with and without hematuria—for example, N30.00, Acute cystitis without hematuria, and N30.01, Acute cystitis with hematuria.

The terminology of benign prostatic hypertrophy or benign prostatic hyperplasia is replaced with the term "enlarged prostate" in category N40.

The chapter ends with the intraoperative and postprocedural complications of the genitourinary system like those found in the preceding chapters. Complications of cystostomy and other external stoma of the urinary system are found in the range of codes N99.510–N99.538. Specific genitourinary conditions, such as postprocedural acute or chronic kidney failure, urethral stricture, and pelvic peritoneal adhesions, can be found in category N99.

Several block and category title changes have been made in Chapter 14. For example, subsection 617–629 in ICD-9-CM is titled "Other disorders of female genital tract," whereas the corresponding section in ICD-10-CM, N80–N98, is titled "Noninflammatory disorders of female genital tract."

Codes have also moved to Chapter 14 from other chapters in ICD-9-CM. For example, ICD-9-CM code 099.40, Other nongonococcal urethritis, unspecified, moved from Chapter 1, but its ICD-10-CM counterpart, code N34.1, Nonspecific urethritis, is in Chapter 14.

Several notes are available to indicate that an additional code should be used. Some examples follow:

- N17, Acute Kidney failure—Code also associated underlying condition
- N18, Chronic kidney disease (CKD)—Code first any associated:
    - diabetic chronic kidney disease (E08.22, E09.22, E10.22, E11.22, E13.22)
    - hypertensive chronic kidney disease (I12.-, I13.-)
    - Use additional code to identify kidney transplant status, if applicable (Z94.0)
- N30, Cystitis—Use additional code to identify infectious agent (B95–B97)
- N31, Neuromuscular dysfunction of bladder, NEC—Use additional code to identify any associated urinary incontinence (N39.3–N39.4-)
- N33, Bladder disorders in diseases classified elsewhere—Code first underlying disease, such as: schistosomiasis (B65.0–B65.9)
- N40.1, Enlarged prostate with lower urinary tract symptoms (LUTS)—Use additional code for associated symptoms, when specified:
    - incomplete bladder emptying (R39.14)
    - nocturia (R35.1)
    - straining on urination (R39.16)
    - urinary frequency (R35.0)
    - urinary hesitancy (R39.11)
    - urinary incontinence (N39.4-)
    - urinary obstruction (N13.8)
    - urinary retention (R33.8)
    - urinary urgency (R39.15)
    - weak urinary stream (R39.12)

## ICD-10-CM Review Exercises: Chapter 13

Assign the correct ICD-10-CM diagnosis codes to the following exercises.

1. Patient was evaluated for proteinuria and hematuria and the final diagnosis established as chronic nephritic syndrome with diffuse membranous glomerulonephritis

   ______________________________

2. Patient complained of frequent urination with pain and was diagnosed with acute suppurative cystitis, with hematuria due to E coli

   ______________________________

3. Patient is currently being treated for chronic kidney disease, stage 3. She has previously undergone a kidney transplant but still continues to suffer from chronic kidney disease. This patient is also treated for hypothyroidism following removal of the thyroid for thyroid carcinoma. At this time, there is no longer evidence of an existing thyroid malignancy.

   ______________________________

4. This male patient complained of lower abdominal pain and the inability to urinate over the past 24 hours. After study, the patient was diagnosed as having acute kidney failure due to acute tubular necrosis, caused by a urinary obstruction. The urinary obstruction was a result of the patient's benign prostatic hypertrophy. The patient was treated with medications and the acute kidney failure was resolved prior to discharge.

   ______________________________

5. Premenopausal menorrhagia

   ______________________________

6. A patient complaining of fever, malaise, and left flank pain has a urinalysis performed that showed bacteria of more than 100,000/ml present in the urine and subsequent urine culture shows Proteus growth as the cause of the urinary tract infection. The patient was treated with intravenous antibiotics. The patient also has a history of repeated UTIs over the past several years. The final diagnosis is urinary tract infection due to Proteus.

   ______________________________

7. Endometriosis of uterus and bilateral fallopian tubes and ovaries

   ______________________________

8. Fibrocystic disease of right breast

   ______________________________

9. Prolapse of cervix (female)

   ______________________________

10. Female Infertility due to fallopian tubal blockage

    ______________________________

Chapter 14

# Complications of Pregnancy, Childbirth and the Puerperium

## Learning Objectives

At the conclusion of this chapter, you should be able to:

1. Describe the organization of the conditions and codes included in Chapter 11 of ICD-9-CM, Complications of Pregnancy, Childbirth and the Puerperium (630–679)
2. Describe the organization of the conditions and codes included in Chapter 15 of ICD-10-CM, Pregnancy, Childbirth and the Puerperium (O00–O9A)
3. Define the terms *abortion, missed abortion, threatened abortion, recurrent pregnancy loss* and identify the different ICD-9-CM and ICD-10-CM categories used to classify the diagnosis of abortion
4. Identify the different ICD-10-CM categories used to classify the diagnosis of abortion.
5. Identify the circumstances in which ICD-9-CM category 639, Complications following abortion and ectopic and molar pregnancies and ICD-10-CM categories O00–O08, Pregnancy with abortive outcome is used to describe a woman's condition
6. Define the phrase *early onset of delivery* and describe circumstances in which ICD-9-CM code 644.21 should be assigned
7. Define the term *pregnancy* and describe the ICD-9-CM guidelines for determining preterm, term, and postterm pregnancies and explain the fifth-digit subclassification numbers used with the ICD-9-CM pregnancy codes.
8. Define the term *puerperium*
9. Define the term *ectopic pregnancy* and explain the meaning of the fifth digits used with the ICD-9-CM codes
10. Define the term *normal delivery* and describe the procedures that can be performed with a normal delivery
11. Identify and describe the ICD-9-CM category V27 codes and describe the circumstances in which these codes are used with a delivery code
12. Identify the ICD-10-CM category Z37 codes and describe the circumstances in which these codes are used with a delivery code

13. Identify and describe the various obstetrical and nonobstetrical conditions included in the ICD-9-CM category codes of 642–649 and ICD-10-CM category codes O20–O29.
14. Briefly describe the ICD-9-CM procedure codes used to identify delivery procedures
15. Briefly describe the pregnancy, labor, and delivery codes described in ICD-9-CM categories 650–659 and categories O80–O82 in ICD-10-CM.
16. Briefly describe the complication codes associated with labor and delivery described in ICD-9-CM categories 660–669 and ICD-10-CM categories O60–O77.
17. Identify and describe the various complication codes described in ICD-9-CM categories 670–679 and in ICD-10-CM categories O85–O92.
18. Assign diagnosis and procedure codes for Chapter 11 of ICD-9-CM
19. Assign diagnosis codes for Chapter 15 of ICD-10-CM

## ICD-9-CM Chapter 11, Complications of Pregnancy, Childbirth and the Puerperium (630–679)

Chapter 11, Complications of Pregnancy, Childbirth and the Puerperium, in the Tabular List in volume 1 of ICD-9-CM includes the following categories and section titles:

| Categories | Section Titles |
|---|---|
| 630–633 | Ectopic and Molar Pregnancy |
| 634–639 | Other Pregnancy with Abortive Outcome |
| 640–649 | Complications Mainly Related to Pregnancy |
| 650–659 | Normal Delivery, and Other Indications for Care in Pregnancy, Labor and Delivery |
| 660–669 | Complications Occurring Mainly in the Course of Labor and Delivery |
| 670–677 | Complications of the Puerperium |
| 678–679 | Other Maternal and Fetal Complications |

A detailed diagram of the female reproductive system is shown in figure 14.1.

### Abortion (Categories 634–639)

The diagnosis of abortion is defined as the expulsion or extraction from the uterus of all or part of the products of conception: an embryo or a nonviable fetus weighing less than 500 grams. When a fetus's weight cannot be determined, an estimated gestation of less than 22 completed weeks is considered an abortion in ICD-9-CM. In ICD-10-CM, an abortion includes early fetal death before completion of 20 weeks of gestation. The procedure also known as abortion is more precisely described as a dilation and curettage, dilation and evacuation, or aspiration curettage.

Abortions, as well as complications following abortion and ectopic and molar pregnancies, are classified to categories 634–639 in ICD-9-CM.

**634 Spontaneous abortion**
**635 Legally induced abortion**
**636 Illegally induced abortion**
**637 Unspecified abortion**
**638 Failed attempted abortion**
**639 Complications following abortion and ectopic and molar pregnancies**

**Figure 14.1.** Structures in the female peritoneal and pelvic cavities

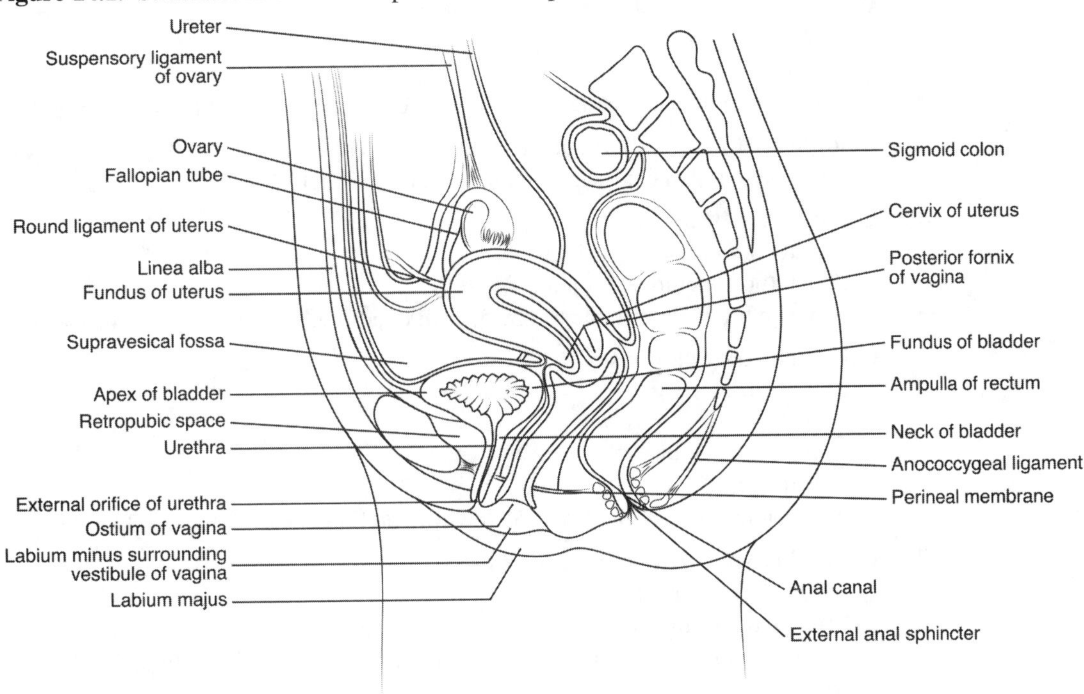




## Fourth-Digit Subcategories

The fourth digits used with categories 634–638 indicate the presence or absence of a complication arising during an admission or an encounter for an abortion. The following list of fourth-digit subcategories is at the beginning of the section "Other Pregnancy with Abortive Outcome" (634–639):

**.0 Complicated by genital tract and pelvic infection**
Endometritis
Salpingo-oophoritis
Sepsis NOS
Septicemia NOS
Any condition classifiable to 639.0, with condition classifiable to 634–638
*Excludes:* *urinary tract infection (634–638 with .7)*

**.1 Complicated by delayed or excessive hemorrhage**
Afibrinogenemia
Defibrination syndrome
Intravascular hemolysis
Any condition classifiable to 639.1, with condition classifiable to 634–638

**.2 Complicated by damage to pelvic organs and tissues**
Laceration, perforation, or tear of:
bladder
uterus
Any condition classifiable to 639.2, with condition classifiable to 634–638

| | |
|---|---|
| **.3** | **Complicated by renal failure** |
| | Oliguria |
| | Uremia |
| | Any condition classifiable to 639.3, with condition classifiable to 634–638 |
| **.4** | **Complicated by metabolic disorder** |
| | Electrolyte imbalance with conditions classifiable to 634–638 |
| **.5** | **Complicated by shock** |
| | Circulatory collapse |
| | Shock (postoperative) (septic) |
| | Any condition classifiable to 639.5, with condition classifiable to 634–638 |
| **.6** | **Complicated by embolism** |
| | Embolism: |
| | NOS |
| | Amniotic fluid |
| | Pulmonary |
| | Any condition classifiable to 639.6, with condition classifiable to 634–638 |
| **.7** | **With other specified complications** |
| | Cardiac arrest or failure |
| | Urinary tract infection |
| | Any condition classifiable to 639.8, with condition classifiable to 634–638 |
| **.8** | **With unspecified complication** |
| **.9** | **Without mention of complication** |

### Fifth-Digit Subclassification

The following three fifth digits are required for use with categories 634–637:

**0** **unspecified**
**1** **incomplete**
**2** **complete**

Fifth-digit assignment is based on the status of the patient at the beginning of the encounter. ICD-9-CM uses the following definitions for complete and incomplete abortions:

- A complete abortion is the expulsion of all of the products of conception from the uterus prior to the episode of care.
- An incomplete abortion is the expulsion of some, but not all, of the products of conception from the uterus. If placenta or secundines remain, the abortion is considered incomplete. A subsequent admission for retained products of conception following a spontaneous or legally induced abortion is assigned the appropriate code from category 634, Spontaneous abortion, or 635, Legally induced abortion, with a fifth digit of 1 for incomplete. This advice is appropriate even when the patient was discharged previously with a discharge diagnosis of complete abortion (CMS 2014).

A review of the pathology report will confirm a complete or an incomplete abortion. A coder would not code an incomplete or complete abortion strictly based on the documentation in the pathology report. The pathology report could be used to initiate an appropriate query to the provider if the provider documentation is not clear on the type of abortion that occurred.

Category 638 does not require the use of a fifth digit because the code describes a failed attempted abortion and, as such, the abortion did not occur.

### Complications

Complications are classified according to the body system involved, such as "complicated by genital tract and pelvic infection" or by the specific type, such as "complicated by shock."

The fourth digit 7 is assigned when a specific complication is stated in the health record but cannot be classified to the previous six subcategories. In these cases, the abortion code is listed first, followed by a code specifying the complication.

The fourth digit 8 is assigned when the documentation indicates the presence of a complication of an abortion without further specification as to type of complication. Avoid assigning the fourth digit 8. There should be documentation in the record that would allow more specific documentation of the type of complication that has occurred. The physician should be queried in these situations. The fourth digit 9 is assigned when a complication is not mentioned.

Codes from categories 640–648 and 651–659 may be used as additional codes with an abortion code to indicate the complication that resulted in the abortion. When a complication of pregnancy is the known cause of the abortion, the fifth digit 3, antepartum condition or complication, should be assigned with the pregnancy code. A fifth digit of 0 is incorrect as it is known at what stage of the pregnancy the antepartum condition occurred. A fifth digit of 1 or 2 is inappropriate on a pregnancy code for a patient who suffers an abortion because the abortion is not a "delivery" by definition.

**A point to remember:** Codes from the 660–669 series must not be used for complications of abortion. Codes from categories 640–648 and 651–659 in the pregnancy chapter may be used and reported with the fifth digit 3, antepartum condition or complication.

### Category 639

Category 639, Complications following abortion and ectopic and molar pregnancies, is used when a complication occurs after the abortion itself was completed during a previous admission. The category is provided for use when it is required to classify separately the complications classifiable to the fourth-digit level in categories 634–638. For example, category 639 is used when the complication itself was responsible for an episode of medical care (the abortion or ectopic or molar pregnancy itself having been dealt with at a previous episode); and there are immediate complications of ectopic or molar pregnancies classifiable to 630–633 that cannot be identified at the fourth-digit level. Note that the fourth-digit subcategories in category 639 parallel those in categories 634–638.

**A point to remember:** A code from categories 634–638 cannot be assigned with a code from category 639.

### Early Onset of Delivery (644.21) Resulting in Live Fetus

The National Center for Health Statistics (NCHS), in consultation with the American Congress of Obstetricians and Gynecologists (ACOG), has confirmed that code 644.21, Early onset of delivery, should be assigned for the delivery of a liveborn infant weighing less than 500 g or having completed less than an estimated 22 weeks of gestation. If the infant is liveborn, regardless of the duration of the pregnancy, the record cannot be coded with an abortion code, but instead an early onset of delivery. If the infant was not liveborn, the situation would be diagnosed by the physician as an abortion because of the infant's weight and the term of pregnancy. (*Coding Clinic* 2nd Quarter 1991, 16). In addition to code 644.21, a code to describe the outcome of delivery (V27) must be assigned. If the delivery or abortion was induced, a code for the procedure performed also should be assigned.

**A point to remember:** A coder cannot assign *both* the diagnosis code for an early onset of delivery (644.21) and an abortion (categories 634–638) on the same patient's record. The outcome of the delivery is either a liveborn infant (644.21) or a nonviable infant (categories 634–638) if the episode of care is during the time period of less than 22 completed weeks. A V27 code is also assigned for the single infant born.

**EXAMPLE:** Spontaneous abortion resulting in liveborn fetus: 644.21, Early onset of delivery; V27.0, Outcome of delivery, single liveborn

**EXAMPLE:** Induced abortion resulting in liveborn fetus; aspiration and curettage: 644.21, Early onset of delivery; V27.0, Outcome of delivery, single liveborn; 69.51, Aspiration curettage of uterus for termination of pregnancy

### Missed Abortion (632)

A missed abortion occurs when the fetus has died before completion of 22 weeks' gestation, with retention in the uterus. ACOG defines a missed abortion as an empty gestational sac, blighted ovum, or a fetus or fetal pole without a heartbeat prior to completion of 20 weeks, 0 days of gestation. ACOG acknowledges the ICD-9-CM definition of missed abortion as any fetal death prior to completion of 22 weeks.

After six weeks in the uterus, dead fetus syndrome (641.3X) may develop, with disseminated intravascular coagulation (DIC) and progressive hypofibrinogenemia. Massive bleeding may occur when delivery is finally completed. During this time, symptoms of pregnancy disappear. A brownish vaginal discharge may occur, but no bleeding.

Missed abortions should be completed by physician intervention as soon as a diagnosis with Doppler ultrasound or other methods is certain. A common method of terminating the pregnancy involves the insertion of laminaria stents to dilate the cervix (69.93), followed by aspiration.

Coders frequently confuse the clinical condition of missed abortion with a different clinical state of spontaneous abortion. A missed abortion is the retention in the uterus of a fetus that has died. The death is indicated by cessation of growth, hardening of the uterus, loss of size of the uterus, and absence of fetal heart tones after they have been heard on previous examinations. In contrast to a spontaneous abortion, no products of conception, fetal parts, or tissue is expelled from the uterus when the patient has a missed abortion. All of the uterine contents remain in the uterus. When a spontaneous abortion occurs, the woman experiences one or more of the classic symptoms, such as uterine contractions, uterine hemorrhage, dilation of the cervix, and presentation or expulsion of all or part of the products of conception.

### Threatened Abortion (640.0)

A threatened abortion is characterized by bleeding of intrauterine origin occurring before the 22nd completed week of gestation, with or without uterine colic, without expulsion of the products of conception, and without dilation of the cervix. ICD-10-CM category O20 states hemorrhage occurs before completion of 20 weeks.

### Recurrent Pregnancy Loss (646.3X and 629.81)

A recurrent pregnancy loss, also known as a habitual or recurrent abortion, is the spontaneous expulsion of a dead or nonviable fetus in three or more consecutive pregnancies at about the same period of development. Coding guidelines for this condition include:

- If the recurrent abortion is current, that is, the patient's admission or encounter is for an abortion, ICD-9-CM offers direction to the abortion codes (634–638).

- If the current hospital admission or encounter involves a pregnancy, assign code 646.3X, Recurrent pregnancy loss.
- If the current hospital admission or encounter does not involve a pregnancy, assign code 629.81, Recurrent pregnancy loss without current pregnancy.

## Exercise 14.1

Assign ICD-9-CM diagnosis and procedure codes to the following:

1. Spontaneous abortion, complete, during the 22nd week of pregnancy, with liveborn infant

   ______________________________

2. Missed abortion, 19 weeks' gestation

   ______________________________

3. Complete legal abortion performed by dilation and curettage (D&C), complicated by excessive hemorrhage

   ______________________________

4. Incompetent cervix resulting in incomplete spontaneous abortion; D&C performed to remove products of conception

   ______________________________

5. Defibrination syndrome following induced abortion 2 weeks ago

   ______________________________

## Pregnancy

Pregnancy is the state of a female after conception until the birth (delivery) of the child. Normal pregnancies are intrauterine and the duration of pregnancy from conception to delivery is about 266 days. The following guidelines may be used in determining preterm, term, and postterm pregnancies:

- Preterm: Delivery before 37 completed weeks of gestation (patient is in her 37th or earlier week of pregnancy)
- Term: Delivery between 38 and 40 completed weeks of gestation (patient is in her 38th, 39th, or 40th week of pregnancy)
- Postterm: Delivery between 41 and 42 completed weeks of gestation (Patient is in her 41st or 42nd week of pregnancy)
- Prolonged: Delivery for a pregnancy that has advanced beyond 42 completed weeks of gestation (patient is in her 43rd or later week of pregnancy)

The postpartum period, or puerperium, begins immediately after delivery and continues for six weeks. In the Alphabetic Index to Diseases, long listings of conditions appear under the following main terms:

**Pregnancy**
**Labor**

**Delivery**
**Puerperium/Puerperal/Postpartum**

Indentations are often used in the Alphabetic Index under these main terms, so extreme care should be taken in locating and selecting the appropriate code.

## Exercise 14.2

Using only the Alphabetic Index (volume 2), assign ICD-9-CM diagnostic codes to the following (*excluding* fifth digits and outcome of delivery):

1. Postpartum varicose veins of legs

   ______________________________

2. 24-week gestation with bleeding

   ______________________________

3. Spontaneous breech delivery

   ______________________________

4. Spontaneous abortion followed by a D&C

   ______________________________

5. Triplet pregnancy, delivered spontaneously

   ______________________________

### Classification of Pregnancy

Pregnancies are classified to the following categories and sections:

| | |
|---|---|
| 633 | Ectopic Pregnancy |
| 640–649 | Complications Mainly Related to Pregnancy |
| 650–659 | Normal Delivery, and Other Indications for Care in Pregnancy, Labor, and Delivery |
| 660–669 | Complications Occurring Mainly in the Course of Labor and Delivery |
| 670–677 | Complications of the Puerperium |
| 678–679 | Other Maternal and Fetal Complications |

Typically, obstetrical cases require assigning codes from categories 630–679 from Chapter 11, which describe complications of pregnancy, childbirth, and the puerperium. However, if the condition being treated is not affecting the pregnancy, assign code V22.2, Incidental pregnancy, rather than a code from Chapter 11. Coders should note that the physician is responsible for indicating that a condition is not affecting the pregnancy.

## Guidelines for Sequencing Codes Related to Pregnancy

In sequencing codes for conditions related to pregnancy, list codes from Chapter 11 first, followed by other codes that further specify the condition or disease.

The following guidelines should be reviewed when selecting the principal diagnosis:

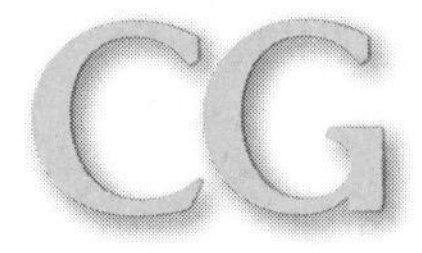

- The circumstances of the encounter or admission should determine the principal diagnosis.
- When an admission does not involve a delivery, the principal diagnosis should identify the principal complication that necessitated the admission. When more than one complication exists that equally meets the definition for principal diagnosis, any one of the complications may be sequenced first.
- When an admission involves delivery, the principal diagnosis should identify the main circumstance or complication of the delivery. In cases where a cesarean delivery was performed, a diagnosis must be included to reflect the reason for it.
- If the reason for the admission/encounter was unrelated to the condition resulting in the cesarean delivery, the condition related to the reason for the admission/encounter should be selected as the principal diagnosis, even if a cesarean was performed.
- In encounters for routine prenatal visits without the presence of any complication, the following codes are appropriate: V22.0, Supervision of normal first pregnancy, and V22.1, Supervision of other normal pregnancy. These codes are not to be assigned with codes from chapter 11.
- In encounters for prenatal visits in high-risk pregnancies, a code from category V23, Supervision of high-risk pregnancy, should be sequenced first. Additional codes from chapter 11 should be assigned to describe specific complications.

A thorough review of the record is necessary to describe the circumstances of the patient's admission or visit to assign the correct principal diagnosis for an inpatient and the first-listed diagnosis code for an outpatient encounter. The type of delivery, the complication of the pregnancy, and the reasons for the obstetrical patient's care are all determining factors in what are the appropriate diagnosis codes to assign.

## Ectopic Pregnancy (633)

An ectopic pregnancy is a pregnancy arising from implantation of the ovum outside the uterine cavity. About 98 percent of ectopic pregnancies are tubal (occurring in the fallopian tube) (Sepilian 2014). Other sites include the peritoneum or abdominal viscera, ovary, or cervix. ICD-9-CM classifies ectopic pregnancy to category 633, with fourth digits identifying the site of the ectopic pregnancy. The fifth digit of 0 or 1 indicates whether or not an intrauterine pregnancy is present with the ectopic pregnancy. With the use of reproductive technology there appears to have been an increase in multiple gestation pregnancies (ectopic pregnancies coexisting with intrauterine pregnancies).

## Fifth-Digit Subclassification

Assignment of the fifth digit centers on the episode of care. An episode of care is an encounter in which a patient receives care. Generally, an inpatient episode of care extends from the time of admission until the time of discharge. An outpatient episode of care involves a visit to a clinic or physician's office, or a home healthcare visit.

The following fifth-digit subclassification is required for use in categories 640–649, 651–659, 660–669, 670–676, and 678–679:

**0 unspecified as to episode of care or not applicable**

**1 delivered, with or without mention of antepartum condition**

Antepartum condition with delivery
Delivery NOS
Intrapartum
obstetric condition
Pregnancy, delivered
} (with mention of antepartum complication during current episode of care)

**2 delivered, with mention of postpartum complication**

Delivery with mention of puerperal complication
during current episode of care

**3 antepartum condition or complication**

Antepartum obstetric condition, not delivered
during the current episode of care

**4 postpartum condition or complication**

Postpartum or puerperal obstetric condition or complication
following delivery that occurred:
during previous episode of care
outside hospital, with subsequent admission for observation or care

The fifth digit 0 is for the rare occurrence in which the episode of care is unspecified or not applicable. Note that the fifth digit 0 is applicable with all the categories (excluding those so stated).

Fifth digits 1 and 2 indicate that the delivery occurred during the same admission. Fifth digit 1 is assigned whenever an antepartum complication is present; fifth digit 2 is assigned when a postpartum complication exists. Because these digits indicate that delivery occurred during the current episode of care, they may be used together on the same record if both an antepartum and a postpartum condition are present.

Fifth digits 3 and 4 both indicate that the delivery did not occur during the current episode of care. Fifth digit 3 is assigned when an antepartum condition is present; fifth digit 4 is assigned when a postpartum condition exists. Because these digits indicate that delivery did not occur during the current admission, they can never be combined with fifth digits 1 and 2. Moreover, they cannot be assigned together because the patient cannot be in both the antepartum state and the postpartum state during the same episode of care.

**A point to remember:** More than one fifth digit can occur in the same patient's health record, but only in the following combinations:

1 only, or with 2, but never with 0, 3, or 4
2 only, or with 1, but never with 0, 3, or 4
3 only, never with 0, 1, 2, or 4
4 only, never with 0, 1, 2, or 3

**Note:** All categories requiring the use of the fifth-digit subclassification have a section marker appearing directly before the category.

## Exercise 14.3

Determine the appropriate fifth digit for the following:

1. Shock during labor and delivery

   ______________________________

2. Pyrexia of unknown origin during the puerperium (postpartum), delivery during previous admission

   ______________________________

3. Retained placenta without hemorrhage, delivery this admission

   ______________________________

4. Prolonged first-stage labor, delivery this admission

   ______________________________

5. Late vomiting of pregnancy, undelivered

   ______________________________

## Normal Delivery (650)

Category 650, Normal delivery, is assigned when all the following criteria are met:

- Delivery of a full-term, single, healthy liveborn infant
- Delivery without prenatal or postpartum complications classifiable to categories 630–679. (This includes antepartum and postpartum conditions such as multiple gestation and breast abscess. Code 650 may be used if the patient had a complication at some point during her pregnancy, but at the time of the admission for the delivery, the complication had been resolved.)
- Cephalic, occipital, or vertex presentation (head first) with spontaneous, vaginal delivery requiring minimal or no assistance, with or without episiotomy, without fetal manipulation (for example, rotation, version) or instrumentation (forceps)

**A point to remember:** Because of these specific criteria, many deliveries cannot be assigned to category 650. No fourth or fifth digits apply to code 650. Code 650 is always a principal diagnosis code. It is not to be used if any other code from chapter 11 is needed to describe a current complication of the antenatal, delivery, or perinatal period. Additional codes from other chapters may be used with code 650 if they are not related to or are not in any way complicating the pregnancy.

The following procedure codes may be reported with code 650:

**73.01 Induction of labor by artificial rupture of membranes**
**73.09 Other artificial rupture of membranes (at time of delivery)**
**73.59 Other manually-assisted delivery**
**73.6 Episiotomy with repair**

**75.34 Other fetal monitoring**
**03.91 Injection into spinal canal, anesthetic agent for anesthesia**

Various procedure codes for sterilization, such as 66.21–66.29 or 66.31–66.39, can also be used with code 650.

## Exercise 14.4

Which of the following obstetrical cases qualify for a code 650 assignment? Delivery of:

1. Liveborn infant, 35 weeks' gestation
2. Liveborn infant, full-term, with cephalic presentation
3. Normal full-term liveborn infant, cephalic presentation with midline episiotomy with repair
4. Liveborn infant, full-term, cephalic presentation with fetal monitoring and epidural block
5. Liveborn infant, twin, with breaking of the water bag to facilitate delivery
6. Liveborn infant, full-term, transverse presentation switched to cephalic by physician before delivery
7. Liveborn infant with artificial rupture of the membranes at 44 weeks' gestation
8. Vaginal birth after cesarean, normal liveborn infant
9. Premature liveborn infant, delivered by low transverse cesarean delivery
10. Stillborn infant, cephalic presentation, unassisted delivery

## Outcome of Delivery (V Codes)

The outcome of delivery, as indicated by a code from category V27, should be included on all maternal delivery records. This is always an additional, not a principal, diagnosis code used to reflect the number and status of babies delivered. Many hospitals rely on these codes to provide more information on obstetrical outcomes. Code V27 is referenced in the Alphabetic Index to Diseases under the main term "Outcome of delivery."

**EXAMPLE:** Normal delivery and pregnancy, single liveborn: 650, Normal delivery; V27.0, Outcome of delivery, single liveborn

## Obstetrical and Nonobstetrical Complications

Many preexisting conditions, including diabetes, hypertension, and anemia, may affect or complicate the pregnancy or its management. In addition, the pregnancy may aggravate the preexisting condition.

For this reason, if the pregnancy aggravates the preexisting or nonobstetrical condition or vice versa, the condition is reclassified to Chapter 11 of ICD-9-CM. The categories representing such conditions are 642–643, 645, 646–649, and 670–677. In some cases, the code in the obstetrical chapter is all that is required to completely describe the condition. In other situations, a secondary code is needed to specify the condition further.

### Category 642

Category 642, Hypertension complicating pregnancy, childbirth, and the puerperium, provides specific subcategories for the type of hypertension; therefore, a secondary code from category 401, Essential hypertension, is not required. According to official coding guidelines, additional codes from other chapters may be used in conjunction with chapter 11 codes to further specify the condition.

**EXAMPLE:** Term pregnancy complicated by benign essential hypertension, delivered: 642.01, Benign essential hypertension complicating pregnancy, childbirth, and the puerperium, Single liveborn infant, V27.0.

### Category 643

Category 643, Excessive vomiting in pregnancy, also provides specific subcategories; therefore, additional codes are not required unless ICD-9-CM notations instruct otherwise. For example, code 643.8 has the note to "Use additional code to specify the cause."

### Category 645

ACOG requested a code for women who are between 40 and 42 weeks' gestation as this may be the primary reason for the obstetrical services being rendered. A pregnancy is not considered postdated until after 42 completed weeks. Women in this group are considered potentially high risk for pregnancy complications.

The title of category 645 was changed from prolonged pregnancy to late pregnancy. Subcategory 645.1 was added to describe postterm pregnancy or pregnancy over 40 completed weeks to 42 completed weeks of gestation. Subcategory 645.2 was added to describe prolonged pregnancy or pregnancy that has advanced beyond 42 completed weeks of gestation.

### Categories 646–649

For the most part, codes in categories 646–649 require the assignment of an additional code to further specify the condition. For example:

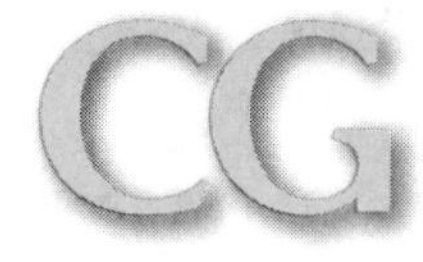

- Subcategory 646.2, Unspecified renal disease in pregnancy, without mention of hypertension, requires assignment of an additional code to specify the type of renal disease.

**EXAMPLE:** Term pregnancy with chronic nephropathy, delivered: 646.21, Unspecified renal disease in pregnancy, without mention of hypertension; 582.9, Chronic glomerulonephritis with unspecified pathological lesion in kidney, Single liveborn infant, V27.0.

- Subcategory 646.3 has been retitled "Recurrent pregnancy loss" in place of the former title of "Habitual aborter." Similarly, code 629.81 has been retitled "Recurrent pregnancy loss without current pregnancy" to describe a woman who is not currently pregnant but has a history of recurrent pregnancy loss.
- Subcategory 646.6, Infections of genitourinary tract in pregnancy, requires assignment of an additional code to specify the infection.
- Subcategory 646.8, Other specified complications of pregnancy, is used when the complication is not classified elsewhere in chapter 11.
- Category 647, Infectious and parasitic conditions in the mother classifiable elsewhere, but complicating pregnancy, childbirth, or the puerperium, is further subdivided to identify the type of infectious or parasitic condition. A second code may be assigned to describe the infectious or parasitic condition.

**EXAMPLE:** Intrauterine pregnancy, 18 weeks with chronic gonorrhea: 647.13, Gonorrhea in the mother classifiable elsewhere, but complicating pregnancy, childbirth, or the puerperium; 098.2, Chronic gonococcal infection of lower genitourinary tract

- Category 648, Other current conditions in the mother classifiable elsewhere, but complicating pregnancy, childbirth, or the puerperium, is further subdivided to include a variety of conditions. This category is quite broad and requires assignment of an additional code to further specify the condition.

**EXAMPLE:** Intrauterine pregnancy, 20 weeks, active cocaine abuse: 648.43, Mental disorders in the mother complicating pregnancy, childbirth, or the puerperium; 305.60, Nondependent cocaine abuse

**EXAMPLE:** Intrauterine pregnancy, 20 weeks, dependence on cocaine: 648.33, Drug dependence in the mother complicating pregnancy, childbirth, or the puerperium; 304.20, Cocaine dependence

Note that ICD-9-CM reclassifies abuse of a drug to mental disorders (648.4) and drug and alcohol addiction to drug dependence (648.3) in the pregnancy chapter of ICD-9-CM. This is another example of why the health record must be reviewed carefully to ensure accurate code assignments.

Other conditions included in category 648 are diabetes mellitus in pregnancy and gestational diabetes. Pregnant women who are diabetic should be assigned code 648.0X with an additional code from category 249 or 250, Diabetes mellitus, to identify the type of diabetes present. Another code, V58.67, Long-term (current) use of insulin, should also be assigned if the type II diabetes is being treated with insulin.

Gestational diabetes can occur during the second and third trimester of pregnancy in women who were not diabetic prior to pregnancy. Gestational diabetes can cause complications in pregnancy similar to those of preexisting diabetes mellitus. It also puts the woman at greater risk of developing diabetes mellitus after the pregnancy. Gestational diabetes is coded to 648.8X, Abnormal glucose tolerance. Codes 648.0X and 648.8X are never used on the same patient's record. In addition, code V58.67, Long-term (current) use of insulin, should also be assigned if the gestational diabetes is being treated with insulin.

- Category 649 includes several common conditions that complicate pregnancy and require specific identification when it occurs. Most of the codes have the directional note "Use additional code to identify . . ." so that a secondary code may be used to add specificity. Included in this category are such factors as smoking, obesity, bariatric surgery status, coagulation defects, epilepsy, spotting, and uterine size date discrepancy. Cervical shortening, a condition that is suspected of being a warning sign of impending premature birth, is included in this category of codes. All of these conditions are known to complicate a pregnancy and frequently require additional monitoring and evaluation of the patient.

### Category 670

Category 670, Major puerperal infection, contains four subcategory codes that include the most serious manifestations of major postpartum infection: puerperal endometritis, puerperal sepsis, puerperal septic thrombophlebitis, and other major puerperal infections such as pelvic cellulitis or peritonitis. Only the fifth digits of 2 and 4 should be used with this category to reflect the episode of care that describes when the puerperal infection occurred, either after delivery but before discharge or during the postpartum period of 42 days after delivery.

Code 670.2X should be assigned for puerperal sepsis with a secondary code to identify the causal organism, for example, a bacterial infection with a code from category 041. A code from category 038, Septicemia, should not be used for puerperal sepsis. The code 995.91, Sepsis, should not be assigned with code 670.2X, as it already describes sepsis. However, if applicable, use the additional code of 995.92 for severe sepsis and any associated acute organ dysfunction when present.

### Category 671

Category 671, Venous complications in pregnancy and the puerperium, is subdivided to identify the types of venous conditions or complications. Some of the codes within this category require an additional code to completely describe the obstetrical condition and associated complication. Under subcategories 671.2, Superficial thrombophlebitis and 671.3 and 671.4, Deep phlebothrombosis, antepartum and postpartum, an additional code from category 453 is required to identify the type of vein thrombosis that exists. Other subcategory codes within 671 are specific and fully describe the associated condition with one code.

**EXAMPLE:** 26-week intrauterine pregnancy, varicose veins of legs: 671.03, Varicose veins of legs complicating pregnancy and the puerperium

### Categories 673–676

For the most part, categories 673–676 also represent conditions or complications that are specific; therefore, no additional codes are required to further specify the conditions. However, subcategory 674.0, Cerebrovascular disorders in the puerperium, requires an additional code to describe the specific cerebrovascular disorder.

### Categories 678–679

Fetal medicine codes are included in categories 678–679. Modern diagnostic testing allows physicians to diagnose fetal anomalies very accurately. These codes describe care provided to the mother as well as the unborn fetus. In recent years, there has been increased use of in utero surgery to correct fetal anomalies. Codes in category 678 describe fetal hematologic conditions as well as fetal conjoined twins. Codes in category 679 identify maternal and fetal complications from in utero procedures. Fifth digits identify the episode of care including antepartum, delivery, and postpartum care.

## Exercise 14.5

Assign ICD-9-CM codes to the following:

1. Hyperemesis gravidarum with dehydration, 12 weeks' gestation

2. Uterine pregnancy, undelivered, with thyrotoxic crisis due to toxic diffuse goiter

3. Uterine pregnancy, delivered this admission, with postpartum superficial thrombophlebitis; single full-term liveborn male infant

4. Mild preeclampsia complicating pregnancy, delivered this admission; single full-term liveborn female infant

5. Failure of lactation, delivered 1 week ago (patient discharged from hospital 5 days ago)

# Labor and Delivery

Labor and delivery refers to the way the female organism functions to expel the products of conception from the uterus through the vagina to the outside world. Labor is divided into four stages:

1. The first stage (stage of dilation) begins with the onset of regular uterine contractions and ends when the os is completely dilated and flush with the vagina, thus completing the birth canal.
2. The second stage (stage of expulsion) extends from the end of the first stage until the expulsion (delivery) of the infant is completed.
3. The third stage (placental stage) extends from the expulsion of the child until the placenta and membranes are expelled.
4. The fourth stage denotes the hour or two after delivery when uterine tone is re-established.

## ICD-9-CM Classification of Obstetrical Procedures

Obstetrical procedures are classified in chapter 13 of the Tabular List in volume 3 of ICD-9-CM. The codes for obstetrical procedures are listed under "Delivery" in the Alphabetic Index to Procedures. A partial listing appears in the following example:

**Delivery** (with)
  assisted spontaneous 73.59
  breech extraction (assisted) 72.52
    partial 72.52
      with forceps to aftercoming head 72.51
    total 72.54
      with forceps to aftercoming head 72.53
    unassisted (spontaneous delivery)
        *—omit code*
  cesarean section—*see* cesarean section
  Credé maneuver 73.59
  DeLee maneuver 72.4

ICD-9-CM classifies delivery procedures to the following categories:

**72 Forceps, vacuum, and breech delivery**
**73 Other procedures inducing or assisting delivery**
**74 Cesarean section and removal of fetus**
**75 Other obstetric operations**

### Category 72, Forceps, Vacuum, and Breech Delivery

Category 72 is subdivided to describe the use of high, mid, or low forceps, the type of breech delivery, and vacuum extraction.

**EXAMPLE:** Delivery with low forceps with episiotomy: 72.1, Low forceps operation with episiotomy

**EXAMPLE:** Partial breech delivery: 72.52, Other partial breech extraction

### Category 73, Other Procedures

Category 73 is subdivided to describe procedures that induce or assist the delivery process. The subdivisions include:

- Subcategory 73.0, Artificial rupture of membranes, is further subdivided to describe induction or augmentation of labor.
- Code 73.1, Other surgical induction of labor, is assigned to indicate all other methods used to surgically induce labor, excluding artificial rupture of membranes.
- Subcategory 73.2, Internal and combined version and extraction, is assigned when the physician externally and internally manipulates the fetus.
- Code 73.3, Failed forceps, is assigned when the physician uses forceps to assist in the delivery of the fetus, but delivery does not result.
- Code 73.4, Medical induction of labor, is assigned when a chemical substance (such as Pitocin) is introduced into the mother's body to stimulate labor. An exclusion note under this code states "medication to augment labor—omit code." In other words, if a chemical substance is administered to augment or "move along" the labor, the code is to be omitted.
- Subcategory 73.5, Manually assisted delivery, is assigned when the hands of the physician or practitioner assist the head of the fetus through the birth canal. This code is further subdivided to specify codes for manual rotation of the fetal head (73.51) and other manually assisted delivery (73.59).
- Code 73.6, Episiotomy, is assigned when the vulvar orifice is incised to facilitate the birthing process. The exclusion note in this code indicates that episiotomies performed with vacuum extraction or forceps are assigned to codes in category 72.
- Code 73.8, Operations on fetus to facilitate delivery, is used to indicate when such procedures are necessary.
- Subcategory 73.9, Other operations assisting delivery, includes external version, replacement of prolapsed umbilical cord, incision of cervix, and pubiotomy.

### Category 74, Cesarean Section

Cesarean section (C-section) or cesarean delivery is the extraction of the fetus, placenta, and membranes through an incision in the abdominal and uterine walls. ICD-9-CM classifies C-sections to category 74, which is subdivided to describe types of C-sections: classical, low cervical, and extraperitoneal. A classical cesarean section, also known as a transperitoneal classical cesarean section, is performed with an incision made in the upper segment or the corpus of the uterus. A lower cervical cesarean section, also known as a lower uterine segment cesarean section, is performed with an incision across the lower uterine segment, either transperitoneally or extrapertioneally. An extraperitoneal cesarean section, also known as a supravesical cesarean section, is performed without an incision of the peritoneum. Instead the peritoneal fold is displaced upward and the bladder displaced downward or to the midline and then the uterus is opened by an incision in its lower segment. Both ICD-9-CM and ICD-10-PCS provide codes for the three types of cesarean deliveries described. (Dorland 2012) Another code within the ICD-9-CM category 76, Cesarean Section is code 74.3, Removal of extratubal ectopic pregnancy, is assigned for removal of an ectopic pregnancy.

### *Category 75, Other Obstetric Operations*

The most commonly used procedure codes within this category are for diagnostic amniocentesis (75.1), other fetal monitoring (75.34), and repair of current obstetric lacerations (75.50–75.69) other than repair of routine episiotomy.

## Exercise 14.6

Assign ICD-9-CM procedure codes to the following:

1. Medical induction of labor

 ______________________

2. Low forceps delivery with episiotomy

 ______________________

3. Total breech delivery

 ______________________

4. Manually-assisted delivery

 ______________________

5. Low cervical cesarean delivery

 ______________________

## Normal Delivery, and Other Indications for Care in Pregnancy, Labor, and Delivery (650–659)

Assignment of the codes in this category is as follows:

- Category 650, Normal delivery, is assigned for deliveries requiring minimal or no assistance.
- Category 651, Multiple gestation, is subdivided to fourth-digit subcategories that identify the number of fetuses. An additional code from category V91, Multiple gestation placenta status, is used with the category 651 codes to indicate the number of placentas and amniotic sacs.
- Category 652, Malposition and malpresentation of fetus, is subdivided to fourth-digit subcategories that identify the types of malposition and malpresentation.
- Category 653, Disproportion, addresses the difference in size between the fetal head and the pelvis. The fourth-digit subcategories identify the type of disproportion and the site.
- Category 654, Abnormality of organs and soft tissues of pelvis, classifies any abnormalities, congenital or acquired, affecting the delivery process.

 **EXAMPLE:** Patient admitted at 39 weeks' gestation for a scheduled repeat cesarean delivery (low cervical) because the patient had a previous cesarean delivery during her last pregnancy: 654.21, Previous cesarean delivery, delivered, with or without mention of antepartum condition; 74.1, Low cervical cesarean section. A V27 category code would also be used to indicate the outcome of delivery

- Category 655, Known or suspected fetal abnormality affecting management of mother, is subdivided to fourth-digit subcategories that describe the type of abnormality.

  **EXAMPLE:** Patient admitted at 38 weeks' gestation for a scheduled cesarean delivery (classical) for known fetal hydrocephalus confirmed on ultrasound: 655.01, Central nervous system malformation in fetus; 74.0, Classical cesarean section. A V27 category code would also be used to indicate the outcome of delivery.

- Category 656, Other fetal and placental problems affecting management of mother, is subdivided to fourth-digit subcategories that describe the specific problem.

  **EXAMPLE:** Patient admitted at 38 weeks' gestation in fetal distress; emergency cesarean delivery performed: 656.81, Other specified fetal and placental problems; 74.99, Other cesarean section of unspecified type. A V27 category code would also be used to indicate the outcome of delivery.

  The code 656.81 in this example for fetal distress is an illustration of using the Alphabetic Index for correct code assignment rather than the code description to select a code. A coder may note the code 656.3X, pregnancy with fetal distress, in the Tabular List. Code 656.3X is a condition that is rarely seen as it is intended to describe fetal acidemia affecting the management of the pregnancy and is not the condition that physicians describe as fetal distress in patients today. This exercise is used to alert the reader that is it important to follow the Alphabetic Index directions and not to select a code based on reading the Tabular List code titles.

**A point to remember:** Codes from categories 655 and 656 are assigned only when the fetal condition is actually responsible for modifying the management of the mother, that is, by requiring diagnostic studies, additional observation, special care, or termination of the pregnancy. The fact that a fetal condition exists does not justify assigning a code from this series to the mother's health record.

- Category 657, Polyhydramnios, identifies an excessive amount of amniotic fluid in the pregnant uterus. This is a three-digit code that requires the use of 0 as a fourth digit in order that the appropriate fifth digit of 0, 1, or 3 can be used to identify the episode of care.
- Category 658, Other problems associated with amniotic cavity and membranes, is subdivided to fourth-digit subcategories that identify the types of conditions, such as oligohydramnios and infection of the amniotic cavity.
- Category 659, Other indications for care or intervention related to labor and delivery, not elsewhere classified, includes several conditions, including:
  - Subcategory 659.0, Failed mechanical induction, is the failure of induction by surgical or other instrumental methods, such as forceps.
  - Subcategory 659.1, Failed medical or unspecified induction, is the failure of the medical induction to stimulate the labor process.

## Complications Occurring Mainly in the Course of Labor and Delivery (660–669)

Complications that can occur in the course of labor and delivery include obstructed labor and trauma to the perineum and vulva, among others.

### Obstructed Labor (660)

Category 660, Obstructed labor, is subdivided to describe the types of obstructed labor, including:

- Subcategory 660.0, Obstruction caused by malposition of fetus at onset of labor, includes a note to assign an additional code from 652.0–652.9 to describe the malposition.
- Subcategory 660.1, Obstruction by bony pelvis, includes a note to assign an additional code from 653.0–653.9 to describe the disproportion.
- Subcategory 660.2, Obstruction by abnormal pelvic soft tissues, includes a note to assign an additional code from 654.0–654.9 to describe the abnormality.

A patient may be admitted to the hospital in labor and after a trial of labor the documentation indicates there is a failure to progress, but the physician does not mention obstructed labor. The patient has a cesarean delivery as a result. However, to the physician, the labor is considered obstructed because the labor fails to progress and the fetus does not descend into the birth canal. A trial of labor may be done to see if the head of the fetus will pass through the pelvic brim. The failure to progress may be due to maternal conditions such as a contracted pelvis, cervical dystocia, or malpresentation, malposition, or disproportion of the fetus. Labor is considered obstructed when the fetus fails to descend through the birth canal in spite of uterine contractions whether the physician documents failure to progress or not. An instructional note in the Tabular List supports the code assignment of both the obstructed labor and the reason for it. Under categories 652, 653, and 654 states "code first any associated obstructed labor (660.0, 660.1, or 660.2.)

For example, the physician documents the patient has cephalopelvic disproportion, failure to progress and these are the reasons for the cesarean delivery. In the Tabular List, there is an instructional note under category 653, Disproportion, "Code first any associated obstructed labor (660.1)" (CDC 2014). Two codes would be assigned, 660.11, Obstruction by bony pelvis and 653.41, Fetopelvic disproportion with an additional code for the outcome of delivery, V27.X.

### Trauma to Perineum and Vulva during Delivery (664)

Category 664, Trauma to perineum and vulva during delivery, includes perineal lacerations. This category is subdivided into eight fourth-digit subcategories. The following six subcategories identify laceration degrees:

- Subcategory 664.0, First-degree perineal laceration, includes lacerations, ruptures, or tears involving the fourchette, hymen, labia, skin, vagina, and/or vulva.
- Subcategory 664.1, Second-degree perineal laceration, includes lacerations, ruptures, or tears (following episiotomy) that involve the pelvic floor, perineal muscles, and/or vaginal muscles.
- Subcategory 664.2, Third-degree perineal laceration, includes lacerations, ruptures, or tears (following episiotomy) that involve the anal sphincter, rectovaginal septum, and/or sphincter, not otherwise specified.
- Subcategory 664.3, Fourth-degree perineal laceration, includes lacerations, ruptures, or tears of sites classifiable to subcategory 664.2 and also involving the anal mucosa and/or the rectal mucosa.

- Subcategory 664.4, Unspecified perineal laceration, is available for use when the extent of the laceration is not specified in the health record.
- Subcategory 664.6, Anal sphincter tear complicating delivery, not associated with third-degree perineal laceration.

### Other Complications of Labor and Delivery (669)

Category 669, Other complications of labor and delivery, not elsewhere classified, includes the following three fourth-digit subcategories:

- Subcategory 669.5, Forceps or vacuum extractor delivery without mention of indication, is assigned when the reason for the forceps or vacuum extraction is not indicated.
- Subcategory 669.6, Breech extraction without mention of indication, is assigned when the reason for the breech extraction is not indicated.
- Subcategory 669.7, Cesarean delivery without mention of indication, is assigned when the reason for the cesarean delivery is not indicated.

**A point to remember:** If the specific reason is documented for the breech extraction or cesarean, forceps, or vacuum extractor delivery, that code is assigned rather than the preceding nonspecific codes.

**A point to remember:** Inexperienced coders often confuse conditions that affect the health of the mother with the conditions that affect the health of the newborn infant. Chapter 11 codes 630–677 are used to describe maternal conditions and are reported only on the mother's record.

Codes from Chapter 15, Certain Conditions Originating in the Perinatal Period (760–779), are used to describe the fetus, newborn, or infant's conditions. The perinatal period is generally accepted as the first 28 days of life. Codes 760–763, Maternal causes of perinatal morbidity and mortality, are reported on the infant's record only when a maternal condition affects the infant's health and treatment. Codes 764–779 reflect other conditions that originate in the infant's perinatal period. These describe conditions that the infant may acquire before birth, at birth, or within the 28 days after birth.

## ICD-9-CM Review Exercises: Chapter 14

Assign ICD-9-CM diagnosis, V, and procedure codes (if applicable) to the following:

1. Intrauterine death at 21 weeks' gestation, undelivered

2. Pregnancy, 26 weeks' gestation, with known Down syndrome of the fetus; patient admitted for further management and evaluation, undelivered

3. Obstructed labor due to a large baby, single liveborn male; classic cesarean delivery

4. Normal pregnancy with spontaneous delivery; first-degree perineal laceration with repair; single liveborn

5. Tubal pregnancy (with no mention of concurrent intrauterine pregnancy); unilateral salpingectomy with removal of tubal pregnancy

6. 25-week pregnancy with urinary tract infection secondary to *E. coli*; patient went home undelivered

7. Blighted ovum

8. Term pregnancy with failure of cervical dilation; lower uterine segment cesarean delivery with single liveborn female

9. Term pregnancy with placenta previa and hemorrhage; single liveborn male; repeat low cervical cesarean section

10. Threatened abortion with hemorrhage at 15 weeks; home undelivered

11. 30-week pregnancy with uncontrolled type I diabetes mellitus; home undelivered

12. 25-week pregnancy with internal hemorrhoids; home undelivered

13. Term pregnancy with cephalic presentation and normal spontaneous vaginal delivery of single liveborn infant

*(Continued on next page)*

## ICD-9-CM Review Exercises: Chapter 14 (Continued)

14. Term pregnancy with postpartum pyrexia; single liveborn male; normal spontaneous vaginal delivery with low midline episiotomy with repair

15. Postpartum deep thrombophlebitis, developing 3 weeks following delivery with the occurrence of an acute DVT in the popliteal vein of the right lower extremity

16. Admission for sterilization with multiparity; tubal ligation with Falope ring

17. 35-week pregnancy with fetal distress; classical cesarean section with delivery of single stillborn infant

18. Low forceps delivery with episiotomy of term pregnancy; single liveborn female

19. Elective abortion (complete) complicated by excessive hemorrhage with acute blood loss anemia; elective abortion via dilation and curettage

20. Spontaneous vaginal cephalic delivery of full-term live infant twins; twin gestation with dichorionic/diamniotic (two placentae, two amniotic sacs)

# ICD-10-CM Chapter 15, Pregnancy, Childbirth and the Puerperium (O00–O9A)

## Organization and Structure of ICD-10-CM Chapter 15

Chapter 15 of ICD-10-CM includes categories O00–O9A arranged in the following blocks:

| | |
|---|---|
| O00–O08 | Pregnancy with abortive outcome |
| O09 | Supervision of high risk pregnancy |
| O10–O16 | Edema, proteinuria and hypertensive disorders in pregnancy, childbirth and the puerperium |
| O20–O29 | Other maternal disorders predominantly related to pregnancy |
| O30–O48 | Maternal care related to the fetus and amniotic cavity and possible delivery problems |
| O60–O77 | Complications of labor and delivery |
| O80, O82 | Encounter for delivery |
| O85–O92 | Complications predominantly related to the puerperium |
| O94–O9A | Other obstetric conditions, not elsewhere classified |

With respect to classification changes, episode of care is no longer a secondary axis of classification for most conditions classified in Chapter 15. Instead ICD-10-CM identifies the trimester in which the condition occurred at the fifth- and sixth-character level.

Code titles have been revised in a number of locations in Chapter 15. For instance, ICD-9-CM's terminology states the indication for care such as inlet contraction of pelvis (653.2). ICD-10-CM terminology is much more descriptive of what the code represents, that is, maternal care for disproportion due to inlet contraction of pelvis (O33.2).

**Other examples of title changes:**

ICD-9-CM: 654, Abnormality of organs and soft tissues of pelvis
ICD-10-CM: O34, Maternal care for abnormality of pelvic organs

ICD-9-CM: 664, Trauma to perineum and vulva during delivery
ICD-10-CM: O70, Perineal laceration during delivery

Codes for elective (legal or therapeutic) abortion are classified with the abortion codes in Chapter 11 of ICD-9-CM. In contrast, the elective abortion (without complication) code has been moved to code Z33.2, Encounter for elective termination of pregnancy, in Chapter 21 of ICD-10-CM. Complications of induced termination of pregnancy are found in category O04.

ICD-10-CM requires the use of a seventh characters to identify the fetus to which certain complication codes apply.

**EXAMPLE:** **O32** **Maternal care for malpresentation of fetus**

One of the following seventh characters is to be assigned to each code under category O32.

0 not applicable or unspecified
1 fetus 1
2 fetus 2
3 fetus 3
4 fetus 4
5 fetus 5
9 other fetus

The ICD-10-CM codes for obstructed labor incorporate the reason for the obstruction into the code therefore only one code is required rather than two as in ICD-9-CM. For example, to code obstructed labor due to face presentation the following two ICD-9-CM codes are required: 660.0X, Obstruction caused by malposition of fetus at onset of labor and 652.4X, Face or brow presentation. In ICD-10-CM, only code O64.2XXX, Obstructed labor due to face presentation, is coded.

## Coding Guidelines and Instructional Notes for ICD-10-CM Chapter 15

At the beginning of Chapter 15 are notes that provide instructions for coding professionals. Codes from this chapter are for use only on maternal records, never on newborn records. An instructional note appears at the beginning of Chapter 15 to remind the coder to use an additional code from category Z3A, Weeks of gestation, to identify the specific week of the pregnancy. This is done on all obstetrical patient's records, not strictly those patients who deliver during a current episode of care.

The postpartum period begins immediately after delivery and continues for six weeks following delivery. A postpartum complication is any complication occurring within the six-week period.

Trimesters are counted from the first day of the last menstrual period. They are defined as follows:

- First trimester—less than 14 weeks 0 days
- Second trimester—14 weeks 0 days to less than 28 weeks 0 days
- Third trimester—28 weeks 0 days until delivery

The NCHS has published chapter-specific guidelines for Chapter 15 in the *ICD-10-CM Official Guidelines for Coding and Reporting:*

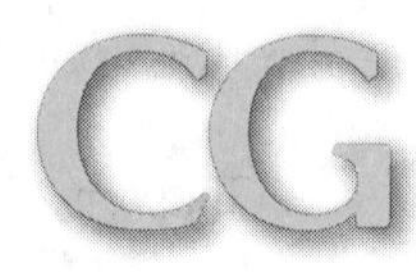


- Guidelines I.C.15.a. General rules for obstetric cases
  These guidelines address the rules that codes from chapter 15 have sequencing priority over codes from other chapters. Additional codes from other chapters can be used with obstetric codes. Chapter 15 codes are only used on the maternal record, not the newborn's record. The majority of codes in Chapter 15 have a final character that indicates the trimester of pregnancy.
- Guidelines I.C.15.b. Selection of OB principal or first-listed diagnosis
  Routine outpatient prenatal visits when no complications are present will be reported with a code from category Z34, encounter for supervision of pregnancy. Prenatal visits for patients with high-risk conditions will be coded from category 009, supervision of high-risk pregnancy with additional codes from Chapter 15 that further specify the condition. When no delivery occurs during an episode of care, the diagnosis codes should describe the complication of pregnancy that necessitated the encounter. When a delivery occurs, the principal diagnosis should describe the main circumstances or complication of the delivery. If a cesarean delivery occurs, the principal diagnosis should be the condition established after study that was responsible for the patient's admission. If the patient was admitted with a condition that resulted in the cesarean procedure, that is the principal diagnosis. However, if the reason for the admission was unrelated to the reason that a cesarean delivery was performed, the condition related to the reason for admission is selected for the principal diagnosis. An outcome of delivery from category Z37, Outcome of delivery, should be assigned to every maternal record when a delivery has occurred.
- Guideline I.C.15.c. Pre-existing conditions versus conditions due to the pregnancy

Certain categories in Chapter 15 distinguish between conditions of the mother that existed prior to the pregnancy, which are pre-existing conditions, and conditions that resulted as a direct result of the pregnancy. It is important to examine the documentation in the record to identify pre-existing conditions and pregnancy related conditions.

- Guideline I.C.15.d. Pre-existing hypertension in pregnancy
  Codes in category 010, Pre-existing hypertension are used to describe the condition as it complicates the pregnancy, childbirth and the puerperium including complications of hypertensive heart and chronic kidney disease.
- Guidelines I.C.15.e. Fetal conditions affecting the management of the mother
  Codes in categories 035 and 036, maternal cause for known or suspected fetal abnormality or other fetal problems are assigned only when the fetal condition Is responsible for modifying the management of the mother. The fact that a fetal condition exists does not justify a code from this series to the mother's record.
- Guideline I.C.15.f. HIV infection in pregnancy, childbirth and the puerperium
  If the obstetrical patient has an HIV-related illness, the principal diagnosis should be 098.7- with additional codes for the HIV-related illnesses. If the patient has asymptomatic HIV infection status, codes from the 098.7- series and Z21, asymptomatic HIV infection status should be used.
- Guideline I.C.15.g. Diabetes mellitus in pregnancy
  An obstetrical patient with diabetes should be coded with a code from category 024, Diabetes mellitus in pregnancy, followed by the appropriate diabetes code(s) (E08-E13) from Chapter 4.
- Guideline I.C.15.h. Long term use of insulin
  Code Z79.4, Long-term (current) use of insulin should be used if the diabetes mellitus is being treated with insulin
- Guideline I.C.15.i. Gestational (pregnancy induced) diabetes
  Codes for gestational diabetes are in subcategory 024.4, gestational diabetes mellitus. No other code

(*Continued*)

(*Continued*)

from category O24 should be used with a code from O24.4.

- Guideline I.C.15.j. Sepsis and septic shock complicating abortion, pregnancy, childbirth and the puerperium
When assigning a Chapter 15 code for sepsis complicating abortion, pregnancy, childbirth and the puerperium, an additional code for the specific type of infection should be assigned. If severe sepsis is present, another additional diagnosis code is assigned.
- Guideline I.C.15.k. Puerperal sepsis
Code O85, Puerperal sepsis is assigned in the postpartum state when present with an additional code to identify the causal organism from category B95-B96, Bacterial infections in conditions classified elsewhere.
- Guidelines I.C.15.l. Alcohol and tobacco use during pregnancy, childbirth and the puerperium
Codes from categories O99.31, Alcohol use complication pregnancy and O99.33, Smoking (tobacco) complication pregnancy should be assigned when a mother uses alcohol or any type of tobacco product during the pregnancy or puerperium. An additional code from F10, Alcohol related disorders and F17, Nicotine dependence or Z72.0, Tobacco use should be assigned to identify the specific situation describing the substance related disorders.
- Guideline I.C.15.m. Poisoning, toxic effects, adverse effects and underdosing in a pregnant patient
A code from subcategory O9A.2, Injury, poisoning and certain other consequences of external causes should be sequenced first with additional codes to identify the injury, poisoning, toxic effect, adverse effect or underdosing situation with other additional codes to specify the conditions caused by these externally caused problems.
- Guidelines I.C.15.n. Normal delivery, code O80
Code O80 is used to describe a delivery that is a full-term normal delivery of a single healthy infant without any complications antepartum, during the delivery, or postpartum during the delivery episode of care. Code O80 is always a principal diagnosis code. Additional codes from other chapters may be used with code O80 if they are not related to or are in any way complicating the pregnancy. Code O80 may be used even if the patient had a complication at some time during the pregnancy but the complication is no longer present at

the time of delivery. Code Z37.0, single live birth, is the only outcome of delivery code that can be used with code 080.

- Guidelines I.C.15.o. The peripartum and postpartum periods
  The guideline defines the time period for peripartum (last month of pregnancy to five months postpartum) and postpartum (begins immediately after delivery and continues for six weeks following delivery.) The guidelines describe coding pregnancy related conditions during these time periods and after the 6 week period.
- Guidelines I.C.15.p. Code 094, sequelae of complications of pregnancy, childbirth and the puerperium
  Code 094, Sequelae of complications of pregnancy, childbirth and pueperium is used when an initial complication develops a sequela requiring care at a future date. This code may be used any time after the initial postpartum period. This code is sequenced following the code that describes the sequelae of the complication.
- Guidelines I.C.15.q. Abortions
  The guideline describes the coding of terminations of pregnancy and coding of spontaneous abortions, including when an abortion results in a liveborn infant and how to code the complications that lead to an abortion.
- Guideline I.C.15.r. Abuse in pregnant patient
  For suspected or confirmed cases of abuse of a pregnant female, code(s) from subcategories 09A.3 through 09A.5 are sequenced first, followed by the appropriate codes, if applicable, to identify any associated current injury due to the physical abuse, sexual abuse and the perpetrator of the abuse.

To gain an understanding of these rules, access the 2014 guidelines from NCHS website (http://www.cdc.gov/nchs/icd/icd10cm.htm) and read Chapter 15, Pregnancy, Childbirth and the Puerperium guidelines I.C.15.a.1–I.C.15.r.

## Coding Overview for ICD-10-CM Chapter 15

Chapter 15, Pregnancy, Childbirth and the Puerperium (O00–O9A), in ICD-10-CM is significantly different from ICD-9-CM. Codes are in the range of O00–O9A (letter O, digit zero, digit zero), a interesting coding coincidence given these letter O codes are for Obstetrics. Codes from Chapter 15 are used only on maternal records and never on newborn infant records.

The majority of codes in Chapter 15 have a final character indicating the trimester of pregnancy. Absent from ICD-10-CM are the equivalent of fifth digits that indicate delivered or undelivered. The time frames for the trimesters are:

- **1st Trimester:** less than 14 weeks, 0 days
- **2nd Trimester:** 14 weeks, 0 days to less than 28 weeks, 0 days
- **3rd Trimester:** 28 weeks, 0 days until delivery

Assignment of the final character for the trimester should be based on the provider's documentation of the trimester or the number of weeks for the current admission or encounter. This applies to the trimester for pre-existing conditions as well as those that develop during or are due to the pregnancy. The coder can use the provider's documentation of the number of weeks of gestation to convert it to a trimester. There are also options for the coder to assign an "in childbirth" open for the obstetric complication being coded instead of a trimester code. This should be done when the delivery occurs during the current admission and an "in childbirth" option exists. There is a choice for "unspecified trimester" final character. This should rarely be used because the documentation of care for an obstetrical patient should always contain the patient's weeks of gestation or trimester. The "unspecified trimester" code is not to be used when poor documentation exists in the obstetrical patient's record.

Assignment of the final character for trimester should be based on the trimester for the current admission or encounter. Whenever delivery occurs during the current admission and there is an "in childbirth" option for the obstetric complication being coded, the "in childbirth" code should be assigned.

For routine prenatal outpatient visits when there is no complication present, a code from category Z34 (the equivalent of the ICD-9-CM V22.0 and V22.1 codes) for the encounter for supervision of normal pregnancy is used as the first-listed code. If the prenatal outpatient visit is to manage a high-risk pregnancy, a code from Chapter 15 category O09, Supervision of high-risk pregnancy, is used as the first-listed code. The high-risk pregnancy supervision codes are in the obstetric code chapter and not in Chapter 21, where the Z34 codes are located.

A code from category Z37, Outcome of delivery, is used on every maternal record when a delivery occurs. This category of codes is equivalent to the ICD-9-CM category V27 codes for the outcome of delivery.

The definition of a normal delivery is the same in ICD-10-CM as in ICD-9-CM: A full-term normal delivery occurs when the woman has no complications during the antepartum period, during delivery, or postpartum during the delivery episode, and delivers a single, healthy infant. Code O80, Encounter for full-term uncomplicated delivery, in ICD-10-CM replaces code 650 in ICD-9-CM. Code O80 code is not used with any other code from Chapter 15.

In ICD-10-CM, the abortion codes are O02.1, Missed abortion, O03, Spontaneous abortion, and O04, Complications following (induced) termination of pregnancy. ICD-10-CM does not contain codes for illegally induced abortions or unspecified abortions. Absent from ICD-10-CM are the equivalent of ICD-9-CM's fifth digits for abortion codes that indicate "complete," "incomplete," or "unspecified" status.

The ICD-10-CM code for an uncomplicated elective termination of pregnancy (Z33.2) is found in Chapter 21, Factors Influencing Health Status and Contact with Health Services, not in with the OB codes found in Chapter 15.

According to the coding guidelines, code O80 should be assigned when a woman is admitted for a full-term normal delivery and delivers a single, healthy infant without any complications antepartum, during the delivery, or postpartum during the delivery episode. Code O80 is always the principal diagnosis. It is not to be used if any other code from Chapter 15 is needed to describe a current complication of the antenatal, delivery, or perinatal period. Additional codes from other chapters may be used with code O80 if they are not related to or are in any way complicating the pregnancy.

When a delivery occurs, the principal diagnosis should correspond to the main circumstances or complication of the delivery. In cases of cesarean delivery, the selection of the principal diagnosis should be the condition established after study that was responsible for the patient's admission. If the patient was admitted with a condition that resulted in the performance of a cesarean procedure, that condition should be selected as the principal diagnosis. If the reason for the admission or encounter was unrelated to the condition resulting in the cesarean delivery, the condition related to the reason for the admission or encounter should be selected as the principal diagnosis

Codes have been moved from other chapters in ICD-9-CM to Chapter 15 in ICD-10-CM, for example, encounter for supervision of high-risk pregnancy has been moved from the Supplementary Classification of Factors Influencing Health Status and Contact with Health Services to ICD-10-CM Chapter 15, to category O09.

The episode of care (delivered, antepartum, postpartum) is no longer the axis of classification, but rather the trimester in which the condition occurred. Because certain obstetric conditions or complications occur during certain trimesters, not all conditions include codes for all three trimesters. Also some codes do not include the trimester classification at all because the condition always occurs in a specific trimester, or the concept of trimester of pregnancy is not applicable.

Codes from this chapter are for use for conditions related to or aggravated by the pregnancy, childbirth, or by the puerperium (maternal causes or obstetric causes).

The time frame for differentiating the abortion and fetal death codes has changed from 22 to 20 weeks (see subcategory O36.4). The time frame for differentiating early and late vomiting in pregnancy has been changed from 22 to 20 weeks (see category O21). Preterm labor is defined as before 37 completed weeks of gestation (see category O60).

Certain codes in Chapter 15 require a seventh character to identify the fetus in a multiple gestation that is affected by the condition being coded. These are the applicable seventh characters:

0—not applicable or unspecified
1—fetus 1
2—fetus 2
3—fetus 3
4—fetus 4
5—fetus 5
9—other fetus

The seventh character 0 is for single gestations and multiple gestations where there are no complications and the affected fetus is unspecified. Seventh characters 1 through 9 are for cases of multiple gestations to identify the fetus for which the code applies, or which there is a complication that is attributable to a specific fetus. A code from category O30, Multiple gestation must also be assigned when assigning these codes.

Multiple notes and coding guidelines apply to this chapter, so a very careful review is necessary to become proficient at coding these conditions.

One of the blocks in Chapter 21, Factors Influencing Health Status and Contact with Health Services is Z30–Z39, Persons encountering health services in circumstances related to reproduction. The following are Chapter 21 codes that are related to the female pregnancy and frequently coded with Chapter 15 codes describing the obstetrical condition:

Z30 Encounter for contraceptive management
Z31 Encounter for procreative management
Z32 Encounter for pregnancy test and childbirth and childcare instruction

Z33 Pregnant state
Z34 Encounter for supervision of normal pregnancy
Z36 Encounter for antenatal screening of mother
Z3A Weeks of gestation
Z37 Outcome of delivery
Z39 Encounter for maternal postpartum care and examination

Outcome of delivery codes (Z37.0–Z37.9) are intended for use as an additional code to identify the outcome of delivery on the mother's record. It is not for use on the newborn record. These codes exclude the situation when the outcome of the delivery is a stillbirth (P95).

Codes in category Z3A, Weeks of gestation, are for use only on the maternal record to indicate the weeks of gestation of pregnancy. These are always used as additional codes as the codes for the pregnancy, childbirth and the puerperium (O00–O9A) are always listed first. Codes in this category range from Z3A.01 for less than 8 weeks of pregnancy to Z3A.49 for a gestation greater than 42 weeks. There is also a code for weeks of gestation of pregnancy not specified (Z3A.00). The majority of the codes end with the last two digits that match the gestation of the pregnancy, for example, Z3A.40 for 40 weeks of gestation. The code for the weeks of gestation is used for all pregnancy patients, not exclusively for the patients who deliver during the current encounter. The date of admission should be used to determine weeks of gestation for inpatient admissions that extend more than one gestational week.

Within the ICD-10-PCS coding system, the coding guidelines addressing the Obstetrics Section describes the procedures performed on the "products of conception." Figure 14.2 a diagram of a pregnant female, shows what is meant by products of conception in ICD-10-PCS, that is, the contents of the uterus during a pregnancy including the fetus, amniotic fluid, umbilical cord and placenta.

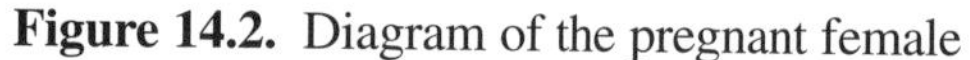

**Figure 14.2.** Diagram of the pregnant female

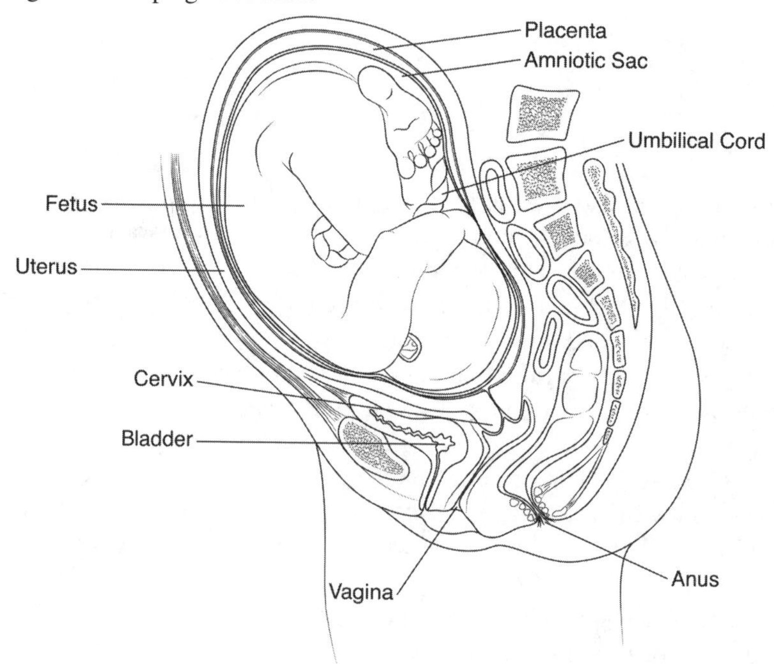

## ICD-10-CM Review Exercises: Chapter 14

Assign the correct ICD-10-CM diagnosis codes to the following exercises.

1. This 25-year-old patient has admitted with difficulty breathing. She has AIDS and is 21 weeks pregnant. Workup reveals Pneumocystis carinii pneumonia due to the AIDS. What is the correct diagnosis code(s)?

 ______________________

2. 16-week pregnancy with mild hyperemesis and urinary tract infection which grew out E. coli

 ______________________

3. The patient is a 40 year old G2 P1 woman who is 26-weeks pregnant and being seen for gestational hypertension. Other than being an elderly, multigravida patient, she is not having any other problems during this pregnancy.

 ______________________

4. Patient is a woman who is G1P0 at 39 weeks with twin gestation. The delivery complicated by nuchal cord, without compression, of fetus 2. Both infants were liveborn and healthy.

 ______________________

5. Patient returns to the office with breast pain. The patient is a 24-year-old woman who is 3 weeks postpartum. Final diagnosis documented as nonpurulent postpartum mastitis.

 ______________________

6. 20-week pregnancy with low weight gain and pre-existing essential hypertension complicating the pregnancy.

 ______________________

7. Patient is a woman, who is G4, P3, 28 weeks, and seen today for continued follow-up of her gestational diabetes. Her diabetes has been well controlled on oral medications.

 ______________________

8. The patient, G1P0, was admitted in active labor at 38 completed weeks of gestation. The patient was dilated to 6 cm approximately 7 hours following admission. Pitocin augmentation was started and she progressed to complete dilation. A second degree perineal laceration occurred during delivery and was repaired. A female infant was delivered with Apgar scores of 9 and 9.

 ______________________

9. The patient is admitted in active labor during week 39 of pregnancy. The patient experienced no complications during her pregnancy. The patient labored for 8 hours and delivered a liveborn male over an intact perineum.

 ______________________

10. The patient, G3P2, was admitted in premature labor at approximately 34 weeks' gestation with a history of contractions for the last 24 hours. She was experiencing contractions every 5 to 8 minutes. An ultrasound showed an intrauterine fetal death of triplet 2 but the other two were progressing normally. The contractions stopped for approximately 24 hours and then started again. It was noted by the physician that the continued contractions were due to fetus 2. The patient was given magnesium sulfate for tocolysis which was unsuccessful. The patient also developed a fever with an infection of the amniotic sac. The patient continued to be in active labor and due to the infection was allowed to spontaneously deliver the three infants, two liveborn and one fetal death. The patient experienced no postpartum complications.

 ______________________

# Chapter 15

# Diseases of the Skin and Subcutaneous Tissue

## Learning Objectives

At the conclusion of this chapter, you should be able to:

1. Describe the organization of the conditions and codes included in Chapter 12 of ICD-9-CM, Diseases of the Skin and Subcutaneous Tissue (680–709)
2. Describe the organization of the conditions and codes included in Chapter 12 of ICD-10-CM, Diseases of the Skin and Subcutaneous Tissue (L00–L99)
3. Define and differentiate between the terms *cellulitis* and *abscess*
4. Define the term *erythema*
5. Describe the different stages of decubitus or pressure ulcers
6. Briefly describe the types of procedures that can be performed on the breast, as well as on skin and subcutaneous tissue
7. Define and differentiate between the terms *excisional* and *nonexcisional* debridement
8. Assign ICD-9-CM diagnosis and procedure codes for diseases of the skin and subcutaneous tissue
9. Assign ICD-10-CM codes for diseases of the skin and subcutaneous tissue

## Chapter 12, Diseases of the Skin and Subcutaneous Tissue (680–709)

Chapter 12, Diseases of the Skin and Subcutaneous Tissue, in the Tabular List in volume 1 of ICD-9-CM, includes conditions such as dermatitis, cellulitis, ulcers of the skin and subcutaneous tissue, urticaria, and diseases of the nails and hair. An image of the layers of the integumentary system is shown in figure 15.1. Chapter 12 of ICD-9-CM contains the following categories and section titles:

| Categories | Section Titles |
|---|---|
| 680–686 | Infections of Skin and Subcutaneous Tissue |
| 690–698 | Other Inflammatory Conditions of Skin and Subcutaneous Tissue |
| 700–709 | Other Diseases of Skin and Subcutaneous Tissue |

**Figure 15.1.** Layers of the integumentary system

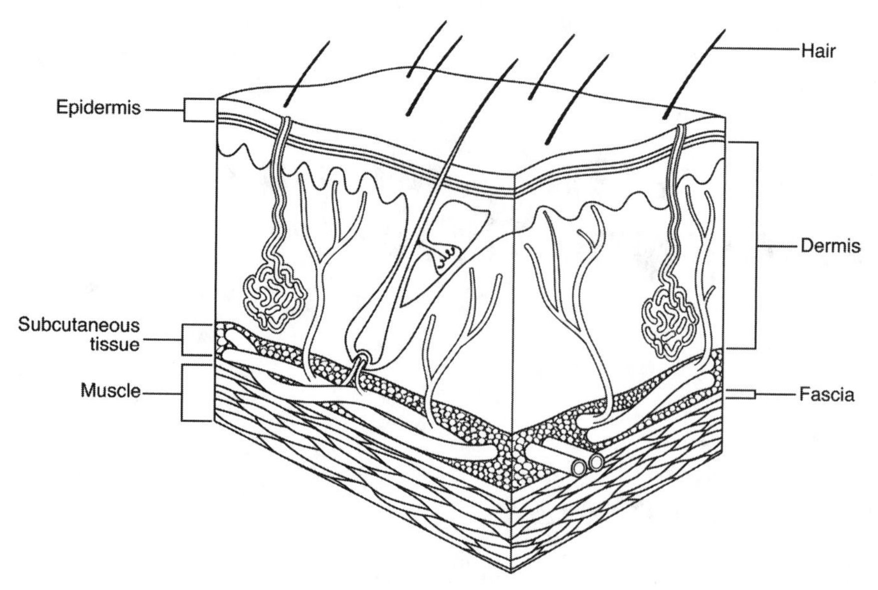




## Cellulitis and Abscess (681 and 682)

Cellulitis is an acute inflammation of a localized area of superficial tissue. Predisposing conditions are open wounds, ulcerations, tinea pedis, and dermatitis, but these conditions need not be present for cellulitis to occur. Physical findings of cellulitis reveal red, hot skin with edema at the site of the infection. The area is tender, and the skin surface has a peau d'orange (skin of an orange) appearance with ill-defined borders. Nearby lymph nodes often become inflamed.

A cutaneous or subcutaneous abscess is a localized collection of pus causing fluctuant soft-tissue swelling surrounded by erythema. These abscesses usually follow minor skin trauma, and the organisms isolated are typically bacterial infection indigenous to the skin of the involved area. Abscesses may occur internally in tissues, organs, and confined spaces. An abscess begins as cellulitis.

Cellulitis will clear within a few days with antibiotic treatment. Although drainage of abscesses may occur spontaneously, some abscesses may require incision and drainage, and possibly antibiotic therapy.

ICD-9-CM classifies cellulitis to categories 681 and 682. Category 681, Cellulitis and abscess of finger and toe, is subdivided to fourth-digit subcategories that identify the site. Category 682, Other cellulitis and abscess, also is subdivided to identify the site. An additional code should be assigned to identify the organism involved.

**EXAMPLE:** Cellulitis of the upper arm due to *Streptococcus*: 682.3, Other cellulitis and abscess of upper arm and forearm; 041.00, *Streptococcus* infection in conditions classified elsewhere and of unspecified site

## Dermatitis (690–694)

Dermatitis is an inflammation of the skin. ICD-9-CM classifies contact dermatitis, which is caused by a reaction to substances, to category 692. Fourth-digit subcategories include specific substances such as detergents, solvents, oils and greases, drugs and medicines in contact with the skin, other chemical products, foods, and plants.

**EXAMPLE:** Contact dermatitis due to detergents: 692.0, Contact dermatitis and other eczema due to detergents

Sunburn and other ultraviolet burns in ICD-9-CM are included in a dermatitis category. Sunburn and tanning bed burns can be equal in severity to second- and third-degree burns. In keeping with the intent of ICD-9-CM to separate sunburn from other burns, fifth-digit codes were added in 2001 to subcategory 692.7, Contact dermatitis and other eczema, due to solar radiation. The codes are 692.71, which includes sunburn, first-degree sunburn, and sunburn NOS; 692.76, Sunburn of second degree; and 692.77, Sunburn of third degree.

Another code, 692.82, was revised to describe dermatitis due to other (ultraviolet) radiation, such as from a tanning bed.

ICD-9-CM classifies dermatitis due to substances taken internally to category 693. Certain medications can cause the condition of dermatitis. Code 693.0, Dermatitis, due to drugs and medications, is assigned when the drug causes the skin reaction. An additional external cause code is assigned to identify the drug, when known. Another code in this category is used to describe the situation when a food taken internally causes a dermatitis.

## Erythematous Conditions (695.0–695.9)

Erythema is redness of the skin due to capillary dilation. Erythematous conditions are skin disorders relating to or marked by erythema. A number of distinct disorders are included in category 695. Erythema multiforme is an acute eruption of macules, papules, or subepidermal vesicles presenting in a multiform appearance. The characteristic lesions appear over the dorsal aspect of the hands and forearms. Its origin may be allergic, drug sensitivity, or it may be caused by herpes simplex infection. The eruption may be self-limited (erythema multiforme minor, 695.11) or recurrent and run a severe and possibly fatal course (erythema multiforme major, 695.12). Stevens-Johnson Syndrome (SJS) (code 695.13) is a bullous form of erythema multiforme that may be extensive over the body and produce serious subjective symptoms and possibly death. Toxic epidermal necrolysis (TEN) may also occur with SJS. TEN is a syndrome in which large portions of skin become intensely erythematous with epidermal necrolysis. The skin peels off the body in a manner of a second-degree burn. This condition may result from a drug sensitivity but often its cause is unknown. Codes are available to describe SJS (code 695.13), SJS with TEN (695.14), and TEN (695.15).

Other codes in category 695 include erythema nodosum, rosacea, lupus erythematosus, Ritter's Disease, and erythema intertrigo. Subcategory codes 695.50–695.59 are used to describe the percentage of body surface that has exfoliation due to erythematosus conditions. A "code first" note appears with subcategory 695.5 to direct the coder to code first the erythematous condition causing the exfoliation, such as Ritter's Disease, SJS, or toxic epidermal necrolysis.

## Pressure (Decubitus) Ulcer (707.00–707.09)

Pressure or decubitus ulcers are caused by tissue hypoxia secondary to pressure-induced vascular insufficiency, and they may become secondarily infected with components of the skin and gastrointestinal flora. The ulceration of tissue usually is at the location of a bony prominence that has been subjected to prolonged pressure against an external object, such as a bed, wheelchair, cast, or splint. Tissues over the elbows, sacrum, ischia, greater trochanters of the hip, external malleoli of the ankle, and heels are most susceptible. Other sites may be involved depending on the patient's positions. Patients may have more than one decubitus, located at different sites on the body. Decubitus ulcers may extend into deeper tissue including muscle and bone. The ulcers may also be referred to as pressure ulcers, pressure sores, or bedsores.

ICD-9-CM contains codes at the fifth-digit level for the more common body sites where decubitus ulcers may occur. A "use additional code" note appears under subcategory 707.0, decubitus ulcer, reminding the coder to assign an additional code(s) to identify the stage(s) of the pressure ulcer(s) as described by the clinician.

## Pressure Ulcer Stages

Pressure ulcers are often identified by their location on the body, shape, depth, and healing status. The depth of the ulcer is identified by stages I–IV. According to the National Pressure Ulcer Advisory Panel (NPUAP 2014), the descriptions of the four stages are:

| | |
|---|---|
| Category/Stage I | Intact skin with nonblanching erythema (a reddened area on the skin). This may be referred to as discoloration of the skin without ulceration. |
| Category/Stage II | Abrasion, blister, shallow open ulcer or crater, or other partial thickness skin loss |
| Category/Stage III | Full-thickness skin loss involving damage or necrosis into subcutaneous soft tissues |
| Category/Stage IV | Full-thickness skin loss with necrosis of soft tissues through to the muscle, tendons, or tissues around underlying bone (NPUAP 2014) |

Pressure ulcers may also be described as "unstageable." This is a specific type of pressure ulcer, and the code for unstageable, code 707.25, should not be used when stages I–IV are not documented. When the documentation is absent, a code for pressure ulcer, stage unspecified is used. An unstageable pressure ulcer has full-thickness tissue loss in which the base of the ulcer is covered by slough and/or eschar in the wound bed or has been treated with a skin or muscle flap. Stages I and II may be described as superficial lesions, with more serious lesions being identified as stages III and IV.

Subcategory codes 707.20–707.24 are used to identify the pressure ulcer stages I–IV as well as a code for an unspecified stage. Two codes are needed to completely describe a pressure ulcer: one code for the location and another code for the stage. The *ICD-9-CM Official Guidelines for Coding and Reporting* contain specific directions for coding pressure ulcers, including the stage, as well as bilateral and multiple pressure ulcers.

Coding of pressure ulcers and their stages can be based on medical record documentation from clinicians other than the patient's healthcare provider or physician. Wound care nurses or rehabilitation therapists often provide specialized services for patients with pressure ulcers. The diagnosis of pressure ulcer must be made by the physician. However, the coder can use the nurse or therapist's documentation of the pressure ulcer stage to assign the additional code for the pressure ulcer stage. The pressure ulcer stage codes can only be reported as secondary diagnoses and must meet the definition of reportable additional diagnosis.

### *Chronic Ulcer of Skin, Lower Limbs, Except Pressure Ulcer (707.1)*

A patient may have a chronic ulcer of the skin of the lower limbs as a sole problem or the ulcer may be the result of another condition. Codes 707.10–707.19 may be used alone when there is no known underlying condition or cause. However, when the causal condition is known, that condition should be coded first with an additional code from the 707.1 subcategory. Common underlying causes may be diabetes, atherosclerosis, chronic venous hypertension, and postphlebitic syndrome.

## Exercise 15.1

Assign ICD-9-CM codes to the following:

1. Pressure ulcer of heel, stage I

2. Acne vulgaris

3. Postinfectional skin cicatrix; scar revision by Z-plasty

4. Cellulitis of the foot; cellulitis due to *Streptococcus* infection

5. Diaper rash

6. Pilonidal cyst with abscess; incision and drainage

7. Allergic urticaria

8. Circumscribed scleroderma

9. Erythema multiforme major

10. Infected ingrowing nail; removal of nail

11. Dermatitis due to animal dander

12. Dermatitis attributed to eating fresh strawberries

13. Stevens-Johnson Syndrome with toxic epidermal necrolysis overlap syndrome with resulting exfoliation of approximately 10 percent of body surface

14. Rosacea acne

15. Acute lymphadenitis due to staphylococcal infection

# Operations on the Integumentary System (Breast, Skin, and Subcutaneous Tissue)

Chapter 15 in the Tabular List in volume 3 of ICD-9-CM includes codes for the following procedures:

- 85, Operations on the breast
- 86, Operations on skin and subcutaneous tissue

## Operations on the Breast

Procedures such as mastectomy, mammoplasty, and insertion of breast tissue expanders and breast implants are subdivisions of category 85. Diagnostic procedures such as biopsies of the breast are also subdivisions of category 85.

Code 85.0, Mastotomy, is used for incision and drainage of a breast abscess. A mastotomy is also performed for the insertion of a breast catheter after a lumpectomy has been performed for carcinoma of the breast. If the catheter is inserted during a session when the radiation seeds were not implanted at the same time, code 85.0 is used for the catheter placement. If the catheter is placed and radioactive seeds are delivered through the catheter for internal radiation to tissue near the lumpectomy site during the same session, only code 92.27, Implantation or insertion of radioactive elements, is assigned. This code assignment includes all the components of the procedure.

Subcategory 85.1 includes diagnostic procedures performed on the breast, such as closed [percutaneous] [needle] biopsy (85.11) or an open biopsy of the breast (85.12).

A lumpectomy of the breast, performed for a benign or malignant breast mass, can be one of three possible procedures. Code 85.21, Local excision of lesion of breast, is the most likely procedure and is the code assignment when the term *lumpectomy* is referenced in the Alphabetic Index to Procedures, volume 3. If physicians perform a more extensive procedure to remove a breast lump, documentation may reveal that a resection of a breast quadrant (85.22) or a partial mastectomy (85.23) was performed. Careful reading of the operative description is recommended.

Subcategory 85.3, Reduction mammoplasty, and subcutaneous mammectomy codes are subdivided to identify the types of procedures performed for breast reductions.

Subcategory 85.4, Mastectomy, is subdivided to identify the extent of the procedure and the side(s) involved (unilateral or bilateral).

Subcategory 85.5, Augmentation mammoplasty, includes unilateral and bilateral breast enlargements, including injection of saline into breast tissue expanders.

A variety of breast reconstruction surgeries are described with a wide range of codes found in subcategory 85.7, Total breast reconstruction, to other repair and plastic operations on the breast identified by codes 85.81–85.99.

## Operations on Skin and Subcutaneous Tissue

Category 86, Operations on skin and subcutaneous tissue, includes subdivisions with procedures such as insertion of infusion pumps and totally implantable vascular access devices, excision of skin, and subcutaneous lesions and skin grafting.

## Debridement

Debridement is the removal of foreign material and contaminated or devitalized tissue from, or adjacent to, a traumatic or infected lesion until the surrounding healthy tissue is exposed (Dorland 2014). ICD-9-CM classifies debridement to the following two codes: 86.22, Excisional debridement of wound, infection, or burn; and 86.28, Nonexcisional debridement of wound, infection, or burn.

The following guidelines apply to coding debridement:

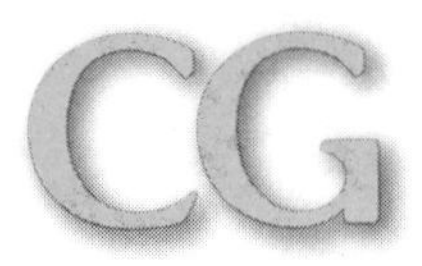

- For coding purposes, excisional debridement, code 86.22, is assigned when it is performed by any healthcare provider. Excisional debridement is the surgical removal, or cutting away, of necrotic tissue or slough, usually performed with a scalpel. Excisional debridement can be performed in the operating room, the emergency department, or at bedside, depending on the extent of the area to be debrided. An article in the first quarter 2008 *Coding Clinic* newsletter encouraged coders to work with their physicians and other healthcare providers to ensure that the documentation in the health record is very specific regarding the type of debridement performed. If there is any question as to whether the debridement is excisional or nonexcisional, the provider should be queried for clarification.
- For coding purposes, nonexcisional debridement performed by a physician or nonphysician healthcare professional is assigned code 86.28. Nonexcisional debridement can include the use of forceps (tweezers), scissors, hydrogen peroxide, wet dressings of water, or whirlpool baths. Nonexcisional debridement often includes the clipping away of loose necrotic tissue fragments.

The term *sharp debridement* may be found in documentation of wound debridements performed by physicians and physical therapists. The use of a sharp instrument does not always mean it is an excisional debridement. Generally debridement performed by a physical therapist is nonexcisional debridement, code 86.28. Only if the documentation of the sharp debridement of skin or subcutaneous tissue is further described as excisional, the procedure should be coded with 86.22. This code does not include the minor removal of loose fragments with scissors or scraping away tissue with a sharp instrument, as both of these procedures would be coded to 86.28. Pulsed or pulsatile lavage, mechanical lavage, mechanical irrigation, or high-pressure irrigation are also examples of nonexcisional debridement.

## ICD-9-CM Review Exercises: Chapter 15

Assign ICD-9-CM diagnosis and procedure codes to the following:

1. Pressure ulcer of sacrum, stage III, with excisional debridement performed by the physician in the operating room

2. Cellulitis of the upper arm with nonexcisional debridement performed by the physical therapist

3. Dermatitis due to detergent

4. Blue nevus of foot; excision of nevus, foot

5. History of breast cancer; status post mastectomy, right breast; insertion of unilateral breast implant

6. Chronic ulcer of left ankle; full-thickness skin graft, left lower leg

7. Benign breast cyst, left; percutaneous needle breast biopsy

8. Adenocarcinoma of right breast, lower inner quadrant; quadrant resection of breast, lower inner quadrant

9. Hypertensive kidney disease with chronic kidney disease, stage V; insertion of totally implantable vascular access device

10. Idiopathic urticaria

# ICD-10-CM Chapter 12, Diseases of Skin and Subcutaneous Tissue (L00–L99)

## Organization and Structure of ICD-10-CM

Chapter 12 of ICD-10-CM includes categories L00–L99 arranged in the following blocks:

| | |
|---|---|
| L00–L08 | Infections of the skin and subcutaneous tissue |
| L10–L14 | Bullous disorders |
| L20–L30 | Dermatitis and eczema |
| L40–L45 | Papulosquamous disorders |
| L49–L54 | Urticaria and erythema |
| L55–L59 | Radiation-related disorders of the skin and subcutaneous tissue |
| L60–L75 | Disorders of skin appendages |
| L76 | Intraoperative and postprocedural complications of skin and subcutaneous tissue |
| L80–L99 | Other disorders of the skin and subcutaneous tissue |

Chapter 12 of ICD-10-CM represents a complete restructuring to bring together groups of diseases that are related. Additionally, greater specificity has been added to many of the codes at either the fourth-, fifth- and even sixth-character level. ICD-9-CM Chapter 12 has only three subchapters which have been expanded in ICD-10-CM to create the nine blocks listed above.

One example of an organizational change to Chapter 12 of ICD-10-CM is a subchapter or block for ICD-10-CM codes for radiation-related disorders of the skin and subcutaneous tissue. The conditions found in this block are not located together in ICD-9-CM.

Some categories in Chapter 12 have undergone title changes to reflect current terminology. For instance, ICD-10-CM uses androgenic alopecia while this term is not used at all in ICD-9-CM.

An example of a classification improvement is the addition of characters in ICD-10-CM to represent the site and severity of the pressure ulcer.

While ICD-9-CM did add a subcategory for pressure ulcer stages in Fiscal Year 2009, two codes are required to code this specificity. ICD-10-CM provides the site (including laterality) and the stage all in one code.

## Coding Guidelines and Instructional Notes for Chapter 12

Instructions for coding dermatitis and eczema have been expanded in Chapter 12. For example, the note "in this block the terms dermatitis and eczema are used synonymously and interchangeably" has been added to categories L20–L30.

Additionally, the excludes note has been expanded in ICD-10-CM for categories L20–L30, compared to categories 690–698 in ICD-9-CM.

ICD-9-CM: **Other Inflammatory Conditions of Skin and Subcutaneous Tissue (690–698)**

*Excludes:* panniculitis (729.30–729.39)

ICD-10-CM: **Dermatitis and Eczema (L20–L30)**

*Excludes:* chronic (childhood) granulomatous disease (D71)
dermatitis gangrenosa (L08.0)
dermatitis herpetiformis (L13.0)
dry skin dermatitis (L85.3)
factitial dermatitis (L98.1)
perioral dermatitis (L71.0)
radiation-related disorders of skin and subcutaneous tissue (L55–L59)
stasis dermatitis (I83.1–I83.2)

With the formation of new categories for allergic (L23) and irritant (L24) contact dermatitis, new instructions on which condition to code first, that is, the drug or substance, have also been created.

**EXAMPLE:**

**L23.3** Allergic contact dermatitis due to drugs in contact with skin.
Use additional code for adverse effect, if applicable, to identify drug (T36–T50 with fifth or sixth character 5)

**L24.4** Irritant contact dermatitis due to drugs in contact with skin.
Use additional code for adverse effect, if applicable, to identify drug (T36–T50 with fifth or sixth character 5)

**L27.0** Generalized skin eruption due to drugs and medicaments taken internally
Use additional code for adverse effect, if applicable, to identify drug (T36–T50 with fifth or sixth character 5)

**L27.1** Localized skin eruption due to drugs and medicaments taken internally
Use additional code for adverse effect, if applicable, to identify drug (T36–T50 with fifth or sixth character 5)

The NCHS has published chapter-specific guidelines for Chapter 12 of ICD-10-CM. For example, Coding Guideline I.C.12.a.1 Pressure Ulcer Stages:

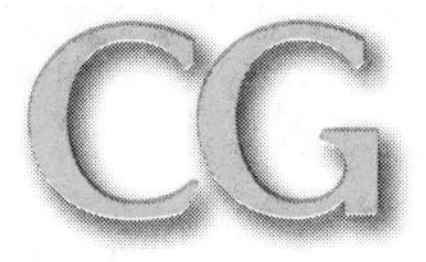

Codes from category L89, Pressure ulcer, are combination codes that identify the site of the pressure ulcer as well as the stage of the ulcer. The ICD-10-CM classifies pressure ulcer stages based on severity, which is designated by stages 1–4, unspecified stage, and unstageable. Assign as many codes from category L89 as needed to identify all the pressure ulcers the patient has, if applicable.

**Coding Guideline I.B.14. Documentation for BMI and Pressure Ulcer Stages**

For the body mass index (BMI) and pressure ulcer stage codes, code assignment may be based on medical record documentation from clinicians who are not the patient's provider (that is, physician or other qualified healthcare practitioner legally accountable for establishing the patient's diagnosis), since this information is typically documented by other clinicians involved in the care of the patient (for example, a dietitian often documents the BMI and nurses often document the pressure ulcer stages). However, the associated diagnosis (such as overweight, obesity, or pressure ulcer) must be documented by the patient's provider. If there is conflicting medical record documentation, either from the same clinician or different clinicians, the patient's attending provider should be queried for clarification.

To gain an understanding of these rules, access the 2014 guidelines from NCHS website (http://www.cdc.gov/nchs/icd/icd10cm.htm) and read Chapter 12, Diseases of the Skin and Subcutaneous Tissue guidelines I.C.12.a.

## Coding Overview for ICD-10-CM Chapter 12

Chapter 12 of ICD-10-CM, Diseases of the Skin and Subcutaneous Tissue (L00–L99), contains specific codes for skin infections, bullous disorders, dermatitis, eczema, papulosquamous disorders, urticaria, erythema, radiation-related skin disorders, as well as intraoperative and postprocedural complications of skin and subcutaneous tissue.

Many codes include laterality, such as L02.522, Furuncle of the left hand, and L03.111, Cellulitis of the right axilla. Codes for unspecified sides of the body, such as L02.639, Carbuncle of unspecified foot, also exist.

Category L89, Pressure ulcer, contains combination codes that identify the site as well as the stage of the pressure ulcer. The same pressure ulcer stages, 1–4, unspecified stage, and unstageable stage, are included in ICD-10-CM as in ICD-9-CM. Laterality is also included in the pressure ulcer codes, as seen in L89.321, Pressure ulcer of left buttock, stage 1. As in ICD-9-CM, no code is assigned in ICD-10-CM if the documentation states that the pressure ulcer is completely healed. Any associated gangrene should be sequenced first.

Chapter 12 has been restructured to bring together groups of diseases that are related to one another in some way, moving from three subsections in ICD-9-CM to nine subsections in ICD-10-CM. In ICD-10-CM, these are referred to as blocks.

Instructional notes have been expanded and have several uses in this chapter. They indicate an additional code should be used to identify the organism or infectious agent. Notes also indicate that the drug or substance, underlying disease, or associated underlying condition should be coded first. Examples are listed here:

- L14, Bullous disorders in diseases classified elsewhere, Code first underlying disease
- L23.3, Allergic contact dermatitis due to drugs in contact with skin, Use additional code for adverse effect, if applicable, (T36–T65) to identify drug or substance
- L97, Non-pressure chronic ulcer of lower limb, not elsewhere classified, Code first any associated underlying condition

A note under block L20–L30, Dermatitis and eczema, indicates that in this block, the terms "dermatitis" and "eczema" are used synonymously and interchangeably.

Non-pressure chronic ulcers of lower limbs NEC (L97) are also specified by site, laterality, and severity. An important note appears with this category:

A code from L97 may be used as a principal or first listed code if no underlying condition is documented as the cause of the ulcer. If one of the underlying conditions listed below is documented with a lower extremity ulcer, a causal condition should be assumed.

Code first any associated underlying condition, such as:

- Atherosclerosis of the lower extremities (I70.23-, I70.24-, I70.33-, I70.34-, I70.43-, I70.44-, I70.53-, I70.54-, I70.63-, I70.64-, I70.73-, I70.74-)
- Chronic venous hypertension (I87.31-, I87.33-)
- Diabetic ulcers (E08.621, E08.622, E09.621, E09.622, E10.621, E10.622, E11.621, E11.622, E13.621, E13.622)
- Postphlebitic syndrome (I87.01-, I87.03-)
- Postthrombotic syndrome (I87.01-, I87.03-)
- Varicose ulcer (I83.0-, I83.2-)
- Code first any associated gangrene (I96)

Coders must be careful to distinguish the documentation in the record of "pressure" and "non-pressure" ulcers treated for the patient. It is possible that one patient has both types of skin ulcers. The codes in category L97, Non-pressure chronic ulcer of lower limb, not elsewhere classified, may also be referred to as a chronic or a non-healing ulcer by the provider. The chronic or non-pressure ulcers are usually caused by another disease, as noted by the "code first" note under category L97, as patients with diabetes, atherosclerosis, and other vascular problems are prone to developing non-pressure ulcers. The codes in category identify the site of the chronic ulcer, such as thigh, calf, ankle, and the laterality, such as right or left. The subcategories are further specified by the depth of the ulcer: limited to breakdown of skin, with fat layer exposed, with necrosis of muscle, with necrosis of bone and one code for unspecified severity. Non-pressure ulcers are not identified with a "stage" like the pressure ulcers are described.

## ICD-10-CM Review Exercises: Chapter 15

Assign the correct ICD-10-CM diagnosis codes to the following exercises

1. Irritant contact dermatitis due to cosmetics; Cystic acne

   The patient was seen with extensive inflammation and irritation of the skin of both upper eyelids and under her eyebrows that was spreading to her temples and forehead. Upon questioning the patient, the physician learned that she had recently used new eye cosmetics. The physician had examined the patient during a prior visit for cystic acne. During this visit, the physician also examined the patient's cystic acne on her forehead and jawline. The patient was advised to continue using the medication previously prescribed. The patient was also advised to immediately discontinue use of any make-up on the face and was given a topical medication to resolve the inflammation which was an adverse effect of the cosmetics that came in contact with the skin on her face.

2. Gangrenous pressure ulcer of the right hip and a pressure ulcer of the sacrum documented by the physician. The nursing assessment indicates a stage 2 pressure ulcer of the sacrum with a stage 3 decubitus ulcer of the right hip.

3. Dermatitis covering entire body due to antibiotics (penicillin) taken correctly as prescribed

4. Abscess of the entire left big toe

5. Atherosclerosis of the native arteries of the right ankle region, with non-healing ulcer, with breakdown of the skin on right ankle

6. The patient was seen for treatment of a fine rash that had developed on the patient's trunk and upper extremities over the last three to four days. The patient was diagnosed with hypertension seven days ago and started on Ramipril 10 mg daily. The physician determined the localized rash to be dermatitis due to the Ramipril. The Ramipril was discontinued and the patient was prescribed a new antihypertensive medication, Captopril. In addition, the physician prescribed a topical cream for the localized dermatitis.

7. Cellulitis in the right lower extremity with streptococcus B organism documented by the physician as the cause of the cellulitis. Patient also has stage 1 decubitus ulcer of the left buttock and stage 2 decubitus ulcer in the right gluteal region

8. Cellulitis of the right anterior neck treated with intravenous antibiotics. The patient is also a known morphine drug abuser and exhibited considerable drug-seeking behavior and continuously requested morphine. All narcotics were discontinued and the patient exhibited no drug withdrawal symptoms.

9. Discoid lupus erythematosus

10. Psoriatic arthritis

# Chapter 16

# Diseases of the Musculoskeletal System and Connective Tissue

## Learning Objectives

At the conclusion of this chapter, you should be able to:

1. Describe the organization of the conditions and codes included in Chapter 13 of ICD-9-CM, Diseases of the Musculoskeletal System and Connective Tissue (710–739)
2. Describe the organization of the conditions and codes included in Chapter 13 of ICD-10-CM, Diseases of the Musculoskeletal System and Connective Tissue (M00–M99)
3. Describe the types of arthritic conditions classified to ICD-9-CM and ICD-10-CM categories and codes
4. Describe the conditions classified as *dorsopathies* using ICD-9-CM and ICD-10-CM categories and codes
5. Define the two types of *compartment syndrome*
6. Define and differentiate between the terms *pathologic, malunion, nonunion,* and *stress* fractures
7. Briefly describe the types of arthroscopic surgery that can be performed in the musculoskeletal system, including the circumstances in which to code "arthroscopy" in ICD-9-CM and in which to omit the ICD-9-CM codes when it serves as the operative approach
8. Assign ICD-9-CM diagnosis and procedure codes for diseases of the musculoskeletal system and connective tissue
9. Assign ICD-10-CM codes for diseases of the musculoskeletal system and connective tissue

## Chapter 13, Diseases of the Musculoskeletal System and Connective Tissue (710–739)

Chapter 13, Diseases of the Musculoskeletal System and Connective Tissue, in the Tabular List in volume 1 of ICD-9-CM is divided into the following categories and section titles:

| Categories | Section Titles |
|---|---|
| 710–719 | Arthropathies and Related Disorders |
| 720–724 | Dorsopathies |
| 725–729 | Rheumatism, Excluding the Back |
| 730–739 | Osteopathies, Chondropathies, and Acquired Musculoskeletal Deformities |

An illustration of the bones of the human skeletal system are shown in figure 16.1 for your reference.

**Figure 16.1.** Anterior and posterior views of the skeletal system

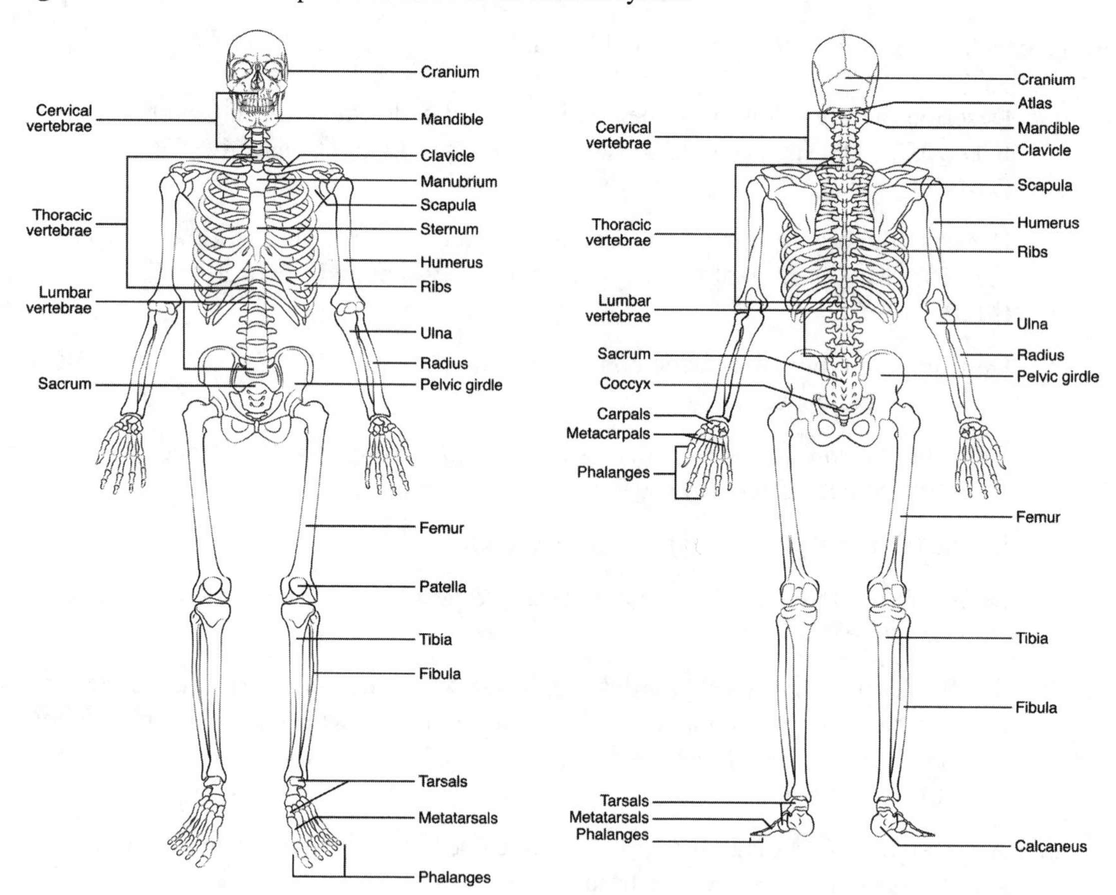




### Fifth-Digit Subclassification

At the beginning of Chapter 13, information on using the fifth-digit subclassification with the following categories is given: 711–712, 715–716, 718–719, and 730. The fifth-digit subclassification is repeated at the beginning of each of those series of codes.

## Systemic Lupus Erythematosus

Systemic lupus erythematosus (SLE) is a chronic generalized connective tissue disorder ranging from mild to fulminating and marked by skin eruptions, arthralgia, fever, leukopenia, visceral lesions, and other constitutional symptoms, as well as many autoimmune phenomena, including hypergammaglobulinemia with the presence of antinuclear antibodies and lupus erythematosus (LE) cells (Dorland 2012).

ICD-9-CM classifies SLE to code 710.0. At the beginning of this code, a note advises use of an additional code to identify manifestations such as nephritis or endocarditis.

## Arthritis

ICD-9-CM classifies arthritic conditions to categories 711–716. It should be noted that many codes in these categories are set in italic type to indicate that they are not intended to be the first-listed code.

### *Rheumatoid Arthritis*

Rheumatoid arthritis, a chronic, crippling condition, affects the joints of the hands, wrists, elbows, feet, and ankles. Periods of remission and exacerbation occur in afflicted patients. Although the exact etiology is unknown, immunologic changes and tissue hypersensitivity, complicated by a cold and damp climate, may have a contributory effect. The synovial membranes are primarily affected. The joints become inflamed, swollen, and painful, as well as stiff and tender. A characteristic sign of rheumatoid arthritis is the formation of nodules over body surfaces. During an active period of rheumatoid arthritis, the patient suffers from malaise, fever, and sweating.

ICD-9-CM classifies rheumatoid arthritis to category 714. Again, a note advises coders to use additional codes to identify any manifestations, such as myopathy and polyneuropathy with code 714.0. Rheumatoid arthritis that affects children is coded to subcategory 714.3, Juvenile chronic polyarthritis.

## Dorsopathies (720–724)

The section Dorsopathies (720–724) contains codes describing intervertebral disc disorders and spondylosis, in addition to other back disorders. It should be noted that categories 721 (Spondylosis and allied disorders) and 722 (Intervertebral disc disorders) have fourth-digit subcategories that designate the presence or absence of myelopathy, which refers to a functional disorder of the spinal cord. Category 724 (Other and unspecified disorders of back) identifies common conditions of the back that occur in the thoracic and lumbar regions. Because spinal stenosis in the lumbar region can produce neurogenic claudication, specific codes exist to identify lumbar region spinal stenosis without neurogenic claudication (724.02) and lumbar region spinal stenosis with neurogenic claudication (724.03) to recognize the different medical treatment requirements for these patients.

## Rheumatism, Excluding the Back (725–729)

The section Rheumatism, Excluding the Back (725–729) includes codes for disorders of muscles, tendons and their attachments, and of other soft tissues. Common conditions such as rotator cuff syndrome of shoulder and allied disorders (codes 726.10–726.19), lateral epicondylitis (726.32) as well as various forms of bursitis, tendinitis, and myositis are included here.

### Compartment Syndrome

A compartment syndrome or compartmental syndrome is a condition in which increased pressure is within an enclosed tissue space. It most often occurs in an extremity but can occur in the abdomen and other sites. There are two types of compartment syndrome—traumatic or nontraumatic. Causes may be external compression or soft tissue swelling such as edema or hematoma. Some specific causes are burns, frostbite, snakebite, postsurgical edema or hemorrhage, hemophilia, and anticoagulant therapy. Compartments are covered by fascia and when pressure in the compartment is measured to be high or elevated, an emergency surgical procedure such as a fasciotomy is indicated. Exertional compartment syndrome, also known as nontraumatic compartment syndrome, is known to occur in individuals who exercise frequently, especially runners who suffer from compartment syndrome in their leg(s). It can also occur in the forearm. These nontraumatic types are usually considered a chronic form of the condition, but a patient can have an acute episode and may require emergency treatment. Nontraumatic compartment syndrome is coded based on its location in the body, that is, 729.71 for upper extremity, 729.72 for lower extremity, 729.73 for abdomen, and 729.79 for other sites. Traumatic compartment syndrome is recognized as an early complication of trauma and is coded within the injury section of ICD-9-CM. Specific codes exist in the range of 958.90–958.99 depending on the location of the compartment syndrome following trauma.

## Osteopathies, Chondropathies, and Acquired Musculoskeletal Deformities (730–739)

The section Osteopathies, Chondropathies, and Acquired Musculoskeletal Deformities (730–739) includes codes describing osteomyelitis, bone cysts, malunion and nonunion of fractures, pathological fractures, acquired deformities of the limbs, and curvature of the spine.

### Osteomyelitis

Category 730, Osteomyelitis, periostitis, and other infections involving bone, is further subdivided to fourth-digit subcategories that describe acute or chronic osteomyelitis, as well as osteopathy or bone infections resulting from other diseases such as poliomyelitis. The fifth-digit subclassification identifies the site involved. An additional code should be assigned that describes the organism involved.

### Pathologic Fractures

Pathologic fractures are classified to subcategory 733.1, with the fifth-digit subclassification identifying the specific site. These types of fractures occur in existing diseases such as osteoporosis or bone metastasis, both of which are capable of weakening the bone. Often pathologic fractures are spontaneous in nature; however, minor injuries can result in a fracture because the bone is already weakened. Pathologic fractures are reported with subcategory 733.1 when the fracture is first diagnosed, and this code continues to be used as long as the patient is receiving active treatment for the fracture. Active treatment includes surgery, emergency department visits, and evaluation and treatment by a new physician.

Pathologic fractures are coded with aftercare codes (subcategories V54.0, V54.2, V54.8 or V54.9) for visits after the patient has completed active treatment for the fracture and the patient is receiving routine care for the fracture during the healing or recovery period. Examples of aftercare include cast changes, cast removal, removal of internal and external fixation devices, medication adjustment, and follow-up visits following fracture treatment.

Stress fractures (733.93–733.98) are excluded from the codes for pathologic fracture. Coders must be cautious not to confuse the pathologic and stress fractures with the traumatic injuries that cause bones to fracture, which are coded with the fracture injury codes in ICD-9-CM.

### Malunion and Nonunion Fractures

Malunion of a fracture (733.81) refers to a fracture that was reduced, but the bone ends did not align properly during the healing process. Malunions are often diagnosed during the healing stages and require surgical intervention.

Nonunion of a fracture (733.82) is the failure of the bone ends to align or heal. This usually requires a reopening of the fracture site, with some type of internal fixation and bone grafting performed. Nonunion fractures are often more difficult to treat than malunions. An additional diagnosis code for late effect of fracture (905.0–905.5) is also assigned.

### Stress Fractures

Bones may develop "fatigue" or stress fractures from repetitive forces applied before the bone and its supporting structures have time to accommodate such force. When a stress fracture is first suspected, x-rays are often negative. Days or weeks may pass before the fracture line is visible. However, a presumptive diagnosis is necessary to begin prompt treatment. The term *stress reactio*n is synonymous with stress fracture.

### Arthroscopic Surgery

An arthroscope is a small, tubular instrument containing magnifying lenses, a light source, and a video camera. Very small instruments are used with the arthroscope to perform surgical procedures on a joint, such as repair or removal of tissue or to take a biopsy. Arthroscopic surgery is commonly performed on most joints, including the knee, shoulder, wrist, and ankle. Arthroscopic surgery is often performed on an outpatient basis, and these procedures cause less damage to the body, minimize pain and scarring, and allow a faster recovery than open joint procedures involving an arthrotomy.

Arthroscopy of a joint is coded with ICD-9-CM volume 3 codes in the range of 80.20–80.29. However, the use of an arthroscope is often the "approach" during a therapeutic or diagnostic joint procedure. When a more definitive procedure is performed through an arthroscope, only the definitive procedure code is assigned. An additional code for the arthroscopy is not needed. For example, if a patient had an arthroscopic arthroplasty of the knee with a chondroplasty and debridement of meniscus performed, only the code 81.47, Other repair of knee, would be assigned. The arthroscopic approach code, 80.26, is not assigned.

### Hip Bearing Surfaces

Four procedure codes exist to describe the different types of bearing surface materials used in hip prosthetic implants. The types of surfaces described in the codes are:

**00.74 Hip bearing surface, metal-on-polyethylene**
**00.75 Hip bearing surface, metal-on-metal**
**00.76 Hip bearing surface, ceramic-on-ceramic**
**00.77 Hip bearing surface, ceramic-on-polyethylene**

These codes are used as additional procedure codes when a hip replacement procedure is coded (81.51 and 81.52), or revision of hip replacement procedure is coded (81.53, 00.70–00.73.) A revision of a hip replacement procedure may be described as a conversion of a hemiarthroplasty to a total joint replacement. Any time a component of a joint that has been previously replaced is revised, the subsequent procedures performed on the same joint would be considered a revision arthroplasty even though part of the joint is being replaced for the first time.

## ICD-9-CM Review Exercises: Chapter 16

Assign ICD-9-CM codes to the following:

1. Displacement of thoracic intervertebral disc and laminectomy with excision of disc
2. Paget's disease of the bone (no bone tumor noted)
3. Chronic juvenile rheumatoid arthritis; total hip revision replacing a previous hemiarthroplasty with both acetabulum and femoral components replaced using metal-on-polyethylene hip bearing surfaces
4. Lumbar spondylosis with myelopathy
5. Chondromalacia of the patella
6. Primary localized osteoarthrosis of the hip; total hip replacement with ceramic-on-ceramic bearing surface
7. Acute osteomyelitis of ankle due to *Staphylococcus aureus*
8. Pathologic fracture of the vertebra due to metastatic carcinoma of the bone from the lung
9. Acquired talipes equinovarus (acquired clubfoot)
10. Systemic lupus erythematosus
11. Postlaminectomy syndrome of the thoracic region
12. Kyphosis due to osteoporosis

## ICD-9-CM Review Exercises: Chapter 16 (Continued)

13. Left knee internal derangement with old medial meniscal tear; arthroscopy of left knee with partial medial meniscectomy

14. Pyogenic arthritis of hand due to group B streptococcus

15. Ankylosing spondylitis

16. Baker's cyst of knee with excision

17. Pathologic fracture of the humerus due to postmenopausal osteoporosis; closed reduction, fracture of humerus

18. Nonpyogenic arthritis of the hip due to staphylococcal infection

19. Aneurysmal bone cyst, left tibia; excision of cyst

20. Slipped upper femoral epiphysis (nontraumatic)

# ICD-10-CM Chapter 13, Diseases of the Musculoskeletal System and Connective Tissue (M00–M99)

## Organization and Structure of ICD-10-CM Chapter 13

ICD-10-CM Chapter 13 contains more subchapters, categories, and codes than ICD-9-CM Chapter 13. Rather than having four subchapters grouping many conditions together, ICD-10-CM organizes the musculoskeletal system and connective tissue in the following blocks:

M00–M02 Infectious arthropathies
M05–M14 Inflammatory polyarthropathies
M15–M19 Osteoarthritis

| | |
|---|---|
| M20–M25 | Other joint disorders |
| M26–M27 | Dentofacial anomalies [including malocclusion] and other disorders of jaw |
| M30–M36 | Systemic connective tissue disorders |
| M40–M43 | Deforming dorsopathies |
| M45–M49 | Spondylopathies |
| M50–M54 | Other dorsopathies |
| M60–M63 | Disorders of muscles |
| M65–M67 | Disorders of synovium and tendon |
| M70–M79 | Other soft tissue disorders |
| M80–M85 | Disorders of bone density and structure |
| M86–M90 | Other osteopathies |
| M91–M94 | Chondropathies |
| M95 | Other disorders of the musculoskeletal system and connective tissue |
| M96 | Intraoperative and postprocedural complications and disorders of musculoskeletal system, not elsewhere classified |
| M99 | Biomechanical lesions, not elsewhere classified |

Almost every code in Chapter 13 of ICD-10-CM has been expanded in some way, with the expansion including very specific sites as well as laterality. Numerous codes have been moved from various chapters in ICD-9-CM to Chapter 13 in ICD-10-CM.

**EXAMPLES:**

- Category 274, Gout in ICD-9-CM Chapter 3: Endocrine, Nutritional and Metabolic Diseases and Immunity Disorders, is classified as M10, Gout, in ICD-10-CM Chapter 13
- Code 268.2, Osteomalacia, unspecified in ICD-9-CM Chapter 3 is classified to category M83, Adult osteomalacia in ICD-10-CM Chapter 13
- Code 524.4, Malocclusion, unspecified, in ICD-9-CM Chapter 9: Diseases of the Digestive System, is classified to code M26.4, Malocclusion, unspecified in ICD-10-CM Chapter 13

Category M80 in ICD-10-CM classifies the type of osteoporosis in addition to the site of a current pathological fracture into one combination code.

Additionally, some categories and subcategories in Chapter 13 require the use of seventh characters, such as A for initial encounter for fracture or S for sequelae of fracture.

## Coding Guidelines and Instructional Notes for ICD-10-CM Chapter 13

The first block of the chapter on diseases of the musculoskeletal system and connective tissue for infectious arthropathies includes arthropathies due to microbiological agents. To assist coding professionals on the correct usage of categories M00–M02, a note appears at the beginning of the section to provide definitions for direct and indirect infection.

Distinction is made between the following types of etiological relationships:

- Direct infection of joint—where organisms invade synovial tissue and microbial antigen is present in the joint
- Indirect infection—which may be of two types: a reactive arthropathy, where microbial infection of the body is established but neither organisms nor antigens can be identified in the joint, and a postinfective arthropathy, where microbial antigen is present but recovery of an organism is inconstant and evidence of local multiplication is lacking

Instructional notes have also been added to different categories or subcategories to explain how codes should be assigned.

| | | |
|---|---|---|
| **EXAMPLE:** | **M21.7** | **Unequal limb length (acquired)**<br>Note: The site used should correspond to the shorter limb |
| | **M50** | **Cervical disc disorders**<br>Note: Code to the most superior level of disorder |

Includes notes have also been used to define terms.

| | | |
|---|---|---|
| **EXAMPLE:** | **M66** | **Spontaneous rupture of synovium and tendon** |
| | Includes | Rupture that occurs when a normal force is applied to tissues that are inferred to have less than normal strength |

The NCHS has published chapter-specific guidelines for Chapter 13 of ICD-10-CM, for example:

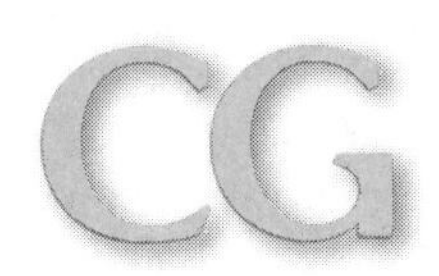


- Guideline I.C.13.a. Site and laterality
  - Most of the codes have site and laterality designations. The site represents either the bone, joint, or muscle involved.
- Guideline I.C.13.b. Acute traumatic versus chronic or recurrent musculoskeletal conditions
- Guideline I.C.13.c. Coding of pathologic fractures
- Guideline I.C.13.d.2. Osteoporosis with Current Pathological Fracture
  - Category M80, Osteoporosis with current pathological fracture, is for patients who have a current pathologic fracture at the time of an encounter. The codes under M80 identify the site of the fracture. A code from category M80, not a traumatic fracture code, should be used for any patient with known osteoporosis who suffers a fracture, even if that patient had a minor fall or trauma, if that fall or trauma would not usually break a normal, healthy bone.

To gain an understanding of these rules, access the 2014 guidelines from NCHS website (http://www.cdc.gov/nchs/icd/icd10cm.htm) and read Chapter 13, Diseases of the Musculoskeletal System and Connective Tissue guidelines I.C.13.a–I.C.13.d.

## Coding Overview of ICD-10-CM Chapter 13

Chapter 13 of ICD-10-CM, Diseases of the Musculoskeletal System and Connective Tissue (M00–M99), describes many of the same conditions found in ICD-9-CM. There is another code alliteration in this chapter: **M** codes for **M**usculoskeletal.

A note at the beginning of Chapter 13 states, "Use an external cause code following the code for the musculoskeletal condition, if applicable, to identify the cause of the musculoskeletal condition" (CDC 2014).

Most of the codes in Chapter 13 include site and laterality. The site indicates the bone, joint, or muscle involved. For example, Stress fracture of right tibia (M84.361), rheumatoid bursitis of left shoulder (M06.212), and muscle spasm of back (M62.830).

Some current musculoskeletal conditions in Chapter 13 are the result of a previous injury or trauma to a site and others are recurrent conditions. Any acute injury is coded using a different chapter in ICD-10-CM. However, some fractures that are included in Chapter 13 are current events. Examples of exceptions are stress fractures (M84.3) and pathological fractures (M84.4–M84.6). These fracture codes require an appropriate seventh character to identify the episode of care. For example, the seventh character A indicates initial encounter for the fracture, and the seventh character D is used for subsequent encounter for fracture with routine healing. The use of these seventh characters for the episode of care is new in ICD-10-CM and is also used for traumatic fractures coded in Chapter 19 of ICD-10-CM.

ICD-10-CM has different categories and subcategories for pathologic fractures: category M80, Osteoporosis with current pathological fractures; subcategory M84,4, Pathological fracture, not elsewhere classified; M84.5, Pathological fracture in neoplastic disease; and subcategory M84.6, Pathological fracture in other disease.

Intraoperative and postprocedural complications of the musculoskeletal system are included in Chapter 13 in ICD-10-CM. In addition to the codes for hemorrhage, hematoma, accidental puncture, or laceration, there are codes specific to musculoskeletal complications, such as subcategory M96.6, Fracture of bone following insertion of orthopedic implant, joint prosthesis, or bone plate. These codes identify the bone, such as femur, and laterality.

A number of block, category, and subcategory title changes have been made in Chapter 13, for example, subsection 710–719 in ICD-9-CM, titled "Arthropathies and related disorders," is called "Arthropathies" in section M00–M25 in ICD-10-CM. Also, a number of conditions have moved to this chapter from other chapters in ICD-9-CM. For example, gout moved from Chapter 3; polyarteritis nodosa has moved from Chapter 7; and categories 524, Dentofacial anomalies, including malocclusion, and 526, Diseases of the jaw, moved from Chapter 9.

Bone, joint, or muscle conditions that are the result of a healed injury and recurrent bone, joint, or muscle conditions are also usually found in Chapter 13. Any current, acute injury should be coded to the appropriate injury code from Chapter 19, Injury, Poisoning and Certain Other Consequences of External Causes; chronic or recurrent conditions should generally be coded with a code from Chapter 13. These instructions are included in the *ICD-10-CM Official Guidelines for Coding and Reporting*, chapter specific guidelines for the musculoskeletal system and connective tissue.

The following seventh character extensions are required for codes in Chapter 13 that represent pathological or stress fractures in category M84.3–M84.6:

A—Initial encounter for fracture
D—Subsequent encounter for fracture with routine healing
G—Subsequent encounter for fracture with delayed healing
K—Subsequent encounter for fracture with nonunion
P—Subsequent encounter for fracture with malunion
S—Sequela

Seventh character A is for use as long as the patient is receiving active treatment for the fracture. Examples of active treatment are: surgical treatment, emergency department encounter, and evaluation and treatment by a new physician. Seventh character D is to be used for encounters after the patient has completed active treatment. Examples of subsequent treatment are: cast change or removal, removal of external or internal fixation device, medication adjustment, other aftercare and follow-up visits. Seventh character letters are defined in the *ICD-10-CM Official Guidelines for Coding and Reporting* specifically in chapter specific guidelines (Chapter 19) for injury, poisoning, and certain other consequences of external causes.

Some terms have been defined in the classification or there is an includes note to identify other disease terminology that is included in a particular block of codes or a category. In category M15, Polyosteoarthritis, there is an includes note that states it includes arthritis of multiple sites. The block of codes from M30–M36, Systemic connective tissue disorders, includes autoimmune disease NOS, collagen (vascular) disease NOS, systemic autoimmune disease and systemic collagen (vascular) disease. Kyphoscoliosis is included in category M41, Scoliosis. Category M47, Spondylosis, includes such conditions as arthrosis or osteoarthritis of spine and degeneration of facet joints. Similarly, in category M50, Cervical disc disorders, includes cervicothoracic disc disorders with or without cervicalgia with the coder assigning the code for the most superior level of the disorder. In category M66, Spontaneous rupture of synovium and tendon a spontaneous rupture is defined as one that occurs when a normal force is applied to tissues that are inferred to have less than normal strength. Soft tissue disorders of occupational origin are included in category M70, Soft tissue disorders related to use, overuse and pressure. Finally, category M87, Osteonecrosis, includes the condition known as avascular necrosis of bone.

## ICD-10-CM Review Exercises: Chapter 16

Assign the correct ICD-10-CM diagnosis codes to the following exercises:

1. Patient with senile osteoporosis is seen for the complaints of severe back pain with no history of trauma. X-rays revealed pathological compression fractures of several lumbar vertebrae.

2. Juvenile rheumatoid arthritis, only occurring in both ankles

3. Patient has left upper lobe carcinoma, diagnosed over five years ago, but is seen now for a fracture of the shaft of the right femur. During this admission, the patient was diagnosed with metastatic bone cancer (from the lung) and this fracture is a result of the metastatic disease. This patient's lung cancer was treated with radiation and there is no longer evidence of an existing primary malignancy.

4. Bacterial septic arthritis, right knee

5. Stress fracture, right tibia, seen in the clinic for a subsequent encounter with routine healing

6. Juvenile idiopathic scoliosis, lumbar region

7. Tear of medial meniscus, anterior horn, due to old injury, left knee

8. Chondromalacia, patellae, bilateral knees

9. Pain in right elbow with joint effusion in right elbow, cause unknown; both symptoms being investigated

10. Ankylosing spondylitis, thoracic spinal region

## Chapter 17

# Congenital Anomalies and Certain Conditions Originating in the Perinatal Period

## Learning Objectives

At the conclusion of this chapter, you should be able to:

1. Describe the organization of the conditions and codes included in ICD-9-CM Chapters 14, Congenital Anomalies (740–759), and 15, Certain Conditions Originating in the Perinatal Period (760–779)
2. Describe the organization of the conditions and codes included in ICD-10-CM Chapters 16, Certain Conditions Originating in the Perinatal Period (P00–P96), and 17, Congenital Malformations, Deformations and Chromosomal Abnormalities (Q00–Q99)
3. Briefly describe the newborn ICD-9-CM coding guidelines, including how to sequence the newborn, congenital, and perinatal codes
4. Describe the newborn or perinatal period
5. Define the term *congenital anomaly*
6. Describe the process for coding a pediatric syndrome that is not listed in the Alphabetic Index of ICD-9-CM or ICD-10-CM
7. Briefly describe the types of common congenital anomalies classified in Chapter 14 of ICD-9-CM
8. Describe the circumstances in which a code from Chapter 15 of ICD-9-CM or Chapter 16 of ICD-10-CM can be assigned in terms of the age of the patient who has the condition
9. Describe the types of conditions classified in ICD-9-CM categories 760–763, Maternal causes of perinatal morbidity and mortality, that may affect the fetus or newborn
10. Describe the circumstances in which codes from ICD-9-CM categories 764 and 765 are used on a newborn or perinatal record, including weeks of gestation and birth weight
11. Define the term *meconium* and describe the conditions associated with the passage of meconium

12. Review the types of respiratory infections and cardiac dysrhythmias that can occur in newborn and perinatal infants
13. Assign ICD-9-CM diagnosis and procedure codes for congenital anomalies and certain conditions originating in the perinatal period
14. Assign ICD-10-CM codes for congenital anomalies and certain conditions originating in the perinatal period

Newborns often suffer from congenital anomalies and certain other conditions that originate in the perinatal period. This chapter addresses the coding of the congenital and perinatal conditions in ICD-9-CM. In the ICD-10-CM classification, two separate chapters are included to address congenital and perinatal conditions. This textbook chapter addresses the ICD-9-CM and ICD-10-CM coding of the congenital and perinatal conditions.

When coding the birth of an infant, a code from categories V30–V39 is used according to the type of birth. This code is assigned once only to a newborn as a principal diagnosis at the time of birth. Instructions on the assignment of the V30–V39 series codes can be found in chapter 23 of this text. The coding of the newborn status with V30–V39 codes should be reviewed prior to beginning this chapter.

## ICD-9-CM Official Newborn Coding Guidelines

The *ICD-9-CM Official Guidelines for Coding and Reporting* contain directions regarding Chapter 14 of ICD-9-CM, Congenital Anomalies, and Chapter 15 of ICD-9-CM, Certain Conditions Originating in the Perinatal Period. The guidelines can be found in appendix H on the website accompanying this text.

The newborn, or perinatal, period is defined as before birth through the first 28 days after birth. All clinically significant conditions noted on routine newborn examinations should be coded. A condition is significant if it requires one or more of the following:

- Clinical evaluation
- Therapeutic treatment
- Diagnostic procedures
- Extended length of hospital stay
- Increased nursing care and/or monitoring
- Implications for future healthcare needs

The perinatal guidelines are identical to the general coding guidelines for the selection of additional diagnoses, with the exception of the final item—implications for future healthcare needs. Codes should be assigned for conditions that have been specified by the provider as having implications for future healthcare needs, for example, it is appropriate to code congenital anomalies when identified by the physician, even when no apparent treatment is provided. Codes from the perinatal chapter should not be assigned unless the provider has established a definitive diagnosis. The physician determines whether a condition is clinically significant.

# Chapter 14, Congenital Anomalies (740–759)

A congenital anomaly is an irregularity or abnormality that is present at, and existing from, the time of birth. Chapter 14 in the Tabular List in volume 1 of ICD-9-CM classifies congenital anomalies. The chapter is organized by body system, beginning with the central nervous system. Because many conditions can be either congenital in origin or acquired, coders must carefully review the subterms in the Alphabetic Index to select the appropriate code to describe congenital conditions.

When a specific abnormality is diagnosed at the time of birth, the congenital anomaly is listed as an additional diagnosis, with the V30–V39 series used to indicate the newborn status. Congenital anomalies may also be the principal or first-listed diagnosis for admissions or encounters subsequent to the newborn admission. Codes for congenital anomalies may be used throughout the life of the patient. For example, a 40-year-old patient with Down syndrome would be assigned code 758.0 at the time of a healthcare visit. If a congenital anomaly has been corrected, a personal history code should be used to identify the history of the anomaly.

## Coding Guidelines

When an anomaly is diagnosed, assign an appropriate code from categories 740–759, Congenital anomalies. Such abnormalities may occur as a set of symptoms or as multiple malformations. ICD-9-CM does not contain a specific code for the many, sometimes rare, pediatric syndromes that are treated by pediatric specialists, for example, Loey-Dietz Syndrome. There may be an occasion when the physician describes an infant as having a particular named syndrome. For all ICD-9-CM coding of disease syndromes, if the coder cannot locate an ICD-9-CM code in the Alphabetic Index under the specific named syndrome, the coder should ask the physician if the condition is known by any other descriptor. If ICD-9-CM does not specifically index the syndrome or condition, a code should be assigned for each presenting manifestation of the syndrome.

### *Principal versus Additional Diagnosis*

If a congenital anomaly is noted during the hospital admission when the infant was born, the code describing the anomaly is assigned as an additional diagnosis. The principal diagnosis is a code from the section Liveborn Infants According to Type of Birth (V30–V39).

**EXAMPLE:** Liveborn male infant born in the hospital with tetralogy of Fallot: V30.00, Single liveborn, delivered in hospital without mention of cesarean delivery; 745.2, Tetralogy of Fallot

However, if the patient was transferred on the day of birth to another hospital for care of the congenital anomaly, the principal diagnosis at the second hospital would be the congenital anomaly.

**EXAMPLE:** Liveborn male infant transferred for care of thoracic spina bifida with hydrocephalus: 741.02, Spina bifida of dorsal [thoracic] region with hydrocephalus

## Common Congenital Anomalies

Congenital anomalies, also known as birth defects, have been the leading cause of infant mortality in the United States over the past several years. Birth defects substantially contribute to childhood morbidity and long-term disability (CDC 2014b). More than 4,500 different birth defects have been identified. Congenital anomalies can affect almost every body system.

There are three major categories of known causes:

- Chromosomal disorders (either hereditary or arising during conception)
- Exposure to an environmental chemical (for example, medications, alcohol, cigarettes, solvents)
- Mother's illness during pregnancy, exposing the infant to viral or bacterial infections

The stage of fetal development at the time of exposure to one of the two latter causes is critical. Fetal development is particularly vulnerable in the first trimester of pregnancy. The life expectancy and quality of life for individuals with many birth defects has improved greatly over the past 40 years. This is a result of pioneering surgery that can correct certain defects before the infant is born, as well as neonatal intensive care units that provide specialized care and advanced technology to treat the infant.

## Central Nervous System Defects

Central nervous system (CNS) defects involve the brain, spinal cord, and associated tissue. These include neural tube defects (anencephaly, spina bifida, and encephalocele), microcephalus, and hydrocephalus.

One of the more common CNS defects is spina bifida. Spina bifida is a defective closure of the vertebral column. It ranges in severity from the occult type revealing few signs to a completely open spine (rachischisis). In spina bifida cystica, the protruding sac contains meninges (meningocele), the spinal cord (myelocele), or both (myelomeningocele). Commonly seen in the lumbar, low thoracic, or sacral region, spina bifida extends for three to six vertebral segments. When the spinal cord or lumbosacral nerve roots are involved, as is usually the case, varying degrees of paralysis occur below the involved level. This may result in orthopedic conditions such as clubfoot, arthrogryposis, or dislocated hip. The paralysis also usually affects the sphincters of the bladder and rectum. In addition, children born with the more severe form of spina bifida have spine and brain problems, such as hydrocephalus or scoliosis (WebMD 2013).

In ICD-9-CM, most types of spina bifida, excluding spina bifida occulta, are assigned to category 741. This category is further subdivided to fourth-digit subcategories that describe the presence or absence of hydrocephalus. The fifth-digit subclassification describes the site of the spina bifida. Spina bifida occulta (756.17), however, is classified to category 756, Other congenital musculoskeletal anomalies.

If surgical repair is deemed necessary, the opening in the vertebral column is closed. If hydrocephalus exists, a shunt (most often a ventriculoperitoneal shunt) also may be necessary.

ICD-9-CM classifies repairs of spina bifida to subcategory 03.5, Plastic operations on spinal cord structures. Code 03.51 is assigned for spinal meningocele; code 03.52, for spinal myelomeningocele; and code 03.59, when the type is not elsewhere classifiable.

## Cardiovascular System Defects

Cardiovascular system defects involve the heart and circulatory system and are the most common group of birth defects in infants. Surgical procedures repair defects and restore circulation to as normal as possible. Some defects can be repaired before birth, whereas others may require multiple surgical procedures after birth. Smaller defects may be repaired in a cardiac catheterization laboratory instead of an operating room. Some of the more commonly occurring cardiovascular defects are patent ductus arteriosus, atrial septal defect, ventricular septal defect, and pulmonary artery anomalies.

Descriptions of cardiovascular system defects and their common abbreviations are as follows:

- Hypoplastic left heart syndrome (746.7) is a condition in which the entire left half of the heart is underdeveloped. This condition may be repaired in a series of three procedures over one year. If not treated, the condition can be fatal within one month.
- Common truncus or persistent truncus arteriosus (PTA) (745.0) is a failure of the fetal truncus arteriosus to divide into the aorta and pulmonary artery. It can be corrected surgically.
- Pulmonary valve atresia (746.01) and stenosis (746.02) are conditions that obstruct or narrow the pulmonary heart valve. Mild forms are relatively well tolerated and require no intervention. More severe forms are surgically corrected.
- Tetralogy of Fallot (TOF) (745.2) is a defect characterized by four anatomical abnormalities within the heart that results in poorly oxygenated blood being pumped to the body. It can be corrected surgically.
- Total anomalous pulmonary venous return (TAPVR) (747.41) is a malformation of all of the pulmonary veins. In this condition, the pulmonary veins empty into the right atrium, or a systemic vein, instead of into the left atrium.
- Transposition of great vessels or great arteries (TGV) (745.10–745.19) is a defect in which the positions of the aorta and the pulmonary artery are transposed. Immediate surgical correction is required.
- Tricuspid valve atresia and stenosis (746.1) is the absence or narrowing of the valve between the right atrium and ventricle. Severe cases are surgically corrected.
- Aortic valve stenosis (AS) (746.3) is the congenital narrowing or obstruction of the aortic heart valve. This can be surgically repaired in some cases.
- Atrial septal defect (ASD) (745.5) is a hole in the wall between the upper chambers of the heart (the atria). The openings may resolve without treatment or require surgical intervention. This condition may also be referred to as patent foramen ovale.
- Coarctation of the aorta (747.10) is a defect in which the aorta is narrowed somewhere along its length. Surgical correction is recommended even for mild defects.
- Endocardial cushion defect is a spectrum of septal defects arising from imperfect fusion of the endocardial cushions in the fetal heart (745.60–745.69). These defects are repaired surgically.

- Patent ductus arteriosus (PDA) is a condition in which the channel between the pulmonary artery and the aorta fails to close at birth (747.0). Many of these close spontaneously and cause no consequences. The condition can also be surgically and medically repaired.
- Ventricular septal defect (VSD) (745.4) is a hole in the lower chambers of the heart, or the ventricles. The openings may resolve without treatment; however, the condition can be surgically corrected.
- Ebstein anomaly (746.2) is a deformation or displacement of the tricuspid valve with the septal and posterior leaflets being attached to the wall of the right ventricle. Only severe cases are corrected surgically.

## Respiratory System Defects

Respiratory system congenital anomalies, mainly in the lungs, trachea, and nose, are life-threatening, but less common than those involving other major organs. The major defect is lung atresia or hypoplasia—the failure to develop or underdevelopment of one or both lungs (748.5).

## Digestive System Defects

Digestive system defects include orofacial defects (for example, choanal atresia, or cleft palate and lip) and gastrointestinal defects (for example, esophageal atresia, rectal and intestinal atresia and stenosis, and pyloric stenosis).

### *Cleft Lip and Cleft Palate*

Cleft lip, cleft palate, and combinations of the two are the most common congenital anomalies of the head and neck. A cleft is a fissure or elongated opening of a specified site, usually occurring during the embryonic stage. A cleft palate is a split in the roof of the mouth (the palate) and a cleft lip is the presence of one or two splits in the upper lip. Cleft lips and palates are classified as partial or complete, and can occur either bilaterally or unilaterally. The most common clefts are left unilateral complete clefts of the primary and secondary palate, and partial midline clefts of the secondary palate involving the soft palate and part of the hard palate. The incisive foramen serves as the dividing point between the primary and the secondary palate.

In ICD-9-CM, cleft palate and cleft lip are classified to category 749. This category is subdivided to describe cleft palate (749.0), cleft lip (749.1), and a combination of the two (749.2). These subcategories are further subdivided to identify unilateral or bilateral and complete or incomplete cleft palate or cleft lip. Documentation in the record should be reviewed to determine whether the cleft is complete or incomplete (partial). The physician should be queried when the documentation is unclear.

Surgical repair of cleft lips and/or palates may occur immediately after birth or delayed for several weeks after birth depending on the individual patient. Sometimes secondary revisions are required to correct any tissue deformities or scars. ICD-9-CM assigns code 27.54 for repair of cleft lip, code 27.62 for correction of cleft palate, and code 27.63 for revision of cleft palate repair.

### Pyloric Stenosis

Pyloric stenosis is a narrowing of the outlet between the stomach and small intestine. It results from hypertrophy of the circular and longitudinal muscularis of the pylorus and distal antrum of the stomach. Typically, the infant feeds well from birth until two or three weeks after birth, at which time occasional regurgitation of food, or spitting up, occurs, followed several days later by projectile vomiting. Dehydration due to the vomiting is common. Surgery is the treatment of choice. Fredet-Ramstedt pyloromyotomy is performed following management of the dehydration.

ICD-9-CM assigns code 750.5 for congenital pyloric stenosis. Code 43.3 describes the pyloromyotomy.

## Genitourinary Tract Defects

Both male and female infants may be afflicted with defects of the reproductive organs and the urinary tract. Some are relatively minor and fairly common defects that can be repaired by surgery. Some of the genitourinary tract defects are as follows:

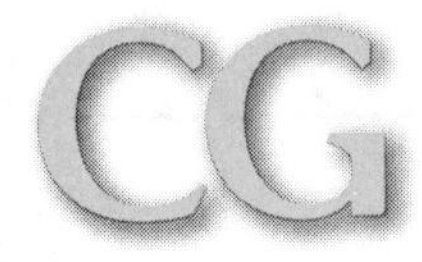


- Abnormalities of uterus codes (752.31–752.39) identify congenital anomalies such as agenesis of uterus, hypoplasia of uterus, unicornuate uterus, bicornuate uterus, septate uterus, arcuate uterus, and other anomalies of uterus. Collectively these conditions may be referred to as Mullerian anomalies of the uterus. Women are likely to be diagnosed with these conditions after seeking medical attention for infertility or repeated pregnancy loss.
- Bladder exstrophy (753.5) is a condition in which the bladder is turned inside out with portions of the abdominal and bladder walls missing. This must be surgically repaired.
- Male epispadias (752.62) is a relatively rare defect in which the urethra opens on the top surface of the penis and surgical correction is needed. Female epispadias is coded to 753.8.
- Hypospadias (752.61) is a relatively common defect that appears as an abnormal penile opening on the underside of the penis rather than at the end. Surgical correction may be needed for cosmetic, urologic, and reproductive reasons.
- Obstructive genitourinary defect is an obstruction of the ureter, renal pelvis, urethra, or bladder neck (753.20–753.29, 753.6). Severity of the condition depends on the level of the obstruction. Urine accumulates behind the obstruction and produces organ damage. This

*(Continued)*

*(Continued)*

condition can be corrected surgically while the fetus is in the uterus or after birth.

- Renal atresia (753.3) is the absence or underdevelopment of the kidneys and may be unilateral or bilateral. Newborns with bilateral renal atresia often expire due to respiratory failure within a few hours of birth. Unilateral renal atresia may not be detected for years.
- Polycystic kidney disease (PKD) is an inherited disorder characterized by multiple, bilateral, grapelike clusters of fluid-filled cysts that grossly enlarge the kidneys, compressing and eventually replacing functioning renal tissue. The infantile form of this condition reveals an infant with pronounced epicanthal folds, a pointed nose, a small chin, and floppy, low-set ears. Signs of respiratory distress and congestive heart failure also may be present. This condition eventually deteriorates into uremia and renal failure.

ICD-9-CM classifies cystic kidney disease to subcategory 753.1, with the following fifth-digit subclassifications:

**753.10 Cystic kidney disease, unspecified**
**753.11 Congenital single renal cyst**
**753.12 Polycystic kidney, unspecified type**
**753.13 Polycystic kidney, autosomal dominant**
**753.14 Polycystic kidney, autosomal recessive**
**753.15 Renal dysplasia**
**753.16 Medullary cystic kidney**
**753.17 Medullary sponge kidney**
**753.19 Other specified cystic kidney disease**

When there is no further specification as to type of polycystic kidney disease, assign code 753.12. In addition, assign other complications that may be present, such as chronic kidney disease (585.1–585.9).

## Musculoskeletal Defects

Musculoskeletal defects are relatively common disorders and range from minor problems to more serious conditions. Clubfoot is the most common musculoskeletal congenital anomaly.

### *Clubfoot*

Clubfoot is a general term that is used to describe a variety of congenital structural foot deformities involving the lower leg, ankle, and foot joints, ligaments, and tendons. Clubfoot deformities include:

- Varus deformities, which are characterized by a turning inward of the feet (codes 754.50–754.59)
- Valgus deformities, which are characterized by a turning outward of the feet (codes 754.60–754.69)
- Talipes cavus, which is recognized by increased arch of the foot (code 754.71)
- Talipes calcaneus or equinus, in which the entire foot exhibits an abnormal upward or downward misalignment (code 754.79)

The generic term *clubfoot* is classified as talipes, unspecified (code 754.70).

## Chromosomal Defects

Chromosomal abnormalities are disorders that arise from abnormal numbers of chromosomes or from defects in specific fragments of the chromosomes. Each disorder is associated with a characteristic pattern of defects that arises as a consequence of the underlying chromosomal abnormality. Congenital heart defects, especially septal defects, are common among these infants and are a major cause of death. The more common chromosomal conditions include the following:

- Down syndrome is associated with the presence of a third number 21 chromosome. It results in intellectual disabilities, distinctive malformations of the face and head, and other abnormalities. The severity of these problems varies widely among the affected individuals. Down syndrome is one of the more frequently occurring chromosomal abnormalities.
- Edward's syndrome is associated with the presence of a third number 18 chromosome. It causes major physical abnormalities and severe intellectual disabilities. Many children with this disorder expire in the first year of life due to the abnormalities of the lungs and diaphragm, heart defects, and blood vessel malformations.
- Patau's syndrome is associated with the presence of a third number 13 chromosome. The infants have many internal and external abnormalities, including profound retardation. Death may occur in the first few days of life due to the respiratory difficulties, heart defects, and severe defects in other organ systems.

Category 758, Chromosomal anomalies, includes syndromes like these stated conditions that are associated with the number and form of the chromosomes. The patient may have additional conditions as a result of the chromosomal anomalies that are reported with an additional code. For example, patients with Down syndrome frequently have congenital heart disease including ventricular septal defect and atrioventricular canal defect. The cardiac conditions would be assigned as an additional code when evaluated and treated in a patient with Down syndrome (Chen 2014).

## Exercise 17.1

Assign ICD-9-CM codes to the following (unless otherwise noted, assume this visit is subsequent to admission for birth):

1. Thyroglossal duct cyst with excision
2. Single liveborn male (born in the hospital) with polydactyly of fingers
3. Unilateral cleft lip and palate; repair of cleft lip
4. Patent ductus arteriosus with repair
5. Single liveborn male (born in the hospital via cesarean delivery) with congenital diaphragmatic hernia and repair of diaphragmatic hernia (abdominal approach)
6. Congenital hydrocephalus with insertion of ventriculoperitoneal shunt
7. Hypoplasia of lung
8. Small omphalocele; open umbilical herniorrhaphy with graft
9. Childhood-type polycystic kidney
10. Congenital talipes equinovalgus; Down syndrome

# Chapter 15, Certain Conditions Originating in the Perinatal Period (760–779)

Chapter 15, Certain Conditions Originating in the Perinatal Period, in the Tabular List in volume 1 of ICD-9-CM includes the following categories and section titles:

| Categories | Section Titles |
|---|---|
| 760–763 | Maternal Causes of Perinatal Morbidity and Mortality |
| 764–779 | Other Conditions Originating in the Perinatal Period |

The perinatal period is defined as beginning before birth and lasting through 28 days after birth.

## Inclusion Notation

The following includes note appears at the beginning of Chapter 15:

> **15. CERTAIN CONDITIONS ORIGINATING IN THE PERINATAL PERIOD (760–779)**
>
> Includes: conditions that have their origin in the perinatal period, before birth through the first 28 days after birth, even though death or morbidity occurs later

Although the perinatal period lasts through 28 days following birth, the codes within Chapter 15 may be assigned beyond that period when the condition still exists. However, the condition must have its origin in the perinatal period, even though it could continue to affect the patient beyond that time.

**EXAMPLE:** Six-month-old was admitted to the hospital with acute respiratory failure due to bronchopulmonary dysplasia: 518.81, Acute respiratory failure; 770.7, Chronic respiratory disease arising in the perinatal period

In the above example, the patient developed bronchopulmonary dysplasia (BPD) during the perinatal period while receiving prolonged and high concentrations of inspired $O_2$. Although this patient is no longer in the perinatal period, the BPD is still present and, as such, should be coded. BPD occurs commonly in infants who had respiratory distress syndrome at birth, as well as those who have required endotracheal intubation and a respirator for many days.

## Coding Guidelines

The following subsections offer guidelines that may be used when coding certain conditions originating in the perinatal period.

### *Categories 760–763*

According to the *ICD-9-CM Official Coding and Reporting Guidelines*, codes from categories 760–763, Maternal causes of perinatal morbidity and mortality, are assigned only when the maternal condition has actually affected the fetus or newborn. The fact that the mother has an associated medical condition or experiences some complication of pregnancy, labor, or delivery does not justify the routine assignment of codes from these categories to the newborn's record.

A number of substances are known to have effects on the development of the fetus when the mother is exposed to the substance during pregnancy. Subcategory 760.7, Noxious influences affecting fetus or newborn via placenta or breast milk, identifies through the use of the fifth digit the substance found to have harmed the fetus or newborn. Some of the substances are legal and illegal drugs, such as narcotics and cocaine, but others include anti-infective agents, anticonvulsants, and antimetabolic agents that must be continued through the pregnancy.

**EXAMPLE:** Liveborn infant born (in hospital) with fetal alcohol syndrome to an alcohol-dependent mother: V30.00, Single liveborn, delivered in hospital without mention of cesarean delivery; 760.71, Alcohol affecting fetus via placenta or breast milk

**EXAMPLE:** Delivery of a normal and healthy infant (in hospital) to a mother who occasionally uses cocaine: V30.00, Single liveborn, delivered in hospital without mention of cesarean delivery

In the first example, the use of alcohol by the mother was manifested in the infant; therefore, a code for fetal alcohol syndrome was assigned.

In the second example, however, the infant was healthy and normal despite the mother's occasional use of cocaine; therefore, the code to describe noxious influences of cocaine affecting the fetus (760.75) was not assigned.

## Categories 764–765

Categories 764 and 765 are classified in the section Other Conditions Originating in the Perinatal Period. Category 764 classifies slow fetal growth and fetal malnutrition. Category 765 classifies disorders related to short gestation and low birth weight.

Most physicians indicate a newborn's weight in grams. However, weight may also be recorded in pounds and ounces. One pound equals approximately 454 grams. A two-pound infant weighs about 907 grams, a five-pound infant weighs about 2,268 grams, and a 10-pound infant weighs about 4,536 grams. The ICD-9-CM system classifies an infant's weight in grams.

At the beginning of this section, the following fifth-digit subclassification, which applies to categories 764, 765.0, and 765.1, is introduced:

**0 unspecified [weight]**
**1 less than 500 grams**
**2 500–749 grams**
**3 750–999 grams**
**4 1,000–1,249 grams**
**5 1,250–1,499 grams**
**6 1,500–1,749 grams**
**7 1,750–1,999 grams**
**8 2,000–2,499 grams**
**9 2,500 grams and over**

These fifth digits are used to identify the weight of the infant at birth, not the weight at subsequent visits.

The birth weight fifth digits are limited for use to category 764 and to subcategories 765.0, Extreme prematurity, and 765.1, Other preterm infants. The inclusion terms for these codes describe only birth weight with no reference to gestational age.

For the premature infant, the weeks of gestation are also valuable information. With codes from category 764 and subcategories 765.0 and 765.1, a code from subcategory 765.2 is to be used as an additional code to specify weeks of gestation as documented by the physician. More than one code in the 765 category should be used to describe the preterm infant; that is, one to describe the birth weight, and a second code to indicate the completed weeks of gestation. Weeks of gestation may allow the physician to predict the probability of developmental problems later.

Codes from category 764 and subcategories 765.0 and 765.1 should not be assigned based solely on recorded birth weight or estimated gestational age, but on the attending physician's assessment of maturity of the infant and statement of the infant's gestational age or birth weight. Because physicians may use different criteria in determining prematurity, the coder should not record a diagnosis of prematurity unless the physician documents this condition.

### Conditions Associated with Meconium

Meconium is a newborn's first stool, consisting of a combination of swallowed amniotic fluid and mucus from the baby. The passage of meconium before birth can be an indication of fetal distress. It is seen in infants small for gestational age, post dates, or those with cord complications or other factors compromising placental circulation. Meconium aspiration syndrome occurs when meconium from amniotic fluid in the upper airway is inhaled into the lungs by the newborn with his or her first breath. This invokes an inflammatory reaction in the lungs, which can be fatal. Meconium staining is not meconium aspiration. Meconium aspiration is not meconium aspiration syndrome. ICD-9-CM provides distinct codes for the different conditions involving meconium:

763.84 Meconium passage during delivery
770.11 Meconium aspiration without respiratory symptoms
770.12 Meconium aspiration with respiratory symptoms
779.84 Meconium staining

### Respiratory Problems in Infants after Birth

Conditions classified to subcategory 770.8, Other respiratory problems after birth, are frequently present in infants. Subcategory 770.8, along with its fifth digits, includes different newborn respiratory conditions that vary in type and severity. Many infants suffer from more than one condition listed under 770.8, for example, code 770.84, Respiratory failure of newborn, which may exist with other respiratory problems. Subcategory 770.8 does not include conditions related to lack of oxygen at birth that are properly indexed to codes within subcategory 768, Intrauterine hypoxia and birth asphyxia.

### Infections

ICD-9-CM classifies perinatal infections to category 771, Infections specific to the perinatal period. According to the includes note that appears under the category heading of 771, Infections specific to the perinatal period, these infections can be acquired before birth, during birth, via the umbilicus, or acquired during the first 28 days after birth. The perinatal period is defined as before birth through the first 28 days after birth.

> Includes: Infections acquired before or during birth or via the umbilicus
> or during the first 28 days after birth

Therefore, an infant who develops a urinary tract infection at the age of 20 days would be assigned code 771.82, Urinary tract infection of newborn. Newborn, neonatal, and perinatal refer to the time period of birth through 28 days of life. If the infection is acquired within the first 28 days of life, the perinatal code is used.

Subcategory 771.8, Other infections specific to the perinatal period, is another series of codes used frequently with newborns. It includes infections ranging from urinary tract infection to septicemia. Unique codes exist for septicemia or sepsis of newborn (771.81) and bacteremia of newborn (771.83.) There is direction under 771.8 to "use additional code to identify organism or specific infection." For newborn sepsis, a code from category 038, Septicemia, should not be assigned because code 771.81 describes the sepsis. If a newborn develops severe sepsis, an additional code of 995.92 is assigned with 771.81, with additional codes to identify any associated acute organ dysfunction.

### Neonatal Cardiac Dysrhythmia

Infants may have either bradycardia or tachycardia after birth that is unrelated to the stress of labor or delivery or other intrauterine complications. These symptoms are almost always a symptom of an underlying condition, but the cause may not be immediately known. Neonatal bradycardia is coded to 779.81, and neonatal tachycardia is coded to 779.82.

## ICD-9-CM Review Exercises: Chapter 17

Assign ICD-9-CM codes to the following (assume this visit is subsequent to the admission for birth, unless otherwise noted, and in the perinatal period):

1. Live newborn (born in hospital) with fetal distress with onset before labor

2. Newborn transferred to hospital B with tetralogy of Fallot; Blalock-Taussig procedure with cardiopulmonary bypass (assign codes for hospital B)

3. Hyperbilirubinemia of prematurity; prematurity (birth weight of 2,000 g with 35 completed weeks of gestation); phototherapy

4. Erb's palsy

5. Hypoglycemia in infant with diabetic mother

6. Erythroblastosis fetalis

7. Premature "crack" baby born in hospital to a mother dependent on cocaine; birth weight of 1,247 g, 32 completed weeks of gestation

8. Newborn readmitted on day 10 of life with pneumonia

9. Newborn transferred to University Hospital for treatment of group B streptococcal septicemia

## ICD-9-CM Review Exercises: Chapter 17 (Continued)

10. Necrotizing enterocolitis, stage I, discovered in a newborn at birth

11. Single newborn delivered via cesarean section; large for gestational age (mother is diabetic)

12. Transferred from hospital A to hospital B with spina bifida involving the dorsal region with hydrocephalus; repair of myelomeningocele with insertion of ventriculoperitoneal shunt (assign codes for hospital B)

13. Newborn (born in hospital) via normal spontaneous vaginal delivery with respiratory failure; 50 hours of mechanical ventilation with endotracheal intubation

14. Disseminated intravascular coagulation in a 15-day-old infant

15. Newborn male, born in hospital via repeat cesarean section, with hypospadias

# ICD-10-CM Chapter 16, Certain Conditions Originating in the Perinatal Period (P00–P96)

## Organization and Structure of ICD-10-CM Chapter 16

Chapter 16 of ICD-10-CM includes categories P00–P96 arranged in the following blocks:

| | |
|---|---|
| P00–P04 | Newborn affected by maternal factors and by complications of pregnancy, labor and delivery |
| P05–P08 | Disorders of newborn related to length of gestation and fetal growth |
| P09 | Abnormal findings on neonatal screening |
| P10–P15 | Birth trauma |
| P19–P29 | Respiratory and cardiovascular disorders specific to the perinatal period |
| P35–P39 | Infections specific to the perinatal period |
| P50–P61 | Hemorrhagic and hematological disorders of newborn |
| P70–P74 | Transitory endocrine and metabolic disorders specific to newborn |
| P76–P78 | Digestive system disorders of newborn |
| P80–P83 | Conditions involving the integument and temperature regulation of newborn |
| P84 | Other problems with newborn |
| P90–P96 | Other disorders originating in the perinatal period |

A number of new subchapters have been added to Chapter 16 for certain conditions originating in the perinatal period. For example, codes for respiratory and cardiovascular disorders specific to the perinatal period are grouped together in block P19–P29.

Chapter 16 of ICD-10-CM contains terminology updates. The terms "fetus" and "newborn" used in many ICD-9-CM code titles have been removed from ICD-10-CM code titles. Additionally, in the first block in ICD-10-CM, newborns affected by maternal factors and by complications of pregnancy, labor, and delivery, the phrase "suspected to be" is included in the code title as a nonessential modifier to indicate that the codes are for use when the listed maternal condition is specified as the cause of confirmed or suspected newborn morbidity or potential morbidity.

| **EXAMPLES:** | P00.3 | Newborn (suspected to be) affected by other maternal circulatory and respiratory diseases |
|---|---|---|
| | P00.4 | Newborn (suspected to be) affected by maternal nutritional disorders |
| | P00.5 | Newborn (suspected to be) affected by maternal injury |

Some revisions to the classification have occurred as well. For instance, the subclassification for 2,500 grams and over for birth weight is no longer an option for category P05.

## Coding Guidelines and Instructional Notes for ICD-10-CM, Chapter 16

Throughout Chapter 16 are notes that help to clarify how codes are to be used. For example, the following note appears under P07: When both birth weight and gestational age of the newborn are available, both should be coded with birth weight sequenced before gestational age. Also, the following note appears under P08.21: Newborn with gestation period over 40 completed weeks to 42 completed weeks.

Codes from this chapter are only for use on the newborn or infant record, never on the maternal record, as indicated by a note that appears at the beginning of Chapter 16. Codes from this chapter are also only applicable for liveborn infants. Further, should a condition originate in the perinatal period and continue throughout the life of the child, the perinatal code should continue to be used regardless of the age of the patient as explained by an introductory note to Chapter 16.

A note at block P00–P04, Newborn affected by maternal factors and by complications of pregnancy, labor, and delivery also provides guidance. These codes are for use when the listed maternal conditions are specified as the cause of confirmed morbidity or potential morbidity which have their origin in the perinatal period (before birth through the first 28 days after birth). Codes from these categories are also used for newborns suspected of having an abnormal condition resulting from exposure from the mother or the birth process, but without signs or symptoms, and which after examination and observation, is found not to exist. These codes may be used even if treatment is begun for a suspected condition that is ruled out.

The NCHS has published chapter-specific guidelines for Chapter 16 of ICD-10-CM:

- Guidelines I.C.16.a. General perinatal rules
- Guideline I.C.16.b. Observation and evaluation of newborns for suspected conditions not found (This section is reserved for future expansion with no current guidelines provided.)

- Guidelines I.C.16.c. Coding additional perinatal diagnoses
- Guideline I.C.16.d. Prematurity and fetal growth retardation
- Guideline I.C.16.e. Low birth weight and immaturity status
- Guideline I.C.16.f. Bacterial sepsis of newborn
- Guideline I.C.16.g. Stillbirth

To gain an understanding of these rules, access the 2014 guidelines from NCHS website (http://www.cdc.gov/nchs/icd/icd10cm.htm) and read Chapter 16, Newborn (perinatal) guidelines.

## Coding Overview of ICD-10-CM Chapter 16

Chapter 16 of ICD-10-CM, Certain Conditions Originating in the Perinatal Period (P00–P96), describes conditions that occur before birth and through the 28th day following birth. Codes from this chapter are used on the neonate's record and may be used throughout the life of the patient as long as the condition that originated in the perinatal period is still present.

Similar to ICD-9-CM, codes in ICD-10-CM Chapter 16 identify newborns affected by maternal factors, disorders related to length of gestation, and fetal growth, birth trauma, and respiratory, cardiovascular, hemorrhagic, endocrine, and digestive conditions of the newborn. Codes from category P07, Disorders of newborn related to short gestation and low birth weight, are similar to the category 765 codes in ICD-9-CM.

The same birth weights are used in ICD-9-CM and ICD-10-CM to identify an extremely low birth weight newborn (999 grams or less) and other low birth weight newborns (1000 to 2499 grams). However, immaturity and prematurity codes in ICD-10-CM have a different structure. ICD-9-CM identifies the weeks of gestation for preterm infants specifically in two week intervals (765.20–765.29)—for example, 29–30 completed weeks of gestation is reported with code 765.25. In ICD-10-CM, the codes are divided into two subcategories. Subcategory P07.2 is used for extreme immaturity of newborn—defined as less than 28 completed weeks, with specific codes for less than 24 completed weeks, 24–26 completed weeks, and 27 completed weeks. Subcategory P07.3 is used for other preterm newborn—defined as 28 completed weeks or more but less than 37 completed weeks, with specific codes for 28–31 completed weeks and 32–36 completed weeks.

The principal diagnosis for coding the birth episode of a newborn is not included in Chapter 16. The birth episode is instead coded with a code from category Z38, Liveborn infants according to place of birth and type of delivery, which is similar to the V30 category codes in ICD-9-CM. Instead of adding fourth and fifth digits to the V30 codes to identify where the baby was born and the type of delivery, ICD-10-CM's Z38 codes specifically identify the number of liveborn infants, where they are born (in hospital, outside hospital), and how they were delivered (vaginally or by cesarean). Other ICD-10-CM codes exist for twin, triplet, quadruplet, quintuplet, and other multiple liveborn infants, For example, the birth record for a single liveborn infant, born in the hospital, and delivered vaginally is ICD-10-CM code Z38.00. A twin liveborn infant, born in the hospital, delivered by cesarean, is ICD-10-CM code Z38.31. Similar to ICD-9-CM, a code from ICD-10-CM category Z38 is assigned to a newborn once, at the time of birth.

Block and category title changes have been made in this chapter, for example, ICD-9-CM subsection 760–763 is titled "Maternal causes of perinatal morbidity and mortality," whereas the ICD-10-CM counterpart, P00–P04, is titled "Newborn affected by maternal factors and by complications of pregnancy, labor, and delivery."

While conditions originating in the perinatal period and congenital anomalies each had a specific chapter in ICD-9-CM, they are listed in a different order in ICD-10-CM.

| ICD-9-CM | ICD-10-CM |
|---|---|
| Chapter 14: Congenital Anomalies (740–759) | Chapter 16, Certain conditions originating in the perinatal period (P00–P96) |
| Chapter 15: Certain Conditions Originating in the Perinatal Period (760–779) | Chapter 17, Congenital malformations, deformations, and chromosomal abnormalities |

The introductory notes at the beginning of the chapter provide clarification. Codes from this chapter are for use on newborn records only, never on maternal records and include conditions that have their origin in the fetal or perinatal period (before birth through the first 28 days after birth) even if morbidity occurs later. Coding Guideline I.C.16.a.1. further states that Chapter 16 codes may be used throughout the life of the patient if the condition is still present. Coding Guideline i.c.16.a.4. clarifies that conditions originating in the perinatal period, and continuing throughout the life of the patient, would have perinatal codes assigned regardless of the patient's age.

Providers utilize different criteria in determining prematurity. A code for prematurity should not be assigned unless it is documented. Assignment of codes in categories P05, Disorders of newborn related to slow fetal growth and fetal malnutrition, and P07, Disorders of newborn related to short gestation and low birth weight, not elsewhere classified, should be based on the recorded birth weight and estimated gestational age. Codes from category P05 should not be assigned with codes from category P07.

According to the *ICD-10-CM Official Coding and Reporting Guidelines*, when both birth weight and gestational age are available, two codes from category P07 should be assigned, with the code for birth weight sequenced before the code for gestational age.

Category Z38 in Chapter 21, Factors Influencing Health Status and Contact with Health Services, classifies liveborn infants according to place of birth and type of delivery. This category is for use as the principal code on the initial record of a newborn baby. It is not to be used on the mother's record. When coding the birth episode in a newborn record, assign a code from category Z38, Liveborn infants according to place of birth and type of delivery, as the principal diagnosis. A code from category Z38 is assigned only once, to a newborn at the time of birth. If a newborn is transferred to another institution, a code from category Z38 should not be used at the receiving hospital. This is a coding guidelines cited in the *ICD-10-CM Official Coding and Reporting Guidelines* for Chapter 16 codes

Also stated in the *ICD-10-CM Official Coding and Reporting Guidelines*, category P36, Bacterial sepsis of newborn, includes congenital sepsis. If a perinate is documented as having sepsis without documentation of congenital or community acquired, the default is congenital and a code from category P36 should be assigned. If the P36 code includes the causal organism, an additional code from category B95, Streptococcus, Staphylococcus, and Enterococcus as the cause of diseases classified elsewhere, or B96, Other bacterial agents as the cause of diseases classified elsewhere, should not be assigned. If the P36 code does not include the causal organism, assign an additional code from category B96. If applicable, use additional codes to identify severe sepsis (R65.2-) and any associated acute organ dysfunction.

# ICD-10-CM Chapter 17, Congenital Malformations, Deformations and Chromosomal Abnormalities (Q00–Q99)

## Organization and Structure of ICD-10-CM Chapter 17

Chapter 17 of ICD-10-CM includes categories Q00–Q99 arranged in the following blocks:

| | |
|---|---|
| Q00–Q07 | Congenital malformations of the nervous system |
| Q10–Q18 | Congenital malformations of eye, ear, face and neck |
| Q20–Q28 | Congenital malformations of the circulatory system |
| Q30–Q34 | Congenital malformations of the respiratory system |
| Q35–Q37 | Cleft lip and cleft palate |
| Q38–Q45 | Other congenital malformations of the digestive system |
| Q50–Q56 | Congenital malformations of genital organs |
| Q60–Q64 | Congenital malformations of the urinary system |
| Q65–Q79 | Congenital malformations and deformations of the musculoskeletal system |
| Q80–Q89 | Other congenital malformations |
| Q90–Q99 | Chromosomal abnormalities, not elsewhere classified |

The arrangement of ICD-10-CM's Chapter 17 is an improvement over ICD-9-CM's Chapter 14. Congenital malformations, deformations, and chromosomal abnormalities have been grouped into subchapters or blocks making it easier to identify the type of conditions classified to chapter 17. Modifications have also been made to specific categories that bring the terminology up-to-date with current medical practice.

**EXAMPLE:** **Q61 Cystic kidney disease**
Q61.0 Congenital renal cyst
Q61.1 Polycystic kidney, infantile type
Q61.2 Polycystic kidney, adult type

Other changes to chapter 17 include classification changes that provide greater specificity than found in ICD-9-CM.

**EXAMPLES:** Q35.1 Cleft hard palate
Q35.3 Cleft soft palate
Q35.5 Cleft hard palate with cleft soft palate
Q35.7 Cleft uvula
Q35.9 Cleft palate, unspecified

## Coding Guidelines and Instructional Notes for ICD-10-CM Chapter 17

Additional modifications were made to specific codes. For example, in ICD-9-CM certain congenital malformations of the anterior segment of the eye do not have any instructions for code usage listed below codes 743.44 or 743.45. In contrast, guidelines for ICD-10-CM code Q13.1 and Q13.81 state to use an additional code for associated glaucoma.

Congenital anomalies or syndromes may occur as a set of symptoms or multiple malformations. If there is no specific code, a code should be assigned for each manifestation of the syndrome, from any chapter in the classification. For syndromes with specific codes, additional codes may be assigned to identify manifestations not included in the specific code.

The NCHS has published chapter-specific guidelines for chapter 17 of ICD-10-CM:

- Guideline I.C.17. Congenital malformations, deformations and chromosomal abnormalities (Q00–Q99)

To gain an understanding of these rules, access the 2014 guidelines from NCHS web site (http://www.cdc.gov/nchs/icd/icd10cm.htm) and read Chapter 17, Congenital Malformations, Deformations and Chromosomal Abnormalities.

## Coding Overview for ICD-10-CM Chapter 17

Chapter 17 of ICD-10-CM, Congenital malformations, deformations and chromosomal abnormalities, contains codes in the range of Q00–Q99. Codes from Chapter 17 may be used throughout the life of the patient as long as the condition is present; the condition is not only coded at birth or when it is first diagnosed. If a congenital malformation or deformity has been corrected, a personal history code should be used to identify the history of the malformation or deformity.

Conditions included in Chapter 17 are organized by body system—for example, Q20–Q28, Congenital malformations of the circulatory system, and Q65–Q79, Congenital malformations and deformations of the musculoskeletal system—and include laterality for limbs and bones. More specific codes are included in ICD-10-CM to further describe the congenital condition. For example, in ICD-9-CM, there is one code for Down syndrome: 758.0. In ICD-10-CM, there are four codes (Q90.0–Q90.9) to identify Down syndrome as Trisomy 21, nonmosaicism, mosaicism, translocation, or unspecified. Updated terminology is also included. For example, in place of Patau's Syndrome and Edward's Syndrome, the same conditions are coded with specific types of Trisomy 18 and Trisomy 13 codes in the range of Q91.0–Q91.7. The older terminology does appear in the Alphabetic Index but directs the coder to the index entry for Trisomy 18 or Trisomy 13.

Many codes for congenital conditions and chromosomal abnormalities have been expanded in ICD-10-CM. For example, chromosomal anomalies are classified to category 758 in ICD-9-CM; however in ICD-10-CM, there are nine categories (Q90, Q91, Q92, Q93, Q95, Q96, Q97, Q98, and Q99) for chromosomal abnormalities, not elsewhere classified.

Again, block, category, subcategory, and code title changes have been made in Chapter 17, for example, in ICD-9-CM, code 758.1 is titled "Patau's syndrome," whereas the counterpart codes in ICD-10-CM (Q91.4–Q91.7) are titled "Trisomy 13."

These codes are assigned when a malformation or deformation or chromosomal abnormality is documented, and the code may be the principal or first listed diagnosis on a record or a secondary diagnosis.

When no unique code is available, assign additional code(s) for any manifestations that may be present. When the code assignment specifically identifies the malformation, deformation, or chromosomal abnormality, manifestations that are an inherent component of the anomaly should not be coded separately. Additional codes should be assigned for manifestations that are not an inherent component.

Codes from Chapter 17 may be used throughout the life of the patient. If the congenital malformation or deformity has been corrected, a personal history code should be used to identify the history of the malformation or deformity. Although present at birth, malformation, deformation, or chromosomal abnormality may not be identified until later in life, and if diagnosed by the physician, it is appropriate to assign a code from codes Q00–Q99.

For the birth admission, the appropriate code from category Z38, Liveborn infants, according to place of birth and type of delivery, should be sequenced as the principal diagnosis, followed by any congenital anomaly codes, Q00–Q89.

## ICD-10-CM Review Exercises: Chapter 17

1. Newborn was delivered by cesarean section. Congenital condition diagnosed was complete transposition of the great vessels with cyanosis.

2. Full-term newborn was delivered four days ago and discharged home. The infant was readmitted to the hospital and diagnosed with hyperbilirubinemia. Phototherapy was initiated and the baby will continue to have phototherapy provided at home after discharge.

3. Full-term female infant was born in this hospital by vaginal delivery. Her mother has been an alcoholic for many years and would not stop drinking during her pregnancy. The baby was born with fetal alcohol syndrome and was placed in the NICU.

4. Premature "crack" baby born in the hospital by cesarean section to a mother dependent on cocaine. The newborn did not show signs of withdrawal. Birth weight of 1,247 g, 31 completed weeks of gestation. Dehydration was also diagnosed and treated.

5. Frontal encephalocele with hydroencephalocele.

6. 20-day-old infant was admitted with Staphylococcus aureus sepsis.

7. Penoscrotal hypospadias.

8. Cleft palate involving both the soft and hard palate, with bilateral cleft lip.

9. Newborn suspected to be affected by maternal use of alcohol during the pregnancy but not found to have fetal alcohol syndrome. Newborn transferred to NICU at another hospital, code for the hospital receiving the infant.

10. Newborn transferred to Children's hospital for delayed closure of the ductus arteriosus of the heart (code for Children's hospital)

# Chapter 18

# Symptoms, Signs, and Abnormal Findings

## Learning Objectives

At the conclusion of this chapter, you should be able to:

1. Describe the organization of the conditions and codes included in Chapter 16 of ICD-9-CM, Symptoms, Signs, and Ill-Defined Conditions (780–799)
2. Describe the organization of the conditions and codes included in Chapter 18 of ICD-10-CM, Symptoms, Signs and Abnormal Clinical and Laboratory Findings, Not Elsewhere Classified (R00–R99)
3. Define and differentiate between the terms *signs* and *symptoms*
4. Describe the coding guidelines for the assignment of a symptom code with an established disease code
5. Explain how symptom codes are organized in ICD-9-CM and ICD-10-CM
6. Describe the types of conditions classified to the categories for nonspecific abnormal findings
7. Identify the Alphabetic Index entries for locating nonspecific abnormal findings in order to code them
8. Referring to the Official Guidelines for Coding and Reporting, briefly describe the use of sign and symptom codes for hospital inpatients as a principal or additional diagnosis
9. Describe the differences in coding of qualified diagnosis, such as possible or probable, when the patient is an inpatient in the hospital as opposed to an outpatient in any healthcare setting
10. Describe when ICD-10-CM codes for coma scale (R40.21–R40.23) are used
11. Assign ICD-9-CM diagnosis and procedure codes for symptoms, signs, and ill-defined conditions
12. Assign ICD-10-CM codes for symptoms, signs, and abnormal findings

# ICD-9-CM Chapter 16, Symptoms, Signs, and Ill-Defined Conditions (780–799)

Chapter 16, Symptoms, Signs, and Ill-Defined Conditions, in the Tabular List in volume 1 of ICD-9-CM contains the following categories and section titles:

| Categories | Section Titles |
|---|---|
| 780–789 | Symptoms |
| 790–796 | Nonspecific Abnormal Findings |
| 797–799 | Ill-Defined and Unknown Causes of Morbidity and Mortality |

## Definitions

A sign is objective evidence of a disease observed by the physician. A symptom is any subjective evidence of disease reported by the patient to the physician.

Some symptoms, such as hives (708.9), gastrointestinal hemorrhage (578.9), menstrual pain (625.3), and low back pain (724.2), have been classified elsewhere in ICD-9-CM. Such symptoms are associated with a given organ system and thus are assigned to the chapter in ICD-9-CM that deals with the corresponding organ system, such as otalgia or earache, is assigned code 388.70 in the diseases of the nervous system and sense organs chapter.

Other symptoms are associated with many systems or are of unknown cause; they are classified to Chapter 16. Examples of these types of symptoms include coma, convulsions, fever, jaundice, chest pain, cough, nausea, vomiting, respiratory arrest, and anorexia.

## When to Use a Code from Chapter 16

Carefully read the long note that appears at the beginning of Chapter 16. It outlines the uses of codes included in this chapter. The conditions, signs, and symptoms included in categories 780–796 consist of:

- Cases for which no more specific diagnosis can be made even after all facts bearing on them have been investigated
- Signs or symptoms existing at the time of initial encounter that proved to be transient and whose causes could not be determined
- Provisional diagnosis in a patient who failed to return for further investigation or care
- Cases referred elsewhere for investigation or treatment before the diagnosis was made
- Cases in which a more precise diagnosis was not available for any other reason
- Certain symptoms that represent important problems in medical care and might be classified in addition to the code for a known cause or disease
- A symptom that was treated in an outpatient setting and did not have the workup necessary to determine a definitive diagnosis

Sign and symptom codes are entirely appropriate to assign when a definitive diagnosis has not been established at the end of an outpatient visit or an inpatient hospital stay. When a specific diagnosis is not supported by available health record documentation, the sign or symptom code is used instead to explain the reason for the visit or the diagnostic testing performed.

### *Symptoms (780–789)*

The first section of Chapter 16 includes a variety of symptoms. In some cases, symptoms may be assigned as additional diagnoses. The following guidelines should be of assistance in determining when to assign a symptom as an additional diagnosis:

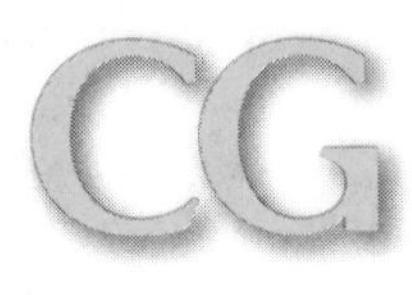


- **Conditions that are an integral part of a disease process:** Signs and symptoms that are integral to the disease process should not be assigned as additional codes.

**EXAMPLE:** Nausea and vomiting with gastroenteritis: 558.9, Other and unspecified noninfectious gastroenteritis and colitis

Only the code for gastroenteritis (558.9) is assigned. The code for nausea and vomiting (787.01) is not assigned because these are symptoms of gastroenteritis.

- **Conditions that are not an integral part of a disease process:** Additional signs and symptoms that may not be routinely associated with a disease process should be coded when present.

**EXAMPLE:** Patient with metastases to brain admitted in comatose state: 198.3, Secondary malignant neoplasm of brain and spinal cord; 780.01, Coma

The code for coma (780.01) should be added as an additional diagnosis; coma is a significant condition that is not routinely associated with brain metastases.

Symptoms and signs are used frequently to describe reasons for service in outpatient settings. Outpatient visits do not always allow for the type of study that is needed to determine a diagnosis. Often the purpose of the outpatient visit is to relieve the symptom rather than to determine or treat the underlying condition. Coders must code the outpatient's condition to the highest level of certainty. The highest level of certainty is often an abnormal sign or symptom code that is assigned as the reason for the outpatient visit.

Most subcategories in the "Symptoms (780–789)" section are grouped by body systems, such as category 781, Symptoms involving nervous and musculoskeletal systems, and category 785, Symptoms involving cardiovascular system. Category 780, however, classifies general symptoms that are not related to one specific body system.

Subcategory 780.3 is subdivided to recognize different forms of seizures or convulsions not identified as epileptic. Two codes exist for febrile seizures. A complex febrile seizure (code 780.32) is defined as a fever-associated seizure that is focal, prolonged (lasting more than 15 minutes), or recurs within 24 hours in children between the ages of six months and five years. These may also be described as "atypical" or "complicated" febrile seizures. Any other fever-associated seizure that does not meet this definition is defined as a "simple" febrile seizure (code 780.31.) A febrile seizure that is not specified as simple or complex will be coded as unspecified to the 780.31 code. Another code is included for post traumatic seizures (code 780.33). The last code under this subcategory, 780.39, includes other or recurrent convulsions that are not related to fever and may also be described as "convulsive seizure or fit" in the diagnostic statement.

Subcategory 780.9 has been further divided to include code 780.91, Fussy infant (baby); and codes 780.92, Excessive crying of infant (baby); 780.93, Memory loss; 780.94, Early satiety; and 780.95, Other excessive crying (for child, adolescent, or adult). Code 780.96 is a symptom code for generalized pain or pain without specificity of site. Code 780.97, Altered mental status, identifies a frequent clinical state that requires investigation. Altered mental status or a change in mental status can be a symptom of many different illnesses. Underlying etiologies may include trauma, infection, neoplasm, or alcohol and drug use, as well as endocrine disorders, neurological disorders, psychiatric disorders and diseases of the kidney. Altered mental status is not to be confused with altered level of consciousness (780.01–780.09) or delirium (780.09). After workup, if a specific cause of the altered mental status is known, that condition should be coded, and the symptom code of 780.97 should not be used.

Other categories in this chapter include codes for symptoms involving different body systems:

**781 Symptoms involving nervous and musculoskeletal system**
**782 Symptoms involving skin and other integumentary tissue**
**783 Symptoms concerning nutrition, metabolism, and development**
**784 Symptoms involving head and neck**
**785 Symptoms involving cardiovascular system**
**786 Symptoms involving respiratory system and other chest symptoms**
**787 Symptoms involving digestive system**
**788 Symptoms involving urinary system**
**789 Other symptoms involving abdomen and pelvis**

Symptom codes, categories 780–789, are frequently used in the outpatient settings to indicate that the patient has a physical complaint for which a definitive diagnosis has not been established. It is possible that a symptom code might be used for an inpatient diagnosis when a reason for the complaint cannot be determined. In addition, symptom codes may be used as additional codes with an established diagnosis to describe the complete story of the patient's illness if the symptom is not an integral or usual part of the disease.

### *Coding Nonspecific Abnormal Findings (790–796)*

Categories 790–796 contain codes for nonspecific abnormal findings from laboratory, x-ray, pathologic, and other diagnostic tests. These nonspecific findings may be referred to as "signs" or "clinical signs." Codes for nonspecific abnormal test results or findings may be found under such Alphabetic Index entries as "abnormal, abnormality, abnormalities," "findings, abnormal, without diagnosis," "decrease, decreased," "elevation," "high," "low," or "positive."

- Abnormal findings from laboratory, x-ray, pathologic, and other diagnostic results are not coded and reported unless the physician indicates their clinical significance. If the findings are outside the normal range and the physician has ordered other tests to evaluate the condition or has prescribed treatment, it is appropriate to ask the physician whether the diagnosis code(s) for the abnormal findings should be added.

- Exclusion notes in this section direct coders to search elsewhere in ICD-9-CM when documentation in the health record states the presence of a specific condition. Codes for these specific conditions are located in the Alphabetic Index under the main term "Findings, abnormal, without diagnosis."

Often abnormal findings are the reason for additional testing to be performed on patients in the outpatient setting. For example, elevated prostate specific antigen (PSA) (code 790.93) may be a reason for continued testing or monitoring of a patient. The code does not provide a specific diagnosis, but indicates an abnormal finding for a specific organ. Abnormal findings recorded in the record may or may not be appropriate to code. If the coder notes an abnormal laboratory finding that appears to have triggered additional testing or therapy, the coder should ask the physician whether the abnormal finding is a clinically-significant condition.

On other occasions, the coder will notice abnormal findings on radiologic studies that may well be incidental to the patient's current condition. For example, an elderly patient with congestive heart failure is given a chest x-ray. A finding of degenerative arthritis is noted in the radiologist's conclusion, but no apparent treatment or further evaluation has occurred. It is unlikely that the arthritis should be coded as it is considered an incidental finding.

The radiologist's findings can be used to identify the specific site of a fracture when the attending or ordering physician's diagnosis statement is nonspecific. For example, the attending physician writes "Fracture, left tibia." However, the radiologist describes the injury as a fracture of the shaft of the tibia. The coder may code 823.20, Fracture, tibia, shaft, based on the specific findings of the radiologist (*Coding Clinic* 1999 for ICD-9-CM and First Quarter 2013 for ICD-10-CM).

The radiologist's findings may also be used to clarify an outpatient's diagnosis or reason for services. For example, a patient comes to the hospital for an outpatient x-ray. The physician's order for the x-ray is "possible kidney stones." The radiologist's statement on the radiology report is "bilateral nephrolithiasis." Based on the fact that the radiologist is a physician, it is appropriate to code the calculus of the kidney, 592.0, as the patient's diagnosis (*Coding Clinic* 2000).

The title of category 793, Nonspecific (abnormal) findings on radiological and other examination of body structure, includes the term "abnormal" in parenthesis, indicating it is a nonessential modifier. This category includes findings that are considered inconclusive and not necessarily abnormal. For example, a routine mammogram may be considered inconclusive due to what is termed "dense breasts." This is not an abnormal condition but a condition that may require further testing—for example, an ultrasound—to conclude that no malignant condition exists that cannot be found on the mammogram. The diagnosis of dense breast or inconclusive mammography is assigned code 793.82, Inconclusive mammogram.

### Coding of Pap Smears

The coding of Pap smears often involves the coding of nonspecific abnormal findings. Because the classification of abnormal Pap smears has become more specific in recent years, ICD-9-CM now includes more code options under categories 795 and 796.

The Bethesda System of Cytologic Examination is used by most of the laboratories in the United States as the preferred method of reporting the results of abnormal Pap smears. In ICD-9-CM, code 795.03 describes Pap smear of cervix with low-grade squamous intraepithelial lesion and code 795.04 describes Pap smear of cervix with high-grade squamous intraepithelial lesion. Other codes describe Pap smear with cervical high-risk human papillomavirus (HPV) DNA test positive (795.05), Pap smear of cervix with cytologic evidence of malignancy (795.06), and with cervical low-risk HPV DNA test positive (795.09). Another code describes an unsatisfactory smear or an inadequate sample (795.08) (Bergeron 2003).

The excludes note for subcategory 795.0 refers the coder to other subcategories for confirmed dysplasia, CIN I–III, or carcinoma in situ conditions.

### Coding of Anthrax Exposure

Another category of nonspecific abnormal findings has emerged as a result of possible bioterrorist activities and the existence of confirmed cases of anthrax. Different degrees of exposure to anthrax may be coded as follows:

- Code 795.31 is used for the asymptomatic patient who tests positive for anthrax by nasal swab.
- Code V01.81 would be used when the individual has been actually exposed to anthrax or has come in contact with anthrax spores but has not tested positive.
- Code V71.82 is used for the individual who seeks medical evaluation with concerns about anthrax exposure but is found not to have been exposed.

### Elevated Tumor-associated Antigens

Testing has become common practice for elevations in tumor-associated antigens (TAA), antigens that are relatively restricted to tumor cells, tumor-specific antigens (TSA), antigens unique to tumor cells, and in the diagnosis of and the follow-up care for many malignancies. A unique code for elevated PSA was created when this test became routine in the monitoring of prostate cancer. Many other TAA and TSA tests have become standard practice and other elevated TAA codes are available for use: 795.81, Elevated carcinoembryonic antigen (CEA); 795.82, Elevated cancer antigen 125 (CA 125); and 795.89, Other elevated tumor-associated antigens.

## *Ill-Defined and Unknown Causes of Morbidity and Mortality (797–799)*

The "Ill-Defined and Unknown Causes of Morbidity and Mortality" section of Chapter 16 includes conditions for which further specification is not provided in the health record or for which the underlying cause is unknown. These codes should not be used when a more definitive diagnosis is available.

Asphyxia once meant the stopping of the pulse, but the term has more recently been associated with hypoxia and hypercapnia. Hypoxia refers to a deficiency of oxygen reaching the tissues of the body, usually due to low inspired oxygen. Hypoxemia is deficient oxygenation of the blood. Hypercapnia refers to elevated levels of carbon dioxide in the arterial blood. Low oxygen levels can be present without asphyxiation. These different conditions have distinct codes in ICD-9-CM:

786.09 Hypercapnia
799.01 Asphyxia
799.02 Hypoxemia

Subcategory 799.2, Signs and symptoms involving emotional state, describe conditions in a patient such as nervousness, irritability, impulsiveness, emotional lability, and demoralization and apathy that cannot be explained by an established diagnosis. These conditions may be explained after study as due to neurological diseases or past head injuries. Another subcategory, 799.5, Signs and symptoms involving cognition, was established to indicate cognitive symptoms that may be associated with traumatic brain injury. These cognitive impairments include attention or concentration deficits, cognitive communication deficits, and visuospatial and psychomotor deficits that may be associated with undiagnosed and/or past traumatic brain injury, as well as patients presenting with symptoms of a neurological disorder.

## Inpatient Coding Guidelines

The *ICD-9-CM Official Guidelines for Coding and Reporting* address the use of sign and symptom codes as a principal diagnosis and when a sign or symptom code should not be used. The guidelines also address the correct use of sign and symptom codes as additional diagnoses.

### Using Signs and Symptoms as Principal Diagnosis for Inpatient Encounters

According to guideline II.A. of the *Official Guidelines for Coding and Reporting*, codes for symptoms, signs, and ill-defined conditions from Chapter 16 are not to be used as principal diagnoses when a related definitive diagnosis has been established. For example, with abdominal pain due to acute gastric ulcer, only the gastric ulcer is coded. However, the symptom can be designated as principal diagnosis when the patient is admitted for the purpose of treating the symptom and there is no treatment or evaluation of the underlying disease. For example, a patient is admitted for dehydration due to gastroenteritis for the purpose of rehydration. The gastroenteritis alone could have been treated on an outpatient basis. In this case, the code for the dehydration can be designated as principal diagnosis even though the cause of the condition is known.

Another reference is made to signs and symptoms in the official coding guidelines in item II.E.: When a symptom(s) is followed by contrasting/comparative diagnoses, the symptom code is sequenced first.

The following coding guideline applies only to the coding of inpatient admissions to short-term, acute, long-term care, and psychiatric hospitals. According to guideline II.H of the *Official Guidelines for Coding and Reporting*, if the diagnosis documented at the time of discharge is qualified as "probable," "suspected," "likely," "questionable," "possible," or "still to be ruled out," or uses other, similar terms indicating uncertainty, code the condition as if it existed or was established. The basis of these guidelines is the diagnostic workup, arrangements for further workup or observation, and initial therapeutic approach that correspond most closely with the established diagnosis. For example, if a patient was admitted to the hospital with fever, cough, and shortness of breath, but after workup the physician was not able to positively diagnose the patient with pneumonia, the discharge diagnosis would be "probable pneumonia." The diagnosis of pneumonia would be coded as if it had been proven to exist.

### Using Signs and Symptoms as Additional Diagnoses

Codes for signs and symptoms are assigned as additional codes only when the sign or symptom is not integral to the underlying condition. It also may be appropriate to code a sign or symptom when its presence is significant in relationship to the patient's condition and/or the care given. When ascites is present in a patient with liver cirrhosis, for example, the ascites often must be treated separately from the cirrhosis.

Signs and symptoms are not coded when they are implicit in the diagnosis or when the symptoms are included in the condition code. For example, with chest pain due to myocardial infarction (MI), no symptom code is assigned for the chest pain because it is implicit in the MI. Another example is the diagnosis of atherosclerosis of the extremities with gangrene. The gangrene is not coded separately because it is included in code 440.24, Atherosclerosis of the extremities with gangrene.

**Note:** The coding guideline for symptoms followed by contrasting/comparative diagnosis applies only to the selection of the principal diagnosis. For example, if the physician lists a secondary diagnosis statement of vertigo due to Meniere's syndrome versus labyrinthitis, only the vertigo is coded (*Coding Clinic* 1998).

In the inpatient setting, abnormal findings included in reports of diagnostic tests are not coded unless the physician has indicated the clinical significance of the findings. The coder can ask the physician if the abnormal condition should be coded, especially when it appears the physician has ordered other tests to evaluate the condition or ordered treatment.

## Outpatient Coding Guidelines

Many outpatient visits are coded with ICD-9-CM codes for signs and symptoms when a definitive diagnosis has not been established. Coders of outpatient and physician visits must follow Section IV: Diagnostic Coding and Reporting Guidelines for Outpatient Services, within the *ICD-9-CM Official Guidelines for Coding and Reporting*:

Signs, symptoms, abnormal test results, or other reasons for the outpatient visit are used when a physician qualifies a diagnostic statement as "possible," "probable," "suspected," "questionable," "rule out," or "working diagnosis," or other similar terms indicating uncertainty. The condition qualified in that statement should not be coded as if it existed. Rather, the condition should be coded to the highest degree of certainty, such as the signs or symptoms the patient exhibits. For example, the physician writes the diagnosis for an outpatient as "rule out pneumonia" and describes the patient as having fever, cough, and malaise. Pneumonia is not coded for this patient. Instead, the symptoms of fever, cough, and malaise are coded, as this is what is known as certain to be occurring in the patient. Pneumonia has not been confirmed.

These guidelines differ from acute care, short-term, long-term, and psychiatric hospital inpatient rules, where a qualified condition is coded as if it exists, because the evaluation and management of the suspected condition in these settings is often equal to the treatment of the same condition that has been confirmed.

The term *ruled out* designates the fact that the condition stated to be ruled out does not exist. This condition, therefore, cannot be coded and the preceding signs, symptoms, or abnormal test results are coded instead.

In the outpatient setting, an abnormal finding included in reports of diagnostic tests interpreted by a physician is coded without the attending physician documenting the same condition. When the final report that contains the abnormal finding is available at the time of coding, it is appropriate to code any confirmed diagnoses contained in the physician's interpretation. In this situation, it is not appropriate to code the related signs and symptoms in addition to the confirmed condition.

## ICD-9-CM Review Exercises: Chapter 18

Assign ICD-9-CM codes to the following outpatient encounters:

1. Office visit conclusion: Rule out diabetes; patient complains of polydipsia and polyuria for several weeks prior to the office visit

2. Sudden infant death syndrome

3. Sleep apnea with insomnia

4. Shortness of breath, cause undetermined

5. An elderly patient was admitted to the hospital through the Emergency Department after being found unconscious at home. The physician's admitting diagnosis was possible CVA. The patient was found to be in a coma due to a cerebral artery occlusion with cerebral infarction. The patient died without regaining consciousness. The physician's final diagnosis was "Cerebral artery occlusion with cerebral infarction and coma." What diagnosis or diagnoses should be coded for this hospital stay?

6. Urgency of urination

7. Pneumonia with cough

8. Elevated blood pressure reading; hypertension not confirmed

9. Stress urinary incontinence in male patient

10. Abnormal Pap smear of the cervix, atypical squamous cell changes of undetermined significance (ASC-US)

11. Convulsive seizures; epilepsy, ruled out

12. Right upper quadrant abdominal pain

13. Chronic fatigue syndrome

*(Continued on next page)*

## ICD-9-CM Review Exercises: Chapter 18 (Continued)

14. Abdominal mass with jaundice

15. Inconclusive mammogram due to dense breasts

16. Abnormal glucose tolerance test

17. Elevated PSA

18. Respiratory arrest of unknown origin

19. Failure to thrive in 2-year-old child

20. Laënnec's cirrhosis of liver with ascites

21. A patient was treated in the Emergency Department and then released to go home. During the visit, the patient complained of an earache and fever. The physician discharged the patient and indicated that the patient should be followed up by the pediatrician for "Possible acute otitis media." What condition(s) should be coded for this Emergency Department visit?

22. A patient was admitted to the hospital with the complaints of severe lower-back pain and weakness in one leg. The patient was discharged after three days, with the final diagnosis documented by the physician as "Probable herniated lumbar disc." What condition(s) should be coded for this hospital stay?

23. A patient was seen in her physician's office with the complaints of itchy eyes and scratchy throat. The physician prescribed a medication and wrote the diagnosis of "Suspected seasonal allergies" in her medical record. What condition(s) should be coded for this office visit?

24. After four days in the hospital following an admission for abdominal pain, the patient's test results were inconclusive. On discharge, the physician documented the following as the final diagnosis: "Acute abdominal pain due to acute cholecystitis or acute pancreatitis." What diagnosis or diagnoses should be coded for this hospital stay?

25. Chest pain, noncardiac in origin

# ICD-10-CM Chapter 18, Symptoms, Signs and Abnormal Clinical and Laboratory Findings, Not Elsewhere Classified (R00–R99)

## Organization and Structure of ICD-10-CM Chapter 18

Chapter 18 of ICD-10-CM includes categories R00–R99 arranged in the following blocks:

| | |
|---|---|
| R00–R09 | Symptoms and signs involving the circulatory and respiratory systems |
| R10–R19 | Symptoms and signs involving the digestive system and abdomen |
| R20–R23 | Symptoms and signs involving the skin and subcutaneous tissue |
| R25–R29 | Symptoms and signs involving the nervous and musculoskeletal systems |
| R30–R39 | Symptoms and signs involving the genitourinary system |
| R40–R46 | Symptoms and signs involving cognition, perception, emotional state and behavior |
| R47–R49 | Symptoms and signs involving speech and voice |
| R50–R69 | General symptoms and signs |
| R70–R79 | Abnormal findings on examination of blood, without diagnosis |
| R80–R82 | Abnormal findings on examination of urine, without diagnosis |
| R83–R89 | Abnormal findings on examination of other body fluids, substances and tissues, without diagnosis |
| R90–R94 | Abnormal findings on diagnostic imaging and in function studies, without diagnosis |
| R97 | Abnormal tumor markers |
| R99 | Ill-defined and unknown cause of mortality |

Chapter 18 of ICD-10-CM has undergone some organizational changes. For example, in ICD-10-CM, codes for general symptoms and signs follow those related specifically to a body system or other relevant grouping.

Symptom codes have been moved from one chapter to another in ICD-10-CM.

| EXAMPLES: | | | |
|---|---|---|---|
| | **Diagnosis: Bradycardia** | | |
| | ICD-9-CM (Chapter 7) | 427.89 | Other specified cardiac dysrhythmias |
| | ICD-10-CM (Chapter 18) | R00.1 | Bradycardia, unspecified |
| | **Diagnosis: Pleurisy** | | |
| | ICD-9-CM (Chapter 8) | 511.0 | Pleurisy without mention of effusion or current tuberculosis |
| | ICD-10-CM (Chapter 18) | R09.1 | Pleurisy |
| | **Diagnosis: Dry Mouth** | | |
| | ICD-9-CM (Chapter 9) | 527.7 | Disturbance of salivary secretion |
| | ICD-10-CM (Chapter 18) | R68.2 | Dry mouth, unspecified |

A fairly substantial classification change was made to hematuria. Various types of hematuria are coded in Chapter 18 unless included with the underlying condition such as acute cystitis with hematuria. In those cases, the code is found in other chapters such as Chapter 14, Diseases of the Genitourinary System.

## Coding Guidelines and Instructional Notes for ICD-10-CM Chapter 18

The following note appears at the beginning of Chapter 18 in ICD-10-CM outlining the conditions classified to this chapter:

Chapter 18 includes symptoms, signs, abnormal results of clinical or other investigative procedures, and ill-defined conditions regarding which no diagnosis classifiable elsewhere is recorded.

Signs and symptoms that point rather definitely to a given diagnosis have been assigned to a category in other chapters of the classification. In general, categories in this chapter include the less well-defined conditions and symptoms that, without the necessary study of the case to establish a final diagnosis, point perhaps equally to two or more diseases or to two or more systems of the body. Practically all categories in the chapter could be designated "not otherwise specified," "unknown etiology," or "transient." The Alphabetical Index should be consulted to determine which symptoms and signs are to be allocated here and which to other chapters. The residual subcategories, numbered .8, are generally provided for other relevant symptoms that cannot be allocated elsewhere in the classification.

The conditions, signs, and symptoms included in Chapter 18 consist of: (1) cases for which no more specific diagnosis can be made even after all the facts bearing on the case have been investigated; (2) signs or symptoms existing at the time of the initial encounter that proved to be transient and whose causes could not be determined; (3) provisional diagnosis in a patient who failed to return for further investigation or care; (4) cases referred elsewhere for investigation or treatment before the diagnosis was made; (5) cases in which a more precise diagnosis was not available for any other reason; (6) certain symptoms, for which supplementary information is provided, that represent important problems in medical care in their own right.

Additionally, notes for code usage appear at the subchapter level.

Many of the new blocks and categories in Chapter 18 have Excludes1 notes such as the one found under R09, Other symptoms and signs involving the circulatory and respiratory system, that directs the coder to locate diagnosis codes that appear in other chapters of ICD-10-CM.

Guidelines that clarify code usage are also found under specific codes. Code R52, Pain unspecified, includes inclusive terms and Excludes1 notes.

The NCHS has published chapter-specific guidelines for Chapter 18 of ICD-10-CM:

- Guideline I.C.18.a. Use of symptom codes
- Guideline I.C.18.b. Use of a symptom code with a definitive diagnosis code
- Guideline I.C.18.c. Combination codes that include symptoms
- Guideline I.C.18.d. Repeated falls
- Guideline I.C.18.e. Coma scale
- Guideline I.C.18.f. Functional quadriplegia
- Guideline I.C.18.g. SIRS due to non-infectious process
- Guideline I.C.18.h. Death NOS

To gain an understanding of these rules, access the 2014 guidelines from the NCHS web site (http://www.cdc.gov/nchs/icd/icd10cm.htm) and read Chapter 18, Symptoms, Signs and Abnormal Clinical and Laboratory Findings.

## Coding Overview for ICD-10-CM Chapter 18

Similar to ICD-9-CM, Chapter 18 of ICD-10-CM, Symptoms, Signs and Abnormal Clinical and Laboratory Findings, Not Elsewhere Classified (R00–R99), includes symptoms, signs, abnormal results of clinical or other investigative procedures, and ill-defined conditions regarding which no diagnosis classifiable elsewhere is recorded. Signs and symptoms that are more specific to a given diagnosis are assigned to the chapter in ICD-10-CM that includes the body system that relates to that sign or symptom.

This chapter contains blocks of codes from R00–R49 that describe symptoms and signs involving certain body systems, such as circulatory, respiratory, and digestive. General symptoms and signs (R50–R69) include symptoms and signs that could be explained by various body systems—for example, fever, unspecified (R50.9), headache (R51), and syncope (R55). Within this chapter are the codes for systemic inflammatory response syndrome (SIRS) of noninfectious origin (R65.10–R65.11) and codes for severe sepsis (R65.20–R65.21). Code first notes appear with these codes to code first the underlying condition and to use an additional code to identify specific acute organ dysfunction when it exists. A welcome addition to ICD-10-CM is the code R29.6, Repeated falls, a statement frequently used by physicians as the explanation of why a patient was receiving a health evaluation. The statement of "repeated falls" cannot be coded with ICD-9-CM.

In addition, this chapter contains abnormal test findings that have not been established as being the result of a certain disease. Codes in the range of R70 to R79, Abnormal findings on examination of blood, without diagnosis, contain such findings as impaired or elevated fasting glucose (R73.01) and abnormal coagulation profile (R79.1) for abnormal or prolonged prothrombin time (PT) or partial thromboplastin time (PTT). Other abnormal test results are reported by codes for abnormal findings on examination of urine and other body fluids, substances and tissues, without diagnosis (R80–R89). For example, abnormal Pap smear findings are contained in this range of codes. Categories R90–R94 identify abnormal findings on diagnostic imaging and in function studies, without diagnosis. Within these codes are such findings as mammographic calcification found on diagnostic imaging of breast (R92.1) and abnormal electrocardiogram (R94.31).

To help the coder locate the symptoms and signs without an established diagnosis, the Alphabetic Index contains such entries as "abnormal, abnormality, abnormalities," "elevated, elevation," "findings, abnormal, inconclusive, without diagnosis," and "positive." These Index entries are similar to those found in ICD-9-CM.

### Glasgow Coma Scale

According to the *ICD-10-CM Official Coding and Reporting Guidelines,* subcategory R40.2, Coma, incorporates the Glasgow coma scale (R40.211–R40.244). The Glasgow coma scale codes can be used in conjunction with traumatic brain injury or sequelae of cerebrovascular disease codes. They are primarily for use by trauma registries and research use, but they may be used in any setting where this information is collected. The Glasgow coma scale codes are sequenced after the diagnosis code(s). These codes, one from each subcategory (R40.21,

R40.22, R40.23), are needed to complete the scale. The seventh character indicates when the scale was recorded, and it should match for all three codes:

0—unspecified time
1—in the field [EMT or ambulance]
2—at arrival to emergency department
3—at hospital admission
4—24 hours or more after hospital admission

At a minimum, report the initial score documented on presentation at the facility. This may be a score from the emergency medicine technician (EMT) or in the emergency department. If desired, a facility may choose to capture multiple Glasgow coma scale scores.

According to direction provided in the First Quarter 2014 *Coding Clinic* for ICD-10-CM and ICD-10-PCS, the Glasgow coma score may be documented by emergency medical personnel prior to arrival at the hospital and non-physician emergency medical personnel in the hospital emergency department after the patient's arrival. It would be appropriate to use the prehospital documentation or the non-physician documentation to determine the Glasgow coma score to code. The coder should note that subcategory R40.24, Glasgow coma scale, total score, is used only when the total score is documented instead of the individual measures for the eyes open, verbal response, and motor response.

## ICD-10-CM Review Exercises: Chapter 18

Assign the correct ICD-10-CM diagnosis codes to the following exercises:

1. Right upper quadrant rebound abdominal tenderness

2. The patient is seen complaining of right upper quadrant abdominal pain. In addition, the patient is having nausea and vomited several times. Patient also has elevated blood pressure readings but a diagnosis of hypertension is not made at this visit.

3. Microcalcification found on breast mammography

4. Sinoatrial bradycardia

5. Assign the Glasgow coma scale code(s) when the patient had the following documented by the EMT: Eyes do not open, no verbal response, with no motor response. The neurologist documented the following on day 2 of the hospital admission: Eyes open to sound, verbal response produced inappropriate words, and motor response with flexion withdrawal."

6. The patient who has experienced a fever of 101 degrees Fahrenheit with chills was brought to the emergency department. Laboratory tests, including a complete blood count and urinalysis, were performed with normal results. The ER physician wrote the final diagnosis as "Fever with chills, possible viral syndrome."

7. The attending physician concluded the patient had "atypical chest pain due to either angina or GERD.

8. Cardiorespiratory arrest

9. Abnormal glucose tolerance test (GTT)

10. Swollen lymph glands in the neck

## Chapter 19

# Injury and Poisoning I

## Learning Objectives

At the conclusion of this chapter, you should be able to:

1. Describe the organization of the conditions and codes included in Chapter 17 of ICD-9-CM, with a focus on injuries, categories 800–959
2. Describe the organization of the conditions and codes included in Chapter 19 of ICD-10-CM, with a focus on injuries, categories S00–T34
3. Define the terms *fracture* and *closed and open fracture*
4. Identify circumstances in which to use the acute traumatic fracture codes and the fracture aftercare codes in ICD-9-CM
5. Define the term *dislocation* and describe closed and open dislocation
6. Define and differentiate between the terms of *sprain* and *strain* and be familiar with the Alphabetic Index entries for both terms
7. Briefly describe the different forms of intracranial injury
8. Identify terminology that is synonymous with the term *open wound*
9. Explain the meaning of *complicated* as it pertains to open wound in ICD-9-CM
10. Briefly describe first-degree, second-degree, third-degree, and deep, full-thickness burns
11. Explain the coding guidelines for assigning diagnosis codes for burns, including the sequela or late-effect conditions of burns
12. Describe the types of injuries that are classified as superficial injuries
13. Identify the correct seventh character required for reporting certain injury codes in ICD-10-CM
14. Assign ICD-9-CM and ICD-10-CM diagnosis codes for injuries

# ICD-9-CM Chapter 17, Injury and Poisoning: Injury Codes (800–959)

Chapter 17, Injury and Poisoning, in the Tabular List in volume 1 of ICD-9-CM includes the following categories and section titles:

| Categories | Section Titles |
|---|---|
| 800–829 | Fractures |
| 830–839 | Dislocation |
| 840–848 | Sprains and Strains of Joints and Adjacent Muscles |
| 850–854 | Intracranial Injury, Excluding Those with Skull Fracture |
| 860–869 | Internal Injury of Thorax, Abdomen, and Pelvis |
| 870–897 | Open Wounds |
| 900–904 | Injury to Blood Vessels |
| 905–909 | Late Effects of Injuries, Poisonings, Toxic Effects and Other External Causes |
| 910–919 | Superficial Injury |
| 920–924 | Contusion with Intact Skin Surface |
| 925–929 | Crushing Injury |
| 930–939 | Effects of Foreign Body Entering through Orifice |
| 940–949 | Burns |
| 950–957 | Injury to Nerves and Spinal Cord |
| 958–959 | Certain Traumatic Complications and Unspecified Injuries |
| 960–979 | Poisoning by Drugs, Medicinal and Biological Substances |
| 980–989 | Toxic Effects of Substances Chiefly Nonmedicinal as to Source |
| 990–995 | Other and Unspecified Effects of External Causes |
| 996–999 | Complications of Surgical and Medical Care, Not Elsewhere Classified |

Chapter 17 of ICD-9-CM encompasses a wide variety of injuries, as well as poisonings and surgical and medical complications. This textbook chapter addresses injuries, and chapter 20 addresses poisonings, adverse effects, and complications of surgical and medical care.

Injuries are traumatic in nature, resulting in damage to a body part. The damage may occur to such an extent that the tissues are destroyed. Various external causes such as blows, falls, guns, knives, industrial equipment, or household items may be responsible for injuries.

ICD-9-CM classifies injuries into well-defined categories such as fractures, dislocations, sprains, and open wounds, which are easier to understand than some disease processes. Traumatic injuries, however, may predispose a person to a nontraumatic disease. For example, bacteria may settle at the site of a bone fracture and cause acute osteomyelitis.

## Main Terms for Injuries

The Alphabetic Index to Diseases in ICD-9-CM classifies injuries according to their general type, such as a wound, fracture, or dislocation. The subterms under the general type of injury identify the anatomical site.

## Instructions for Coding Injuries

ICD-9-CM uses fifth digits in the injury section to provide data on level of consciousness, specific anatomical site, and severity of injury. Fifth digits must be used as indicated in the ICD-9-CM system. When coding injuries, a separate code should be used to identify each specific injury. The code for the most severe injury is usually coded as the principal or first listed and should be identified as the most serious condition by the provider and evidenced by the treatment performed. This chapter contains all types of injuries, from superficial abrasions and contusions on the skin to intracranial and spinal injuries that can be life changing and life threatening. The coder must review the *ICD-9-CM Official Guidelines for Coding and Reporting* for the coding of injuries, especially the rules addressing the coding of fractures and burns.

### Exercise 19.1

Describe the data the fifth digit provides for each of the following codes:

1. 832.04

2. 811.12

3. 942.14

4. 866.01

5. 800.06

## Fractures (800–829)

A traumatic fracture is a break in the bone due to a traumatic injury. Tenderness and swelling develop at the site of the break, with a visible or palpable deformity, pain, and weakness. X-rays show a partial or an incomplete break at the site of the fracture.

In ICD-9-CM, traumatic fractures are classified to categories 800–829. At the fourth-digit level, fractures are identified as closed or open. In closed fractures, the skin remains intact; in open fractures, a break in the skin occurs. At the beginning of the section "Fractures" (800–829), the following list of terms synonymous with open and closed appears:

> The descriptions "closed" and "open" used in the fourth-digit subdivisions include the following terms:
>
> closed (with or without delayed healing):
>
> | | |
> |---|---|
> | comminuted | impacted |
> | depressed | linear |
> | elevated | simple |
> | fissured | slipped epiphysis |
> | fracture NOS | spiral |
> | greenstick | |
>
> open (with or without delayed healing):
>
> | | |
> |---|---|
> | compound | puncture |
> | infected | with foreign body |
> | missile | |

When there is no indication as to whether the fracture is open or closed, the code describing a closed fracture is assigned.

According to the *ICD-9-CM Official Guidelines for Coding and Reporting*, traumatic fractures are coded using the acute traumatic fracture codes (categories 800–829) as long as the patient is receiving active treatment for the fracture. Examples of active treatment are surgery, emergency department visits, and evaluation and treatment by a new physician.

Traumatic fractures are coded using the aftercare codes (subcategories V54.0, V54.1, V54.8, or V54.9) for patient care encounters when the patient has completed active treatment and is receiving routine care for the fracture during the healing or recovery period. Examples of fracture aftercare are cast changes or removals, removal of internal or external fixation devices, medication adjustment, and follow-up visits following fracture treatment. Aftercare codes are not assigned when treatment is directed at a current acute injury.

Coders are permitted to use an x-ray report to assign a more specific fracture diagnosis code. The physician may not list the specific site of the fracture, but an x-ray report in the health record shows the precise site. It is appropriate for the coder to assign the more specific code from the x-ray report without consulting the physician. However, if there is any question as to the appropriate diagnosis, the coder must contact the physician.

A fifth-digit subclassification often is used in fracture coding to identify the specific site involved.

**816 Fracture of one or more phalanges of hand**

Includes: finger(s) thumb

The following fifth-digit subclassification is for use with category 816:

**0 phalanx or phalanges, unspecified**
**1 middle or proximal phalanx or phalanges**
**2 distal phalanx or phalanges**
**3 multiple sites**

**816.0 Closed**

**816.1 Open**

In the preceding example, the fourth digit describes a closed or open fracture of the phalanges, with the fifth digit identifying the specific site of the fracture.

Remember that pathologic fractures due to underlying bone disease are not considered traumatic and, as such, are not classified to Chapter 17 of ICD-9-CM with the traumatic fracture codes. Pathologic fractures, codes 733.10–733.19, are located in Chapter 13 of ICD-9-CM.

## Exercise 19.2

Assign ICD-9-CM codes to the following:

1. Simple greenstick fracture, shafts of tibia and fibula

2. Comminuted fracture of humerus

3. Compound fracture of lower end of ulna

4. Fracture of femur due to gunshot wound

5. Fracture of right fibula due to osteogenesis imperfecta

### Multiple Fractures

Whenever possible, separate codes should be assigned for multiple fractures unless the Alphabetic Index or Tabular List provides instructions to the contrary.

**EXAMPLE:** Closed fracture of the distal radius with closed fracture of the metacarpal bone. Two codes are assigned: 813.42, Other fractures of distal end of radius (alone) and 815.00, Closed fracture of unspecified metacarpal bone(s)

Combination categories for multiple fractures are provided for use in the following situations:

- When the health record contains insufficient detail

  **EXAMPLE:** "Multiple fractures of right upper limb" is the only information provided in the health record: 818.0, Ill-defined fractures of upper limb

  In this example, no additional information is provided in the health record as to the specific sites of the upper limb involved; therefore, code 818.0 is assigned.

- When the reporting form limits the number of codes that can be assigned

  **EXAMPLE:** Patient had many traumatic injuries, including several fractures of the hand bones, which were identified in the health record. Because of all the other more critical injuries, space was not available on the form to code each metacarpal fracture separately: 817.0, Closed multiple fractures of hand bones

  In this example, the single code 817.0 would be assigned for the multiple fractures of the hand bones.

## Exercise 19.3

Assign ICD-9-CM codes to the following:

1. Open frontal fracture with subarachnoid hemorrhage with brief loss of consciousness

   ______________________________

2. Multiple fractures of the right lower extremity

   ______________________________

3. Open fracture of the patella

   ______________________________

4. Supracondylar fracture of the right humerus and fracture of the olecranon process of the right ulna

   ______________________________

5. Infected shaft of the tibia fracture

   ______________________________

## Dislocation and Subluxation (830–839)

Dislocation is the displacement of a bone from its joint. The joints most commonly affected are in the fingers, thumbs, and shoulders. Pain and swelling occur, as well as the loss of use of the injured part. To promote healing, the dislocation can be reduced and the joint immobilized by applying a cast.

A dislocation that occurs with a fracture is included in the fracture code. The reduction of the dislocation is included in the code for the fracture reduction.

A subluxation is an incomplete dislocation with the contact between the joint surfaces remaining in place. A subluxation commonly seen in children under the age of five is "nursemaid's elbow." This injury occurs when a small child is lifted, yanked, or swung by the hand or wrist or falls on an outstretched arm. The injury is a subluxation of the radial head from the annular ligament. The ligament is trapped in the elbow joint and causes acute pain. By manipulating the elbow joint to release the trapped tissue, the subluxation can be corrected, and the pain is immediately relieved.

ICD-9-CM classifies the dislocation of a joint without associated fracture to categories 830–839. These categories also include subluxation, that is, an incomplete or a partial dislocation. The fourth-digit classification differentiates between open and closed dislocations.

**EXAMPLE:**

**832 Dislocation of elbow**

The following fifth-digit subclassification is for use with category 832:

**0 elbow unspecified**
**1 anterior dislocation of elbow**
**2 posterior dislocation of elbow**
**3 medial dislocation of elbow**
**4 lateral dislocation of elbow**
**9 other**

**832.0 Closed dislocation**

**832.1 Open dislocation**

**832.2 Nursemaid's elbow**
**Subluxation of the radial head**

At the beginning of the section "Dislocation" (830–839), the following list of terms synonymous with open and closed appears:

The descriptions "closed" and "open," used in the fourth-digit subdivisions, include the following terms:

| closed: | open: |
|---|---|
| complete | compound |
| dislocation NOS | infected |
| partial | with foreign body |
| simple | |
| uncomplicated | |

"Chronic," "habitual," "old," or "recurrent" dislocations should be coded as indicated under the entry "Dislocation, recurrent;" and "pathological" as indicated under the entry "Dislocation, pathological."

When a dislocation is not indicated as closed or open, it should be classified as closed. As with fractures, ICD-9-CM uses the fifth digit to identify the specific site.

Once a dislocation of a joint has occurred, it takes less provocation or effort to produce another dislocation. Only the initial occurrence of the joint dislocation is coded to the injury code. All subsequent dislocations of the same joint are coded as recurrent dislocation. For example, a college athlete was brought to the emergency department with an anterior dislocation of the shoulder that occurred while he was wrestling at a sporting event. The athlete stated he has had dislocated shoulders previously. The physician describes the dislocation as "recurrent." This is coded as 718.31, Recurrent dislocation of joint, shoulder, from the ICD-9-CM chapter on musculoskeletal diseases. It is not coded with an acute dislocation code for the shoulder, 831.01.

## Sprains and Strains (840–848)

A sprain is an injury of the supporting ligaments of a joint resulting from a turning or twisting of a body part. Sprains are extremely painful and are accompanied by swelling and discoloration. They require rest for the injury to heal. Whiplash is a specific type of sprain, usually due to a sudden throwing of the head forward and then backward. It results in a compression of the cervical spine that involves the bones, joints, and intervertebral discs.

A strain is simply an overstretching or overexertion of some part of the musculature. Strains usually respond to rest.

Codes within the categories 840–848 are current injuries. Patients also may suffer from chronic strains of the neck or back or derangements of different joints. The physician may describe these conditions as chronic, old, or recurrent. Using terms such as "sprain/strain" or "derangement," the coder should refer to the subterm for the site and use another subterm to describe the chronic or old condition. The coder will be referred to codes within the "Diseases of the Musculoskeletal System" section, categories 710–739.

### Exercise 19.4

Assign ICD-9-CM codes to the following:

1. Acute lumbosacral strain

2. Dislocation of the first and second cervical vertebrae

3. Compound dislocation of the hip

4. Sprain of the lateral collateral ligament of knee

5. Anterior dislocation of the elbow

## Intracranial Injury, Excluding Those with Skull Fracture (850–854)

At the beginning of this section on intracranial injury, a note appears that the section includes traumatic brain injury, without skull fracture. Another statement is included to instruct the coder: "The description 'with open intracranial wound,' used in the fourth-digit subdivisions, includes those specified as open or with mention of infection or foreign body."

As mentioned in chapter 1 of this book, the notes in ICD-9-CM often provide a definition that must be applied to that section, category, or subcategory. The purpose of the note in this section is to offer information that when a diagnostic statement includes the terms *open, infected,* or *foreign body,* the fourth-digit code describing an open intracranial wound should be assigned.

In addition to this section note, a fifth-digit subclassification for categories 851–854 is provided.

### Cerebral Concussion

A concussion is a type of minor brain injury that is a short loss of normal brain function in response to a head injury. Concussions can be caused by any blow to the head from sports or assaults, from motor vehicle accidents or could be the result of hitting the head on the ground after a fall. The jarring of the brain that occurs can cause the person to lose consciousness. How long a person is unconscious may be a sign of the severity of the concussion. But not all people with a concussion lose consciousness, even though they may describe visual disturbances immediately like "seeing stars." A person can have a concussion and not realize it. Symptoms of a concussion may occur immediately or can be delayed by days or weeks later. Symptoms may include a headache, neck pain, loss of consciousness for a short period of time, nausea, ringing in the ears, dizziness, or tiredness. More serious symptoms that require a return to the physician or emergency department are changes in alertness and consciousness seizures, trouble waking and sleeping, muscle weakness, lack of coordination, trouble walking, repeated vomiting, nausea, confusion and slurred speech (CDC 2014c and NLM 2014).

A computerized axial tomography (CT) scan or magnetic resonance imaging (MRI) study may be performed to rule out intracranial bleeding or swelling. Codes for cerebral concussion range from 850.0–850.9, based on the exact injury that occurred and the amount of time the patient had loss of consciousness. If the physician describes the patient's condition as a "head injury" with no loss of consciousness, the condition is classified to 959.01, Head injury, unspecified. Coders should not assume the diagnosis of "head injury" is equivalent to cerebral concussion without concurrence by the documenting physician. The diagnosis of "traumatic brain injury" should not be assumed to be concussion either. The Alphabetic Index entry of "injury, brain, traumatic," NEC directs the coder to *see also* Injury, intracranial. However if no additional injury is available from the physician, the code for traumatic brain injury, not otherwise specified is included under category 854, Intracranial injury of other and unspecified nature.

### Cerebral Contusion

Often caused by a blow to the head, a cerebral contusion is a more severe injury involving a bruise of the brain with bleeding into brain tissue, but without disruption of the brain's continuity. The loss of consciousness that occurs often lasts longer than that of a concussion. A laceration or fracture often accompanies the contusion. Any type of laceration of the brain results in some destruction of brain tissue and a subsequent scarring that may cause posttraumatic epilepsy. Codes for cerebral laceration and contusion range from 851.0–851.9, with fifth digits added to indicate whether a loss of consciousness or concussion occurred.

### Subdural Hematoma

A subdural hematoma is the formation of a hematoma between the dura and the leptomeninges. Often resulting from a tear in the arachnoid, the acute form of subdural hematoma is associated with a laceration or contusion. Chronic subdural hematomas may result from closed head injuries such as falls. Symptoms include headache, increasing drowsiness, hemiparesis, and seizures. A subdural hematoma may also be a non-traumatic condition so the coder should not assume that all patients with a diagnosis of subdural hematoma has a traumatic brain injury. The Alphabetic Index directs the coder to see also Hemorrhage, subdural when the entry for Hematoma, subdural, nontraumatic is located.

## Internal Injury of Thorax, Abdomen, and Pelvis (860–869)

Internal injuries of the thorax, abdomen, and pelvis are classified to categories 860–869. Codes in this section include injuries to the internal organs such as blunt trauma, contusion, crushing, hematoma, laceration, puncture, tear or traumatic rupture. The fourth-digit subcategories describe the presence or absence of an open wound. The fifth-digit subclassification identifies the specific site, the specific type of injury, or the severity of the injury.

**861.0 Heart, without mention of open wound into thorax**

**861.00 Unspecified injury**
**861.01 Contusion**
Cardiac contusion
Myocardial contusion
**861.02 Laceration without penetration of heart chambers**
**861.03 Laceration with penetration of heart chambers**

**861.1 Heart, with open wound into thorax**

**861.10 Unspecified injury**
**861.11 Contusion**
**861.12 Laceration without penetration of heart chambers**
**861.13 Laceration with penetration of heart chambers**

**864 Injury to liver**

The following fifth-digit subclassification is for use with category 864:

**0 unspecified injury**
**1 hematoma and contusion**
**2 laceration, minor**
Laceration involving capsule only or without significant involvement of hepatic parenchyma [i.e., less than 1 cm deep]
**3 laceration, moderate**
Laceration involving parenchyma, but without major disruption of parenchyma [i.e., less than 10 cm long and less than 3 cm deep]
**4 laceration, major**
Laceration with significant disruption of hepatic parenchyma [i.e., 10 cm long and 3 cm deep]
Multiple moderate lacerations, with or without hematoma
Stellate lacerations of liver
**5 laceration, unspecified**
**9 other**

**864.0 Without mention of open wound into cavity**

**864.1 With open wound in cavity**

## Exercise 19.5

Assign ICD-9-CM codes to the following:

1. Traumatic hemothorax with open wound into thorax and concussion with loss of consciousness

 ____________________

2. Cerebral contusion with brief loss of consciousness

 ____________________

3. Traumatic laceration of the liver, moderate

 ____________________

4. Traumatic subdural hemorrhage with open intracranial wound; loss of consciousness, unknown time

 ____________________

5. Traumatic duodenal injury

 ____________________

## Open Wound (870–897)

ICD-9-CM classifies open wounds to categories 870–897. An open wound is an injury of the soft tissue parts associated with rupture of the skin. Open wounds may be animal bites, avulsions, cuts, lacerations, puncture wounds, and traumatic amputation. In addition, an open wound may be a penetrating wound, which involves the passage of an object through tissue, which leaves an entrance and exit, as in the case of a knife or gunshot wound. Finally, a fractured tooth or one broken due to trauma is classified to an open wound code, either 873.63 or 873.73, as the code for bone fractures does not include a code for teeth.

The seriousness of an open wound depends on its site and extent. If a major vessel or organ is involved, a wound may be life-threatening. For example, the rupture of a large artery or vein may cause blood to accumulate in one of the body cavities, which is referred to as hemothorax, hemopericardium, hemoperitoneum, or hemarthrosis, depending on the body cavity involved. The significance of the hemorrhage rests on the volume of the blood loss, the rate of loss, and the site of hemorrhage. Large losses may induce hemorrhagic shock.

Crushing wounds are excluded from these categories and, instead, are classified to categories 925–929.

### *Instructional Notes*

Three instructional notes appear at the beginning of the section "Open Wound" (870–897).

**OPEN WOUND (870–897)**

Includes: animal bite, laceration, avulsion, puncture wound, cut, traumatic amputation

*Excludes:* *burn (940.0–949.5)*
*crushing (925–929.9)*
*puncture of internal organs (860.0–869.1)*
*superficial injury (910.0–919.9)*
*that incidental to:*
*dislocation (830.0–839.9)*
*fracture (800.0–829.1)*
*internal injury (860.0–869.1)*
*intracranial injury (851.0–854.1)*

Note: The description "complicated" used in the fourth-digit subdivisions includes those with mention of delayed healing, delayed treatment, foreign body, or infection.

In the preceding example, the includes note identifies wounds that are classified to categories 870–897 and the excludes note identifies wounds that are classified elsewhere in ICD-9-CM. The third note defines the term "complicated." The definition contains specific criteria that must be documented in the health record before a code is selected to describe a complicated wound.

**EXAMPLE:** Delayed healing of open wound of foot: 892.1, Complicated open wound of foot except (toes) alone

In this example, the wound was considered complicated because the diagnostic statement included the terminology "delayed healing;" therefore, code 892.1 was assigned.

The description "complicated" used in the fourth-digit subdivisions includes those with mention of delayed healing, delayed treatment, foreign body, or infection.

## Fourth- and Fifth-Digit Subdivisions

ICD-9-CM uses the fourth-digit subcategories and the fifth-digit subclassification to identify the type of open wound, the site of the wound, complicated or uncomplicated wounds, and involvement of tendon.

**874 Open wound of neck**

**874.0 Larynx and trachea, without mention of complication**

874.00 Larynx with trachea
874.01 Larynx
874.02 Trachea

**874.1 Larynx and trachea, complicated**

874.10 Larynx with trachea
874.11 Larynx
874.12 Trachea

**880 Open wound of shoulder and upper arm**

The following fifth-digit subclassification is for use with category 880:

**0 shoulder region**
**1 scapular region**
**2 axillary region**
**3 upper arm**
**9 multiple sites**

**880.0 Without mention of complication**
**880.1 Complicated**
**880.2 With tendon involvement**

### Repair of Open Wounds

Open wounds, such as laceration of skin, are typically repaired by the suturing of skin and subcutaneous tissue or by the use of the newer tissue adhesives. Procedure code 86.59, closure of skin and subcutaneous tissue of other sites, includes the repair of open wound by suturing, as well as the application of Dermabond, a tissue adhesive.

## Exercise 19.6

Assign ICD-9-CM codes to the following:

1. Laceration of external ear

2. Traumatic below-knee amputation with delayed healing

3. Open wound of buttock

4. Open wound of wrist involving tendons

5. Avulsion of eye

## Burns (940–949)

Burns are assigned to categories 940 through 949 in ICD-9-CM and include burns due to electrical heating appliances, electricity, flames, hot objects, lightning, radiation, chemicals, and scalding.

Burns also are classified by depth, extent, and, where needed, agent (external cause or E code). By depth, burns are classified as first degree (erythema), second degree (blistering), third degree (full-thickness), and fourth degree (deep full-thickness), as described below:

- A first-degree burn is the least severe and includes damage to the epidermis or outer layer of skin alone. The burn may also be described as superficial. The skin appears pink to red and painful. There is some edema, but no blisters or eschar. Dead skin may peel away two to three days after the burn.
- A second-degree burn involves the epidermis and dermis. There is mild to moderate edema and the burn will blister but there is no eschar. The burn may also be described as either superficial partial thickness or deep partial thickness. Superficial partial thickness burns extend into the upper dermal layer and leave the skin pink to red. Because the nerve endings are exposed, any stimulation causes extreme pain. Deep partial thickness burns extend into the deeper layers of derma, leaving the skin red to pale with moderate edema. Blisters are infrequent but there will be soft, dry eschar. The patient will experience pain but not as severe as in a superficial partial thickness burn because some of the nerve endings have been destroyed.
- A third-degree burn is more severe and includes all three layers of skin: epidermis, dermis, and subcutaneous. A third-degree burn is also known as a full-thickness burn. The skin may appear black, brown, yellow, white, or red. Edema is severe. The burn penetrates the derma and may reach the subcutaneous fat. Pain is minimal because nerve endings are almost completely destroyed. There are no blisters but there is hard eschar.
- Physicians, particularly in specialty burn centers, will describe deep full-thickness burns. These fourth-degree burns are the most severe. The burn extends deep through the skin into the underlying fascia and may damage the tendons and bones. The skin is black with no edema, and the eschar is hard. Because the nerve endings are destroyed, pain is minimal. The Alphabetic Index directs the coder to codes for fourth-degree burns with the entry: Burn, fourth degree—see Burn, by site, third degree, deep.

### Guidelines for Coding Burns and Encounters for Late Effects of Burns

The following official guidelines apply when coding burns and encounters for the late effects of burns:

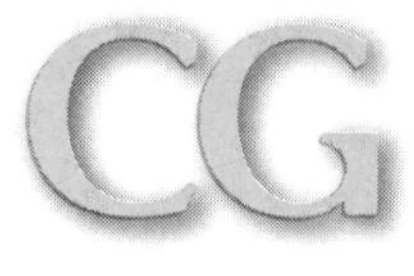


- Code all burns with the highest degree of burn sequenced first.
- Classify burns of the same local site (a three-digit category level [940–947]), but of different degrees, to the subcategory identifying the highest degree recorded in the diagnosis.
- Code nonhealing burns as acute burns. Code necrosis of burned skin as a nonhealed burn.
- Assign code 958.3, Posttraumatic wound infection, not elsewhere classified, as an additional code for any documented infected burn site.

- When coding multiple burns, assign separate codes for each burn site. Category 946, Burns of multiple specified sites, should be used only if the locations of the burns are not documented.
- Category 949, Burn, unspecified, is extremely vague and should seldom be used.
- Assign codes from category 948, Burns classified according to extent of body surface involved, when the site of the burns is not specified or when there is a need for additional data. Use category 948 as additional coding when it is necessary to provide data for evaluating burn mortality, such as that needed by burn units. Also, use category 948 as an additional code for reporting purposes when there is mention of a third-degree burn involving 20 percent or more of body surface. In assigning a code from category 948, observe the following criteria:
    - Fourth-digit codes are used to identify the percentage of total body surface involved in a burn (all degrees).
    - Fifth digits are assigned to identify the percentage of body surface involved in a third-degree burn.
    - The fifth digit 0 is assigned when less than 10 percent of body surface or no body surface is involved in a third-degree burn.
- Category 948 is based on the classic "rule of nines" in estimating body surface involved: head and neck are assigned 9 percent; each arm, 9 percent; each leg, 18 percent; the anterior trunk, 18 percent; the posterior trunk, 18 percent; and the genitalia, 1 percent. Physicians may change these percentage assignments, where necessary, to accommodate infants and children who have proportionately larger heads than adults, as well as patients whose buttocks, thighs, or abdomens are proportionately larger than normal. The assignment of the percent of body surface involved in a burn is based only on physician documentation.
- Code encounters for the treatment of the late effects of burns (for example, scars or joint contractures) to the residual condition (sequela), followed by the appropriate late effect code (906.5–906.9). A late effect E code also may be used, if desired.
- When appropriate, both a sequela with a late effect code and a current burn code may be assigned on the same record.

Sunburn is caused by overexposure to the ultraviolet rays from sunlight. Sunburns can be described as first, second, or third degree, depending on the depth of the burn. Sunburns are not classified in the range of 940–949 with traumatic burns due to flames or other sources of heat. Instead, sunburns are classified to codes 692.70–692.79, contact dermatitis due to solar radiation.

## Coding Debridements of Wounds, Infections, or Burns

Excisional debridement, 86.22, is assigned when the procedure is performed by physicians, nurses, therapists, or physician assistants. Nonexcisional debridement performed by a physician or other healthcare professional is assigned to 86.28. Documentation in the health record must be very specific regarding the type of debridement performed and the provider queried if there is any question as to whether the procedure was excisional or nonexcisional. Additional information about the coding of excisional and nonexcisional debridement is included in chapter 15 of this textbook.

### Exercise 19.7

Assign ICD-9-CM codes to the following:

1. Second-degree burn of chest wall and first-degree burn of face
2. Full-thickness burns of back
3. Third-degree burns of back involving 20 percent of body surface
4. Thirty percent body burns with 10 percent third degree
5. Deep third-degree burn of forearm
6. Nonhealing second-degree burns of right upper arm and right hand
7. Infected second-degree burn of left thigh
8. First- and second-degree burns on multiple sites of legs
9. First- and second-degree burns of palm
10. First- and second-degree burns of scalp with third-degree burns of shoulder

## Superficial Injury, and Contusion with Intact Skin, and Crushing Injury (910–929)

Superficial injuries such as abrasions or contusions are not coded when associated with more severe injuries (for example, fractures, open wounds) of the same site. The following subsections describe the conditions for coding superficial injury, contusion with intact skin surface, and crushing injury.

### *Superficial Injury (910–919)*

Superficial injuries are classified to categories 910–919. This section includes a variety of superficial injuries, from abrasions to superficial foreign bodies. The fourth-digit subcategories specify type of injury and presence or absence of infection.

**910 Superficial injury of face, neck, and scalp, except eye**

- **910.0 Abrasion or friction burn without mention of infection**
- **910.1 Abrasion or friction burn, infected**
- **910.2 Blister without mention of infection**
- **910.3 Blister, infected**
- **910.4 Insect bite, nonvenomous, without mention of infection**
- **910.5 Insect bite, nonvenomous, infected**
- **910.6 Superficial foreign body (splinter) without major open wound and without mention of infection**
- **910.7 Superficial foreign body (splinter) without major open wound, infected**
- **910.8 Other and unspecified superficial injury of face, neck, and scalp without mention of infection**
- **910.9 Other and unspecified superficial injury of face, neck, and scalp, infected**

### *Contusion with Intact Skin Surface (920–924)*

Contusions are injuries of the soft tissue. Although the skin is not broken, the small vessels or capillaries are ruptured and the result is bleeding into the tissue. When the blood becomes trapped in the interstitial spaces, the result is a hematoma. A bruise without a fracture or an open wound is also coded to the condition of contusion with intact skin surface. The codes in this section do not include a contusion, bruise, or hematoma of an internal organ, intracranial location, or a nerve. A contusion, bruise, or hematoma are incidental if occurring at the same site as a crushing injury, dislocation, fracture, internal injury, intracranial injury, nerve injury or open wound and are not coded separately. Inside the more serious injury described in the previous sentence is coded and the contusion, bruise, or hematoma is part of that same injury.

ICD-9-CM classifies these types of contusions to categories 920 through 924. The fourth-digit subcategories are subdivided to identify the specific site involved.

### *Crushing Injury (925–929)*

Crushing injuries usually occur when part or all of an extremity is pulled into, and compressed by, rollers in a machine, such as those found in industrial plants. A crushing injury also may occur in a nonindustrial setting. Avulsion of skin and fat or a friction burn of the tissues may result. Abrasion burns are often severe, including third degree. Vessels, nerves, and muscles may be avulsed, and bones may be dislocated or fractured. A common complication is secondary congestion, which can lead to paralysis and to severe muscle fibrosis and joint stiffness. Muscle compartments may need decompression, and muscles and ligaments may need to be sectioned. Often the overall circulation of the extremity is of greater concern than definitive management of specific structures. These types of injuries may be called wringer, compression, crush, crushed, or crushing injuries.

A directional note appears under the section heading, Crushing injury (925–929): Use additional code to identify any associated injuries, such as:

- Fractures (800–829)
- Internal injuries (860.0–869.1)
- Intracranial injuries (850.0–854.1)

## Injury to Blood Vessels (900–904), Nerves and Spinal Cord (950–957)

This subsection describes the conditions for coding injury to blood vessels and the nerves and spinal cord.

**A point to remember:** When a primary injury results in minor damage to peripheral nerves or blood vessels, list the primary injury first, with additional code(s) from categories 950–957, Injury to nerves and spinal cord, and/or from categories 900–904, Injury to blood vessels. Also, when the primary injury is to the blood vessels or nerves, list the primary injury first.

### *Injury to Blood Vessels (900–904)*

The codes for injuries to blood vessels include arterial hematomas, avulsions, cuts, lacerations, ruptures, and traumatic aneurysms or fistulas that are secondary to other injuries such as fractures or open wounds. Codes from categories 900–904 are usually assigned as additional diagnoses, with the underlying injury listed first.

**EXAMPLE:** Open wound of the forearm with injury to the ulnar blood vessel: 881.00, Open wound of forearm without mention of complication; 903.3, Injury to ulnar blood vessels

### *Injury to Nerves and Spinal Cord (950–957)*

The codes for injury to nerves and the spinal cord include injuries with or without the presence of an open wound. The includes note that appears at the heading of this section states that a division of a nerve, traumatic neuroma, or traumatic transient paralysis that occurs with an open wound is included in the codes here. Category 952, Spinal cord injury without evidence of spinal bone injury, is subdivided at the fourth- and fifth-digit levels to identify the specific sites involved.

### *Certain Traumatic Complications and Unspecified Injuries (958–959)*

Certain conditions are considered consequences of external causes or injuries that stem from forces or circumstances that arise outside the body. This section contains several complications of injuries as well as other and unspecified, relatively minor, injuries of different body sites.

Within this range of codes is code 958.3, Posttraumatic wound infection, not elsewhere classified. This code is not used to describe an infected open wound. which is coded to a complicated open wound by site. However, code 958.3 can be used as an additional code to describe an infected burn. The code for the burn site would be listed as well. A different code exists for postoperative or surgical wound infections, 998.59.

Traumatic compartment syndrome of an extremity, abdomen, or other body location can occur as the result of trauma; for example, a burn or compression injury. Compartment syndrome occurs when increased pressure occurs in an enclosed space, which leads to decreased circulation and, potentially, to tissue loss. If the pressure is markedly elevated it represents a medical emergency that requires immediate surgical intervention, such as a fasciotomy. Traumatic compartment syndrome is coded based on the body part involved with codes 958.90–958.99.

Category 959, Injury, other and unspecified, is intended for use when there is no other information available to classify the condition elsewhere, such as injuries to blood vessels, nerves, internal organs, or intracranial sites. Emergency physicians may use the term "head injury" to describe a traumatic event. ICD-9-CM classifies head injury to different categories based on whether or not the patient suffered a loss of consciousness as a result of the head injury. The diagnosis of "head injury" with no documentation of loss of consciousness is classified to code 959.01. If the head injury produced a loss of consciousness, the Alphabetic Index directs the coder to subcategory 850.5. Other codes within category 850 may be used to describe a patient who had a head injury or cerebral concussion with loss of consciousness of a specified or unspecified amount of time. The coder should examine the documentation closely for specific descriptions of the type of head injury in order to code correctly. Cerebral concussion and head injury may be used interchangeably by physicians but coders should not make the assumption that the terminology is equal. When there is doubt, the coder should ask the documenting physician for clarification as to the nature of the injury.

## Exercise 19.8

Assign ICD-9-CM codes to the following:

1. Open wound of the lower leg with tendon involvement and injury to the anterior tibial artery

   ______________________

2. Nonvenomous insect bite, elbow, infected

   ______________________

3. Contusion of the lower leg and knee

   ______________________

4. Crushing injury of left hand and wrist

   ______________________

5. Spinal cord injury, C1–C4

   ______________________

## Effects of Foreign Body Entering through Orifice (930–939)

Foreign objects often are found in various body openings in the pediatric population. Children sometimes put small items in their noses or ears or swallow coins or marbles.

Foreign bodies also can lodge in the larynx, bronchi, or esophagus, usually during eating. Foreign bodies in the larynx may produce hoarseness, coughing, and gagging, and partially obstruct the airway, causing stridor. A grasping forceps through a direct laryngoscope can remove foreign bodies from the larynx.

Foreign bodies in the bronchi usually produce an initial episode of coughing, followed by an asymptomatic period before obstructive and inflammatory symptoms occur. Foreign bodies are removed from the bronchi through a bronchoscope.

Foreign bodies in the esophagus produce immediate symptoms of coughing and gagging, with the sensation of something being "stuck in the throat," as well as causing difficulty in swallowing. Foreign bodies in the esophagus can be removed through an esophagoscope. Intraocular foreign bodies require removal by an ophthalmic surgeon.

ICD-9-CM classifies foreign bodies in orifices to categories 930–939. These categories are further subdivided to fourth-digit subcategories that identify the specific site or orifice. These codes can be found in the Alphabetic Index by referencing the main term "Foreign body" and the subterm "entering through orifice." When the foreign body is associated with an open wound, it is coded as an open wound, complicated, by site. A foreign body inadvertently left in an operative wound is considered to be a complication of a procedure and is coded 998.4.

## Chapter 19 ICD-9-CM Review Exercises

Assign ICD-9-CM codes to the following:

1. Q-Tip stuck in ear

2. Foreign body in eye

3. Marble in colon

4. Bean in nose

5. Removal of coin from bronchus

6. Compound fracture of the tibia with open reduction and internal fixation

7. Contusion of the cheek and forearm

8. Left Colles' fracture with closed reduction

9. Open wound of the forearm with tendon involvement

10. Concussion with no loss of consciousness, with abrasion of the elbow and foot

# ICD-10-CM Chapter 19, Injury, Poisoning and Certain Other Consequences of External Causes (S00–T88)

## Organization and Structure of ICD-10-CM Chapter 19

In this chapter of the textbook, the focus will be on the injury codes that were created in ICD-10-CM. with codes in the range of S00–T34. Chapter 19 of ICD-10-CM also includes the coding of drug related illnesses such as poisoning, adverse effect and underdosing of drug. Codes in the range of T36–T88 will be addressed in chapter 20 of the textbook.

A significant modification was made to the organization of Chapter 19 in ICD-10-CM. Type of injury is the first axis of classification for the injuries in ICD-9-CM whereas specific types of injuries found in categories S00–S99 of ICD-10-CM are arranged by body region beginning with the head and concluding with the ankle and foot. This results in the grouping of injury types together under the site where it occurred.

| | |
|---|---|
| S00–S09 | Injuries to the head |
| S10–S19 | Injuries to the neck |
| S20–S29 | Injuries to the thorax |
| S30–S39 | Injuries to the abdomen, lower back, lumbar spine, pelvis and external genitals |
| S40–S49 | Injuries to the shoulder and upper arm |
| S50–S59 | Injuries to the elbow and forearm |
| S60–S69 | Injuries to the wrist, hand and fingers |
| S70–S79 | Injuries to the hip and thigh |
| S80–S89 | Injuries to the knee and lower leg |
| S90–S99 | Injuries to the ankle and foot |
| T07 | Injuries involving multiple body regions |
| T14 | Injury of unspecified body region |
| T15–T19 | Effects of foreign body entering through natural orifice |
| T20–T32 | Burns and corrosions |
| T33–T34 | Frostbite |

In addition, generally the listings of conditions that follow the site are as follows:

- Superficial injury
- Open wound
- Fracture
- Dislocation and sprain
- Injury of nerves
- Injury of blood vessels

- Injury of muscle and tendon
- Crushing injury
- Traumatic amputation
- Other and unspecified injuries

Some categories in Chapter 19 have undergone title changes to reflect terminology in use today. For example, ICD-10-CM uses the terms displaced and nondisplaced in the code descriptors for fractures, while these terms were not used in ICD-9-CM.

In ICD-10-CM, codes from blocks T20–T32 classify burns and corrosions. The addition of the term *corrosion* is new in ICD-10-CM. The burn codes identify thermal burns, except for sunburns, that come from a heat source. The burn codes are also for burns resulting from electricity and radiation. Corrosions are burns due to chemicals.

## Coding Guidelines and Instructional Notes for Chapter 19

The following guideline appears at the beginning of Chapter 19: Use secondary code(s) from Chapter 20, External Causes of Morbidity, to indicate cause of injury. However, the *ICD-10-CM Official Guidelines for Coding and Reporting*, Part II.20, states "There is no national requirement for mandatory ICD-10-CM external cause code reporting. Unless a provider is subject to a state-based external cause code reporting mandate or these codes are required by a particular payer, reporting of ICD-10-CM codes in Chapter 20, External Causes of Morbidity, is not required. In the absence of a mandatory reporting requirement, providers are encouraged to voluntarily report external cause codes, as they provide valuable data for injury research and evaluation of injury prevention strategies." There are codes within the T section that include the external cause do not require an additional external cause code, for example, an accident poisoning or an adverse effect of a specific drug.

Instructions for coding open wounds have changed in ICD-10-CM. The note in ICD-9-CM defined "complicated" used in the fourth-digit subdivisions to include those open wounds with infection. ICD-10-CM contains a note under the different categories for open wounds and directs the coding professional to use an additional code for associated wound infection and other related injuries.

A similar change has occurred to the instruction for complications of surgical and medical care, not elsewhere classified (T80–T88). In ICD-9-CM, there is no guideline under this subchapter. However, ICD-10-CM includes a note stating to use additional code (Y62–Y82) to identify devices involved and details of circumstances.

Most categories in Chapter 19 have seventh characters that identify the encounter:

A initial encounter
D subsequent encounter
S sequela

Additional seventh characters are available to identify specific encounters for fracture coding. Fracture seventh characters are unique to each type of bone and type of fracture. It is necessary to review the fracture seventh characters carefully before assigning a seventh character.

There are chapter-specific guidelines for Chapter 19 of ICD-10-CM that must be reviewed in their entirety. Examples of the direction provided in these guidelines are as follows:

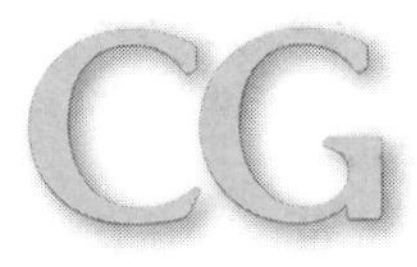


- Guideline I.C.19.a. Application of 7th characters in Chapter 19

Most codes in this chapter require the use of a seventh character for each applicable code.

The three main seventh characters are:

"A" is used for initial encounter to identify when the patient is receiving active treatment. Active treatment is defined as emergency department encounters, surgical treatment and evaluation and management by a new physician (new compared to a previous physician who examined the patient for the same injury previously).

"D" is used for subsequent encounters when the patient is receiving routine care for the condition during the healing or recovery phase after the active treatment is finished. Subsequent encounters may be visits for cast or immobilizer changes and removal, removal of internal or external fixation devices, medication adjustments or other care required during the healing phase. This may also be the period of time described as fracture aftercare. There are aftercare Z codes in ICD-10-CM but these are not used for injuries and poisoning conditions when aftercare or recovery care is provided.

"S" is used for a sequela situation when a complication or condition arises as a direct result of the original injury, such as a scar that remains after a burn heals. When a patient has a sequela condition after an injury both the injury that caused the sequela is coded and the sequela condition is coded. The "S" is added only on the code for the original injury. It is not added to the sequela condition that remains. The specific type of sequela that exists, such as a scar, is sequenced first, followed by the code for the injury with the seventh character of S.

- Guidelines I.C.19.b. Coding of injuries

The coder should assign separate codes for each injury whenever possible. If a combination code is provided for the injuries, it is assigned. Code T07 for unspecified multiple injuries should not be used in the inpatient setting. The only time it would be used is if no information is available to assign a more specific code. The codes for traumatic injuries (S00-T14) should not be used for normal or complicated healing surgical wounds.

When a patient has multiple injuries, the code for the most serious injury, as determined by the provider and the focus of the treatment, is sequenced first.

Superficial injuries are not coded when associated with a more severe injury. For example, abrasions and contusions that occur with a fracture are not coded separately with the fracture.

(*Continued*)

(*Continued*)

An open wound or other injury may result in injuries to nerves and blood vessels. When the primary injury causes minor damage to a peripheral nerve or blood vessel, the primary injury such as the open wound is sequenced first with additional codes for the injuries to the nerves or blood vessels. However, when the primary injury is to the blood vessel or to the nerve, that injury should be sequenced first.

- Guidelines I.C.19.c. Coding of traumatic fractures

When a fracture is not described as open or closed it should be coded to a closed fracture. When a fracture is not described as displaced or not displaced or non-displaced, it should be coded to displaced in ICD-10-CM.

The principles of multiple coding of injuries applies to fracture coding. Fractures are coded individually to specific sites as provided in the fracture code categories. Multiple fracture codes are sequenced according to the severity of the fracture. If a complication of the fracture care or surgical treatment exists, additional codes should be applied. Complications such as malunion fractures and nonunion fractures are reported with the appropriate seventh character for the particular site.

- Guidelines I.C.19.d. Coding of burns and corrosions

The ICD-10-CM guidelines contain numerous directions on the coding of burns and corrosions. For example, burns are defined in ICD-10-CM as originating from a thermal source such as heat or flame as well as from electricity and radiation. Corrosions in ICD-10-CM are burns produced by chemicals. The guidelines for coding burns and corrosions are the same.

The highest degree burn is sequenced first when more than one burn is present. When the patient suffers from external burns, internal burns and/or other related conditions such as smoke inhalation, the circumstances of the admission determine the principal or first listed diagnosis. If a patient has multiple burns of different degrees on the same site, however, only the highest degree burn is coded. When a patient has multiple burns on different sites, codes are assigned for each site, with the highest degree reported for each site. There is a code for site unspecified, T30, that should not be used if at all possible. If a burn is not healing or described as a non-healing burn, it is coded in ICD-10-CM as a current, acute burn. If a burn is infected, an additional code is used to identify the infection.

Assign an additional code from category T31, Burns classified according to extent of body surface involved, or T32, Corrosions classified according to extent of body surface involved, when the site is not specified or when there is a need for additional detail on the percentage of the body surface burned, for example, for acute care settings with burn care units. The coding guidelines state it is advisable to use category T31 when there is a mention of a third-degree burn involving 20 percent or more of the body surface.

Burns often produce sequela conditions such as scars or joint contractures. When coding for visits that describe the care of a sequela, the code for the burn should be reported with the seventh character of "S." Patients may have both current and healed burns as the injuries may heal at different intervals. It is possible to code a patient with both acute and sequela of burns by using the burn codes with different sites coded with a seventh character of "A," "D," and "S" depending on the patient's conditions.

To review the entire set of guidelines for this chapter, access the 2014 guidelines from NCHS website (http://www.cdc.gov/nchs/icd/icd10cm.htm) and read Chapter 19, Injury, Poisoning and Certain Other Consequences of External Causes guidelines I.C.19.a–I.C.19.d.

## Coding Overview for ICD-10-CM Chapter 19

In ICD-10-CM, injuries are grouped by body part rather than by categories of injury, so that all injuries of the specific site (such as head and neck) are grouped together rather than groupings of all fractures or all open wounds. For example, categories in ICD-9-CM are grouped by injury such as fractures (800–829), dislocations (830–839), and sprains and strains (840–848). In ICD-10-CM, categories are grouped by site, such as injuries to the head (S00–S09), injuries to the neck (S10–S19), and injuries to the thorax (S20–S29).

Chapter 19 encompasses two alpha characters. The S section provides codes for the various types of injuries related to single body regions; the T section covers injuries to unspecified body regions as well as poisonings and certain other consequences of external causes.

The following note refers to the entire chapter: Use secondary code(s) from Chapter 20, External Causes of Morbidity, to indicate cause of injury. However, codes within the T section that include the external cause do not require an additional external cause code.

Many codes, such as fractures, include much greater specificity in ICD-10-CM. For example, some of the information that may be found in fracture codes includes the type of fracture, specific anatomical site, whether the fracture is displaced or not, laterality, routine versus delayed healing, nonunions, and malunions. Laterality and identification of type of encounter (initial, subsequent, sequela) are significant components of the codes. Previous Coding Clinical advice that applied to the use of the radiology report that could be used for the specificity of a condition applies to ICD-10-CM as well. If the radiology report provides additional information regarding the site for an injury or condition that the provider has already diagnosed, the specificity described in the report can be used to assign a code.

ICD-10-CM uses a placeholder character "x" for certain codes. The "x" is used as a placeholder at certain codes to allow for future expansion or to fill empty characters in order to add the seventh character for the episode of care. An example of this is S28.0XXA, crushed chest, initial encounter.

Seventh characters are assigned in this chapter, and are identified at the category level to indicate initial encounter, subsequent encounter or sequela.

Fracture seventh characters are expanded to include:

A—Initial encounter for closed fracture
B—Initial encounter for open fracture
D—Subsequent encounter for fracture with routine healing
G—Subsequent encounter for fracture with delayed healing
K—Subsequent encounter for fracture with nonunion
P—Subsequent encounter for fracture with malunion
S—Sequela

Some fracture categories provide for seventh characters extensions to designate the specific type of open fracture. (These designations are based on the Gustilo open fracture classification):

B—Initial encounter for open fracture type I or II (open NOS or not otherwise specified)
C—Initial encounter for open fracture type IIIA, IIIB, or IIIC
E—Subsequent encounter for open fracture type I or II with routine healing
F—Subsequent encounter for open fracture type IIIA, IIIB, or IIIC with routine healing
H—Subsequent encounter for open fracture type I or II with delayed healing
J—Subsequent encounter for open fracture type IIIA, IIIB, or IIIC with delayed healing
M—Subsequent encounter for open fracture type I or II with nonunion
N—Subsequent encounter for open fracture type IIIA, IIIB, or IIIC with nonunion
Q—Subsequent encounter for open fracture type I or II with malunion
R—Subsequent encounter for open fracture type IIIA, IIIB, or IIIC with malunion

According to the *ICD-10-CM Official Guidelines for Coding and Reporting*, a fracture not indicated as displaced or nondisplaced should be coded to displaced and a fracture not designated as open or closed should be coded to closed.

The seventh characters for "initial encounter" are used while the patient is receiving active treatment for the injury, for example, surgical treatment, emergency department encounter, and evaluation and treatment by a new physician. Coding Clinic advice published in Fourth Quarter 2012 stated that the seventh character for initial encounter can be applied when a patient seeks initial care even after a period of time has elapsed. The fact that it is the initial encounter to treat the injury is the important information for coding, not the amount of time that has passed between the time the injury occurred and the time the patient sought treatment.

The seventh characters for "subsequent encounter" are used for encounters after the patient has received active treatment of the injury and is receiving routine care for the injury during the healing or recovery phase. For example, cast change or removal, removal of external or internal fixation device, medication adjustment, other aftercare, and follow-up visits following injury treatment.

The seventh character of S, sequela, is for use for complications or conditions that arise as a direct result of an injury, such as scar formation after a burn. The scars are sequela of the burn. When using seventh character extension S, it is necessary to use both the injury code that precipitated the sequela and the code for the sequela itself. The S is added only to the injury code, not the sequela code or the condition the patient currently has as a result of the injury. The S seventh character identifies the injury responsible for the sequela. The specific type of sequela (for example, scar) is sequenced first, followed by the injury code with the seventh character of S.

The aftercare Z codes should not be used for aftercare for injuries according to the *ICD-10-CM Official Guidelines for Coding and Reporting*. For aftercare of an injury, assign the acute injury code with the appropriate seventh character for "subsequent encounter."

## ICD-10-CM Review Exercises: Chapter 19

Assign the correct ICD-10-CM diagnosis codes to the following exercises:

*Chapter 19 will provide practice coding Chapter 19 codes. External cause codes will be discussed and coded in another chapter. For Lesson 19, assign only diagnosis codes, not external cause codes.*

1. Two (2) cm laceration of the left heel with foreign body. This is a current injury. (Do not assign the external cause codes.)

2. This patient is seen for increased pain in her ankle. She has previous trimalleolar fracture of the left ankle. After evaluation she was found to have a nonunion of her left trimalleolar fracture. (Do not assign the external cause codes.)

3. Displaced, compound comminuted fracture of the right radial shaft. It is a type II open fracture. (Do not assign the external cause code.)

4. The 6-month-old is seen for increased fussiness and vomiting. After significant study, the patient is diagnosed with shaken baby syndrome. (Do not assign the external cause codes.)

5. Delayed healing of his traumatic mandible fracture. The fracture was at the angle of the jaw. (Do not assign the external cause codes.)

6. Frontal skull fracture with a subsequent subdural hemorrhage. There was a 45-minute loss of consciousness at the time of the accident. (Do not assign the external cause codes.)

7. Patient is a complete paraplegic due to a traumatic L2 vertebral fracture five years ago. At this time, she is experiencing no new problems. (Do not assign the external cause codes.)

8. Follow-up of patient's traumatic lateral epicondyle fracture of the right elbow. This is healing normally. (Do not assign the external cause codes.)

9. Patient had a right-sided fracture of 3 ribs, a right chest contusion and a fractured right wrist. None of his injuries required surgical intervention. (Do not assign the external cause codes.)

10. Patient is seen in the physician's office for removal of sutures placed for a laceration of the scalp. The wound has healed and the sutures are removed during this visit.

# Chapter 20

# Injury and Poisoning II

## Learning Objectives

At the conclusion of this chapter, you should be able to:

1. Describe the organization of the conditions and codes included in Chapter 17 of ICD-9-CM, Injury and Poisoning, with a focus on poisoning, adverse effects of drugs, and complications, categories 960–999
2. Describe the organization of the conditions and codes included in Chapter 19 of ICD-10-CM, Injury and Poisoning, with a focus on poisoning and certain other consequences of external causes, categories T36–T88
3. Describe the circumstances in which an *adverse effect* of a drug can occur in a patient
4. Explain the instructions for coding current and late effect or sequela of the adverse effects of drugs
5. Define the term *poisoning*
6. Explain the instructions for coding current and late effect or sequela of poisonings
7. Define the term *underdosing*
8. Describe the organization of the Table of Drugs and Chemicals in ICD-9-CM and identify which E codes are used with poisonings and which E codes are used to report adverse effects of drugs
9. Describe the organization of the ICD-10-CM Table of Drugs and Chemicals and identify which codes are used for which of the following circumstances: poisoning, adverse effect, and underdosing
10. Describe the circumstances in which a complication of surgical and medical care code may be used
11. Explain the instructions for coding complications to identify the various main terms found in the Alphabetic Index to locate the codes

12. Identify the correct seventh characters required for reporting certain codes in ICD-10-CM
13. Assign ICD-9-CM diagnosis and procedure codes for poisoning and adverse effects of drugs, poisoning, and complications of surgical and medical care
14. Assign ICD-10-CM codes for adverse effects, poisonings, underdosing, and complications of surgical and medical care

# ICD-9-CM Chapter 17, Injury and Poisoning: Poisoning, Adverse Effects of Drugs, and Complications (960–999)

Chapter 20 in this textbook provides further explanation of Chapter 17, Injury and Poisoning, in ICD-9-CM.

## Alphabetic Index

ICD-9-CM provides two different sets of code numbers to differentiate between poisonings and adverse effects or adverse reactions to substances. Codes 960–979 are used to identify poisoning by drugs and medicinal and biological substances. These codes are found through a separate index known as the Table of Drugs and Chemicals. This table also is used to classify the appropriate E code for the drug or chemical involved with an adverse reaction, while the actual condition identified as the adverse effect is coded with disease codes. The Table of Drugs and Chemicals follows the Alphabetic Index to Diseases.

## Table of Drugs and Chemicals

The Table of Drugs and Chemicals provides an alphabetic listing of drugs and other agents. The first column identifies the specific substance. The second column, titled "Poisoning," is used when a particular case meets the criteria for poisoning (criteria follow). The remaining five columns describe the circumstance under which the adverse reaction or poisoning occurred.

## Adverse Effects of Drugs

Adverse effects can occur in situations in which medication is administered properly and prescribed correctly in both therapeutic and diagnostic procedures. An adverse effect can occur when everything is done right—right drug, right dose, right patient receiving it, right route of administration—but a physical reaction is experienced. A brief discussion of common causes of adverse effects follows:

- Cumulative effects result when the inactivation and/or excretion of the drug is slower than the rate at which the drug is being administered. This is often documented as drug toxicity in the health record.
- Hypersensitivity or allergic reaction is a qualitatively different response to a drug acquired only after re-exposure to the drug.

- Synergistic reaction is enhancing the effect of a prior or concurrent administration of another drug.
- The effectiveness of a drug may change as the result of interaction with another prescribed medication.
- Side effects are the unwanted predictable pharmacologic effects that occur within therapeutic code ranges.

### Instructions for Coding Adverse Effects

The following instructions apply when coding adverse effects:

1. Code the manifestation or the nature of the adverse effects, such as urticaria, vertigo, gastritis, and so forth.
2. Locate the drug in the "Substance" column of the Table of Drugs and Chemicals in the Alphabetic Index to Diseases.
3. Select the E code for the drug from the "Therapeutic Use" column of the Table of Drugs and Chemicals. Use of the E code is mandatory when coding adverse effects.

   **EXAMPLE:** Atrial tachycardia due to digitalis glycosides intoxication: 427.89, Other specified cardiac dysrhythmias (atrial tachycardia); E942.1, Cardiotonic glycosides and drugs of similar action causing adverse effects in therapeutic use (adverse effect of digitalis)

4. If the adverse effect is the result of the interaction between two or more prescription drugs, assign E codes for both drugs.

   **EXAMPLE:** Premature supraventricular beats due to the interaction of digitalis glycosides and Valium, both correctly prescribed and administered: 427.61, Supraventricular premature beats; E942.1, Cardiotonic glycosides and drugs of similar action causing adverse effects in therapeutic use (adverse effect of digitalis); E939.4, Benzodiazepine-based tranquilizers causing adverse effects in therapeutic use (adverse effect of Valium)

5. Late effect of an adverse effect of a correct substance properly administered is coded as follows:
   - First code the residual or late effect, such as blindness or deafness.
   - Assign code 909.5, Late effect of adverse effect of drug, medicinal or biological substance, to identify a late effect of an adverse reaction. Use the Alphabetic Index to Diseases and see "Late, effect(s) (of), adverse effect of drug, medicinal or biological substance" to locate code 909.5.
   - No specific E code is provided to identify the external cause of a late effect of an adverse reaction to a correct substance properly administered. The residual effect will differ from the immediate reaction. However, the E code is the same as the original code selected from the Therapeutic Use column of the Table of Drugs and Chemicals.

**EXAMPLE:** Hearing loss occurring as a result of previously administered streptomycin therapy: 389.9, Unspecified hearing loss; 909.5, Late effect of adverse effect of drug, medicinal or biological substance; E930.6, Antimycobacterial antibiotics causing adverse effects in therapeutic use

See figure 20.1 for assistance in coding adverse reactions to correct substances properly administered.

**Figure 20.1.** Coding adverse reactions to correct substances properly administered

| Current Condition | | Late Effect |
|---|---|---|
| Code effect:<br>Coma, vertigo, etc. | ←Principal Diagnosis→ | Code effect:<br>Deafness, blindness, etc. |
| | | ***Plus*** |
| | | Late effect 909.5 |
| **And** | | **And** |
| E code from "Therapeutic Use" column of Table of Drugs and Chemicals (E930–949) | ←Other Diagnosis→ | E code from "Therapeutic Use" column of Table of Drugs and Chemicals (E930–949) |

**Use of codes E930–E949 is mandatory when coding adverse effects.**

## Exercise 20.1

Assign ICD-9-CM diagnosis codes to the following clinical situations where the drug involved was taken as prescribed by the physician and produced the adverse effect:

1. Excessive drowsiness due to adverse effects of Periactin

2. Vertigo from dye administered for intravenous pyelogram

3. Constipation from Oncovin injected for Hodgkin's disease

4. Ataxia due to the interaction of carbamazepine and erythromycin

5. Hemiplegia resulting from previous adverse reaction to Enovid

## Unspecified Adverse Effects of Drugs

Sometimes an adverse effect of a drug is unknown or, more often, not documented in the health record. Normally, unspecified adverse effects of drugs are indicated by diagnostic statements such as:

- Toxic effect of
- Drug toxicity
- Drug intoxication
- Drug allergy/hypersensitivity

### *Instructions for Coding Other and Unspecified Adverse Effects of Drugs and Allergies*

Certain coding instructions apply when coding unspecified adverse effects of drugs and allergies. These include:

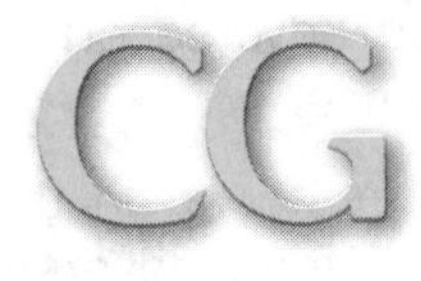


- In the inpatient setting, the health record documentation should provide enough information to determine the specific adverse effect or reaction of a particular medication. In such circumstances, the information previously discussed for coding adverse reactions applies.
- In the event specific information is unavailable and the documentation states toxicity or intoxication to a particular drug with no specific reaction or physical manifestation identified, assign code 796.0, Nonspecific abnormal toxicological findings. First, the physician should be queried to determine whether the toxicity, allergy, or intoxication is either an adverse effect or a poisoning. Then, the applicable E code from the Table of Drugs and Chemicals is assigned to describe the drug or medicinal substance causing the adverse effect.

**EXAMPLE:** While hospitalized, patient developed paroxysmal supraventricular tachycardia secondary to digitalis intoxication. The medication was prescribed and administered correctly: 427.0, Paroxysmal supraventricular tachycardia; E942.1, Cardiotonic glycosides and drugs of similar action causing adverse effects in therapeutic use (adverse effect of digitalis)

**EXAMPLE:** Documentation in the health record of an inpatient states aminophylline toxicity: 796.0, Nonspecific abnormal toxicological findings

*(Continued)*

(*Continued*)

In this example, the coder should query the physician as to whether the toxicity is a poisoning or an adverse reaction (effect), as well as whether there are any associated reactions or manifestations. In the example above for the aminophylline toxicity, if the physician confirms that the toxicity is an adverse effect, E945.7, Anti-asthmatics causing adverse effects in therapeutic use (adverse effect of aminophylline), would be added. However, if the physician declares the toxicity to be a poisoning, then it would be coded as a poisoning. The coding of poisoning is discussed later in this chapter.

- In the outpatient setting there may be instances in which the physician documents an adverse effect to a substance but does not include a description of the adverse effect. In such cases, unspecified adverse effects or reactions may be reported with a code from subcategory 995.2, Other and unspecified adverse effect of drug, medicinal and biological substance. In the inpatient setting, the expectation is that there should be sufficient documentation to describe the type of adverse effect. In the outpatient setting, unspecified adverse effects or reactions may be reported with subcategory codes 995.20–995.29, Other and unspecified adverse effect of drug, medicinal and biological substance.
- Subcategory codes 995.20–995.29 are found in the Alphabetic Index to Diseases under "Effect, adverse, NEC, drugs and medicinals NEC or Allergy, drug." Although the reaction is unspecified, some of the codes in 995.21–995.29 identify the drug, medicinal or biological substance involved.
- Code 995.20 is used for the rare events in which the documentation does not specify the type of adverse effect and does not specify which drug or medicinal or biological substance was involved.
- Code 995.21, Arthus phenomenon or Arthus reaction, is the development of an inflammatory lesion a few hours after an intradermal injection of an antigen. This may also be referred to as a local form of an immune complex disease, the local effect of anaphylaxis or a Type III allergic reaction, or hypersensitivity reaction. Codes 995.22 and 995.23 are used to describe an unspecified adverse effect of anesthesia and insulin, respectively.
- Code 995.24, Failed moderate sedation during procedure, is used to describe the circumstance when moderate or conscious sedation does not

produce adequate sedation for the procedure, or other unexpected consequences of moderate sedation occur. When this situation occurs during a procedure, urgent interventions are necessary to ensure a safe outcome for the patient and completion of the procedure if possible. It may be necessary to obtain the services of an anesthesiologist to maintain adequate sedation in order to complete the procedure or treat the patient. For future procedures that require moderate sedation once a patient experiences failed sedation, different sedation procedures may be necessary. Code V15.80, personal history of failed moderate sedation, would be used to describe the past event when a patient receives future healthcare requiring moderate sedation.

- Code 995.27 is used to describe a "drug allergy" or "drug hypersensitivity," not otherwise specified. Note the specific terminology of allergy is used in this code.
- Code 995.29 is used to describe an unspecified adverse effect of other drug, medicinal and biological substance. For the code, the drug has been identified but is not included in the other codes in this subcategory. In addition, an E code from the "Therapeutic Use" column of the Table of Drugs and Chemicals is assigned to describe the drug or medicinal substance causing the adverse effect.

**EXAMPLE:** Drug reaction to penicillin: 995.29, Unspecified adverse effect of drug, medicinal and biological substance; E930.0, Penicillin causing adverse effects in therapeutic use (adverse effect of penicillin)

**Note:** Codes 995.20, 995.22–995.29 are permissible in the outpatient setting in rare circumstances, when no further documentation is available (*Coding Clinic* 1997). If the drug reaction was described as penicillin toxicity with no specific reaction identified, it would be assigned code 796.0. If the drug causing the unspecified adverse reaction was unknown, code E947.9, Unspecified drug or medicinal substance, would be assigned. This code is indexed under the main term "Drug" in the Table of Drugs and Chemicals.

- Code 995.3, Allergy, unspecified is used to describe the situation in which a patient has an allergy or suffers an allergic reaction to an unspecified substance (other than drug) and the type of reaction is unspecified. This code is not used when the patient has an allergic reaction not otherwise specified to a correct drug or medicinal substance that was properly administered (995.27) or an allergy to existing dental restorative material (525.66).

(*Continued*)

*(Continued)*

- Late effect of an unspecified adverse effect is coded in a similar manner to late effects of specified adverse effects.
  - Since the specific residual is not identified, first code 909.5.
  - Code 909.5, Late effect of adverse effect of drug, medicinal or biological substance, is assigned to identify a late effect of an unspecified adverse reaction. Code 909.5 is found in the Alphabetic Index to Diseases under "Late effect(s) (of), adverse effect of drug, medicinal or biological substance."
  - Select the appropriate code from the "Therapeutic Use" column of the Table of Drugs and Chemicals to identify the drug involved.

**EXAMPLE:** Residuals of previous severe allergic reaction to chemotherapy (fluorouracil), which was discontinued 6 months ago: 909.5, Late effect of adverse effect of drug, medicinal or biological substance; E933.1, Antineoplastic and immunosuppressive drugs causing adverse effects in therapeutic use (adverse effect of fluorouracil)

## Exercise 20.2

Assign ICD-9-CM codes to the following:

1. Rash due to unspecified drug

   ______________________

2. Residuals from previous episode of acute hypersensitivity to sulfonamide

   ______________________

3. Inpatient took Dilantin as prescribed by the doctor but was found to have asymptomatic Dilantin toxicity

   ______________________

4. Emergency department patient with diagnosis of "drug allergy" but the drug name or type is unknown

   ______________________

## Poisonings

Poisoning refers to conditions caused by drugs, medicinal substances, and other biological substances only when the substance involved is not used according to a physician's instructions. A poisoning occurs when something is done wrong—wrong drug, wrong dose, wrong route of administration, wrong person receiving the drug, or the drug should not have been used. A poisoning can occur with prescription drugs, over-the-counter purchased medications, illegal drugs, or when drugs are taken with alcohol beverages. Poisonings can occur in the following ways:

- The wrong dosage of medication given in error during a diagnostic or therapeutic procedure, or during the course of medical care
- The wrong dosage of medication given in error by nonmedical personnel, such as a mother to an infant or a child to an elderly parent
- Medication given to the wrong person by medical or nonmedical personnel
- Medication taken by the wrong person
- The wrong dosage of medication self-administered
- Intoxication (other than cumulative effect)
- Overdose
- Medications (prescription or nonprescription) taken in combination with alcoholic beverages
- Over-the-counter medications taken in combination with prescribed medications without consulting a physician

### Instructions for Coding Poisonings

The following instructions apply when coding poisonings:

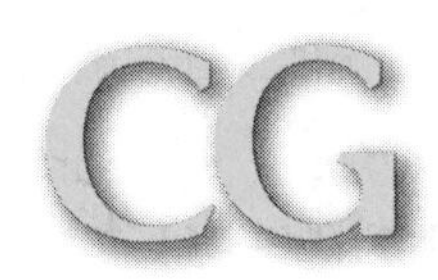


1. Use the Table of Drugs and Chemicals in the Alphabetic Index to Diseases to locate the drug or other agent.
2. Assign the code from the "Poisoning" column.
3. Code the specified manifestation or effect of the poisoning, such as coma, vertigo, drowsiness, that might be experienced.
4. If there is also a diagnosis of drug abuse or dependence to the drug, the abuse or dependence is coded as an additional diagnosis.
5. Identify the external cause of poisoning from the appropriate column of the Table of Drugs and Chemicals. If the intent (accident, self-harm, or assault) of the cause of an injury or poisoning is unknown or unspecified, code the intent as undetermined, E980–E989. If the intent (accident, self-harm, or assault) of the cause of an injury or poisoning is questionable, probable, or suspected, code the intent as undetermined, E980–E989 (Official Coding Guidelines). Use of the E codes is optional for many facilities; however, some states mandate the coding of external causes (E codes).

(*Continued*)

(*Continued*) **EXAMPLE:** Overdosed on aspirin, suicide attempt: 965.1, Poisoning by salicylates (overdose on aspirin); E950.0, Suicide and self-inflicted poisoning by analgesics, antipyretics, and antirheumatics (suicide attempt)

6. Late effect of a poisoning is coded as follows:
   - First code the residual (specified effect), such as deafness or blindness.
   - Assign a code to identify a late effect of poisoning by drugs: 909.0, Late effect of poisoning due to drug, medicinal or biological substance; or 909.1, Late effect of toxic effects of nonmedical substances.
     - Code 909.0 is found in the Alphabetic Index to Diseases under "Late, effect(s) (of), poisoning due to drug, medicinal or biological substance."
     - Code 909.1 is found in the Alphabetic Index to Diseases under "Late effect(s) (of), toxic effect of, nonmedical substance."
   - Use the Alphabetic Index to External Causes to assign one of the following E codes to describe the late effect of an external cause:
     - E929.2, Late effects of accidental poisoning: Found in the Index to External Causes under "Late effect of, poisoning, accidental"
     - E959, Late effects of self-inflicted injury: Found in the Index to External Causes under "Late effect of, suicide, attempt (any means)"
     - E969, Late effects of injury purposely inflicted by other person: Found in the Index to External Causes under "Late effect of, assault"
     - E977, Late effects of injuries due to legal intervention: Found in the Index to External Causes under "Late effect of, legal intervention"
     - E989, Late effects of injury, undetermined whether accidentally or purposely inflicted: Found in the Index to External Causes under "Late effect of, injury undetermined whether accidentally or purposely inflicted"

**Note:** Although E codes are usually optional, it is best to double-check the requirements of the particular state or facility where the coding is being done.

See figure 20.2 for assistance in coding poisonings.

**Figure 20.2.** Coding poisonings

| Current Injury | | Late Effect |
|---|---|---|
| Code from 960–979 | ←Principal Diagnosis→ | Specified effect—deafness, blindness, etc. |
| ***Plus*** | | ***Plus*** |
| Specified effect—tachycardia, coma | ←Other Diagnosis→ | Late effect 909.0 or 909.1 |
| **And** | | **And** |
| E code from one of the following "External Cause" columns of Table of Drugs and Chemicals:<br>accident<br>suicide attempt<br>assault<br>undetermined | ←Other Diagnosis→ | E929.2 or<br>E959 or<br>E969 or<br>E977 or<br>E989 |

**In general, E codes for poisonings are optional, although many healthcare facilities and some states mandate their use.**

Codes 960–979 are never used in combination with codes E930–E949 because codes 960–979 identify poisonings and codes E930–E949 identify the external cause of adverse reactions to correct substances properly administered.

## Exercise 20.3

Assign ICD-9-CM codes to the following:

1. Accidental ingestion of mother's oral contraceptives

2. Lead poisoning from eating paint, accidental injury by a child

3. Listlessness from prescribed Valium and six-pack of beer (grain alcohol). The intent is undetermined.

4. Stricture of esophagus due to accidental lye ingestion 3 years ago

5. Carbon monoxide poisoning from car exhaust in a suicide attempt; victim found in car parked in garage

## Complications of Surgical and Medical Care, Not Elsewhere Classified (996–999)

When a causal relationship is stated between a condition and the surgical or medical care, a code from categories 996–999 may be assigned. A time limit has not been identified because some complications may occur during or directly following surgery, while others may occur later during the same hospitalization or even days, weeks, or months after discharge. In some cases, documentation in the record will clearly state a complication, such as colitis due to radiation therapy. In other cases, documentation in the record will identify symptoms that may refer to a complication. The coder should not make the assumption that all conditions that occur after a medical or surgical procedure are complications as classified by ICD-9-CM in the range of 996–999. Specific documentation in the health record must state the causal relationship between the condition and the complication code(s). When there is a doubt as to the intent of the physician's documentation, the physician must be asked for clarification, including additional documentation entered into the patient's record. This section of ICD-9-CM, categories 996–999, contains numerous includes and excludes notes as well as directions to use additional codes that are intended to aid the coder in locating the most complete and accurate codes. For example, postoperative pain is classified to Diseases of the nervous system and sense organs chapter, category 338, Pain, not elsewhere classified.

The section "Complications of Surgical and Medical Care, Not Elsewhere Classified" is subdivided into the following categories:

**996 Complications peculiar to certain specified procedures**
**997 Complications affecting specified body systems, not elsewhere classified**
**998 Other complications of procedures, not elsewhere classified**
**999 Complications of medical care, not elsewhere classified**

## Classification of Complications

Complications specific to one anatomical site are classified in the chapter of ICD-9-CM for that anatomical site. All other complications are included in codes 996–999.

The following large exclusion note appears at the beginning of the complications section:

**Complications of Surgical and Medical Care,**
**Not Elsewhere Classified** (996–999)

*adverse effects of medicinal agents (001.0–799.9, 995.0–995.8)*
*burns from local applications and irradiation (940.0–949.5)*
*complications of:*
*conditions for which the procedure was performed*
*surgical procedures during abortion,*
*labor, and delivery (630–676.9)*
*poisoning and toxic effects of drugs and chemicals (960.0–989.9)*
*postoperative conditions in which no complications*
*are present, such as:*
*artificial opening status (V44.0–V44.9)*
*Closure of external stoma (V55.0–V55.9)*
*fitting of prosthetic device (V52.0–V52.9)*
*specified complications classified elsewhere*
*anesthetic shock (995.4)*
*electrolyte imbalance (276.0–276.9)*
*postlaminectomy syndrome (722.80–722.83)*
*postmastectomy lymphedema syndrome (457.0)*
*postoperative psychosis (293.0–293.9)*
*any other condition classified elsewhere in the Alphabetic*
*Index when described as due to a procedure*

The excludes note lists many complications/conditions that are not classified to this section. For example, adverse effects of medicinal agents are assigned to codes 001.0–799.9 and 995.0–995.89.

### Category 996

Category 996 includes codes that identify complications in the use of artificial substitutes or natural sources. The large inclusion note at the beginning of this category describes procedures in which artificial substitutes or natural sources are used.

Codes 996.00–996.59 identify mechanical complications of prosthetic devices, implants, and grafts. Complications include the mechanical breakdown, displacement, leakage, mechanical obstruction, perforation, or protrusion of the device, implant, or graft.

Total joint replacement (TJR) is one of the most commonly performed and successful operations in orthopedic surgery. The American Academy of Orthopaedic Surgeons (AAOS) states that "most hip and knee replacement procedures will perform well for the remainder of the patient's life. Current hip and knee replacements are expected to function at least 10 to 20 years in 90 percent of patients" (AAOS 2007).

As the population in the United States ages, and advances in technology lead to the expansion of the indications for TJR to include younger and more active patients, the prevalence of TJR is expected to increase over the next decade. Although most hip and knee replacements last for 15 to 20 years or longer, some hip and knee replacements can fail, necessitating revision surgery. Common reasons for revision joint replacement surgery include mechanical loosening of the prosthesis, dislocation of the prosthetic joint, fracture of the bone around the implant, and implant fracture or failure. To classify the mechanical reasons for revision joint replacement, ICD-9-CM diagnosis codes 996.40–996.49 are provided. In addition to one of these codes, the patient should also be assigned a code from the V43.60–V43.69 range to identify the joint previously replaced by prosthesis.

Other reasons for revision joint replacement surgery are infection or inflammatory reactions due to internal joint prosthesis (996.66) or other complications, such as pain due to the presence of the internal joint prosthesis (996.77).

**996.4 Mechanical complication of internal orthopedic device, implant, and graft**

Mechanical complications involving:
- external (fixation) device utilizing internal screw(s), pin(s), or other methods of fixation
- grafts of bone, cartilage, muscle, or tendon
- internal (fixation) device such as nail, plate, rod, etc.

Use additional code to identify prosthetic joint with mechanical complication (V43.60–V43.69)

*Excludes:* *complications of external orthopedic device, such as: pressure ulcer due to cast (707.00–707.09)*

Subcategory 996.6 identifies infection and inflammatory reaction due to an internal prosthetic device, implant, and graft. The fifth-digit subclassification identifies the type of device, implant, or graft, or the organ system involved. Included under this subcategory heading is a directional note: Use additional code to identify specified infections.

> **996.61 Due to cardiac device, implant, and graft**
> Cardiac pacemaker or defibrillator:
> electrode(s), lead(s)
> pulse generator
> subcutaneous pocket
> Coronary artery bypass graft
> Heart valve prosthesis

Subcategory 996.7 classifies other complications of internal prosthetic devices, implants, and grafts, such as embolism, fibrosis, hemorrhage, pain, stenosis, and thrombus, as well as complications not otherwise specified. Again, the fifth-digit subclassification identifies the specific device or organ system involved. However, problems that occur at the end of life of a mechanical device are an expected outcome and not a complication coded to subcategory 996.7. For example, a prosthetic heart valve may develop stenosis at the end of its expected life or functional duration. The heart valve must be replaced. If the physician documented prosthetic valve stenosis due to end of life of the prosthetic valve, the principal diagnosis code for this example would be V53.39, Fitting and adjustment of other device, other cardiac device. A frequently used code from this subcategory identifies a common complication of renal dialysis grafts:

> **996.73 Due to renal dialysis device, implant, and graft**

Codes under subcategory 996.8 classify both complications and rejection of transplanted organs. A transplant complication code is only assigned if the complication affects the function of the transplanted organ. Two codes are required to fully describe a transplant complication. The specific organ is identified at the fifth-digit subclassification of 996.8. An additional code should be assigned to identify the nature of the complication, such as cytomegalovirus infection.

**EXAMPLE:** **996.81 Complications of transplanted kidney**
**078.5 Cytomegaloviral disease**

Code 996.9 classifies complications of a reattached extremity or body part. The fifth-digit subclassification identifies the specific extremity or body part.

> **996.92 Complications of reattached hand**

## Category 997

Category 997 includes complications of specified body systems not classified elsewhere in ICD-9-CM. The subcategories and subclassifications identify the organ system involved or the specific complication, such as hepatic failure resulting from a surgical procedure (997.49).

**997.4 Digestive system complications**

Complications of:

intestinal (internal) anastomosis and bypass, not elsewhere classified, except that involving urinary tract

Hepatic failure
Hepatorenal syndrome
Intestinal obstruction NOS
} specified as due to a procedure

Excludes: *specified gastrointestinal complications*

*complications of gastric band procedure (539.01–539.09)*
*complications of other bariatric procedure (539.81–539.89)*
*specified gastrointestinal complications classified elsewhere, such as:*
*blind loop syndrome (579.2)*
*colostomy and enterostomy complications (569.60–569.69)*
*complications of intestinal pouch (569.71–569.79)*
*gastrojejunal ulcer (534.0–534.9)*
*gastrostomy complications (536.40–536.49)*
*infection of esophagostomy (530.86)*
*infection of external stoma (569.61)*
*mechanical complication of esophagostomy (530.87)*
*pelvic peritoneal adhesions, female (614.6)*
*peritoneal adhesions (568.0)*
*peritoneal adhesions with obstruction (560.81)*
*postcholecystectomy syndrome (576.0)*
*postgastric surgery syndromes (564.2)*
*pouchitis (569.71)*
*vomiting following gastrointestinal surgery (564.3)*

A note at the beginning of category 997 states "Use additional code to identify complications." It serves as a reminder that an additional code should be assigned to further identify the specific complication.

**EXAMPLE:** **997.1 Cardiac complications**
**427.31 Atrial fibrillation**

Hospital-acquired pneumonia is the second-most-common hospital-associated infection, after catheter-associated urinary tract infections. The primary risk factor for developing hospital-associated bacterial pneumonia is mechanical ventilation with endotracheal intubation or tracheostomy. Mechanical ventilation provides the necessary respiratory support for critically ill patients who are unable to breathe on their own, but the mechanical ventilation puts patients at risk for ventilator-associated pneumonia (VAP). The Centers for Disease Control and Prevention (CDC), as well as other medical specialty organizations, have guidelines related to the prevention, diagnosis, and management of VAP. A unique code to identify VAP (997.31) appears in ICD-9-CM under subcategory 997.3, Respiratory complications. A "use additional code" note appears under code 997.31 to remind the coder to assign an additional code to identify the infectious organism associated with VAP. A code from categories 480–484 should not be assigned to identify the type of pneumonia. Code 997.31 also should not be assigned for a patient with pneumonia who is placed on a mechanical ventilator when the physician has not specifically stated that the pneumonia is VAP.

### Category 998

Category 998 includes other complications of procedures not classified elsewhere in ICD-9-CM. The subcategories identify the type of complication, such as postoperative shock, hemorrhage or hematoma, accidental puncture or laceration, foreign body accidentally left in operation wound or body cavity, postoperative infection, postoperative fistula, and reaction to foreign body accidentally left in operation wound or body cavity. Disruption of operation wound (wound dehiscence) is classified according to whether it is an internal or external operation wound. There is a code for an unspecified type of wound disruption in cases where the physician does not describe the disruption as internal or external. An additional code exists to classify the disruption of a traumatic injury wound repair for a previously closed traumatic laceration.

### Category 999

Category 999 includes complications of medical care not elsewhere classified. The inclusion note at the beginning of this category identifies the types of complications included in this category. Similarly, it identifies complications classified elsewhere in ICD-9-CM. Some of the complications classified in category 999 are complications that can be acquired during hospital stays. Some of these conditions can be very serious and even life threatening. An example of one of these is air embolism, ICD-9-CM code 999.1.

Other conditions are less threatening and are manageable with proper care. An infection due to the presence of a central line catheter is coded with ICD-9-CM code 999.31–999.33, depending on the type of infection. Central line catheters, such as triple lumen, Hickman, and peripherally-inserted central catheter (PICC), are used for long-term intravenous (IV) infusions.

Infusion reactions including extravasation of vesicant chemotherapy or other vesicant agents can occur when there is leakage of the IV drug from the vein into surrounding tissue. Vesicants can produce pain at the site, cause blistering and discoloration on the skin or mucous membrane tissue, and produce significant tissue destruction. These serious reactions that produce injury or damage are coded according to the type of vesicant involved: 999.81, Extravasation of vesicant chemotherapy, and 999.82, Extravasation of other vesicant agent. Not all IV infiltrations or extravasations need to be coded because they usually do not produce injury or damage to the patient. However, when IV infiltrations produce a complication such as infection (999.39), phlebitis (999.2), or sloughing of skin (999.9), and the care of the complication results in an increase in the length of stay or intensity of care, the specific complication should be coded.

Other conditions classified in this category are blood transfusion reactions. A hemolytic transfusion reaction (HTR) is a reaction of increasing destruction of red blood cells due to incompatibility between blood donor and blood recipient. The reaction is noted by such clinical signs as fever, chills, and rigors and laboratory testing signs of hemoglobinuria, presence of antibiotics to RBC antigens, and ABO and non-ABO incompatibility. Hemolytic reactions can be either acute or delayed depending on the timing of occurrence. Acute reactions occur within 24 hours of a transfusion. Delayed reactions can appear between 24 hours and one month after a blood transfusion. The reactions can be due to either blood type A, B, or O (ABO), or non-ABO incompatibility. Non-ABO incompatibility may be due to an Rh incompatibility. HTRs are the leading cause of transfusion-related deaths, but these complications are relatively rare.

Due to advances in donor screening, improved viral marker tests, automated data systems, and changes in transfusion medicine practices, the risks associated with blood transfusion continue to decrease. Overall, the number of transfusion-related fatalities reported to the US Food and Drug Administration (FDA) remains small in comparison to the total number of transfusions. For example, according to the FDA, in 2011, there were approximately 21 million components transfused. During 2011, there were 58 reported transfusion-related and potentially transfusion-related fatalities, with subsequent reports of 65 deaths in 2012, and 59 deaths in 2013 (FDA 2014).

ICD-9-CM diagnosis coding distinguishes between ABO and non-ABO HTRs and between acute and delayed HTRs and other forms of transfusion-related reactions. Codes 999.60–999.69 identify ABO incompatibility reactions due to transfusions of blood or blood products. Codes 999.70–999.79 identify Rh and non-ABO incompatibility reactions. For less specific forms of transfusion reactions, codes 999.80–999.89 are available, but the coder is advised to seek more information about the reaction from the attending physician so as to assign the most specific code available for each patient. Other forms of transfusion reactions include transfusion-related acute lung injury (TRALI) (ICD-9-CM code 518.7), transfusion-associated circulatory overload (TACO) (code 276.61), and febrile nonhemolytic reaction (FNHTR) (code 780.66).

**999 Complications of medical care, not elsewhere classified**

Includes: complications, not elsewhere classified, of:
- dialysis (hemodialysis) (peritoneal) (renal)
- extracorporeal circulation
- hyperalimentation therapy
- immunization
- infusion
- inhalation therapy
- injection
- inoculation
- perfusion
- transfusion
- vaccination
- ventilation therapy

Use additional code, where applicable, to identify specific complication

*Excludes:* *specified complications classified elsewhere such as:*
- *complications of implanted device (996.0–996.9)*
- *contact dermatitis due to drugs (692.3)*
- *dementia dialysis (294.8)*
  - *transient (293.9)*
- *dialysis disequilibrium syndrome (276.0–276.9)*
- *poisoning and toxic effects of drugs and chemicals (960.0–989.9)*
- *postvaccinal encephalitis (323.51)*
- *water and electrolyte imbalance (276.0–276.9)*

### Instructions for Coding Complications

The following instructions apply when coding complications:

1. After confirming that there is a causal relationship between the patient's condition and the surgical or medical care provided, locate the main term for the complication in the Alphabetic Index to Diseases (for example, malabsorption).
2. Check for a subterm indicating that the condition is a result of a complication of medical or surgical care.

| | |
|---|---|
| **Malabsorption** | 579.9 |
| postgastrectomy | 579.3 |
| postsurgical | 579.3 |

3. If a specific code is not identified, consult the main term "Complications" to locate an appropriate code by condition or system.

| | |
|---|---|
| **Complications** | |
| aortocoronary (bypass) graft | 996.03 |

4. When no appropriate code can be found, assign the following nonspecific complication codes only if documentation in the health record supports their assignment. However, the coder should be cautious in assigning these nonspecific codes. If the documentation in the health record is vague, these codes should not be assigned without clarification with the documenting physician.

| | |
|---|---|
| **Complications** | |
| medical care NEC | 999.9 |
| surgical procedures | 998.9 |

5. A second code may be assigned for more specificity if the complication code is too general.

**997.1 Cardiac complications**

Cardiac
  arrest
  insufficiency
Cardiorespiratory failure
Heart failure

} during or resulting from a procedure

*Excludes:* *the listed conditions as long-term effects of cardiac surgery or due to the presence of cardiac prosthetic device (429.4)*

In the preceding example, a second code would be assigned to further describe the cardiac complication, such as cardiac arrest or heart failure.

## Exercise 20.4

Assign ICD-9-CM codes to the following:

1. Infection from ventriculoperitoneal shunt

2. Postmastoidectomy complication

3. Leakage of mitral valve prosthesis

4. Postoperative superficial thrombophlebitis of the right leg

5. Displaced breast prosthesis

## ICD-9-CM Review Exercises: Chapter 20

Assign the appropriate ICD-9-CM codes to the following:

1. Urticaria due to tetracycline, prescribed by physician

2. Operative wound dehiscence

3. Methadone overdose, suicide attempt

4. Air embolism

5. Patient mixed Diuril and alcoholic beverage, which resulted in syncope, described as an accident

6. Severe vomiting due to Cytoxan, which is being administered for bone metastasis with unknown primary site

7. Dislocated hip prosthesis with closed reduction

*(Continued on next page)*

## ICD-9-CM Review Exercises: Chapter 20 (Continued)

8. Postoperative wound infection with cellulitis, lower leg; cellulitis due to *Staphylococcus aureus* infection

9. Chronic cholecystitis with cholelithiasis with postoperative atelectasis; cholecystectomy with intraoperative cholangiogram

10. Attempted suicide with 15 Tylenol (acetaminophen) and 10 ampicillin; depression

11. Ventilator-associated pneumonia

12. Superficial disruption of external operative wound (skin)

13. Thrombophlebitis following intravenous infusion, right arm

14. Transfusion reaction

15. PICC (central venous) line infection

# ICD-10-CM Chapter 19, Injury, Poisoning and Certain Other Consequences of External Causes (S00–T88)

## Organization and Structure of ICD-10-CM Chapter 19

This chapter's discussion of ICD-10-CM, Chapter 19 will focus on the poisoning and certain other consequences of external cause codes.

The codes within this subject are:

| | |
|---|---|
| T36–T50 | Poisoning by, adverse effect of and underdosing of drugs, medicaments and biological substances |
| T51–T65 | Toxic effects of substances chiefly nonmedicinal as to source |
| T66–T78 | Other and unspecified effects of external causes |

T79 Certain early complications of trauma

T80–T88 Complications of surgical and medical care, not elsewhere classified

A significant classification change was made to poisonings by and adverse effects of drugs, medicaments, and biological substances (T36–T50). ICD-10-CM does not provide different category codes to identify poisonings versus adverse effect. Instead, under a single category for a specific drug are codes for poisonings, adverse effects and underdosing of drugs, medicaments and biological substances. Underdosing is a new terminology in ICD-10-CM and is defined as taking less of a medication than is prescribed by a provider or the manufacturer's instructions with a resulting negative health consequence.

**EXAMPLE:** **T46.1 Poisoning by, adverse effect of, and underdosing of calcium-channel blockers**

T46.1X1 Poisoning by calcium-channel blocker, accidental (unintentional)

T46.1X2 Poisoning by calcium-channel blocker, intentional self-harm

T46.1X3 Poisoning by calcium-channel blocker, assault

T46.1X4 Poisoning by calcium-channel blocker, undetermined

T46.1X5 Adverse effect of calcium-channel blocker

T46.1X6 Underdosing of calcium-channel blocker

Sequencing issues are eliminated because poisonings, adverse effects, and underdosing are combination codes.

## Coding Guidelines and Instructional Notes for Chapter 19

A change has occurred to the instruction for complications of surgical and medical care, not elsewhere classified (T80–T88). In ICD-9-CM, there is no guideline under this subchapter. However, ICD-10-CM includes a note stating to use additional code (Y62–Y82) to identify devices involved and details of circumstances.

There are chapter-specific guidelines for Chapter 19 of ICD-10-CM:

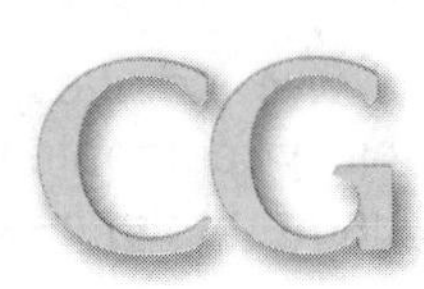


- Guidelines I.C.19.e. Adverse effects, poisoning, underdosing and toxic effects
    - Codes in categories T36–T65 are combination codes that include the substances related to adverse effects, poisonings, toxic effects, and underdosing, as well as the external cause (intent). No additional external cause code is required for poisonings, toxic effects, adverse effects, and underdosing codes.
    - When coding an adverse effect of a drug that has been correctly prescribed and properly administered, assign the appropriate code for the nature of the

*(Continued)*

(*Continued*)

adverse effect followed by the appropriate code for the adverse effect of the drug (T36–T50.) The code for the drugs should have a fifth or sixth character 5. Examples of the nature of an adverse effect are diarrhea, vomiting, and renal or respiratory failure.

When coding a poisoning or reaction to the improper use of a medication such as an overdose or the wrong drug administered, first assign the appropriate code from categories T36–T50. The poisoning code should have the fifth or sixth character for the associated intent (accidental, intentional self-harm, assault, and undetermined). Additional codes should be assigned for all manifestations of poisonings. If there is also a diagnosis of abuse or dependence of the substance, the abuse or dependence code is also assigned as an additional code.

- Underdosing refers to taking less of a medication than is prescribed by a provider or a manufacturer's instruction. For underdosing, assign the code from categories T36–T50 (fifth or sixth character 6). Codes for underdosing should never be assigned as principal or first-listed codes. If a patient has a relapse or exacerbation of the medical condition for which the drug is prescribed because of the reduction in dose, then the medical condition itself should be coded.
- Noncompliance (Z91.12-, Z91.13-) or complication of care (Y63.61, Y63.8–Y63.9) codes are to be used with an underdosing code to indicate intent, if known.

There are additional coding guidelines published for this chapter including:

- Guideline I.C.19.f. Adult and child abuse, neglect and other maltreatment
- Guideline I.C.19.g. Complications of care

To gain a complete understanding of these rules, access the 2014 guidelines from NCHS website (http://www.cdc.gov/nchs/icd/icd10cm.htm) and read Chapter 19, Injury, poisoning and certain other consequences of external causes guidelines I.C.19.e through I.C.19.g.

## Coding Overview for ICD-10-CM, Chapter 19

Chapter 19 encompasses two alpha characters. The S section provides codes for the various types of injuries related to single body regions; the T section covers injuries to unspecified body regions as well as poisonings and certain other consequences of external causes.

Poisoning by, adverse effects of and underdosing of drugs, medicaments and biological substances (T36–T50) includes the following instructions:

| | |
|---|---|
| *Includes:* | adverse effect of correct substance properly administered<br>poisoning of overdose of substance<br>poisoning by wrong substance given or taken in error<br>underdosing by (inadvertently) (deliberately) taking less substance than prescribed or instructed<br>Code first, for adverse effects, the nature of the adverse effect, such as:<br>adverse effect NOS (T88.7)<br>aspirin gastritis (K29.-) blood disorders (D56–D76)<br>contact dermatitis (L23–L25)<br>dermatitis due to substance taken internally (L27.-)<br>nephropathy (N14.0–N14.2) |
| Note: | The drug giving rise to the adverse effect should be identified by use of codes from categories T36–T50 with fifth or sixth character 5.<br>Use additional code(s) to specify:<br>manifestations of poisoning<br>underdosing or failure in dosage during medical and surgical care (Y63.6, Y63.8–Y63.9)<br>underdosing of medication regimen (Z91.12-, Z91.13-)<br>There are also two excludes notes appearing at the start of the section T36–T50. |

There are combination codes for poisonings and the associated external cause (accidental, intentional self-harm, assault, undetermined), and the table of Drugs and Chemicals groups all poisoning columns together, followed by adverse effect and underdosing. When no intent of poisoning is indicated, code to accidental. Undetermined intent is only for use when there is specific documentation in the record that the intent of the poisoning cannot be determined.

Toxic effects of substances chiefly nonmedicinal as to source (T51–T65) provides direction to use additional code(s) for all associated manifestations of toxic effect, such as:

> Use additional code(s) for all associated manifestations of toxic effect, such as:
> personal history of foreign body fully removed (Z87.821)
> respiratory conditions due to external agents (J60–J70)
> to identify any retained foreign body, if applicable (Z18.-)

A note also appears that states when no intent is indicated, the condition should be coded to accidental intent. Undetermined intent is only for use when there is specific documentation in the record that the intent of the toxic effect cannot be determined.

ICD-10-CM's Chapter 19, Injury, Poisoning and Certain Other Consequences of External Causes (S00–T88), represents a substantial reorganization from ICD-9-CM. Codes in categories T36–T50 are combination codes. The codes identify whether the condition is a poisoning, adverse effect, or underdosing of drugs or biological substances. The external cause is included within the codes themselves and not coded separately.

In addition, the seventh character indicates whether the episode of care is the initial encounter (A), subsequent encounter (D), or sequela (S) of the past poisoning, adverse effect or underdosing. An example of a combination code is T36.0X1A, Poisoning by penicillins, accidental (unintentional, initial encounter). Although poisoning and adverse effects of drugs are defined similarly to the ICD-9-CM definition, underdosing is a new concept in ICD-10-CM. The terms are described as follows:

- Poisoning is an overdose of a substance or the wrong substance given or taken in error.
- An adverse effect is a hypersensitivity or reaction to a substance correctly prescribed and properly administered.
- Underdosing is taking less of a medication than is prescribed or instructed by the provider or manufacturer, whether inadvertently or deliberately.

In ICD-10-CM, contrary to rules in ICD-9-CM, when no intent of poisoning is indicated, the poisoning is coded to accidental intent. Undetermined intent is only for use when there is specific documentation that the intent of the poisoning cannot be determined.

When coding an adverse effect of a drug properly prescribed and administered, the code for the nature of the adverse effect is coded first, followed by the code for the adverse effect of the drug (T36–T50.) When coding a poisoning or reaction to the improper use of a medication given or taken in error, the code from categories T36–T50 is assigned first with additional codes used for all manifestations of the poisoning.

This instruction does not apply to the coding of underdosing events. When coding an episode of care where underdosing is diagnosed and the patient has a relapse or exacerbation of the medical condition for which the drug is prescribed because of the reduction in dose, the medical condition is coded first. A code from categories T36–T50 is sequenced as an additional code after the medical condition, followed by an additional code for intent of underdosing—that is, failure in dosage during medical and surgical care (Y63.61, Y63.8, Y63.9) or patient's underdosing of medication regime (Z91.12-, Z91.13-). The underdosing code should never be principal or first-listed codes. If a patient has a relapse or exacerbation of the medical condition for which the drug was prescribed because of the reduction in dose, then the medical condition should be coded first.

The ICD-10-CM Table of Drugs and Chemicals is organized into seven columns with rows for the substances involved. The first, left-most column contains the name of the drug, chemical, or biologic substance. The next six columns contain:

- Poisoning, accidental (unintentional)
- Poisoning, intentional self-harm
- Poisoning, assault
- Poisoning, undetermined
- Adverse effect
- Underdosing

T codes in ICD-10-CM are also available for coding the toxic effect of substances that are chiefly nonmedicinal in nature. For example, the code for toxic effect of carbon monoxide from motor vehicle exhaust, accidental (unintentional), initial encounter, is T58.01XA. Note that this is an example of a code that requires a seventh character but is less than six characters long (T58.01). In this code, a placeholder character of **X** is used to fill the missing sixth character. The seventh character must always be a valid seventh-character in a code; it cannot take the place of a missing sixth character. As discussed earlier, the placeholder character concept is new to ICD-10-CM.

## ICD-10-CM Coding Exercises: Chapter 20

Assign the correct ICD-10-CM diagnosis codes to the following exercises (Do not assign external cause codes).

1. Child is seen emergently for an accidental overdose of acetaminophen. He inadvertently ate several of these when he found an open bottle at home.

2. The woman is admitted for an intentional overdose of marijuana and cocaine. She sustained a fall which resulted in a left cheek and scalp laceration. After she is stabilized medically, she will be transferred to a psychiatric unit. (Do not assign external cause codes.)

3. This patient is seen in the hospital with a diagnosis of congestive heart failure due to hypertensive heart disease. Patient also has stage 5 chronic kidney failure. The patient had been prescribed Lasix previously but admits that he forgets to take his medication every day. This is due to his advanced age. What are the correct diagnosis codes? (Do not assign external cause codes.)

4. A patient has been taking Digoxin and is experiencing nausea and vomiting and profound fatigue. The patient indicates that he has been taking the drug appropriately. The evaluation and treatment was focused on adjustment of medication only. (Do not assign external cause codes.)

5. This elderly woman is seen for increased right hip pain. She has a right hip prosthesis. After extensive evaluation, she is found to have an infection of the prosthesis. She will be scheduled for surgery. (Do not assign external cause codes.)

6. The patient was in the cardiac cath lab for insertion of a dual chamber pacemaker to treat his sick sinus syndrome. During the procedure the pacemaker electrode broke upon insertion. The procedure was abandoned and will be rescheduled. (Do not assign external cause codes.)

7. Allergic Urticaria due to oral tetracycline, prescribed by physician, properly prescribed and administered

8. Patient admits he forgets to take his anticoagulant as prescribed because of his age related senility and developed a recurrent acute vein thrombosis in the iliac vein of his right lower leg as a result of the underdosing of his anticoagulant.

9. The patient was admitted to the intensive care unit in acute respiratory failure due to an intentional overdose of a large amount of lorazepam according to a note left by the patient. The patient was known to suffer from anxiety and depression.

10. The patient was treated for an infection of her intraperitoneal dialysis catheter.

# Chapter 21

# Supplementary Classification of External Causes of Injury and Poisoning (ICD-9-CM, E000–E999) and External Causes of Morbidity (ICD-10-CM, V00–Y99)

## Learning Objectives

At the conclusion of this chapter, you should be able to:

1. Describe the organization of the codes in the External Causes of Injury and Poisoning (E000–E999) in ICD-9-CM and in the External Causes of Morbidity (V00–Y99) in ICD-10-CM
2. Define what the external cause codes represent
3. Be familiar with the separate ICD-9-CM Alphabetic Index to External Causes of Injury and Poisoning and the ICD-10-CM Alphabetic Index to External Causes of Morbidity and identify the terminology used as main terms
4. Explain the sequencing of external cause codes in comparison with diagnosis codes
5. Describe the multiple-cause coding guidelines for external cause codes, focusing on the priority given to particular E codes in terms of sequencing and reporting
6. Assign ICD-9-CM E codes from the supplementary classification to describe the external cause of injury, including the place of occurrence
7. Assign ICD-10-CM codes for external causes of morbidity

## ICD-9-CM Supplementary Classification of External External Causes of Injury and Poisoning (E000–E999)

External causes of injury and poisoning or **E codes** classify environmental events, circumstances, and other conditions as the cause of injuries and other adverse effects. Coding external causes of injuries and poisonings provides data for research and evaluation of injury prevention strategies. E codes capture how the injury, poisoning, or adverse effect happened (cause), the intent (intentional, such as an assault; or unintentional, such as an accident), the person's status (for example, civilian, military), the associated activity, and the place where the event occurred.

The E Codes Supplementary Classification in the Tabular List in Volume 1 of ICD-9-CM includes the following categories and section titles:

| Categories | Section Titles |
|---|---|
| E000 | External Cause Status |
| E001–E030 | Activity |
| E800–E848 | Transport Accidents |
| E849 | Place of Occurrence |
| E850–E858 | Accidental Poisoning by Drugs, Medicinal Substances, and Biologicals |
| E860–E869 | Accidental Poisoning by Other Solid and Liquid Substances, Gases, and Vapors |
| E870–E876 | Misadventures to Patients during Surgical and Medical Care |
| E878–E879 | Surgical and Medical Procedures as the Cause of Abnormal Reaction of Patient, or Later Complication, without Mention of Misadventure at the Time of Procedure |
| E880–E888 | Accidental Falls |
| E890–E899 | Accidents Caused by Fire and Flames |
| E900–E909 | Accidents Due to Natural and Environmental Factors |
| E910–E915 | Accidents Caused by Submersion, Suffocation, and Foreign Bodies |
| E916–E928 | Other Accidents |
| E929 | Late Effects of Accidental Injury |
| E930–E949 | Drugs, Medicinal and Biological Substances Causing Adverse Effects in Therapeutic Use |
| E950–E959 | Suicide and Self-Inflicted Injury |
| E960–E969 | Homicide and Injury Purposely Inflicted by Other Persons |
| E970–E978 | Legal Intervention |
| E979 | Terrorism |
| E980–E989 | Injury Undetermined Whether Accidentally or Purposely Inflicted |
| E990–E999 | Injury Resulting from Operations of War |

## E Codes as Additional Codes Only

An E code cannot be assigned as the principal, first-listed, or the only listed diagnosis code. E codes from the supplementary classification are used in addition to a code from the main chapters of ICD-9-CM classification that identifies the nature of the illness or injury. E codes provide additional information that may be extremely useful to public health agencies and may assist healthcare planners to determine the kinds of accidents a particular facility treats. E codes can identify patients who were injured in transportation accidents, fires, or national disasters, as well as in a wide variety of other situations.

## Alphabetic Index

The Alphabetic Index to External Causes of Injury and Poisoning (E Codes) is a separate index that follows the Table of Drugs and Chemicals in volume 2 of ICD-9-CM. The E code index is organized by main terms describing the accident, circumstance, event, or specific agent that caused the injury or other adverse effect, such as a collision, earthquake, or dog bite.

**Fall, falling** (accidental) E888.9
  building E916
    burning E891.8
      private E890.8
  down
    escalator E880.0
    ladder E881.0
      in boat, ship, watercraft E833
    staircase E880.9
    stairs, steps—*see* Fall, from, stairs
  earth (with asphyxia or suffocation (by pressure)
      (*see also* Earth, falling) E913.3

## Exercise 21.1

Identify the external event that caused the following injuries and assign E codes only:

1. Fractured radius resulting from accidental fall into hole

   ______________________

2. Fracture of humerus due to fall from cliff

   ______________________

3. Hematoma of buttocks from tackle during football game

   ______________________

4. Burn of left palm from splashing grease

   ______________________

5. Firecracker injury with second-degree burn of face

   ______________________

## Use of E Codes

There is no national requirement for mandatory external causes (E) code reporting. Unless a provider is subject to a state-based E code reporting mandate, for example, reporting of certain patients treated in a hospital trauma center or if the codes are required by a specific payer, reporting of E codes is not required. In the absence of a mandatory reporting requirement, providers are encouraged to report E codes as it provides valuable data for injury research and evaluation of injury prevention strategies.

For these reasons, the use of E codes in many healthcare facilities is optional, except for categories E930–E949, Drugs, Medicinal and Biological Substances Causing Adverse Effects in Therapeutic Use in ICD-9-CM. (Refer to chapter 20 in this textbook for the use of these E codes in those circumstances). Each healthcare facility must decide whether it needs the information the E codes provide. Today, information on industrial accidents may be of great value to hospitals planning to market healthcare plans to employers in their market area.

**A point to remember:** Some states mandate the use of some or all E codes. Always check with the policy of the facility or state mandate where the coding is being done to confirm the use of external causes codes.

An E code may be used as an additional code in any category if documentation in the health record supports that use. However, an E code cannot be assigned as a principal or first-listed diagnosis.

## Guidelines for Coding External Causes of Injury, Poisoning, and Adverse Effects of Drugs (E Codes)

The guidelines discussed in the following subsections apply when coding and collecting E codes from health records in hospitals, outpatient clinics, emergency departments, other ambulatory care settings, and physicians' offices.

### *General E Code Guidelines*

An E code from categories E800–E999 may be used with any code in the range of 001–V91 that indicates an injury, poisoning, or adverse effect due to an external cause. An activity E code (categories E001–E030) may be used with a code in the range of 001–V91 that indicates an injury or other health condition that resulted from an activity, or the activity contributed to the condition. General guidelines include:

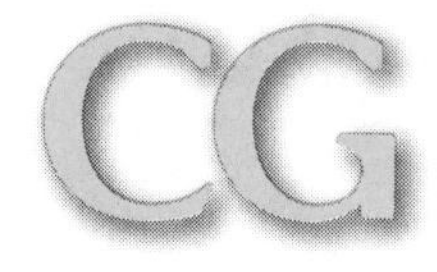


- Assign the appropriate E code for all initial encounters or treatments of an injury, poisoning, or adverse effect of drugs—but not for subsequent treatment.
- Use a late effect E code for subsequent visits when a late effect of the initial injury or poisoning is being treated. There is no late effect E code for adverse effects of drugs.
- Do not use a late effect E code for subsequent visits for follow-up care (for example, to assess healing or to receive rehabilitative treatment) of the injury or poisoning when no late effect of the injury has been documented.
- Use the full range of E codes to completely describe the cause, intent, and place of occurrence, if applicable, for all injuries, poisonings, and adverse effects of drugs.
- Assign as many E codes as necessary to fully explain each external cause. If only one E code can be recorded, assign the one most related to the principal diagnosis.
- Select appropriate E codes by referring to the Index to External Causes and by reading inclusion and exclusion notes in the Tabular List.

## Multiple-Cause Coding Guidelines for E Codes

More than one E code is required to fully describe the external cause of an illness, injury, or poisoning. The assignment of E codes should be sequenced in the following priority.

If two or more events cause separate injuries, an E code should be assigned for each cause. The E code to be listed first will be selected on the following basis:

1. E codes for child and adult abuse take priority over all other E codes, except as described in the child and adult abuse guidelines below.
2. E codes for terrorism events take priority over all other E codes except child and adult abuse.
3. E codes for cataclysmic events take priority over all other E codes, except for child and adult abuse and terrorism.
4. E codes for transport accidents take priority over all other E codes, except for cataclysmic events and for child and adult abuse and terrorism.
5. Activity and external cause status codes are assigned following all causal (intent) E codes.

If the reporting format limits the number of E codes that can be used in reporting clinical data, the E code reported should be the one that is most related to the principal diagnosis. If the format permits reporting of additional E codes, the cause/intent—including medical misadventures—of the additional events should be reported rather than the codes for place, activity, or external status.

## Child and Adult Abuse Guidelines for E Codes

When the cause of an injury or neglect is intentional child or adult abuse (995.50–995.59, 995.80–995.85), the first E code listed should be assigned from categories E960–E968, Homicide and Injury Purposely Inflicted by Other Persons (except category E967). An E code from category E967, Child and adult battering and other maltreatment, should be added as an additional E code to identify the perpetrator, if known. The title of category E967 is "Perpetrator of Child and Adult Abuse." Additionally, inclusion terms for codes E967.0 and E967.2 include the partner of the child's parent or guardian. An inclusion term for code E967.3 was added to better explain the relationship between perpetrator and victim. E967.3 is used when the perpetrator is the spouse, ex-spouse, partner, or ex-partner of the victim.

In cases of neglect when the intent is determined to be accidental, the first E code listed should be E904.0, Abandonment or neglect of infants and helpless persons.

## Guidelines for Unknown or Suspected Intent

If the intent (accident, self-harm, assault) of the cause of an injury or poisoning is unknown or unspecified, assign codes from categories E980–E989, Injury Undetermined Whether Accidentally or Purposely Inflicted.

If the intent (accident, self-harm, assault) of the cause of an injury or poisoning is questionable, probable, or suspected, also assign codes from categories E980–E989.

### Undetermined Cause

When the intent of an injury or poisoning is known, but the cause is unknown, use code E928.9, Unspecified accident; E958.9, Suicide and self-inflicted injury by unspecified means; or E968.9, Assault by unspecified means. These E codes should be used only rarely because documentation in the health record, in both inpatient and outpatient settings, should normally provide sufficient detail to determine the cause of the injury.

## Definitions and Instructions Related to Transport Accidents

At the beginning of the E code supplementary classification in the Tabular List, definitions and examples related to transport accidents are given. Carefully review this material to ensure accurate E code assignment.

### Exercise 21.2

Using the definitions and instructions in the E code supplementary classification related to transport accidents, classify the following:

1. Parachute

   ______________________________

2. Person changing a tire on a vehicle

   ______________________________

3. Snowmobile

   ______________________________

4. Tractor accident on the highway

   ______________________________

5. Baby carriage

   ______________________________

## Place of Occurrence E Codes

Category E849, Place of occurrence, is provided to note the place where an injury or poisoning occurred. This category describes only the place where the event occurred, not the patient's activity at the time of the event.

The E code identifying the cause of the accident, event, or adverse effect must be assigned first, followed by the place of occurrence E code, where applicable.

Do not use E849.9 if the place of occurrence is not stated. Only code the specific place of occurrence as documented in the patient's record.

Place of occurrence E codes can be located in the Index to External Causes under the main term "Accident (to), occurring (at) (in)."

## Exercise 21.3

Assign all the appropriate E codes to the following:

1. Hit by falling tree in forest
2. Hit by baseball on baseball field
3. Slipped on slippery surface at store
4. Choked on food at riding school
5. Developed swimmer's cramp in swimming pool of private home

## Classification of Death and Injury Resulting from Terrorism

The use of these E codes is described in the terrorism guidelines in the *ICD-9-CM Official Guidelines for Coding and Reporting*.

When the cause of an injury is identified by the Federal Bureau of Investigation (FBI) as terrorism, the first-listed E code should be a code from category E979, Terrorism. The definition of terrorism used by the FBI is found in the inclusion note at E979 in the Tabular List. The terrorism E code is the only E code that should be assigned. Additional E codes from the assault categories should not be assigned.

An E code for terrorism should not be assigned if the cause of an injury is only suspected to be the result of terrorism. Instead, a code in the range of E codes should be assigned based on the circumstances as documented.

Code E979.9 is assigned for the secondary effects of terrorism for conditions occurring subsequent to the terrorist event. This code should not be assigned for conditions that are due to the initial terrorist act.

The terrorism subclassification includes the following E codes:

**E979.0 Terrorism involving explosion of marine weapons**
**E979.1 Terrorism involving destruction of aircraft**
**E979.2 Terrorism involving other explosions and fragments**
**E979.3 Terrorism involving fires, conflagration, and hot substances**
**E979.4 Terrorism involving firearms**
**E979.5 Terrorism involving nuclear weapons**
**E979.6 Terrorism involving biological weapons**
**E979.7 Terrorism involving chemical weapons**
**E979.8 Terrorism involving other means**
**E979.9 Terrorism, secondary effects**

Codes E999.0, Late effect of injury due to war operations, and E999.1, Late effect of injury due to terrorism, can also be used as applicable.

## Fourth-Digit Subdivisions

Fourth digits are provided in many E code categories to identify the injured person. Those categories requiring fourth digits are preceded by different book publishers' notations that a fourth digit is required. Fourth-digit subdivisions for the E code appear immediately after the Alphabetic Index to External Causes.

The fourth-digit subdivisions are specific to each of the following E code category groups:

**Railway Accidents (E800–E807)**
**Motor Vehicle Traffic and Nontraffic Accidents (E810–E825)**
**Other Road Vehicle Accidents (E826–E829)**
**Water Transport Accidents (E830–E838)**
**Air and Space Transport Accidents (E840–E845)**

For example, the fourth digit for a pedestrian is 2 in E800–E807 and 0 in E826–E829.

### Exercise 21.4

Assign all appropriate E codes to the following:

1. Fall while getting off the train by railway passenger

 ____________________

2. Pedestrian knocked down by an animal-drawn vehicle

 ____________________

3. Passenger fell from ship gangplank onto dock

 ____________________

4. Passenger hit by boat while waterskiing

 ____________________

5. Rider thrown from horse

 ____________________

## E Codes for Late Effects

When the condition being coded is a late effect of an illness or injury, the E code for the late effect must be assigned rather than a current E code, if the healthcare facility assigns E codes. The E codes for external cause of late effects include:

**E929** **Late effects of accidental injury**
**E959** **Late effects of self-inflicted injury**
**E969** **Late effects of injury purposely inflicted by other person**
**E977** **Late effects of injury due to legal intervention**

**E989 Late effects of injury, undetermined whether accidentally or purposely inflicted**

**E999 Late effects of injury due to war operations and terrorism**

## Coding Guidelines for Late Effects of External Causes

The following guidelines apply when coding late effects of external causes:

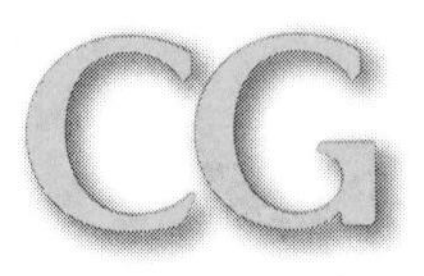

- Late effect E codes exist for injuries and poisonings, but not for adverse effects of drugs, misadventures, and surgical complications.
- A late effect E code (E929, E959, E969, E977, E989, or E999.1) should be used with any report of a late effect or sequela resulting from a previous injury or poisoning (905–909).
- A late effect E code should never be used with a related current nature of injury code.
- Use a late effect E code for subsequent visits when a late effect of the initial injury or poisoning is being treated. There is no late effect E code for adverse effect of drugs. Do not use a late effect E code for subsequent visits for follow-up care (for example, to assess healing, to receive rehabilitative therapy) of the injury or poisoning when no late effect of the injury has been documented.

## Coding of Late Effects

Typically, patients with late effects are coded according to the following criteria:

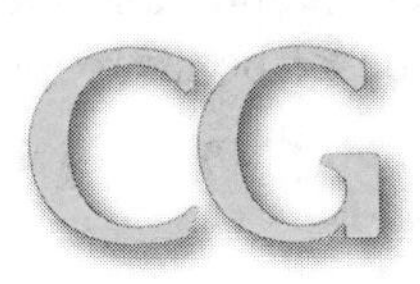

- Residual effect or the condition the patient has at present, found in the Alphabetic Index to Diseases
- Late effect or the condition the patient originally had that produced the residual effect, found in the Alphabetic Index to Diseases under the term "Late effect"
- E code for late effect of original accident or event, found in the Index to External Causes under the term "Late effect"

A detailed discussion of the coding of late effects is presented in chapter 22 of this textbook.

## Exercise 21.5

Assign all appropriate ICD-9-CM codes, including E codes, to the following:

1. Osteomyelitis of femur due to an old compound fracture resulting from an automobile accident 6 months ago in which patient was the driver

   ______________________________

2. Headaches due to an old skull fracture sustained when patient fell from a ladder 1 year ago

   ______________________________

3. Scars of arm due to an old burn sustained in a house fire 3 years ago

   ______________________________

4. Deviated nasal septum due to an old nasal fracture; patient hit with a ball while playing baseball

   ______________________________

5. Anoxic brain damage due to gunshot wound of the head sustained 4 years ago; reported as a homicide attempt

   ______________________________

## Never Events/Serious Reportable Events

ICD-9-CM contains external cause codes to identify and track the occurrence of wrong site surgery, wrong surgery, and wrong patient having surgery to support the collection of data related to the National Quality Forum's "never events." A complete list of the never events and the work of the Department of Health and Human Services' Agency for Healthcare Research and Quality can be found at http://www.ahrq.gov/downloads/pub/advances/vol4/Kizer2.pdf. A wealth of other articles for both consumers and patients, particularly related to patient safety, can be found at http://www.ahrq.gov/consumer/cc/cc102108.htm.

The wrong site, wrong surgery, and wrong patient never events or serious reportable events are among the list of adverse medical events that are serious, largely preventable, and of concern to patients and healthcare providers. The Joint Commission, the Federal government, and state governments use the never events list as the basis for quality indicators and state-based reporting systems. Listed next are examples of E codes that can be used to describe the external cause of several of these factors:

| | |
|---|---|
| E871.0–E871.9 | Foreign object left in body during procedure |
| E876.5 | Performance of wrong operation (procedure) on correct patient |
| E876.6 | Performance of operation (or procedure) on patient not scheduled for surgery |
| E876.7 | Performance of correct operation (procedure) on wrong side/body part |

Some of these events—such as stage 3 and 4 pressure ulcers acquired after admission to the healthcare facility and intravascular air embolism that occurs while being cared for in a healthcare facility—can be captured by ICD-9-CM diagnosis codes and present-on-admission indicators. Other of these events cannot be captured using ICD-9-CM codes because the event is beyond the scope of the classification system. An example of a never event that cannot be coded is an infant discharged to the wrong patient or the abduction of a patient of any age.

## External Cause Status

A code from category E000 should be assigned whenever any other external cause code(s) are assigned, including an activity E code. A code from category E000, External cause status, is assigned to indicate the work status of the person at the time the event occurred. The E code for external cause status identifies the status of the person seeking healthcare for an injury or health condition. The status code indicates whether the event occurred during civilian activity done for income or pay, during military activity, or whether the individual, including a student or volunteer, was involved in a non-work activity such as leisure or hobby activity at the time the causal event produced the injury or condition. Category E000 contains the subcategories of:

E000.0 Civilian activity done for income or pay
E000.1 Military activity
E000.2 Volunteer activity
E000.8 Other external cause status
E000.9 Unspecified external cause status

A code from category E000 should be assigned when applicable with other external cause codes, such as transport accidents. However, the category E000 codes are not applicable to poisonings, adverse effects, misadventures, or late effects. A category E000 code is not assigned if no other E codes are applicable to the encounter. In addition, do not assign code E000.9, Unspecified external cause status, if the status is not stated or documented in the health record.

## Activity Codes

Activity codes (categories E001–E030) identify the activity of the person seeking healthcare for an injury or health condition when the injury or other health condition resulted from an activity or the activity contributed to a condition. These codes can be used with external cause codes from cause and intent code categories if identifying the activity would provide additional information on the event.

External cause codes for activity are mutually exclusive from all other external cause codes. Activity codes are used with external cause codes as appropriate. For example, a strained back resulting from riding a bike would require an activity E code for bike riding. If a bike rider is hit by a car that is a transport accident for E-coding purposes. If the bike rider falls off the bike and suffers an injury, that external event is a fall and would be coded as such with an E code for a fall. Based on the current sequencing guidelines for E codes, the hierarchy of sequencing would be that a transport accident resulting in a fall would be classified as a transport accident.

Activity E codes categories range from E001 to E030. These codes are appropriate for use for both acute injuries and for conditions that are due to long-term cumulative effects of an activity, such as musculoskeletal and connective tissue disorders. These codes also could be used in conjunction with other external cause codes for external cause status (E000) and place of occurrence (E849). This section contains the following categories with corresponding subcategories:

E001 Activities involving walking, marching, hiking and running
E002 Activities involving water and watercraft
E003 Activities involving ice and snow
E004 Activities involving climbing, rappelling and jumping off
E005 Activities involving dancing and other rhythmic movements
E006 Activities involving sports and athletics played individually
E007 Activities involving sports and athletics played as a team or group
E008 Activities involving other specified sports and athletic activities
E009 Activities involving cardiorespiratory exercise
E010 Activities involving muscle strengthening exercise
E011 Activities involving computer technology and electronic devices
E012 Activities involving arts and handcrafts
E013 Activities involving personal hygiene and household maintenance
E014 Activities involving person providing caregiving
E015 Activities involving food preparation, cooking, and grilling
E016 Activities involving property and land maintenance, building and construction
E017 Activities involving roller coasters and other types of external motion
E018 Activities involving playing musical instruments
E019 Activities involving animal care
E029 Other specified activity
E030 Unspecified activity

## Military Operations

The U.S. Department of Defense initiated the addition and expansion of E codes for the identification of the causes of injuries among the military population to assist with the prevention of such injuries. Among the air, space, and water transport vehicles listed, there is also a fourth digit to identify a military type vehicle that is involved in a transport accident. Categories E990–E999, Injuries resulting from operations of war, include specific identification of the cause of injury from military operations.

Examples of specific E codes to identify injuries from military operations are:

E991.6 Injury due to war operations by fragments from vehicle-borne improvised explosive device (IED)
E992.3 Injury due to war operations by explosion of sea-based artillery shell
E993.2 Injury due to war operations by explosion of mortar
E994.0 Injury due to war operations by destruction of aircraft due to enemy fire or explosives
E998.1 Injury due to war operations but occurring after cessation of hostilities by explosion of bombs

## Exercise 21.6

Assign all appropriate E codes for never events/serious reportable events, external cause status, activity codes, and military operations to the following:

1. US Marine captain was killed in war zone by the explosion of an aerial bomb falling on his tent.

2. Patient complained of a stiff back after performing gardening activity in own yard on her day off from work.

3. Patient complained of hearing loss after performing with his rock band during a noisy concert where he was a paid performer as the drummer in the band.

4. Patient had right hip replacement surgery when the left hip was consented to be replaced due to osteoarthritis.

5. Patient found to have a foreign body (4×4 sponge) left in operative wound after abdominal hysterectomy.

## ICD-9-CM Review Exercises: Chapter 21

1. Assign only the external cause codes for this case: The patient injured was an 18-year-old driver of a car that collided with a pickup truck on the interstate highway. The driver confessed to using his cell phone to send a text message to his girlfriend.

2. Assign only the external cause codes for this case: The patient is an army officer who was injured while driving a truck on patrol on a highway outside the military base where he was stationed in Afghanistan when explosive material fragments hit him from an improvised explosive device on the road.

3. Assign only the external cause codes for this case: The patient was bitten by a dog while attempting to rescue it from a barn building on a farm while performing his job as a county animal control officer.

4. Assign only the external cause codes for this case: The patient was a cook in a restaurant and was accidentally burned with hot liquids while cooking on a stove while working.

*(Continued on next page)*

## ICD-9-CM Review Exercises: Chapter 21 (Continued)

5. Assign only the external cause codes for this case: The patient is a 20-year-old man who died in the emergency room in spite of being actively treated for a gunshot wound to his chest that appeared to be the result of an attempted homicide by another man with a handgun. The patient was walking across a store parking lot when he was shot.

 ______________________________

6. Assign both the diagnosis codes for the injuries and the external cause codes for this case: The patient is a 55-year-old man who fell from a ladder outside his single-family home while performing property maintenance by cleaning the gutters on his house. He was found to have a non-displaced femoral neck fracture of his right hip. At this time, no surgical Intervention was needed.

 ______________________________

7. Assign both the diagnosis codes for the injuries and the external cause codes for this case: The patient is a 4-year-old child who had third degree burns on his left lower leg and his back as a result of his clothes catching fire while playing with a candle in his own home (single-family residence).

 ______________________________

8. Assign both the diagnosis codes for the injuries and the external cause codes for this case: The patient is a 30-year-old woman who was the driver of a motor vehicle who was injured in a collision with another motor vehicle on a city street. She was treated for a severe cervical neck strain and a displaced, open fracture of the shaft of her left radius and ulna and will have surgery on the arm the next day.

 ______________________________

9. Assign both the diagnosis codes for the injuries and the external cause codes for this case: The patient is a 12-year-old female who suffered a displaced fracture of her elbow, in particular, the lower end of the humerus at the olecranon process. She fell off her in-line skates at a roller rink while skating for pleasure with her friends.

 ______________________________

10. Assign both the diagnosis codes for the injuries and the external cause codes for this case: The patient is a 60-year-old female, the homeowner, who was shoveling snow off her front stairs when she fell down the icy steps and suffered a trimalleolar fracture of the medial and lateral malleolus of her left ankle. The patient was scheduled for an open reduction and internal fixation the next day at the ambulatory surgery center.

 ______________________________

# ICD-10-CM Chapter 20, External Causes of Morbidity (V00–Y99)

## Organization and Structure of ICD-10-CM

Chapter 20 of ICD-10-CM includes categories V00–Y99 arranged in the following blocks:

V00–V99 Transport accidents
V00–V09 Pedestrian injured in transport accident

| | |
|---|---|
| V10–V19 | Pedal cycle rider injured in transport accident |
| V20–V29 | Motorcycle rider injured in transport accident |
| V30–V39 | Occupant of three-wheeled motor vehicle injured in transport accident |
| V40–V49 | Car occupant injured in transport accident |
| V50–V59 | Occupant of pick-up truck or van injured in transport accident |
| V60–V69 | Occupant of heavy transport vehicle injured in transport accident |
| V70–V79 | Bus occupant injured in transport accident |
| V80–V89 | Other land transport accidents |
| V90–V94 | Water transport accidents |
| V95–V97 | Air and space transport accidents |
| V98–V99 | Other and unspecified transport accidents |
| W00–X58 | Other external causes of accidental injury |
| W00–W19 | Slipping, tripping, stumbling and falls |
| W20–W49 | Exposure to inanimate mechanical forces |
| W50–W64 | Exposure to animate mechanical forces |
| W65–W74 | Accidental non-transport drowning and submersion |
| W85–W99 | Exposure to electric current, radiation and extreme ambient air temperature and pressure |
| X00–X08 | Exposure to smoke, fire and flames |
| X10–X19 | Contact with heat and hot substances |
| X30–X39 | Exposure to forces of nature |
| X52–X58 | Accidental exposure to other specified factors |
| X71–X83 | Intentional self-harm |
| X92–Y09 | Assault |
| Y21–Y33 | Event of undetermined intent |
| Y35–Y38 | Legal intervention, operations of war, military operations and terrorism |
| Y62–Y84 | Complications of medical and surgical care |
| Y62–Y69 | Misadventures to patients during surgical and medical care |
| Y70–Y82 | Medical devices associated with adverse incidents in diagnostic and therapeutic use |
| Y83–Y84 | Surgical and other medical procedures as the cause of abnormal reaction of the patient, or of later complication, without mention of misadventure at the time of the procedure |
| Y90–Y99 | Supplementary factors related to causes of morbidity classified elsewhere |

Codes for external causes are no longer found in a supplemental classification in ICD-10-CM. The causes currently located in the ICD-9-CM E code chapter have been disseminated to Chapter 19, Injury, Poisoning and Certain Other Consequences of External Causes, or Chapter 20, External Causes of Morbidity. Codes in Chapter 20 capture the causes of the injury or health condition, the intent (unintentional or accidental; or intentional, such as suicide or assault), the place where the event occurred, the activity of the patient at the time of the event, and the person's status (namely civilian, military).

There is no national requirement for mandatory external causes code reporting. Unless a provider is subject to a state-based external cause code reporting mandate, for example, reporting of certain patients treated in a hospital trauma center or if the codes are required by a specific payer, reporting of external causes codes are not required. In the absence of a mandatory reporting requirement, providers are encouraged to report external cause codes as it provides valuable data for injury research and evaluation of injury prevention strategies.

Changes in terminology were also necessary due to the revisions made overall to this chapter. For example, ICD-10-CM category V45 is titled "Car occupant injured in collision with railway train or railway vehicle" while the title of ICD-9-CM category E810 is "Motor vehicle traffic accident involving collision with train."

In numerous instances, conditions included as subcategory codes in ICD-9-CM have been given a specific category code in ICD-10-CM allowing expansion of the codes at the fourth-, fifth-, or sixth-character level.

| **EXAMPLE:** | ICD-9-CM: | E884.0 | Accidental fall from playground equipment | |
|---|---|---|---|---|
| | ICD-10-CM: | W09 | Fall on and from playground equipment | |
| | | | W09.0 | Fall on or from playground slide |
| | | | W09.1 | Fall from playground swing |
| | | | W09.2 | Fall on or from jungle gym |
| | | | W09.8 | Fall on or from other playground equipment |

## Coding Guidelines and Instructional Notes for ICD-10-CM Chapter 20

New notes have been added in Chapter 20 to show which categories require the seventh character extensions to indicate whether the episode of care being identified was the initial, subsequent or a secondary encounter, or the condition is a result of an event or sequelae. The category codes that require a seventh character include a note box that lists the instruction "The appropriate 7th character is to be added to code"

A initial encounter
D subsequent encounter
S sequela

While there is an instructional note found at the start of category E849, place of occurrence, in ICD-9-CM, it has been expanded in ICD-10-CM. The instructional note with ICD-10-CM category Y92, Place of occurrence of the external cause, states to use Y92 in conjunction with the activity code. The place of occurrence should be recorded only at the initial encounter for treatment. Also, the coder will use an activity code from category Y93 in addition to the place of occurrence code from category Y92. Category Y93, Activity codes, indicate the activity of the person seeking healthcare for an injury or health condition. The Y93 codes provide additional information on the event.

The National Center for Health Statistics (NCHS) has published chapter-specific guidelines for Chapter 20 of ICD-10-CM:

- Guidelines I.C.20.a. General external cause coding guidelines
- Guideline I.C.20.b. Place of occurrence guideline
- Guideline I.C.20.c. Activity code
- Guideline I.C.20.d. Place of occurrence, activity, and status codes used with other external cause code

- Guideline I.C.20.e. If the reporting format limits the number of external cause codes
- Guideline I.C.20.f. Multiple external cause coding guidelines
- Guideline I.C.20.g. Child and adult abuse guideline
- Guideline I.C.20.h. Unknown or undetermined intent guideline
- Guidelines I.C.20.i. Sequela (late effects) of external cause guidelines
- Guidelines I.C.20.j. Terrorism guidelines
- Guideline I.C.20.k. External cause status

To gain an understanding of these rules, access the 2014 guidelines from NCHS website (http://www.cdc.gov/nchs/icd/icd10cm.htm) and read Chapter 20, External Causes of Morbidity guidelines I.C.20.a–I.C.20.k.

## Coding Overview for ICD-10-CM Chapter 20

This chapter permits the classification of environmental events and circumstances as the cause of injury, and other adverse effects. Where a code from this section is applicable, it is intended that it will be used secondary to a code from another chapter of the Classification indicating the nature of the condition. Most often, the condition will be classifiable to Chapter 19, Injury, Poisoning, and Certain Other Consequences of External Causes (S00–T88). Other conditions that may be stated to be due to external causes are classified in Chapters 1 to 18. For these conditions, codes from Chapter 20 should be used to provide additional information as to the cause of the condition.

Chapter 20 of ICD-10-CM, External Causes of Morbidity (V00–Y99), contain codes that have the first character of **V, W, X,** and **Y** (V00–Y99). Chapter 20 of ICD-10-CM contains a massive expansion from ICD-9-CM. It is helpful to review the Tabular List to gain an understanding of all of the possible codes available.

ICD-10-CM contains an Index to External Causes with main terms identifying the event with such entries as accident, drowning, exposure, forces of nature, falling, slipping, and other events that can cause an injury. Other entries exist for assignment of the activity of the person, place of occurrence, and status of external cause, such as civilian activity, leisure activity, student activity, and such.

According to the *ICD-10-CM Official Guidelines for Coding and Reporting*, an external cause code may be used with any code in the range of A00.0–T88.9, Z00–Z99, classification that is a health condition due to an external cause. Though they are most applicable to injuries, they are also valid for use with such things as infections or diseases due to an external source, and other health conditions, such as a heart attack that occurs during strenuous physical activity.

The external cause code, with the appropriate seventh character (initial encounter, subsequent encounter or sequela) is assigned for each encounter for which the injury or condition is being treated. This is new to ICD-10-CM because E codes in ICD-9-CM were only assigned for the initial encounter for an injury, poisoning or adverse effect.

Many, but not all, of the V00–Y99 codes require a seventh character to indicate whether the healthcare encounter was the initial encounter (A), subsequent encounter (D), or sequela (S). Late effects of external causes of morbidity in ICD-10-CM are reported using the external cause code with the seventh-character S for sequela. These codes should be used with any report of a late effect or sequela resulting from a previous injury. Certain external cause codes are only used once, at the initial encounter for treatment, such as the place of occurrence codes and the activity code(s).

The transport accidents section (V00–V99) is structured in 12 groups. Those relating to land transport accidents (V00–V89) reflect the victim's mode of transport and are subdivided to identify the victim's "counterpart" or the type of event. The vehicle of which the injured person is an occupant is identified in the first two characters since it is seen as the most important factor to identify for prevention purposes. A transport accident is one in which the vehicle involved must be moving or running or in use for transport purposes at the time of the accident. The definitions of transport vehicles are provided in the classification and should be reviewed.

Chapter 20 of ICD-10-CM contains the following blocks of codes:

- V00–V99, Transport accidents
  Structured into 12 groups, such as pedestrian, pedal cyclist, motorcyclist, occupant of three-wheeled motor vehicle, car occupant, occupant of pick-up truck or van, occupant of heavy transport vehicle, bus occupant injured in a transport accident as well as water transport accidents, air and space transport accidents, and other and unspecified transport accidents
- W00–W19, Slipping, tripping, stumbling, and falls
- W20–W49, Exposure to inanimate mechanical forces
  For example, struck by thrown object, contact with sharp glass, or contact with different types of machinery
- W50–W64, Exposure to animate mechanical forces
  For example, accidental hit or strike by another person, contact with dog (bitten or struck), or crushed, pushed, or stepped on by crowd or human stampede
- W65–W74, Accidental nontransport drowning and submersion
- W85–W99, Exposure to electric current, radiation, and extreme ambient air temperature and pressure
- X00–X08, Exposure to smoke, fire, and flames
- X10–X19, Contact with heat and hot substances
- X30–X39, Exposure to the forces of nature
- X52, X58, Accidental exposure to other specified factors
- X71–X83, Intentional self harm
- X92–Y08, Assault
- Y21–Y33, Event of undetermined intent
- Y35–Y38, Legal intervention, operations of war, military operations, and terrorism
- Y62–Y84, Complications of medical and surgical care
- Y62–Y69, Misadventures to patients during surgical and medical care
- Y70–Y82, Medical devices associated with adverse incidents in diagnostic and therapeutic use
- Y83–Y84, Surgical and other medical procedures as the cause of abnormal reaction of the patient, or of later complication, without mention of misadventure at the time of the procedure

- Y90–Y99, Supplementary factors related to causes of morbidity classified elsewhere For example, evidence of alcohol involvement determined by blood alcohol level (Y90), place of occurrence codes (Y92), activity codes (Y93), nosocomial condition (Y95), and external cause status (Y99)

Category Y92, Place of occurrence of the external cause, is for use, when relevant, to identify the place of occurrence. It is to be used in conjunction with an activity code if the activity is stated by the healthcare provider. Place of occurrence should be recorded only at the initial encounter for treatment. Only one code from Y92 should be recorded on a medical record. Do not use place of occurrence code Y92.9 if the place is not stated or is not applicable.

A note at the beginning of category Y93 in the Tabular, states the activity code is provided for use to indicate the activity of the person seeking healthcare for an injury or health condition, such as a heart attack while shoveling snow, which resulted from the activity or was contributed to by the activity. These codes are appropriate for use for both acute injuries, such as those from Chapter 19, and conditions that are due to the long-term, cumulative effects of an activity, such as those from Chapter 13. They are also appropriate for use with external cause codes for cause and intent if identifying the activity provides additional information on the event. These codes should be used in conjunction with codes for external cause status (Y99) and place of occurrence (Y92). The activity code is used only once, at the initial encounter for treatment. Only one code from Y93 should be recorded on the encounter.

The activity codes are not applicable to poisonings, adverse effects, misadventures, or late effects. Do not assign Y93.9, unspecified activity, if the activity is not stated.

This section contains the following broad activity categories:

| | |
|---|---|
| Y93.0 | Activities involving walking and running |
| Y93.1 | Activities involving water and water craft |
| Y93.2 | Activities involving ice and snow |
| Y93.3 | Activities involving climbing, rappelling, and jumping off |
| Y93.4 | Activities involving dancing and other rhythmic movement |
| Y93.5 | Activities involving other sports and athletics played individually |
| Y93.6 | Activities involving other sports and athletics played as a team or group |
| Y93.7 | Activities involving other specified sports and athletics |
| Y93.a | Activities involving other cardiorespiratory exercise |
| Y93.b | Activities involving other muscle strengthening exercises |
| Y93.c | Activities involving computer technology and electronic devices |
| Y93.d | Activities involving arts and handcrafts |
| Y93.e | Activities involving personal hygiene and interior property and clothing maintenance |
| Y93.f | Activities involving caregiving |
| Y93.g | Activities involving food preparation, cooking, and grilling |
| Y93.h | Activities involving exterior property and land maintenance, building, and construction |
| Y93.i | Activities involving roller coasters and other types of external motion |
| Y93.j | Activities involving playing musical instrument |
| Y93.k | Activities involving animal care |

Y93.8 Activities, other specified
Y93.9 Activity, unspecified

Category Y99, External cause status codes should be assigned whenever any other external cause code is assigned for an encounter, including an activity code, except for the events noted below. Assign a code from category Y99, External cause status, to indicate the work status of the person at the time the event occurred. The status code indicates whether the event occurred during military activity, whether a non-military person was at work, whether an individual including a student or volunteer was involved in a non-work activity at the time of the causal event.

A code from Y99, External cause status, should be assigned, when applicable, with other external cause codes, such as transport accidents and falls. The external cause status codes are not applicable to poisonings, adverse effects, misadventures, or late effects.

According to the *ICD-10-CM Official Guidelines for Coding and Reporting*, do not assign a code from category Y99 if no other external cause codes (cause, activity) are applicable for the encounter. Do not assign code Y99.9, Unspecified external cause status, if the status is not stated. An external cause status code is used only once, at the initial encounter for treatment. Only one code from Y99 should be recorded on a health record.

## ICD-10-CM Review Exercises: Chapter 21

Assign the correct ICD-10-CM diagnosis codes to the following exercises:

1. This patient is a 28-year-old male, admitted through the emergency department after the motorcycle he was driving (for leisure) collided with an elk on a mountain highway. The patient was wearing a helmet and suffered a minor head injury with just a short loss of consciousness reported at 15 minutes. His major injury was a displaced, cervical, C2 fracture with complete transection of the spinal cord. Upon evaluation by neurosurgery, the patient had no feeling below his shoulders, although he did admit to tingling in his arms and hands. The patient had no other apparent fractures. The patient's family was notified and arrived two days later.

   Due to problems in the OR, it was necessary to transfer the patient to complete surgical stabilization. The physician's final diagnosis was stated as quadriplegia secondary to C2 vertebral fracture with spinal cord injury. What diagnosis and external cause codes are assigned?

   ________________________________________

2. Assign external cause codes for this case: An army officer was injured while on patrol on the military base in Afghanistan by an explosion of an IED. Assign the external cause codes only.

   ________________________________________

3. Assign external cause codes for this case: The patient was bitten by a dog while attempting to rescue it from a barn while performing his job at animal control. Assign the external cause codes only.

   ________________________________________

4. Assign external cause codes for this case: A cook in a fast food restaurant was accidently burned with hot oil while cooking fried foods while on duty. Assign the external cause codes only.

   ________________________________________

## ICD-10-CM Review Exercises: Chapter 21 (Continued)

5. This 50-year-old male, working on his own home improvement projects, fell from a ladder outside of his single-family home. After evaluation, it was determined that he had a non-displaced femoral neck fracture on the left side. At this time, no surgical intervention is planned. What diagnosis and external cause codes are assigned?

6. A patient fell from a ladder in the garage four weeks ago while working on replacing a garage door switch. The injury resulted in a fracture of L1 and L2 vertebral bodies. He is receiving physical therapy for this routine healing injury. What diagnosis and external cause codes are assigned?

7. Assign external cause codes for this case: An 18-year-old driver of a car that collided with a pickup truck on the interstate highway. The driver confessed to using his cell phone to send a text message to his girlfriend. Assign the external cause codes only.

8. This 62-year-old female was burned by hot grease in her condo's kitchen. She is seen in the hospital's outpatient clinic for large dressing change on her left forearm. She was treated for second-degree burns to her left arm several days ago. What diagnosis and external cause codes are assigned?

9. This 30-year-old female patient was a driver involved in an automobile accident when she was rear-ended by another car on the interstate highway. She was seen in the emergency room complaining of pain in the arm and neck. She was brought into the hospital by the EMTs on a backboard and after proper splinting to the right arm it was evident that there was a compound fracture present. After CT scan of the head and neck, the patient was removed from the backboard. She was treated for a displaced, open fracture type I of the shaft of the right radius and ulna. She also received a collar for her cervical strain. What diagnosis and external cause codes are assigned?

10. A child has second- and third-degree burns of the left calf and second- and third-degree burns of the back. The patient was burned when he was running and fell into the lit fire-place in his parent's bedroom. What diagnosis and external cause codes are assigned?

11. This 28-year-old female was seen for an infection due to a laceration on the palm of her right hand. Apparently, this laceration occurred five days ago but this is the first time she is being treated for the injury. The patient reports that her hand was cut by broken glass at a restaurant, where she was a customer, drinking heavily. She is a chronic alcohol abuser and also a chronic abuser of meth. The wound will not be sutured due to the late presenta-tion for treatment. She will, however, be placed on antibiotics to treat the infection. What diagnosis and external cause codes are assigned?

*(Continued on next page)*

## ICD-10-CM Review Exercises: Chapter 21 (Continued)

12. This patient is an 18-year-old college student who is brought to the emergency department by ambulance, found to be the victim of a random beating. This patient was walking in his neighborhood park when he was pulled down and then beaten during a fight. The patient was comatose when found by the paramedics but did open his eyes in response to pain; however, has no verbal or motor response. The patient was in a coma upon admission but regained consciousness within 40 minutes of arriving in the ED, less than an hour after being found. The MRI is negative for fractures or internal bleeding. The physician describes the injury as a closed head injury with loss of consciousness of less than 1 hour. What diagnosis and external cause codes are assigned?

    ______________________________

13. This is a 59-year-old female who fell down the icy front steps of her single-family house and sustained trauma to her head as well as a nondisplaced closed trimalleolar fracture of the medial and lateral malleolus of her left leg. The patient denies any loss of consciousness. Attention was directed to her head injury which, after CT scan, revealed a basilar skull fracture and a small subdural hematoma. The neurosurgeon felt that the hematoma currently did not require surgical intervention. Serial CT scans showed shrinking of the hematoma after several days. What diagnosis and external cause codes are assigned?

    ______________________________

14. This 12-year-old female is seen for continued pain related to her elbow fracture. Six weeks ago, this patient injured her elbow when she fell while skating at the local roller rink. After further evaluation, the attending physician found a nonunion of the previously displaced right distal humerus fracture. She will be scheduled for surgery in the next two days. What diagnosis and external codes are assigned?

    ______________________________

15. The patient, a 20-year-old male, was seen in the trauma clinic for a follow-up visit after being discharged from the hospital for treatment of a laceration of his right renal artery which was the result of an intentional assault with a handgun. He was shot one month ago while he was standing on the sidewalk outside his apartment building. The patient was making satisfactory recovery from his injury.

    ______________________________

# Chapter 22
# Late Effects

## Learning Objectives

1. Define the terms *late effect, sequela,* and *residual effect*
2. Identify the minimum of two codes that are usually required to report a late effect condition
3. Identify the late effect conditions that are frequently associated with cerebrovascular disease
4. Give examples of medical terminology used in health records to describe the fact that a patient has a late effect condition
5. Explain what period of time is associated with the occurrence of late effect conditions
6. Identify the thirteen ICD-9-CM category codes that describe late effects
7. Examine the ICD-9-CM Alphabetic Index entry under the main term "Late" and the subterm "effect(s) (of)"
8. Examine the ICD-10-CM Alphabetic Index entry under the main term "Sequela"
9. State the coding guidelines for the coding and sequencing of codes to describe late effect conditions
10. Describe the coding guideline exceptions
11. Explain how to code the residual effect when it is not stated in the physician's written diagnostic statement
12. Describe the ICD-9-CM Alphabetic Index rule that requires different sequencing of the codes for the residual condition and the late effect condition
13. Practice assigning late effect codes from the various chapters of ICD-9-CM to describe the residual condition and the late effect condition
14. Assign late effect or sequela codes from various chapters of ICD-10-CM

# ICD-9-CM Coding of Late Effects

This chapter examines the coding of conditions described as late effects of a previous illness or injury. The coder must understand the definition of late effects in order to code such conditions. Physicians may use different terminology to describe a condition that is present today as the result of a condition the patient had in the past. Rarely will a coder see the physician document "late of" of a condition but instead use other terminology in the diagnostic statement to describe the patient's problem today. There is no definite time period between the first condition the patient has until the time the late effect condition is present as this depends on the original condition and the patient.

## Definition of Late Effects

A **late effect** is the **residual effect,** or condition produced and currently present, that remains after the acute phase of an illness or injury has terminated. This residual effect (also referred to as the "residual") is the temporary or permanent health condition that follows the acute phase of an illness or injury. The code for the acute phase of an illness or injury that led to the late effect condition is never used with a code for the late effect.

Coding of late effects generally requires two codes sequenced in the following order: The code for the condition or nature of the late effect currently present, known as the residual, is sequenced first. The code for the late effect or the cause of the residual is sequenced second.

**EXAMPLE:** Hemiplegia following old cerebral thrombosis

Scarring following third-degree burn

Traumatic arthritis following fracture

The hemiplegia, scarring, and traumatic arthritis represent residuals of a previous illness or injury. The cerebral thrombosis, third-degree burn, and fracture represent the causes of the residuals, or what is referred to as the late effect.

An exception to the above guideline would apply in those instances in which the code for late effect is followed by a manifestation code identified in the Tabular List and title or the late effect code has been expanded (at the fourth- and fifth-digit levels) to include the manifestation(s). The code for the acute phase of an illness or injury that led to the late effect is never used with a code for the late effect.

## Late Effects of Cerebrovascular Disease

Coding of late effects of cerebrovascular disease is an example of an exception to the general rule that late effects require two codes as listed above. This includes cerebrovascular accident (CVA), such as cerebral thrombosis or intracranial hemorrhage. Category 438, Late effects of cerebrovascular disease, provides combination codes that identify both the residual (cognitive deficits, aphasia, hemiplegia) and the cause (the CVA), which was previously coded to categories 430–437 when the acute episode occurred. To locate the combination codes for late effects following CVAs, the main term to be used in the Alphabetic Index to Diseases is "Late, effects, (of) cerebrovascular disease," with numerous subterms that identify the current residual condition. More than one code in category 438 may be used to describe a patient with multiple residual conditions present after the acute phase of the CVA is treated.

## Late Effect Terminology

The following are examples of terminology found in diagnostic statements that indicate late effects:

- Residuals of
- Old
- Sequela of
- Late
- Due to or following previous illness or injury

## Passage of Time and Residual Effects

Sometimes the diagnosis will indicate that sufficient time has passed from the occurrence of the acute illness or injury to the development of the residual effect. For example, a fracture in a young person should heal in 4 to 6 weeks; in an older person, in 6 to 12 weeks. When healing does not occur, the physician may indicate the patient has a nonunion fracture that requires a late effect code.

There is no time limit or set period during which a condition may be designated a residual effect. It may be apparent early, as in a CVA, or it may occur months or years later, as with a previous injury, such as a fracture.

### Exercise 22.1

Circle the residual and write in the cause below for each of the following diagnoses:

1. Aphasia due to old CVA

   ______________________

2. Mild intellectual disability following viral encephalitis

   ______________________

3. Seizure disorder secondary to intracranial abscess

   ______________________

4. Contracture of left heel tendon sheath due to poliomyelitis

   ______________________

5. Paralysis of arm due to old radial nerve injury

   ______________________

## Coding of Late Effects

ICD-9-CM contains the following limited number of late effect categories and subcategories to identify the cause of the late effect:

| | |
|---|---|
| **137** | **Late effects of tuberculosis** |
| **138** | **Late effects of acute poliomyelitis** |
| **139** | **Late effects of other infectious and parasitic diseases** |
| **268.1** | **Rickets, late effects** |
| **326** | **Late effects of intracranial abscess or pyogenic infection** |
| **438** | **Late effects of cerebrovascular disease** |
| **677** | **Late effect of complication of pregnancy, childbirth, and the puerperium** |
| **905** | **Late effects of musculoskeletal and connective tissue injuries** |
| **906** | **Late effects of injuries to skin and subcutaneous tissues** |
| **907** | **Late effects of injuries to the nervous system** |
| **908** | **Late effects of other and unspecified injuries** |
| **909** | **Late effects of other and unspecified external causes** |
| **997.6** | **Amputation stump complication** |

Late effects of specific diseases may be found in chapters in ICD-9-CM on specific diseases. For example, late effects of cerebrovascular disease, category 438, is included in the chapter on diseases of the circulatory system.

## Alphabetic Index Entry

The code for the cause of the late effect can be located in the Alphabetic Index to Diseases under the main term "Late" and the subterm "effect(s) (of)."

**Late**—*see also* condition
effect(s) (of)—*see also* condition
cerebrovascular disease (conditions classifiable to 430–437) 438.9
with
alterations of sensations 438.6
aphasia 438.11
apraxia 438.81
ataxia 438.84
cognitive deficits 438.0
disturbances of vision 438.7
dysarthria 438.13
dysphagia 438.82
dysphasia 438.12
facial droop 438.83
facial weakness 438.83
fluency disorder 438.14
hemiplegia/hemiparesis
affecting
dominant side 438.21
nondominant side 438.22
unspecified side 438.20

## Coding Guideline

The residual condition or nature of the late effect is sequenced first, followed by the cause of the late effect. However, in a few instances the code for the late effect is followed by a manifestation code identified in the Tabular List. In these instances, the title or the late effect code has been expanded at the fourth- and fifth-digit levels to include the manifestations.

**EXAMPLE:** Scar of the right hand secondary to a laceration sustained 2 years ago: 709.2, Scar conditions and fibrosis of skin; 906.1, Late effect of open wound of extremities, without mention of tendon injury

**EXAMPLE:** Dysphasia secondary to old CVA sustained 1 year ago: 438.12, Late effect of cerebrovascular disease, speech and language deficits, dysphasia

## Coding Guideline Exceptions

Exceptions to the preceding coding guideline are as follows:

1. If the health record does not identify the specific residual effect, code only the late effect code.

   **EXAMPLE:** Documentation in the health record states "late effect of polio:" 138, Late effects of acute poliomyelitis

2. If the Alphabetic Index to Diseases indicates a different sequence, follow the directions of the index.

   **EXAMPLE:** Scoliosis due to poliomyelitis during childhood

   The following entries appear in the Alphabetic Index to Diseases:

**Scoliosis** (acquired) (postural) 737.30
congenital 754.2
due to or associated with .
poliomyelitis 138 *[737.43]*

The Alphabetic Index directs the coder to sequence first the late effect code (138), followed by the residual *[737.43],* which is in italicized print and, therefore, should not be reported as the principal diagnosis or first-listed code.

138 **Late effects of acute poliomyelitis**
***737.43*** ***Scoliosis associated with other conditions***

3. If ICD-9-CM does not provide a code to describe the cause of the late effect, assign a code only for the residual. Conditions that are stated to be due to previous surgery are not considered late effects. Depending on the circumstances, a "history of" code or surgical complication code may be reported.

### Residual Effect Not Stated

The late effect code can be assigned by itself when the diagnostic statement indicating a late effect does not include the residual condition.

**EXAMPLE:** Late effect of rickets (Rickets developed in childhood, patient is now an adult.)

Only code 268.1, Rickets, late effect, is assigned because the specific effect(s) is (are) not identified.

### Residual Effect Directed by Alphabetic Index

In some cases, when the residual is referenced in the Alphabetic Index to Diseases, the code for a late effect is listed first, followed by a manifestation code in italics and within slanted brackets. In such an instance, the Alphabetic Index takes precedence, with the code for the late effect sequenced first, followed by the code for the residual.

**EXAMPLE:** Kyphosis due to poliomyelitis during childhood
**Kyphosis** (acquired) (postural) 737.10
due to or associated with .
poliomyelitis 138 *[737.41]*

Codes 138, Late effects of acute poliomyelitis, and *737.41, Kyphosis associated with other conditions,* are assigned. The code for the residual (kyphosis) is sequenced after the late effect code as indicated in the Alphabetic Index.

## ICD-9-CM Review Exercises

Assign ICD-9-CM codes to the following residuals and late effects. It is not necessary to assign E codes in these exercises.

1. Recurrent seizures due to previous encephalitis
2. Deformity of uterus acquired as a result of a complication of a previous cesarean delivery
3. Residuals of old gunshot wound of leg
4. Paraplegia from previous laceration of spinal cord
5. Malunion fracture of humerus due to old fracture
6. Hemiplegia affecting nondominant side due to CVA 1 year ago
7. Traumatic arthritis following fracture of left ankle

## ICD-9-CM Review Exercises (Continued)

8. Keloid of arm due to old crushing injury

9. Contracture of right wrist due to poliomyelitis

10. Irradiation hypothyroidism following previous radiation therapy for carcinoma of the head and neck [Do not code the carcinoma in this example.]

11. Scarring due to third-degree burn of left leg

12. Wrist drop due to old injury to radial nerve of right lower arm

13. Mixed conductive and sensorineural hearing loss, unilateral, due to old temporal bone fracture

14. Dysarthria due to previous CVA

15. Unilateral double vision due to old CVA

# ICD-10-CM Sequelae Codes (Late Effects)

## Organization and Structure of ICD-10-CM Sequela Codes

ICD-10-CM does not contain a single chapter for the coding of late effects or sequelae of conditions. These codes are defined into the various body system chapters. For example, codes in category I69, Sequelae of cerebrovascular disease, are found in Chapter 9, Diseases of the Circulatory System.

In the ICD-10-CM Index to Diseases and Injuries, the main term of "Late, effect(s)" directs the coder to see another main term, "Sequelae." The terminology has changed in ICD-10-CM with the words "late effect" in a diagnosis replaced generally by the term "sequela."

## Coding Guidelines and Instructional Notes for ICD-10-CM Late Effect or Sequelae Codes

The NCHS has published guidelines for Late Effect or Sequela codes:

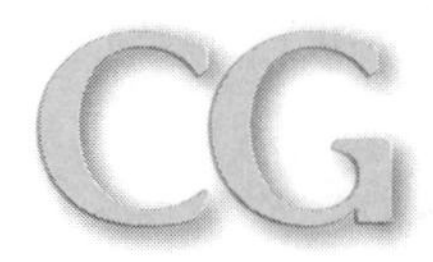

Guidelines I. B. 10. Sequela (Late Effects)

A sequela is the residual effect (condition produced) after the acute phase of an illness or injury has terminated. There is no time limit on when a sequela code can be used. The residual may be apparent early, such as in cerebral infarction, or it may occur months or years later, such as that due to a previous injury. Coding of sequela generally requires two codes sequenced in the following order: the condition or nature of the sequela is sequenced first. The sequela code is sequenced second.

An exception to the above guideline are those instances where the code for sequela is followed by a manifestation code identified in the Tabular List and title, or the sequela code has been expanded (at the fourth, fifth or sixth character levels) to include the manifestations(s). The code for the acute phase of an illness or injury that led to the sequela is never used with a code for the late effect.

Guidelines I. C. 9. d. Chapter specific guidelines, Chapter 9, Diseases of the circulatory system:

(1) Category I69, sequelae of cerebrovascular disease

Category I69 is used to indicate conditions classifiable to categories I60-I67 as the causes of sequela (neurologic deficits), themselves classified elsewhere. These “late effects” include neurological deficits that persist after initial onset of conditions classifiable to categories I60-I67. The neurologic deficits caused by cerebrovascular disease may be present from the onset or may arise at any time after the onset of the condition classifiable to categories I60-I67.

(2) Codes from category I69 may be assigned on a health record with codes from I60-I67, if the patient has a current cerebrovascular disease and deficits from an old cerebrovascular disease.

Guidelines I. C. 15, p. Chapter specific guidelines, Chapter 15, Pregnancy, childbirth and the puerperium:

(1) Code O94

Code O94, sequelae of complication of pregnancy, childbirth and the puerperium, is for use in those cases when an initial complication of a pregnancy develops a sequelae requiring care and treatment at a future date.

(2) This code may be used at any time after the initial postpartum period.

(3) This code, like all late effect codes, is to be sequenced following the code describing the sequelae of the complication.

Guidelines I. C. 19. a. Chapter specific guidelines, Chapter 19, Injury, poisoning, and certain other consequences of external causes:

Most categories in Chapter 19 have a 7th character extensions that are required for each applicable code. Most categories in this chapter have three 7th character values extensions (with the exception of fractures): A, initial encounter, D, subsequent encounter, and S, sequela. Depending on the fracture code, 7th characters exist as A, initial encounter for closed fracture, B, initial encounter for open fracture, D, subsequent encounter for fracture with routine healing, G, subsequent encounter for fracture with delayed healing, K, subsequent encounter for fracture with nonunion, P, subsequent encounter for fracture with malunion, and S, sequela.

a. Application of seventh characters

Seventh character "S", sequela, is for use for complications or conditions that arise as a direct result of an injury, such as scar formation after a burn. The scars are sequela of the burn. When using the 7th character "S," it is necessary to code both the injury code that precipitated the sequelae and the code for the sequela itself. The "S" is added only to the injury code, not the sequela code. The "S" extension identifies the injury responsible for the sequela. The specific type of sequela (that is, scar) is sequenced first, followed by the injury code.

d. 8. Coding of burns and corrosions, sequela with a late effect code and current burn

When appropriate, both a code for a current burn or corrosion with 7th character extension "A" or "D" and a burn or corrosions code with 7th character "S" may be assigned on the same record (when both a current burn and sequela of an old burn exist). Burns and corrosions do not heal at the same rate and a current healing wound may still exist with sequela of a healed burn or corrosion.

To gain an understanding of these rules, access the 2014 guidelines from NCHS website (http://www.cdc.gov/nchs/icd/icd10cm.htm) and search for the term "sequela" or sequelae" and find specific references to these types of codes. The general coding guideline for sequela states these conditions usually require two codes sequenced in the following order. First coded is the condition or nature of the sequela that is present today followed by the sequela code to identify the original condition that produced it. There are two exceptions to that sequencing rule that are described in the general coding guidelines for sequela. It is especially important for the coder to review the coding guidelines for common scenarios such as the coding of sequelae of cerebrovascular disease with the I69 category. Other commonly used sequelae codes are B90-B94, Sequelae of Infectious and Parasitic Diseases, O94, Sequelae of Complications of

Pregnancy, Childbirth, and the Puerperium and the injury and poisoning codes in categories S00-T88.9 that use the seventh character of S to indicate a sequela is present. Again to gain an understanding of these rules, the coder should refer all references to the coding of sequela conditions in the 2014 guidelines.

## Coding Overview: ICD-10-CM Sequelae Codes

In the ICD-10-CM Index to Diseases and Injuries, the main term of "Late, effect(s)" directs the coder to see another main term, "Sequelae." The terminology has changed in ICD-10-CM with the words "late effect" in a diagnosis replaced generally by the term "sequela." In the Index, the coder is directed to either a specific sequela code or to an injury code with the extension or seventh character of **S.**

For example, see the Index entry:

- Sequelae amputation—code to injury with seventh character **S**
- Sequelae, fracture—code to injury with seventh character **S**

These are combination codes that identify the specific original injury and the fact that the healthcare encounter is treating the sequela condition, not the acute injury.

Other entries under the main term of sequelae refer the coder to a specific ICD-10-CM diagnosis code, some with instructional notes at the category or code level.

For example, consider the following Index entries:

Sequelae, disease, cerebrovascular, dysphagia, I69.991

This code appears in the chapter for diseases of the circulatory system. When referencing the I69 code in the Tabular List, the coder is directed to use an additional code with I69.991 to identify the type of dysphagia (R13.1-). This code is somewhat the equivalent to the category 438 codes in ICD-9-CM that indicates the fact that a past stroke caused the patient's current problem. However, there is an expansion of the sequelae of stroke codes in ICD-10-CM and more options are available to describe the full extent of the patient's condition as the result of a stroke.

Sequelae, tuberculosis, pulmonary, B90.9

This code appears in the chapter for infectious and parasitic conditions (which includes active tuberculosis). When the coder turns in the Tabular List to category B90, a code first note directs the coder to code first the condition resulting from the infectious or parasitic condition. This code is equivalent to the rule in ICD-9-CM that directs that the condition the patient has now as a result of the former condition should be coded first, followed by the code for the original disease.

ICD-10-CM allows for coding of sequela of external cause. Sequela are reported using the external cause code with the seventh character extension S for sequela. These codes are used with any report of a late effect or sequela resulting from a previous condition. The sequela external cause code is used for subsequent healthcare visits when a late effect of the initial injury is being treated. See chapter 21 of this textbook for the coding of external cause of morbidity events.

The coder should examine the Alphabetic Index entry of "Sequelae" to review all the possible conditions for which late effect or sequelae codes exist.

## ICD-10-CM Review Exercises: Late Effect or Sequelae Codes

Assign the correct ICD-10-CM diagnosis codes to the following exercises. Do not assign external cause codes to these exercises.

1. Hemiplegia that remains three years after a non-traumatic intracerebral hemorrhage, affecting the right dominant side of the body.

   ______________________________

2. Aphasia due to old cerebral infarction

   ______________________________

3. Malunion fracture of right humerus due to old fracture, follow-up visit

   ______________________________

4. Keloid scar due to old third degree burn of right hand

   ______________________________

5. Adult with contracture of muscle tendon sheath, left lower leg, as a consequence of having poliomyelitis as a child

   ______________________________

6. Chronic gingivitis, nonplaque induced, as a sequela of Vitamin C deficiency

   ______________________________

7. Acquired deformity due to old crushing injury of left foot that is now healed

   ______________________________

8. Cognitive deficits as a result of an old stroke

   ______________________________

9. Visual disturbance as a late effect of a non-traumatic subarachnoid hemorrhage.

   ______________________________

10. Liver damage as the result of a previous viral hepatitis B

   ______________________________

## Chapter 23

# Supplementary Classifications—V Codes (ICD-9-CM, V01–V91) and Factors Influencing Health Status and Contact with Health Services (ICD-10-CM, Z00–Z99)

## Learning Objectives

At the conclusion of this chapter, you should be able to:

1. Describe the organization of the ICD-9-CM supplementary classification of factors influencing health status and contact with health services (V01–V91)
2. Describe the organization of the codes included in Chapter 21 of ICD-10-CM, Factors Influencing Health Status and Contact with Health Services (Z00–Z99)
3. Assign V codes from ICD-9-CM to describe the reason for a healthcare encounter and patient care
4. Assign ICD-10-CM codes for factors influencing health status and contact with health services
5. Describe the types of healthcare situations in which ICD-9-CM V codes and ICD-10-CM Z codes are intended to be used

## Supplementary Classification of Factors Influencing Health Status and Contact with Health Services (ICD-9-CM V01–V91)

Commonly referred to as **V codes,** categories V01–V91 of ICD-9-CM are included in Supplementary Classification of Factors Influencing Health Status and Contact with Health Services in the Tabular List in volume 1.

V code classifications are available for the following situations:

- When a person who is currently not sick uses health services for some purpose, such as acting as a donor, receiving prophylactic care such as an inoculation or vaccination, or receiving counseling on health-related issues.

  **EXAMPLE:** Physician office visit for prophylactic flu shot: V04.81, Need for prophylactic vaccination and inoculation against influenza

- When a person with a resolving disease or injury or one with a chronic long-term condition requiring continuous care encounters the healthcare system for specific aftercare of that disease or injury (for example, dialysis for renal disease, chemotherapy for malignancy, or cast change). A diagnosis or symptom code should be used whenever a current, acute diagnosis is being treated or a sign or symptom is being studied.

  **EXAMPLE:** Patient is admitted for chemotherapy for acute lymphocytic leukemia: V58.11 Encounter for antineoplastic chemotherapy; 204.00, Acute lymphocytic leukemia; 99.25, Chemotherapy

- When circumstances or problems influence a person's health status but are not in themselves a current illness or injury.

  **EXAMPLE:** Patient visits physician's office with a complaint of chest pain with an undetermined cause; patient is status post open-heart surgery for mitral valve replacement, 6 months ago: 786.50, Chest pain, unspecified; V43.3, Heart valve replaced by other means

- For newborns, to indicate birth status.

  **EXAMPLE:** Single newborn delivered via cesarean section: V30.01, Single liveborn delivered by cesarean delivery

V codes are assigned more frequently in hospital ambulatory care departments and other primary care sites, such as physicians' offices, than in acute inpatient facilities. V codes may be used as either a first-listed (principal diagnosis code in the inpatient setting) or secondary code depending on the circumstances of the encounter. Certain V codes may only be used as first listed, others only as secondary codes.

V codes are diagnosis codes and indicate a reason for a healthcare encounter. They are not procedure codes. A procedure code must be assigned in addition to the diagnosis V code to indicate that a procedure was performed.

The *ICD-9-CM Official Guidelines for Coding and Reporting* include an extensive section addressing the use of V codes and their intended purposes.

## V Code Categories and Section Titles

The V code supplementary classification contains the following categories and section titles:

| Categories | Section Titles |
|---|---|
| V01–V06 | Persons with Potential Health Hazards Related to Communicable Diseases |
| V07–V09 | Persons with Need for Isolation, Other Potential Health Hazards and Prophylactic Measures |

| | |
|---|---|
| V10–V19 | Persons with Potential Health Hazards Related to Personal and Family History |
| V20–V29 | Persons Encountering Health Services in Circumstances Related to Reproduction and Development |
| V30–V39 | Liveborn Infants According to Type of Birth |
| V40–V49 | Persons with a Condition Influencing Their Health Status |
| V50–V59 | Persons Encountering Health Services for Specific Procedures and Aftercare |
| V60–V69 | Persons Encountering Health Services in Other Circumstances |
| V70–V82 | Persons without Reported Diagnosis Encountered during Examination and Investigation of Individuals and Populations |
| V83–V84 | Genetics |
| V85 | Body Mass Index |
| V86 | Estrogen Receptor Status |
| V87 | Other Specified Personal Exposures and History Presenting Hazards to Health |
| V88 | Acquired Absence of Other Organs and Tissue |
| V89 | Other Suspected Conditions Not Found |
| V90 | Retained Foreign Body |
| V91 | Multiple Gestation Placenta Status |

Coders should review the multiple guidelines in *ICD-9-CM Official Guidelines for Coding and Reporting*. Within Section I, ICD-9-CM Conventions, General Coding Guidelines, and Chapter-Specific Guidelines, specific guidelines appear for V codes. Detailed information about the intent and appropriate use of V codes is provided in Section I, C-18, Supplemental Classification of Factors Influencing Health Status and Contact with Health Services (V Codes).

## Main Terms

V codes are indexed in the Alphabetic Index to Diseases along with codes for diseases, conditions, and symptoms. It is necessary, however, to become familiar with the main terms in the Alphabetic Index to Diseases that are related to V codes. First, look for terms that describe the reason for the encounter or admission. (The terms documented in the health record will often not lead to the appropriate code.) Then ask: "Why is the patient receiving services?"

**EXAMPLE:** The health record states closure of colostomy: V55.3, Attention to colostomy; 46.52, Closure of stoma of large intestine

The statement in the preceding example requires a V code (V55.3) because the patient was admitted for attention to an artificial opening. In addition, a procedure code (46.52) should be assigned for the closure.

Figure 23.1 shows how the main terms in the Alphabetic Index to Diseases lead to V codes.

**Figure 23.1.** Main terms leading to V codes

| | | |
|---|---|---|
| Admission (encounter) | Donor | Pregnancy |
| Aftercare | Encounter for | Problem |
| Attention to | Examination | Prophylactic |
| Boarder | Exposure | Replacement by artificial or mechanical device or prosthesis of |
| Care (of) | Fitting (of) | Resistance, resistant |
| Carrier (suspected) of | Follow-up | Screening |
| Checking | Health | Status (post) |
| Chemotherapy | Healthy | Supervision (of) |
| Contact | History (personal) of | Test(s) |
| Contraception, contraceptives | Maintenance | Therapy |
| Convalescence | Maladjustment | Transplant(ed) |
| Counseling | Newborn | Unavailability of medical facilities |
| Dependence | Observation | Vaccination |
| Dialysis | Outcome of delivery | |

## Persons with Potential Health Hazards Related to Communicable Diseases (V01–V06) and Persons with Need for Isolation, Other Potential Health Hazards and Prophylactic Measures (V07–V09)

Categories V01–V06 of the V code supplementary classification are assigned when a patient has come in contact with, or has been exposed to, a communicable disease or is in need of prophylactic vaccination and inoculation against a disease. The person does not show any signs or symptoms of the disease he or she was exposed to or came in contact with.

### *Category V01, Contact with or Exposure to Communicable Diseases*

The V01 category codes for contact and exposure to communicable disease may be used as the first-listed code to explain an encounter for testing. However, these codes may be used more commonly as secondary codes to identify a potential health risk.

### *Category V02, Carrier or Suspected Carrier of Infectious Diseases*

The V02 category codes describe colonization status or the presence on or in the body of a particular organism without it causing an illness in the patient. Codes within this category recognize carrier status for cholera, typhoid, amebiasis, gastrointestinal pathogens, diphtheria, specific bacterial diseases, viral hepatitis, and gonorrhea and other venereal and infectious diseases. Some of the commonly used codes in this category are V02.51, Group B Streptococcus carrier, V02.53, Methicillin-susceptible Staphylococcus aureus (MSSA) carrier, V02.54, Methicillin-resistant Staphylococcus aureus (MRSA) carrier, and V02.62, Hepatitis C carrier. Many hospitals test patients routinely for MRSA colonization by performing a nasal swab test upon admission that can identify positive or negative MRSA colonization in the patient.

The **status codes** in category V02 indicate that the patient is either a carrier or suspected carrier of an infectious disease but currently does not exhibit the symptoms of the disease. Status codes in the V code classification are informational because the conditions they describe may affect the course of treatment. Remember, "status" is different from "history" in ICD-9-CM. The history codes in the V code classification indicate the patient no longer has the disease.

### Categories V03–V06, Need for Prophylactic Vaccination and Inoculation

Categories V03–V06 are typically used to describe outpatient encounters for inoculations and vaccinations. The patient is being seen to receive a prophylactic inoculation against a disease. A procedure code must also be used to show the inoculation occurred. Vaccinations and inoculation codes may be used as secondary codes during well-baby or well-child care visits if the service was given as part of routine preventive healthcare.

These codes are located in the Alphabetic Index under the main terms "Prophylactic" and "Vaccination."

**EXAMPLE:** Vaccination against diphtheria: V03.5, Need for prophylactic vaccination and inoculation against diphtheria alone

### Category V07, Need for Isolation and Other Prophylactic or Treatment Measures

Within this category are V codes used to identify the reason for an encounter that could take place in an outpatient setting or identify a reason for a specific prophylaxis administration while the patient was in a hospital. Code V07.2, Prophylactic immunotherapy, is used to describe the administration of an immune gamma globulin, a tetanus antitoxin, or RhoGAM. Codes within the subcategory V07.5 identify the use of agents affecting estrogen receptors and estrogen levels. Immediately following this subcategory heading is a note to "use additional code to identify" the fact that the patient has a personal history of breast or prostate cancer, family history of breast cancer, has estrogen receptor positive status, has postmenopausal status, or has a genetic susceptibility to cancer. The more commonly used code within this subcategory is V07.51, Use of selective estrogen receptor modulators (SERMS), which include raloxifene (Evista), tamoxifen (Nolvadex), and toremifene (Fareston). Women receive these drugs following breast cancer treatment to prevent recurrence and metastasis of the disease. Women may receive these drugs during the course of their chemotherapy, which would then require the additional coding of the active cancer code, such as category 174 for Malignant neoplasm of the breast. A code from subcategory V07.5 could also be used once the patient qualifies as having a history of cancer, in which case the additional code from category V10 would be used to identify the completion of cancer treatment. The long-term use of a drug that falls under subcategory V07.5 would not require the continued use of an active cancer code. A code from subcategory V07.5 could also be used with a V67 category code, Follow-Up Examination.

### Category V08, Asymptomatic Human Immunodeficiency Virus (HIV) Infection Status

Category V08, Asymptomatic human immunodeficiency virus [HIV] infection status, is also discussed in chapter 4 of this textbook. The V08 code indicates the patient has tested positive for the HIV virus but has not manifested symptoms of HIV or acquired immune deficiency syndrome (AIDS).

### Category V09, Infection with Drug-Resistant Microorganisms

Category V09, Infection with drug-resistant microorganisms, should be used as an additional code to indicate the presence of drug resistance of an infectious organism for infectious conditions classified elsewhere. Sequence the infection code first and then the V09 code. V09 codes are to be used when the documentation in the health record indicates that a patient's infection has a known causative bacteria or other organism that is resistant to the medication therapy administered. Subcategory V09.8 is used frequently to identify patients with an infection with microorganisms resistant to other specified drugs, such as vancomycin-resistant organisms. Examples of this are vancomycin (glycopeptide) intermediate *Staphylococcus aureus* (VISA/GISA), vancomycin-resistant enterococcus (VRE), or vancomycin-resistant *Staphylococcus aureus* (VRSA/GRSA). The infection resistance codes are indexed under the main term "Resistance, resistant (to)" followed by the drug name.

**EXAMPLE:** Pulmonary tuberculosis (011.90) with infection resistant to Rifampin (V09.70)

## Persons with Potential Health Hazards Related to Personal and Family History (V10–V19)

The word "history" as used with all V codes may not be consistent with the intent of the word "history" when used by a physician to describe a patient's condition.

**Personal history** in ICD-9-CM means the patient's past medical condition no longer exists and the patient is not receiving any treatment for the condition. However, the information is important because the condition has the potential for recurrence and the patient may require continued monitoring. A physician may use the word "history" to describe a current condition the patient is being treated for, such as history of diabetes mellitus or history of hypertension. If the patient is receiving treatment for the condition, it would not be classified as a history code in ICD-9-CM.

**Family history** codes in ICD-9-CM, categories V16–V19, are used when a patient's family member(s) has a particular disease that puts the patient at higher risk of contracting the same condition. Physicians generally mean the same thing when using the term "family history."

Personal history codes are frequently used in conjunction with follow-up V codes and family history V codes, as well as screening V codes, to explain the reason for the visit or diagnostic testing. These codes are important information as their presence may alter the type of treatment the patient receives.

Categories V10–V19 include codes for personal and family histories of malignant neoplasms and other health problems.

The personal history of malignant neoplasm (V10) category includes primary cancer sites only. **Note:** There are no personal history of secondary neoplasm sites or carcinoma in situ sites. The instructional notes listed under each subcategory refer to specific code ranges for primary malignancies categories (categories 140–195.) Secondary and CA in situ malignancies are excluded from this range of codes.

A patient with leukemia or lymphoma in remission should be classified to the 200–208 categories instead of the V codes in this range. The history of leukemia or lymphatic or hematopoietic neoplasms codes in the V10.6 and V10.7 subcategories means the patient is completely cured of the disease.

Category V12, Personal history of certain other diseases has been expanded to include specific conditions that have the potential to affect future healthcare services.

History of infections of the central nervous system (V12.42), history of circulatory disorders (V12.50–V12.59), and history of pneumonia (V12.61) codes enable the tracking of specific conditions over the lifetime of the patient.

History of urinary (tract) infections (V13.02) and history of nephrotic syndrome (V13.03) can be relevant when similar conditions are currently present. Codes within the V13.1 and V13.2 subcategories describe a woman who has had a problem during previous pregnancies but currently is not pregnant. History of pathological fracture and stress fractures are included in codes V13.51 and V13.52. A code for history of a traumatic fracture is included in code V15.51. Other codes in the V13 category should be used cautiously because the word "history" may be misinterpreted. For example, rarely does a person have a history of arthritis (V13.4). Instead, usually this is a lifelong condition that the physician may document as "history" while actually intending to describe the patient's current health status. But subcategory V13.6, Congenital (corrected) malformations do reflect a historical condition. The codes V13.61–V13.69 are used to identify a patient who has a personal history of a congenital malformation that is no longer present. Many congenital conditions can be repaired and leave no residual condition. However, the fact the patient once had the anomaly is an important consideration during future healthcare encounters.

Most of the category V14 codes and subcategory V15.0 are exceptions to the general rule that history codes mean the condition is no longer present. A person who has had an allergic reaction to food or a substance is always considered allergic to that substance. These V codes indicate that the person is not currently exhibiting an allergic reaction but, instead, has the potential for a reaction if exposed to the substance in the future.

Other codes in category V15 identify the fact that the patient has a personal history that presents hazards to health. Examples of commonly used codes in this category are surgery to the heart and great vessels (V15.1), psychological trauma (V15.41–V15.49), personal history of retained foreign body fully removed (V15.53), noncompliance with medical treatment (V15.81), and history of tobacco use (V15.82.).

A patient with a history of fall(s) or identified as at risk for falling can be classified with code V15.88. This code is used to identify patients at risk for falling or who have a history of falls with or without subsequent injuries. Falls are an important public health problem affecting about one third of adults age 65 years and older annually. About 20 to 30 percent of those who fall will suffer moderate to severe injuries, including hip and other fractures and head trauma. Adults age 75 years or older who fall are more likely to be admitted to a long-term care facility for one year or longer. In this same population, more than 60 percent of deaths are from falls. The code V15.88 can be used to identify patients who require closer monitoring to prevent falls, to justify specific diagnostic or therapeutic services to identify causes of falling, or to order preventive evaluation or services.

Category V16 describes a family history of malignant neoplasm. This risk factor is an important medical fact about a patient and may be the reason for increased monitoring and diagnostic testing of the patient with a family history of cancer. Category V17 identifies family history of certain chronic disabling diseases, such as V17.41, Family history of sudden cardiac death.

Category V18 codes identify a family history of certain other specific conditions that may describe a patient's reason for a healthcare encounter. For example, V18.51, Family history of digestive disorders, colonic polyps, may be the reason a patient has a screening colonoscopy performed at an earlier age or with more frequency than individuals with average risk. Certain individuals are at greater risk of developing colon polyps if they have a family member in whom colon polyps have been diagnosed.

These V codes are indexed under "History (personal) of" in the Alphabetic Index. Note the subterm "family" is indented under "history (personal) of" and is the point of reference for familial conditions.

**EXAMPLE:** Personal history of breast carcinoma: V10.3 (describes a condition coded to 174 or 175 when present and treated)

**EXAMPLE:** Personal history of allergy to penicillin: V14.0, Personal history of allergy to penicillin

**EXAMPLE:** Family history of diabetes: V18.0, Family history of diabetes mellitus

**EXAMPLE:** Personal history of noncompliance with medical treatment: V15.81, Personal history of noncompliance with medical treatment

## Persons Encountering Health Services in Circumstances Related to Reproduction and Development (V20–V29)

Categories V20–V29 include codes for health supervision of infant or child, including routine or subsequent newborn check (V20), constitutional states in development (V21), supervision of normal and high-risk pregnancies (V22 and V23), postpartum care (V24), contraceptive management (V25), procreative management (V26), outcome of delivery (V27), antenatal screening (V28), and observation and evaluation of newborn for suspected condition not found (V29).

### *Category V20, Health Supervision of Infant or Child*

Category V20 codes identify outpatient clinic or doctor office encounters with newborns and young children. V20.2, Routine infant or child health check, identifies a "well baby" or "well child" visit in the office or clinic when the infant or child does not have an illness but is seen for developmental testing, immunizations, or routine health check-ups. Two other codes, V20.31, Health supervision for newborn under eight days, and V20.32, Health supervision for newborn 8 to 28 days, were created for specific post-hospital newborn care visits in the doctor's office or clinic. Most healthy newborns are discharged from the hospital less than 48 hours after birth. Pediatric care standards recommend an examination by the physician within two days of that discharge or no later than 28 days after birth. During this encounter the infant is evaluated for feeding, jaundice, hydration, and elimination problems; the clinician also assesses how well mother and infant are interacting, reviews the newborn's laboratory and screening tests, and communicates the plan for healthcare maintenance, future immunizations, and periodic examinations.

### *Category V22, Normal Pregnancy*

Category V22 is assigned for supervision of a pregnancy. Codes V22.0, Supervision of normal first pregnancy, and V22.1, Supervision of normal subsequent pregnancies, are generally used in outpatient settings and for routine prenatal visits. When a complication of the pregnancy is present, the code for that condition is assigned rather than a code from category V22. These codes are not used with any other pregnancy code in Chapter 11 of ICD-9-CM because the V22 code indicates the patient is pregnant and healthy, whereas the Chapter 11 codes indicate an obstetrical problem or condition exists. Codes V22.0 and V22.1 are indexed under "Pregnancy, supervision (of) (for)" in the Alphabetic Index to Diseases.

Code V22.2, Pregnant state, incidental, would be assigned as an additional code only if a pregnant patient was seen for a reason unrelated to the pregnancy. It is the physician's responsibility to document that the pregnancy is in no way complicating the reason for the visit or the nonobstetrical condition currently being treated. However, it is not a common occurrence for the physician to state the pregnancy is unaffected, no matter how minor the injury or condition. For this reason, a code from Chapter 11 in ICD-9-CM is more frequently used than the V22.2. Code V22.2 is indexed under the main term "Pregnancy" in the Alphabetic Index.

**EXAMPLE:** Patient seen in the emergency department with a sprained wrist; doctor documents that the patient is 30 weeks pregnant, but specifically states the pregnancy is incidental to the encounter: 842.00, Sprains and strains of unspecified site of wrist; V22.2, Pregnant state, incidental

### Category V23, Supervision of High-Risk Pregnancy

Category V23 provides information on conditions that may add risk to a present pregnancy. A code from V23 can be assigned as a principal or first-listed diagnosis or as an additional code. A code from Chapter 11 in ICD-9-CM can be assigned with a code from category V23. Typically, these codes are used for prenatal outpatient visits. Code V23.7, Insufficient prenatal care, may be assigned to patients who had little or no prenatal care. Healthcare providers must define "insufficient" prenatal care and consistently capture this code for the information to be valuable. Codes within the V23.8 subcategories identify elderly (35 years or older at expected date of delivery) or very young (younger than 16 years at expected date of delivery) pregnant females whose age and current pregnancy make them high risk for problems and thus worthy of close monitoring. Codes V23.85 and V23.86 identify the fact that the patient is pregnant as a result of assisted reproductive technology or is pregnant with a history of an in utero procedure during a previous pregnancy.

The V23 category codes are indexed under the main terms "Pregnancy, supervision (of) (for)" and "Pregnancy, management affected by" in the Alphabetic Index.

**EXAMPLE:** Pregnancy, 19-week gestation with history of infertility: V23.0, Pregnancy with history of infertility

**EXAMPLE:** Full term with intrauterine death, spontaneous delivery; no prenatal care received during pregnancy: 656.41, Intrauterine death; V23.7, Insufficient prenatal care; V27.1, Single stillborn; 73.59, Other manually assisted delivery

### Category V24, Postpartum Care and Examination

Category V24 is used primarily in the outpatient setting for uncomplicated follow-up during the postpartum period. Code V24.0 is the principal diagnosis when the mother delivers outside the hospital prior to admission and is admitted for routine postpartum care and no complications are noted. If a postpartum complication is found, however, the appropriate pregnancy diagnosis code is assigned rather than a code from category V24. Category V24 codes are indexed under "Postpartum, observation" or "Lactation" in the Alphabetic Index.

**EXAMPLE:** Visit to physician for routine postpartum examination; no complications were noted: V24.2, Routine postpartum follow-up

**EXAMPLE:** Patient delivered at home and was admitted to hospital with postpartum hemorrhage: 666.14, Other immediate postpartum hemorrhage

### Category V25, Encounter for Contraceptive Management

Category V25 includes codes for contraceptive management, such as general contraceptive counseling and advice, insertion of an intrauterine contraceptive device (IUD), menstrual extraction, and surveillance of previously prescribed contraceptive methods. Codes from this category are indexed under "Contraception, contraceptive" in the Alphabetic Index.

**EXAMPLE:** Visit to physician for prescription of birth control pills: V25.01, Prescription of oral contraceptives

Codes in subcategory V25.1 are used to report an encounter for insertion or removal of an IUD. These codes are frequently used for office visits when the encounter is for the insertion of an IUD (V25.11), for removal of an IUD (V25.12), and for removal and reinsertion of an IUD (V25.13). An encounter for routine checking of an IUD would be reported with code V25.42, Surveillance of previously prescribed contraceptive methods, intrauterine contraceptive device.

Code V25.2, Sterilization, is often assigned as an additional diagnosis when a sterilization procedure is performed during the same admission as a delivery. It may also be assigned as a principal diagnosis when the admission is solely for sterilization.

**EXAMPLE:** Spontaneous delivery of full-term live infant with tubal ligation performed the day after delivery: 650, Normal delivery; 27.0, Outcome of delivery, single liveborn; V25.2, Sterilization; 73.59, Other manually assisted delivery; 66.39, Other bilateral destruction or occlusion of fallopian tube

**EXAMPLE:** Patient desires sterilization; tubal ligation performed: V25.2, Sterilization; 66.39, Other bilateral destruction or occlusion of fallopian tube

### Category V26, Procreative Management

Procreative management describes healthcare services related to producing an offspring. Services related to genetic testing and infertility services can be described with these codes. Screening for genetic carrier status is becoming more commonplace to identify individuals for certain serious genetic disease. For example, a couple may be screened either preconception or early in pregnancy to determine carrier status. If both partners are carriers, different pregnancy management may be instituted. Carrier status screening has become the professional standard of care for cystic fibrosis, Canavan disease, hemoglobinopathies, and Tay-Sachs disease. Because most of the individuals are noncarriers, it is inappropriate to use disease codes to describe the screening encounter; instead, code V26.31 is used to identify the testing of the female partner and V26.34 is used to identify the testing of the male partner for genetic disease carrier status. Other codes within subcategory V26.3 identify encounters for genetic counseling and other genetic testing. If genetic testing is performed for reasons other than procreative management, the coder is referred to screening codes V82.71 and V82.79, Screening for genetic disease carrier status or other genetic screening.

Healthcare encounters for reversal of a previous tubal ligation or vasectomy, artificial insemination, investigation and testing, and genetic counseling are included here. Codes V26.51 and V26.52 describe sterilization status for both men and women and are frequently confused with code V25.2. The "status" codes, V26.51 and V26.52, describe past treatment to acquire sterilization, whereas a person who desires sterilization during the current episode of care is coded with V25.2, Admission for sterilization. The Alphabetic Index to Diseases should be followed closely so as not to confuse these different episodes of healthcare.

Fertility preservation encounters are also included in this category. Individuals in their child-bearing years diagnosed with a malignant condition may seek to preserve fertility before and after cancer treatment and are referred to a fertility specialist to be made aware of what options are available to them before they start cancer treatment. Options may include trying to conceive before treatment or storing sperm, eggs, ovarian tissue, or embryos in a tissue or gamete bank to be used for future conception. Code V26.42 is used to identify the encounter for fertility preservation counseling. When a fertility preservation procedure is performed, the diagnosis code of V26.82 is used to describe the encounter.

**EXAMPLE:** A female patient undergoes fertility testing by fallopian insufflation, V26.21

**EXAMPLE:** A male patient is seen in an encounter for fertility preservation prior to beginning cancer therapy, V26.42

## *Category V27, Outcome of Delivery*

A code from Category V27, Outcome of delivery, should be included on every maternal record when a delivery has occurred. These codes are not to be used on subsequent postpartum records or on the newborn record. They are always secondary codes on the maternal record at the time of delivery. The V27 code indicates whether the delivery produced a single or multiple birth and whether the infants were liveborn or stillborn. The unspecified code, V27.9, should not be used because the maternal health record will identify the details of the delivery. Codes in category V27 are indexed under "Outcome of delivery" in the Alphabetic Index.

**EXAMPLE:** Spontaneous delivery of full-term live infant: 650, Normal delivery; V27.0, Outcome of delivery, single liveborn; 73.59, Other manually assisted delivery

**A point to remember:** Category V27 codes are only assigned to the mother's health record. These codes should not appear on the baby's health record. The V27 maternal codes should not be confused with the V30 newborn codes that are used to describe the newborn's birth status.

## *Category V28, Encounter for Antenatal Screening of the Mother*

Codes within category V28 describe the testing of the female during pregnancy for a variety of conditions and abnormalities. These codes, which are intended to describe the female, not the fetus, are used to indicate the screening was planned. Some of these screening procedures have become common during the antepartum period. If the screening test results are returned with abnormal findings or determine that a condition is present, the abnormal finding or condition should be coded as an additional code with the V28 screening category code. The V28 code is not used if the testing of the female is to rule out or confirm a suspected diagnosis because the patient has some sign or symptom. That is a diagnostic examination and the sign or symptom code is used to explain the reason for the test. The V28 code also indicates that the screening examination was planned. A procedure code is required to confirm that the screening was performed.

### Category V29, Observation and Evaluation of Newborns for Suspected Condition Not Found

Category V29 codes are available for situations in which a newborn (the first 28 days of life) is suspected of having a particular condition that is ruled out after examination and observation. Do not assign a code from category V29 when the patient has identified signs or symptoms of a suspected problem; instead, in these cases code the sign or symptom. V29 codes are used only for healthy newborns and infants for whom no condition after study is found to be present. V29.0 can be a principal or secondary diagnosis code when the newborn is an inpatient. At the time of birth, if a suspected condition is not found, category V29 is used as an additional code because the V30–V39 category code must be listed first to indicate the status of the birth. However, category V29 may be used as a principal code for readmissions or encounters when the V30 code no longer applies. Additional diagnosis codes may be used in addition to the observation code on the newborn record, but only if the additional codes describe a condition unrelated to the suspected condition being evaluated.

Codes for this category are located in the Alphabetic Index under the main term "Observation (for), suspected, condition, newborn."

**EXAMPLE:** Five-day-old newborn is admitted to the hospital with suspected sepsis; following blood cultures, the sepsis was ruled out: V29.0, Observation for suspected infectious conditions

**EXAMPLE:** Single liveborn infant delivered by cesarean delivery in the hospital, suspected of having a neurological condition that is ruled out after observation and study: V30.01, Single liveborn, born in hospital, delivered by cesarean delivery; V29.1, Observation for suspected neurological condition

## Liveborn Infants According to Type of Birth (V30–V39)

A code from categories V30–V39 is used to identify all types of births and is always the first code listed on the health record of the newborn at the time of birth. The V30–V39 codes are used once when the infant is born. If the newborn is transferred to another institution, the V30 series is not used at the second institution or on the infant's subsequent admissions or outpatient visits to any healthcare provider. The V30–V39 categories describe single or multiple liveborns, and single or multiple stillborns. Codes for these categories are indexed under "Newborn" in the Alphabetic Index. Using the Alphabetic Index and the main term "Newborn," the next information to be reviewed is the birth status of the infant: single, twin, or multiple for three or more infants born to the same mother. If the infant was a single birth, the next information needed is whether the baby was born in hospital or outside hospital. If the infant was born inside the hospital, was the birth a vaginal or cesarean delivery? If the infant was a twin birth, the next information needed is the status of the mate—liveborn or stillborn. If the twin's mate was liveborn, for example, the next information needed is whether the infant was born in hospital or outside hospital. If the twin was born in the hospital, a fifth digit will be added to identify it as a cesarean delivery or no mention of cesarean delivery. When coding an infant that was part of a multiple birth, such as triplets or more, the next most important subterm the coder should reference is the status of the "mates all liveborn," "mates all stillborn" or "mates liveborn and stillborn." By correctly accessing the Alphabetic Index with specific subterms that describe the infant's birth, the coder can avoid the unspecified and inaccurate codes of V33, Twin, Unspecified or V37, Other Multiple, Unspecified or V39, Unspecified Infant. In addition to the V30–V39 type of birth code, any disease or birth injury should also be coded as additional diagnoses, if applicable.

### Fourth- and Fifth-Digit Subdivisions

At the beginning of categories V30–V39, instructions for fourth and fifth digits are given.

**.0 Born in hospital (requires a fifth digit)**
**.1 Born before admission to hospital**
**.2 Born outside hospital and not hospitalized**

The fourth digit .0 is assigned when a baby is born in the hospital. The following fifth-digit subclassification is used with the fourth digit .0:

**0 delivered without mention of cesarean delivery**
**1 delivered by cesarean delivery**

**EXAMPLE:** Exceptionally large liveborn male infant delivered in hospital via low cervical cesarean section: V30.01, Single liveborn, delivered in hospital by cesarean delivery; 766.0, Exceptionally large baby

The fourth digit .1 is assigned when a baby is admitted to the hospital immediately following birth. These codes are not assigned to newborns transferred from other hospitals.

**EXAMPLE:** Infant admitted to hospital following birth at home: V30.1, Single liveborn, delivered before admission to hospital

**EXAMPLE:** Infant transferred to hospital B from hospital A with a congenital heart defect—tetralogy of Fallot. Hospital B would assign the following: 745.2, tetralogy of Fallot

The fourth digit .2 is assigned when a baby is born outside the hospital and is not hospitalized. Therefore, this fourth digit should not be used in the acute care setting.

**EXAMPLE:** Single liveborn infant, examined at home after birth. Physical examination essentially normal. Infant will remain at home. Home visit is coded: V30.2, Single liveborn, born outside hospital and not hospitalized

## Exercise 23.1

Assign ICD-9-CM diagnosis and procedure codes (when applicable) to the following:

1. Antenatal screening for chromosomal anomalies by amniocentesis; amniocentesis

2. Admission for sterilization; bilateral endoscopic ligation and division of fallopian tubes

3. Exposure to tuberculosis

4. Twin with stillborn mate delivered in the hospital via cesarean delivery

5. Family history of colon carcinoma

## Persons with a Condition Influencing Their Health Status (V40–V49)

At the beginning of this section for categories V40–V49, a note states: "These categories are intended for use when these conditions are recorded as 'diagnoses' or 'problems.'" (CDC 2014)

Typically, the codes in these categories are assigned as additional diagnoses. Categories V40–V49 are "status" codes that indicate that a patient is a carrier of a disease, has the sequelae or residual of a past disease or condition or has another factor influencing a person's health status. The codes may indicate a transplanted organ or tissue or the presence of an artificial opening such as a colostomy. Postsurgical states are described with these codes to indicate the presence of a mechanical or prosthetic device such as a cardiac pacemaker or an IUD. Other codes in this section describe postprocedural status to indicate a certain procedure has been performed in the past, such as a coronary bypass or angioplasty. A status code is informative because the patient's condition or status may influence the course of treatment he or she receives in the future.

### *Category V42, Organ or Tissue Replaced by Transplant*

Category V42 is used for homologous or heterologous (animal or human) organ transplants. These codes are indexed under "Status (post), transplant" in the Alphabetic Index.

**EXAMPLE:** Status post kidney transplant (human donor):
V42.0, Kidney replaced by transplant

Code, V49.83, Awaiting organ transplant status, is included in another category of ICD-9-CM. Some patients who are on a waiting list for a heart transplant may be hospitalized due to the severity of their illness. V49.83 is a status code to distinguish patients who are hospitalized while awaiting a new heart from patients who are hospitalized for direct treatment of their heart disease. This code could also be used to indicate that the patient is on the heart transplant waiting list.

### Category V43, Organ or Tissue Replaced by Other Means

Category V43 is used when coding replacement of an organ with an artificial device, mechanical device, or prosthesis. Codes in this category are indexed under "Status (post), organ replacement, by artificial or mechanical device or prosthesis of" in the Alphabetic Index.

**EXAMPLE:** Status post hip replacement with a prosthetic device: V43.64, Hip joint replaced by other means

### Category V44, Artificial Opening Status

Category V44 is subdivided to identify the presence of an artificial opening, such as a tracheostomy (V44.0), ileostomy (V44.2), colostomy (V44.3), cystostomy (V44.5), and so forth. These codes are indexed under "Status (post)" in the Alphabetic Index.

**EXAMPLE:** Status post colostomy: V44.3, Colostomy status

The exclusion note at the beginning of category V44 instructs coders to use a code from categories V55.0–V55.9 when the encounter or admission is for attention to or management of that artificial opening.

### Category V45, Other Postprocedural States

Category V45 includes codes for a variety of postprocedural states, such as cardiac pacemaker in situ (V45.01); automatic implantable cardiac defibrillator (V45.02); renal dialysis status (V45.11); noncompliance with renal dialysis (V45.12); presence of cerebrospinal fluid drainage device (V45.2); intestinal bypass or anastomosis status (V45.3); presence of cerebrospinal fluid drainage device (V45.2); cataract extraction status (V45.61); aortocoronary bypass status (V45.81); percutaneous transluminal coronary angioplasty status (V45.82); and bariatric surgery status (nonobstetrical patient) (V45.86).

V45.7, Acquired absence of organ, was created to indicate the status of an acquired absence of an organ in contrast to a congenital absence. This status is useful in describing the reason for the visit when a patient is seen for reconstructive surgery. The code is intended to be used for patient care in which the absence of an organ affects treatment. Subcategory V45.7 includes codes to describe the acquired absence, through surgery or other medical intervention, of breast, intestine, kidney, lung, stomach, urinary sites, genital organs excluding cervix and uterus, as well as other organs.

Code V45.87, Transplant organ removal status, is used to indicate that a transplanted organ has been previously removed. This code is not assigned during the hospital stay when the surgical removal procedure is performed. For that encounter, the reason or complication that necessitated removal of the transplanted organ should be coded instead.

Code V45.88, Status post administration of tPA (rtPA) in a different facility within the last 24 hours prior to admission to current facility, is used by the hospital or physician that receives the patient for continued care. A typical scenario involves a patient in Hospital 1, diagnosed with an acute myocardial infarction or acute ischemic stroke, who receives tissue plasminogen activator (tPA) (usually within three hours of the onset of the symptoms) and is transferred to Hospital 2 for specialized cardio- or cerebrovascular treatment. Only Hospital 2 uses code V45.88 to identify that the patient has received the tPA, even if the tPA infusion is ongoing at the time of the transfer.

Codes from category V45 are indexed under "Status (post)" in the Alphabetic Index.

**EXAMPLE:** Two-year-old admitted for hernia repair of right inguinal hernia; patient also has ventriculoperitoneal shunt: 550.90, Unilateral or unspecified (not specified as recurrent) inguinal hernia, without mention of obstruction or gangrene; V45.2, Presence of cerebrospinal fluid drainage device; 53.00, Unilateral repair of inguinal hernia, not otherwise specified

### *Category V46, Other Dependence on Machines and Devices*

Codes from category V46 are assigned to cases in which patients become dependent on machines or equipment, such as respirators, aspirators, wheelchairs, and supplemental or long-term oxygen therapy. Patients who are dependent on ventilators may be admitted to a healthcare facility when their mechanical ventilator at home has equipment malfunctions or when a power outage causes their machine to fail. A specific code in this category, V46.12, indicates the encounter is associated with the patient's need for medical care due to his respirator dependence during power failure. Patients are often admitted to long-term care facilities specifically to be weaned from a ventilator. Code V46.13 is used to identify an encounter for weaning from a respirator or ventilator. These codes are indexed under "Dependence on" in the Alphabetic Index.

**EXAMPLE:** Patient in acute respiratory failure dependent on respirator: 518.81, Acute respiratory failure; V46.11, Dependence on respirator

## Persons Encountering Health Services for Specific Procedures and Aftercare (V50–V59)

The following important note for categories V51–V58 appears at the beginning of this section:

> Categories V51–V58 are intended for use to indicate a reason for care in patients who may have already been treated for some disease or injury not now present, or who are receiving care to consolidate the treatment, to deal with residual states, or to prevent recurrence.

The word **aftercare** may not be used commonly by the physician to describe this particular episode of care for a patient. Instead, the physician may use terminology such as **follow-up** or *status post* or use an action word to describe the procedure to be performed, such as *closure* of a colostomy. Again, the language of physicians may not always coincide perfectly with the language of ICD-9-CM, and the coder must identify that situation and make the necessary language adjustments in order to code the episode correctly.

Aftercare visit codes describe the patient who has received the initial treatment for a disease or injury but requires continued care during the health or recovery phase. The aftercare may also describe the long-term consequences of the disease.

The aftercare V codes are not used if treatment is being given for a current or acute disease or injury. The diagnosis code should be used in this case.

Typically, aftercare codes are listed first to explain the specific reason for the visit or encounter. An aftercare code may also be used as an additional code when some type of aftercare is provided in addition to the reason for the admission or visit. Aftercare codes should be used with any diagnosis or any other aftercare code to provide specific details of the encounter. The sequencing of multiple aftercare codes is discretionary.

Categories V50–V59 are subdivided to describe the type of service provided. Codes in categories V50–V59 are indexed in the Alphabetic Index under "Admission (encounter), for," "Aftercare," and "Attention to." Typically, codes from these categories are assigned as a principal diagnosis.

### Category V54, Other Orthopedic Aftercare

Category V54 is subdivided to describe particular orthopedic aftercare. Subcategory V54.0, Aftercare involving internal fixation device, identifies the reason for the encounter by describing the type of procedure to be performed: removal of a device or lengthening or adjusting a growth rod. Other codes describe the healing phase of fracture care. Coding guidelines for ICD-9-CM require that an acute fracture code be used while the patient is receiving active treatment for the fracture. Examples of active treatment include surgery, emergency department visits, and evaluation and treatment by a new physician. Subsequent encounters require the use of an aftercare code. Aftercare codes are used to describe the encounters after the patient has completed active treatment of the fracture and is receiving routine care for the fracture during the healing or recovery period. Aftercare includes cast changes or removal, removal of external or internal fixation devices, medication adjustments, and follow-up visits following fracture treatment. Subcategories V54.1, Aftercare for healing traumatic fracture, and V54.2, Aftercare for healing pathologic fracture, exist to describe the services related to the healing process with the fracture site identified. A specific code, V54.81, describes aftercare following a joint replacement.

**EXAMPLE:** Removal of screw from healed fracture of arm: V54.01, Aftercare involving removal of fracture plate or other internal fixation device

**EXAMPLE:** A patient comes to the family physician's office for cast removal. The patient had suffered the fracture and received treatment while away at college, but healing has occurred and the cast needs to be removed. Code V54.89, Other orthopedic aftercare, describes the reason for the visit.

### Category V55, Attention to Artificial Openings

Unlike category V44, Artificial opening status, category V55 describes attention to the artificial opening, which may include the following services:

- Adjustment or repositioning of catheter
- Closure
- Passage of sounds or bougies
- Reforming
- Removal or replacement of catheter
- Toileting or cleansing

Category V55 codes may be first-listed diagnoses or used as additional diagnosis codes. These codes identify encounters for catheter cleaning, fitting, and adjustment services, and other care that is distinct from actual treatment. These codes are not used when there is a complication of the device or catheter.

**EXAMPLE:** Emergency department visit for a patient who needs a replacement of a clogged gastrostomy tube: V55.1, Attention to gastrostomy

**EXAMPLE:** A patient is admitted for a scheduled closure of a colostomy: V55.3, Attention to colostomy

**EXAMPLE:** Encounter for replacement of cystostomy tube: V55.5, Attention to cystostomy

### Category V56, Encounter for Dialysis and Dialysis Catheter Care

V56 codes are used to identify the main reason for the encounter, for example, extracorporeal or peritoneal dialysis and related services. The note "Use additional code to identify the associated condition" appears at the beginning of category V56. The associated condition, that is, the reason for the dialysis or dialysis catheter care, is listed second. Codes in subcategory V56.0 and V56.8 are indexed under "Dialysis" in the Alphabetic Index.

**EXAMPLE:** Visit for renal dialysis for patient with end-stage renal disease: V56.0, Encounter for extracorporeal dialysis; 585.6, End-stage renal disease

### Category V57, Care Involving Use of Rehabilitation Procedures

Category V57 includes codes describing admissions or encounters for physical therapy, speech therapy, occupational therapy, and other rehabilitation procedures. When a patient is admitted for a rehabilitation procedure, the first code listed is the V57 category code, Care involving the use of rehabilitation procedures. The code for the disease or condition requiring rehabilitation should be reported as an additional diagnosis. The fourth digit of the V57 code indicates the focus of treatment, for example, physical therapy, or speech therapy. Only one code from category V57 is required. Code V57.89, Other specified rehabilitation procedures, should be assigned if more than one type of rehabilitation is performed during a single encounter. A procedure code should be reported to identify each type of rehabilitation therapy actually performed.

Since the implementation of Medicare's rehabilitation prospective payment system in 2002, coders have been required to assign a code for the etiologic diagnosis to indicate the condition for which the patient is receiving rehabilitation. The etiologic diagnosis is required on the data collection instrument called the Inpatient Rehabilitation Facility–Patient Assessment Instrument (IRF-PAI).

However, this does not change the official ICD-9-CM coding guidelines with regard to rehabilitation coding. The principal diagnosis for inpatient services or the first-listed diagnosis for outpatient services that must appear on the UB-04 claim form will still be a code from category V57, Care involving use of rehabilitation procedures, when the patient is receiving rehabilitation services.

Codes in category V57 are indexed under "Therapy" in the Alphabetic Index.

**EXAMPLE:** Admission for physical therapy for hemiplegia due to CVA that occurred two weeks ago: V57.1, Care involving other physical therapy; 438.20, Late effect of cerebrovascular disease, hemiplegia

### Category V58, Encounter for Other and Unspecified Procedures and Aftercare

Category V58 includes codes for admissions or encounters for radiotherapy, antineoplastic chemotherapy, antineoplastic immunotherapy, attention to surgical dressings and sutures, other aftercare following surgery, long-term (current) drug use, therapeutic drug monitoring, and so forth.

Aftercare codes describe patient encounters that take place after the initial treatment of a disease has been completed and the patient now requires continued care during the healing or recovery process. Patients may be admitted to skilled nursing facilities or long-term care hospitals for recovery or they may be receiving home care services. The aftercare codes describe services received during such a continuing phase of healthcare.

Aftercare codes are generally the first-listed code to describe the reason for the encounter. However, an aftercare code may be used as an additional code when the aftercare is provided during an admission for treatment of an unrelated condition. In addition, multiple aftercare codes can be used together to fully identify the reason for the aftercare services.

Aftercare codes are not used if treatment is directed at a current acute disease or injury. The diagnosis code is used for these patients. Exceptions to this rule include codes V58.0, Radiotherapy, V58.11, Chemotherapy, and V58.12, Immunotherapy. These codes are always listed first, followed by the malignancy diagnosis code, when the patient's encounter is solely to receive radiation therapy or chemotherapy. Either code can be listed first if the patient is receiving both therapies during the same visit.

**EXAMPLE:** Admission for chemotherapy for patient with metastasis to bone; patient has history of breast carcinoma with mastectomy performed eight years ago: V58.11, Antineoplastic chemotherapy; 198.5, Secondary malignant neoplasm of bone; V10.3, Personal history of malignant neoplasm of breast; procedure 99.25, Injection or infusion of cancer chemotherapeutic substance

Subcategory V58.3 would be used for a follow-up visit for change of surgical or other dressings, checking the wound for healing, or removal of sutures or staples when there is no mention of any wound infection or other complications. Specific codes exist for these types of encounters. Typically, these encounters occur in a physician's office, in an ambulatory clinic or center, or during a home healthcare visit. Code V58.30 is intended to describe the encounter for the change or removal of a nonsurgical wound dressing. The encounter for the change or removal of a surgical wound dressing or packing is code V58.31. An encounter for the purpose of removing sutures or staples would be reported with code V58.32.

Broad categories exist for aftercare following surgery for neoplasms (V58.42), aftercare following surgery for injury and trauma (V58.43), and aftercare following surgery for specific body systems (V58.71–V58.78). The aftercare codes are usually reported outside the acute care hospital setting to identify the postsurgical treatment after the initial treatment and surgery is completed. This postsurgical care may be received in a long-term care hospital or facility or through home care services. These codes should be used with other V codes for postoperative wound dressing care, ostomy care, or other similar V codes to completely describe the services. However, some codes should not be used together. For example, V58.43 should not be reported with one of the V54.1 codes when the surgical aftercare is for the treatment of a healing traumatic fracture because the fracture care code is more specific and there is an excludes note under V58.43. Inclusion terms appear under these aftercare codes to indicate the original disease or injury that was treated, for which aftercare is now being provided. For example:

| | |
|---|---|
| V58.42 | Aftercare following surgery for neoplasm<br>Conditions classifiable to 140–239. |

Generally, one code from subcategories V54.1 or V54.2 is used per patient, unless the patient is recovering from multiple procedures and conditions.

Subcategory V58.6, Long-term (current) drug use, contains status codes that are intended to be used in addition to V58.83, Encounter for therapeutic drug monitoring, or other diagnosis codes. Subcategory V58.6 codes only state that a patient is on a prescribed drug for an extended period of time. There is no definition or timeframe for long term. If a patient receives a drug on a regular basis and has multiple refills available for a prescription, it is appropriate to document long-term drug use. The code indicates a patient's continuous use of a prescribed drug for long-term treatment of a condition or for prophylactic use.

Subcategory V58.6 codes are not used to describe patients who have addictions to drugs. This category also is not used to describe the administration of medications to prevent withdrawal symptoms in patients with drug dependence—for example, methadone maintenance programs. Instead, assign the appropriate code for the drug dependence for this type of visit.

Subcategory V58.6 codes are used for long term drug treatment as a prophylactic measure (for example, to prevent the recurrence of deep vein thrombosis), to treat a chronic disease (such as insulin for diabetes), or for treatment of a disease that requires long-term drug therapy (such as arthritis). Codes from subcategory V58.6 are not assigned for medications administered for a brief period of time to treat an acute illness or injury or to bring a chronic condition under better control. For example, a type II diabetic patient may receive insulin for a period of time when hospitalized to control the blood sugar while the patient is recovering from surgery or another illness. The use of insulin during this hospital stay is not coded with V58.67.

Code V58.83, Encounter for therapeutic drug monitoring, is the correct code to use when a patient visit is for the purpose of undergoing a laboratory test to measure the drug level in the patient's blood or urine or to measure a specific function to assess the effectiveness of a drug. V58.83 may be used alone if the monitoring is for a drug that the patient is on for only a brief period, not long term. However, there is a "use additional code" note after code V58.83 to remind the coder to use an additional code for any associated long-term (current) drug use (V58.61–V58.69) to indicate what drug is being monitored.

**EXAMPLE:** Patient was seen in the physician's office for removal of sutures from healed open wound of the forearm: V58.32, Encounter for removal of sutures

**EXAMPLE:** Admission for chemotherapy for patient with metastasis to liver; patient has history of large intestine/colon carcinoma: V58.11, Encounter for chemotherapy; 197.7, Secondary neoplasm of the liver; V10.05, Personal history of malignant neoplasm of large intestine/colon; 99.25, Injection or infusion of cancer chemotherapeutic substance

**EXAMPLE:** Encounter for radiotherapy for patient with adenocarcinoma of the breast: V58.0, Encounter for radiotherapy; 174.9, Malignant neoplasm of breast

**EXAMPLE:** The patient is on anticoagulants and the physician orders a prothrombin time (PT) to be obtained in the outpatient department: V58.83, Encounter for therapeutic drug monitoring; V58.61, Long-term (current) use of anticoagulants

### Category V59, Donors

Codes from Category V59, Donors, are used for living individuals who are donating blood, tissue, or an organ to be transplanted into another individual. V59 codes are not used when a patient donates his or her own blood to possibly receive during an upcoming scheduled surgery; instead, the reason for the patient's surgery is coded. V59 codes are not used when the potential donor is examined (code V70.8). Also, these codes are not used for cadaveric donations, that is, when a patient's organ(s) are harvested at the time of death according to the patient's stated wishes.

The American College of Obstetricians and Gynecologists (ACOG) requested new codes for egg donors that identify the age of the donor and whether the eggs are intended to be used for anonymous donations or for a designated recipient. Codes V59.70–V59.74 identify the age of the egg or oocyte donor (either younger than age 35 years or age 35 years or older) and specify whether the intended recipient is anonymous or designated.

A sperm donor is indexed in ICD-9-CM to code V59.8, Donor, other specified organ or tissue.

## Exercise 23.2

Assign ICD-9-CM diagnosis and procedure codes to the following:

1. Encounter for fitting of artificial leg; fitting of prosthetic leg (below the knee)

2. Encounter for removal of cast; cast removal

3. Admitted to donate bone marrow; bone marrow aspiration

4. Status post unilateral kidney transplant, human donor

5. Reprogramming of cardiac pacemaker

6. Routine circumcision of 10-year-old boy; circumcision

7. Encounter for chemotherapy for patient with Hodgkin's lymphoma; chemotherapy

8. Encounter for renal dialysis for patient with end-stage renal disease (ESRD); hemodialysis

9. Encounter for occupational therapy for patient with cognitive deficits secondary to an old CVA; occupational therapy

10. Replacement of tracheostomy tube; tracheostomy tube replaced

## Persons Encountering Health Services in Other Circumstances (V60–V69)

Categories V60–V69 include a variety of codes that describe reasons for healthcare encounters and explain circumstances regarding healthcare services that do not fall into other categories. Certain V codes identify the reasons for the encounter, but others are used as additional codes to provide more details about the patient's healthcare services.

### *Category V60, Housing, Household, and Economic Circumstances*

Codes in category V60, Housing, household, and economic circumstances, are used strictly as additional diagnosis codes to further explain the socioeconomic factors that may be influencing the patient's need for healthcare services. The codes in this category may be used to describe circumstances that lead to the disruption of the family unit and create the need for specific healthcare services. For example, code V60.81 identifies a minor child in foster care and may be used to identify the point when this situation impacts the care and management of the child by the healthcare provider.

### *Category V61, Other Family Circumstances*

Category V61, Other family circumstances, is one of several categories in ICD-9-CM that may be used when a patient or family member receives counseling services after an illness or injury, or when support is required to cope with family and social problems. These codes are not used in conjunction with a diagnosis code when counseling is considered integral to the treatment for the condition. Subcategory codes V61.0 identify family disruption situations that may occur due to military deployment, divorce or separation, parent-child estrangement, or an extended absence or death of a family member. Subcategory codes V61.1, Counseling for marital and partner problems, and code V61.21, Counseling for victim of child abuse, allow identification of counseling for family conflict and abuse-related issues, for both the victim and the perpetrator of parental child abuse. Alcoholism (V61.41) or substance abuse (V61.42) in a family member may be a circumstance that causes another family member to seek healthcare or counseling services. A different V code is used, V62.83, when counseling services are provided to the perpetrator of physical or sexual abuse. These counseling codes are used when only counseling services, not medical treatment, is rendered.

### *Category V62, Other Psychosocial Circumstances*

Category V62 includes codes that classify those circumstances, or fear of them, affecting the person directly involved or others, mentioned as the reason for seeking or receiving medical advice or care. Rather than medical conditions, these are psychosocial conditions that often require counseling or other services to improve the individual's status or functioning. These codes may be listed as the only reason for an encounter or the codes may be used in addition to other diagnoses or reasons for visits to provide useful information on circumstances that may affect a patient's care or treatment. Examples of V62 codes include V62.0, Unemployment; V62.6, Refusal of treatment for reasons of religion or conscience; V62.84, Suicidal ideation; and V62.85, Homicidal ideation.

### Category V63, Unavailability of Other Medical Facilities for Care

Category V63, Unavailability of other medical facilities for care, describes circumstances when a certain type of medical facility or service is not available and a patient has to be taken elsewhere or provided services in a facility that would not normally care for this type of patient. Code V63.1, Medical services in home not available, may be a first-listed or additional diagnosis code to explain the occasion when a home healthcare provider is not available and the patient may need to be admitted to an acute care hospital or long-term care facility.

### Category V64, Persons Encountering Health Services for Specific Procedures, Not Carried Out

Category V64, Persons encountering health services for specific procedures, not carried out, was introduced in Chapter 2 of this textbook as it further explains why a procedure or service was not performed. Codes in category V64 can only be used as additional diagnosis codes. The first four subcategory codes identify the circumstance when a particular procedure cannot be performed for different reasons.

Codes V64.00–V64.09 describe specific reasons why an immunization or vaccination was not given. Tracking why an immunization was not given can be as important as tracking those that are given, according to the American Academy of Pediatrics. These codes identify the multiple reasons why a patient did not receive a routine immunization.

V64.1 and V64.2 state that a surgical or other procedure cannot be carried out because of a contraindication or a patient's decision. A contraindication is any medical condition that renders some form of treatment improper or undesirable. For example, the patient may have an infection, cardiac condition, or abnormal diagnostic test that would make performing the surgical procedure unsafe until the contraindication is resolved. The patient may also decide, sometimes at the last minute before surgery begins, that he or she does not want the surgery or procedure performed at this time and the procedure is cancelled. This code may also be used when a patient is recommended to have a procedure during the hospital stay and refuses. For example, the patient refuses coronary artery bypass surgery after a coronary arteriogram demonstrates significant coronary atherosclerosis. V64.2, Surgical or other procedure not carried out because of patient's decision, is used as an additional code to explain this event.

Code V64.3 is used when another circumstance causes the surgery or procedure to be cancelled. Such circumstances may be equipment failure in the surgery or procedure suite, unplanned absence of the surgeon or other necessary medical personnel, or lack of necessary medications or supplies.

Codes within subcategory V64.4, Closed surgical procedure converted to open procedure, are frequently used as additional diagnosis codes to explain when a planned endoscopic procedure cannot be completed and the physician must perform an open or invasive surgical procedure instead. Individual codes exist to explain the conversion of a laparoscopic, thoracoscopic, or arthroscopic procedure to a procedure using open surgical techniques. In each of these events, only the open surgical procedure is coded in ICD-9-CM. An additional code is not required for the initially-attempted endoscopic procedure.

### Category V65, Other Persons Seeking Consultation

Codes from category V65, Other persons seeking consultation, are used to report services sought by one person on behalf of another person not in attendance, to describe an apparently healthy person who feigns illness to obtain medical care, or to classify a variety of counseling services not listed elsewhere. Codes within category V65 may be first-listed or additional diagnosis codes.

**EXAMPLE:** A patient frequently comes to the emergency department or a physician's office with a variety of vague complaints that usually include pain of some type. The doctor documents the patient as having "drug-seeking behavior." The patient's complaints or a code for unspecified drug abuse is listed first with an additional code of V65.2, Person feigning illness.

The counseling sessions that may be reported with a code from this category include dietary counseling, health education, counseling on substance use or abuse, HIV counseling (usually related to HIV testing), and training on the use of insulin pumps. Codes such as V65.49 and V65.8 may explain patient visits to physicians when the patient has no sign or symptom. For example, a patient may have a physician's office appointment to discuss her desire to have an elective bilateral removal of breast implants when there is no medical indication for the procedure. Code V65.8, Other reasons for seeking consultation, would be the principal or first-listed diagnosis because no abnormal symptoms or findings have prompted the surgery.

### Category V66, Convalescence and Palliative Care

Category V66 is used primarily for patients seeking convalescence, often in a long-term care facility or hospice, following surgery, radiotherapy, or chemotherapy. This category is subdivided to describe the reason for the convalescence. The convalescence codes are indexed in the Alphabetic Index under "Convalescence" and "Admission (encounter), for, convalescence following."

Code V66.7 describes an encounter for palliative care, hospice care, or end-of-life care. Code V66.7 is always a secondary code for the patient receiving palliative care for a terminal condition. The terminal condition, such as carcinoma, chronic obstructive pulmonary disease, Alzheimer's disease, or AIDS, should be the principal diagnosis. Code V66.7 is used as a secondary diagnosis code during an inpatient admission or in any other healthcare setting when it is determined that palliative care should be initiated and no further treatment for the terminal illness is desired. There is no time limit or minimum for the use of this code assignment.

**EXAMPLE:** Seventy-year-old patient is admitted to a long-term care facility for convalescence following repair of hip fracture: V66.4, Convalescence following treatment of fracture

**EXAMPLE:** Fifty-year-old patient is admitted to the hospital for management of pain that is caused by her widespread metastatic carcinoma of the liver, lungs, and bones, which spread from her breast carcinoma initially treated more than 10 years ago. After consultation with her physicians and family, the patient elects to discontinue further treatment and receive hospice care with pain management services at home. The metastatic sites and history of breast cancer codes are listed first (according to the circumstances of the admission), with a secondary code, V66.7, Encounter for palliative care.

### *Category V67, Follow-up Examination*

Carefully read the includes note under the category V67 title. It states "surveillance only following completed treatment." (CDC 2011)

The term "follow-up" as it is intended in ICD-9-CM can be different from what a physician intends to describe when he uses the same phrase. The physician may be describing ongoing medical treatment or a recovery phase of the illness or recent surgery. Category V67, Follow-up examination, is to be used only to describe an encounter where the treatment of the condition is completed, and the patient is undergoing surveillance or a checkup to determine if his or her disease-free status continues. When a physician states "follow-up" for hypertension that remains under treatment or "follow-up" after recent cardiac surgery, the V67 category is unlikely to be the appropriate set of codes to use. In these circumstances described by the physician, the hypertension under treatment is likely to be coded or a surgical aftercare code may be more appropriate to describe the healing or recovery phase after surgery.

#### Coding Guidelines

A code from category V67 is assigned as the principal diagnosis, or first-listed diagnosis code, to explain the reason for the encounter when the patient is admitted for the purpose of surveillance after the initial treatment for a disease or injury has been completed. The use of V67 means the condition has been fully treated and no longer exists. It means the patient has no complaints or symptoms of a disease. Following the V67 code, a second code can be used to indicate the reason for the follow-up, such as a personal history of a malignant neoplasm. If, during the follow-up examination, a recurrence, extension, or related condition is identified, the code for that condition is assigned as the principal diagnosis, or first-listed diagnosis code, rather than a code from category V67.

Category V67 is subdivided to describe the completed treatment, such as surgery, radiotherapy, or chemotherapy. Codes in this category are indexed under "Follow-up" and "Admission (encounter), for, follow-up examination" in the Alphabetic Index.

**EXAMPLE:** Patient admitted for follow-up cystoscopy to rule out recurrence of malignant neoplasm of the urinary bladder; patient had a transurethral resection of the bladder 1 year ago and has been cancer free to date; cystoscopy revealed no recurrence: V67.09, Follow-up examination following surgery; V10.51, History of malignant neoplasm of the urinary bladder; 57.32, Other cystoscopy

**EXAMPLE:** Patient admitted for follow-up colonoscopy to rule out recurrent adenoma of the colon; patient had removal of adenoma 3 years ago; colonoscopy was positive for recurrence and adenoma was removed: 211.3, Benign neoplasm of colon; 45.43, Endoscopic destruction of other lesion or tissue of large intestine

## Other Supplementary V codes (V70–V91)

The following note appears at the beginning of this section: Nonspecific abnormal findings disclosed at the time of these examinations are classifiable to categories 790–796.

### Category V70, General Medical Examination

Like the codes in category V20.2, Routine infant or child health check, the codes in category V70 describe reasonably healthy children and adults who seek healthcare services for routine examinations, such as a general physical examination, or examinations for administrative purposes, such as a preschool examination. With the exception of code V70.7, the codes are only used as first-listed diagnoses. These codes are not used if the examination is for the diagnosis of a suspected illness or for treatment of a disease. In these cases, the diagnosis code or possibly a category V71 code is used instead. If a diagnosis or condition is identified during the course of the general medical examination, it should be reported as an additional diagnosis code. Preexisting or chronic conditions, as well as history codes, may also be used as additional diagnoses as long as the examination was for the administrative purpose and not focused on treatment of the medical condition.

**EXAMPLE:** Fifty-five-year-old man has an appointment at his primary care physician's office for his annual physical examination. The patient has mild eczema that is treated with over-the-counter lotions, and he had an inguinal hernia repaired during the past year.

V70.0, Routine general medical examination at a healthcare facility; eczema, 692.9. The hernia is not coded because it no longer exists.

### Category V71, Observation and Evaluation for Suspected Conditions Not Found

Codes from the category V71 are assigned as principal diagnoses for encounters or admissions to evaluate the patient's condition under the following circumstances:

- Some evidence suggests the existence of an abnormal condition.
- A health problem occurs following an accident or other incident that ordinarily results in such a problem.
- No supporting evidence for the suspected condition is found, and no treatment is currently required.

The fact that the patient may be scheduled for continuing observation in the office or clinic setting following discharge does not limit the use of this category.

Code V71.81, Observation for suspected child abuse or neglect, is used when child abuse is suspected but not found after the observation and evaluation is completed. This situation is most likely to occur during a visit to a physician's office, an emergency department, or a primary care clinic.

The observation codes are for use in very limited situations in which a person is being observed for a suspected condition that is ruled out. The observation codes are not for use if an injury or illness or any signs or symptoms related to the suspected condition are present. In such cases, the diagnosis or symptom code should be assigned.

The category V71 observation code is to be used as the first-listed code or as principal diagnosis only. Additional codes may be used in addition to the observation code, but only if they are unrelated to the suspected condition being observed.

Codes in category V71 are indexed in the Alphabetic Index under "Admission (encounter), for, observation (without need for further medical care)" and "Observation (for)."

**EXAMPLE:** A patient is admitted to the hospital for observation following an automobile accident because serious head trauma is suspected; all diagnostic tests are negative for head injury: V71.4, Observation following other accident

## Category V72, Special Investigations and Examinations

Category V72 includes codes to describe ancillary services provided to the patient, such as radiological examinations, laboratory examinations, and preoperative examinations. These codes are indexed in the Alphabetic Index under "Admission (encounter), for, examination" and "Examination."

### Coding Guidelines

When only diagnostic services are provided during the outpatient encounter, sequence first the diagnosis, condition, problem, or other reason that is identified as chiefly responsible for the outpatient encounter. Codes for other appropriate diagnoses then should follow.

A code from category V72, Special investigations and examinations, is assigned as the reason for an encounter only when no problem, diagnosis, or condition is identified as the reason for the examination. Codes from the V72 category can reflect "routine" services, or services that may be ordered without medical necessity. For example, code V72.62, Laboratory examination ordered as part of a routine general medical examination, is used when the patient does not have any medical reasons for the tests but instead the test results provide a baseline for future tests or rule out any unsuspected condition. Another code in this category describes the encounter for laboratory tests to be performed prior to a treatment or procedure such as surgery (V72.63). Code V72.61, Antibody response examination, is used to describe the reason for the prevaccination serologic testing that may be ordered to determine immunity as an alternative to unnecessary vaccinations. Frequently insurance companies do not pay for laboratory or other testing services without a patient's diagnosis or physical symptom or complaint or other evidence of medical necessity for the services. When the patient does not have a medical reason for the testing, a code from the V72 category, such as V72.60 or V72.69, is used. If routine testing of an outpatient is performed during the same visit as a test to evaluate a sign, symptom, or diagnosis, it is appropriate to assign both V code, V72.5 or V72.6x, and the code for the reasons for the diagnostic tests performed to evaluate the sign, symptom or disease. For example, the patient may have a routine chest x-ray done in a patient with no symptoms for screening purposes, and a urinalysis done for a urinary tract infection. Codes V72.5, Radiological examination, not elsewhere classified, and 599.0, Urinary tract infection, site not specified, are assigned for this example. A radiological examination done as part of preprocedural testing is coded to V72.81–V72.84 instead of using code V72.5. Codes from category V72 are rarely used for inpatient coding. A diagnosis code from category V72 reflects the reason for the service, which may be a procedure or a test. The procedure performed on the patient may also be coded with ICD-9-CM or Current Procedural Terminology (CPT). It is likely that the CPT codes are stored in the facility's charge description master and printed directly on the patient's file or bill.

**EXAMPLE:** Patient visits the radiology department for chest x-ray. Because the patient has no other complaints and the x-ray is part of a routine physical examination, only the V code is appropriate: V72.5, Radiology examination, NEC

**EXAMPLE:** Patient visits the radiology department for chest x-ray to rule out pneumonia. Patient complains of cough and fever. Either of these symptoms should be listed first, rather than the V code. The pneumonia is not coded because it was not established during the encounter: 786.2, Cough; 780.60, Fever, unspecified.

**EXAMPLE:** Patient visits the laboratory department for routine blood work as part of his routine general medical examination. Because the patient has no other complaints documented, only the V code is appropriate: V72.62, Laboratory examination ordered as part of a routine general medical examination.

**EXAMPLE:** Patient visits the laboratory department with complaints of polydipsia. A blood glucose test is performed to rule out diabetes. The symptom code for polydipsia is listed first. Because the diabetes has not been established during this encounter, it is not coded: 783.5, Polydipsia

Several codes for women's health visits are included in category V72. For example, subcategory V72.3, Gynecological examination, offers two choices to describe a visit by a woman to her primary care or specialist physician. Code V72.31 is intended to describe a routine gynecological examination for a healthy woman that may include a Pap cervical smear with pelvic examination. Code V72.32 is used to describe the continued monitoring of a woman who makes a visit to the physician's office for a Pap smear to confirm findings of a recent normal smear following an initial abnormal smear. Another common reason for a young woman's visit to a physician is to have a pregnancy test. Usually the test results are known at the conclusion of the visit. A positive test result is assigned a code from category V72.42, Pregnancy examination or test, positive result. If the pregnancy test is negative, code V72.41 is used to report the visit. If the results of the pregnancy test are not available or the pregnancy has not yet been confirmed, code V72.40 is used to report the visit.

During a pregnancy, it may be necessary to test a patient's Rh status. If a pregnant woman's blood group is Rh negative, knowing whether the father is Rh positive or Rh negative will help find the risk of Rh sensitization and whether or not the woman should receive Rh immunoglobulin to prevent sensitization for the rest of the pregnancy. The code V72.86, Encounter for blood typing, would be used for this type of encounter.

Frequently, patients are referred to physicians for consultations or to hospital outpatient departments for preoperative evaluations or clearances. For preoperative evaluations, the visits are coded and sequenced as follows:

1. Code from subcategory V72.8, Other specified examinations, or V72.63 to identify the preoperative consultation or visit. Subcategory V72.8 includes preoperative cardiovascular examinations, preoperative respiratory examinations, other specified preoperative examinations, and unspecified preoperative evaluations. Code V72.63 is the code for pre-procedural laboratory examination.
2. Code to describe the condition for which the surgery is being performed.
3. Code to describe any conditions found during the preoperative evaluation.

## Categories V73–V82, Special Screening Examinations

The codes in categories V73–V82 are used to identify screening examinations for specific conditions and disorders that are currently not active.

Screening is the testing for a disease or condition in reasonably healthy individuals so that early detection and treatment can be provided. The screening code may be the first-listed code if the reason for the visit is specifically the screening examination. It may be an additional code if the screening is done during a visit for other health problems.

If a patient has a physical sign or symptom and is referred for a test to rule out or to confirm a suspected condition, this is a diagnostic examination, not a screening. The screening codes should not be used for this situation. Rather, the patient's physical sign or symptom(s) could be coded as the reason for the test.

When the principal diagnosis is a code from category V72, an additional code from categories V73–V82 may also be assigned to identify any special screening test performed. Should a condition be discovered during the screening, then the code for the condition may be assigned as an additional code. The first listed code is the screening code.

Codes in categories V73–V82 are referenced in the Alphabetic Index under "Screening (for)."

**EXAMPLE:** Patient visits the laboratory department for a routine chemistry profile as well as special screening for diabetes mellitus: V72.60, Laboratory examination; V77.1, Special screening for diabetes mellitus

## Categories V83–V84, Genetic Carrier Status and Genetic Susceptibility to Disease

Codes in category V83, Genetic carrier status, are intended to describe a patient who is known to carry a particular gene that could cause a disease to be passed on to his or her children. The code does not mean the patient has this particular disease. It does not mean there is 100 percent certainty that the disease would be passed on genetically to the next generation. The code could be used to explain why a patient is receiving additional monitoring or testing.

Codes in category V84, Genetic susceptibility to disease, are intended to describe a patient who has a confirmed abnormal gene that makes the patient more susceptible to a particular disease. A patient who has a genetic susceptibility to a disease, particularly if it is a malignancy, may request prophylactic removal of an organ to prevent the disease from occurring. These codes can be used to identify encounters for prophylactic organ removal, including breast, ovary, prostate, endometrium, or other anatomical site.

## Category V85, Body Mass Index (BMI)

The body mass index (BMI) is the determination of a patient's weight in proportion to height. BMI measures are calculated as kilograms per meters squared. BMI can be used to characterize underweight as well as overweight status. For overweight individuals, codes in this category are used in conjunction with a code from category 278, Overweight and obesity, to provide specific information about the patient's status.

The BMI adult codes are for use for individuals older than 20 years. The codes for pediatric BMI use the value ranges for children currently represented in the Centers for Disease Control and Prevention (CDC) growth charts. The age group represented in the year 2000

CDC growth charts is 2 to 20 years old. The pediatric codes report percentiles as used on the growth charts.

For coding of the body mass index measurement, code assignments may be based on documentation from clinicians in addition to the patient's physician or provider. Typically a dietitian will document the BMI number in a nutritional evaluation progress note. However, the dietitian's documentation can only supplement, not replace, the physician's documentation. The physician must document the medical diagnosis of overweight, obesity, or other nutritional problems to be coded. The BMI is reported as an additional diagnosis to the condition being evaluated. As with all additional diagnoses, the BMI should only be reported when it meets the definition of a reportable additional diagnosis.

The BMI codes are:

| | |
|---|---|
| V85.0 | Body Mass Index less than 19, adult |
| V85.1 | Body Mass Index between 19–24, adult |
| V85.21–V85.25 | Body Mass Index between 25–29, adult |
| V85.30–V85.39 | Body Mass Index 30–39, adult |
| V85.41–V85.45 | Body Mass Index 40 and over, adult |
| V85.51–V85.54 | Body Mass Index, pediatric |

### Category V86, Estrogen Receptor Status

The status codes V86.0, Estrogen receptor positive status [ER+] or V86.1, Estrogen receptor negative status [ER–] are used as an additional code for patients who have been diagnosed with breast cancer, both females and males, and have had their estrogen receptor status determined.

About two thirds of breast cancer patients have an estrogen receptor positive [ER+] tumor. The incidence is greater among postmenopausal women. These patients are more likely to benefit from endocrine therapy, so knowledge of their receptor status is important in the selection of adjuvant or palliative therapy. Oral hormones, such as tamoxifen, and estrogen ablation by oophorectomy have proven effective to prolong the duration of disease-free survival, as well as for palliation in the patient with advanced disease when the patient's tumor was estrogen receptor positive.

### Category V87, Other Specified Personal Exposures and History of Presenting Hazards to Health

Codes within subcategories V87.0–V87.3 can be used to describe patients who seek medical care due to exposure or contact with substances that pose a threat to their health. Such substances include arsenic, aromatic amines, benzene, mold, algae bloom, and other potentially hazardous substances. These patients may be without symptoms due to the exposure but have other injuries from the same event. Also within this category are codes to identify the patient's personal history of antineoplastic chemotherapy (V87.41), personal history of monoclonal drug therapy (V87.42), personal history of estrogen therapy (V87.43), personal history of inhaled steroid therapy (V87.44), personal history of systemic steroid therapy (V87.45), personal history of immunosuppressive therapy (V87.46), and personal history of other drug therapy (V87.49). Other codes for history of the particular condition for which the patient received chemotherapy or drug therapy could be used with these codes.

### Category V88, Acquired Absence of Other Organs and Tissue

Some of the codes within this category are important for tracking Pap smear necessity. Women who have had a total hysterectomy with removal of the cervix (V88.01) no longer require cervical Pap smears but do require vaginal smears to test for vaginal malignancies. Women with a cervical stump (V88.02) following a hysterectomy still require cervical Pap smears. Code V88.03 would identify the woman who has a surgically absent cervix but in whom the uterus remains.

### Category V89, Other Suspected Conditions Not Found

Codes within this category are typically used to identify the outpatient encounter in which a pregnant female is referred to a maternal-fetal or fetal medicine specialist when an initial screening ultrasound indicates a possible abnormality. Frequently no abnormality or suspected condition is found after the detailed examination is conducted by the specialist. The V89 codes identify the fetal-maternal condition that was suspected but not found after study. If a fetal-maternal condition is found during the study, the coder is directed to code the confirmed condition, such as a known fetal abnormality that is affecting the management of the mother (655.00–655.93) or other appropriate diagnosis codes on the maternal record. The V89 codes are not to be used if an illness or any signs or symptoms related to the suspected condition or problem are present.

### Category V90, Retained Foreign Body

The US Department of Defense requested new codes be created for embedded fragment status to identify the type of embedded material. The codes were requested primarily to identify military personnel who have had an injury, most likely from an explosion, that resulted in embedded fragments remaining in the body because the location of the fragment makes it too difficult to remove. Any embedded object has the potential to cause infection due to the object itself or any organism present on it when it entered the body. An embedded magnetic object is a contraindication to certain imaging studies and can pose long-term toxicological hazards. Codes in the range of V90.0–V90.9 identify radioactive, metal, plastic, organic, and other types of foreign body fragments. Another code, V15.53, identifies the personal history of a retained foreign body having been removed.

### Category V91, Multiple Gestation Placenta Status

Codes V91.00–V91.99 are status codes for multiple gestations. They indicate the number of placentas and amniotic sacs. Depending on the number, the risk of complications is higher for the pregnant female, and therefore the treatment plan differs. Each code identifies whether the patient has a twin, triplet, quadruplet, or other specified multiple gestation and whether there is one or more placentas and one or more amniotic sacs.

## Sequencing of V Codes

V codes can be used in both inpatient and outpatient settings. V codes may be used as either a first-listed code or secondary code, depending on the circumstances of the visit. Some V codes may only be principal or first-listed diagnosis codes.

V codes often describe the reason for the visit to be the performance of a particular procedure or service. V codes are diagnosis codes. The procedure or service must also be coded with a procedure code to fully describe the visit.

The list below describes the recommended sequencing of V codes according to the *ICD-9-CM Official Guidelines for Coding and Reporting*.

**V Codes That May Only Be Principal or First-Listed Diagnosis**

The list of V codes and categories below may only be reported as the principal or first-listed diagnosis, except when there are multiple encounters on the same day and the health records for the encounters are combined, or when there is more than one V code that meets the definition of principal diagnosis. However, these codes should not be reported if the code does not meet the definition of principal or first-listed diagnosis.

**(Codes listed with an "X" in the fourth digit space indicate all codes in this category are first-listed):**

| | |
|---|---|
| V20.X | Health supervision of infant or child |
| V22.0 | Supervision of normal first pregnancy |
| V22.1 | Supervision of other normal pregnancy |
| V24.X | Postpartum care and examination |
| V26.81 | Encounter for assisted reproductive fertility procedure cycle |
| V26.82 | Encounter for fertility preservation procedure |
| V30.X–V39.X | Liveborn infants according to type of birth |
| V46.12 | Encounter for respirator dependence during power failure |
| V46.13 | Encounter for weaning from respirator [ventilator] |
| V51.0 | Encounter for breast reconstruction following mastectomy |
| V56.0 | Extracorporeal dialysis |
| V57.X | Care involving the use of rehabilitation procedures |
| V58.0 | Radiotherapy |
| V58.11 | Encounter for antineoplastic chemotherapy |
| V58.12 | Encounter for antineoplastic immunotherapy |
| V59.X | Donors |
| V66.X | Convalescence and palliative care (except V66.7, Encounter for palliative care) |
| V68.X | Encounters for administrative purposes |
| V70.X | General medical examination (except V70.7, Examination of participant in clinical trial) |
| V71.X | Observation and evaluation for suspected conditions not found |

## Nonspecific V Codes

Certain V codes are so nonspecific or potentially redundant with other codes that there can be little justification for their use in the inpatient setting. Their use in the outpatient setting should be limited to those instances when there is no further documentation to permit more precise coding. Otherwise, any sign or symptom or any other reason for visit that is captured in another code should be used.

V11.X Personal history of mental disorder. A code from the mental disorders chapter with an in-remission fifth digit should be used instead.

V13.4 Personal history of arthritis

V13.6 Personal history of congenital malformations

V15.7 Personal history of contraception

V23.2 Pregnancy with history of abortion

V40.X Mental and behavioral problems (except V40.31, Wandering in diseases classified elsewhere)

V41.X Problems with special senses and other special functions

V47.X Other problems with internal organs

V48.X Problems with head, neck, and trunk

V49 Problems with limbs and other problems

Exceptions:

- V49.6 Upper limb amputation status
- V49.7 Lower limb amputation status
- V49.81 Asymptomatic postmenopausal status
- V49.82 Dental sealant status
- V49.83 Awaiting organ transplant status
- V49.86 Do not resuscitate status
- V49.87 Physical restraints status

V51.8 Other aftercare involving the use of plastic surgery

V58.2 Blood transfusion, without reported diagnosis

V58.9 Unspecified aftercare

## ICD-9-CM Review Exercises: Chapter 23

Assign ICD-9-CM diagnosis and procedure codes to the following questions. Note: many of the scenarios in these questions are likely to be provided to hospital outpatients or patients seen in a physician's office or ambulatory center. ICD-9-CM, volume 3 procedure codes are not required to be reported for hospital outpatients or physician office visits, as CPT coding is the required procedural coding system for reporting outpatient services. The procedure codes in the following questions may be coded strictly for practice purposes and the answers are included in the answer key. Otherwise, the procedures can be disregarded in this exercise and not coded.

1. Office visit for routine gynecological examination including Pap smear; gynecological examination with Pap smear of the cervix

 ______________________

2. Visit to emergency department after falling 10 feet at work; examination reveals no injuries

 ______________________

3. Encounter for chemotherapy; breast carcinoma, upper inner quadrant; chemotherapy

 ______________________

*(Continued on next page)*

## ICD-9-CM Review Exercises: Chapter 23 (Continued)

4. Visit to radiology department for barium swallow; abdominal pain of right lower quadrant; barium swallow performed and the findings are negative

5. Follow-up examination of colon adenocarcinoma with colon resection 1 year ago, no recurrence found; colonoscopy

6. Encounter for observation of suspected malignant neoplasm of the cervix; Pap smear performed and the findings are negative

7. Routine general medical examination

8. Examination of eyes

9. Admission to inpatient hospice for palliative care for giant cell glioblastoma of brain; patient determined by doctor to be terminal

10. Encounter for laboratory test; patient complains of fatigue

11. Screening for osteoporosis

12. Infant to clinic for developmental handicap screening

13. Status post artificial heart valve

14. Kidney donor; left nephrectomy

15. Encounter for physical therapy; status post below-knee amputation 6 months ago; physical therapy

# ICD-10-CM Chapter 21, Factors Influencing Health Status and Contact with Health Services (Z00–Z99)

## Organization and Structure of ICD-10-CM Chapter 21

What are known as "V" codes in ICD-9-CM are "Z" codes in ICD-10-CM. Codes included in ICD-10-CM's Chapter 21, Factors Influencing Health Status and Contact with Health Services (Z00–Z99), represent reasons for encounters. Z codes are diagnosis codes. If a procedure is performed, a corresponding procedure code must be used with the Z code that identifies the reason for the encounter. As with ICD-9-CM V codes, ICD-10-CM Z codes are provided for encounters when circumstances other than a disease or injury are recorded in the health record as the "diagnosis"—the problem or reason for the encounter.

Coding professionals will find the listing of codes for factors influencing health status and contact with health services a bit different in ICD-10-CM than what is currently found in ICD-9-CM. The following blocks represent the ICD-10-CM arrangement:

| | |
|---|---|
| Z00–Z13 | Persons encountering health services for examinations |
| Z14–Z15 | Genetic carrier and genetic susceptibility to disease |
| Z16 | Resistance to antimicrobial microorganisms drugs |
| Z17 | Estrogen receptor status |
| Z18 | Retained foreign body fragments |
| Z20–Z28 | Persons with potential health hazards related to communicable diseases |
| Z30–Z39 | Persons encountering health services in circumstances related to reproduction |
| Z40–Z53 | Encounters for other specific healthcare |
| Z55–Z65 | Persons with potential health hazards related to socioeconomic and psychosocial circumstances |
| Z66 | Do not resuscitate status |
| Z67 | Blood type |
| Z68 | Body mass index (BMI) |
| Z69–Z76 | Persons encountering health services in other circumstances |
| Z77–Z99 | Persons with potential health hazards related to family and personal history and certain conditions influencing health status |

Some categories in Chapter 21 have rephrased titles to better reflect the situations the codes classify. For example, the description for Z08 is "Encounter for follow-up examination after completed treatment for malignant neoplasm" compared to the ICD-9-CM code title for V67.2 "Follow-up examination following chemotherapy."

An example of decreased specificity in ICD-10-CM is code Z23, Encounter for immunization. This code is not further classified. In ICD-9-CM, category codes V03, V04, V05, and V06 are used to identify the types of immunizations.

## Coding Guidelines and Instructional Notes for ICD-10-CM Chapter 21

The note at the beginning of this chapter has been modified from what it states in ICD-9-CM. All codes in Chapter 21 are affected by these revised guidelines.

Instructional notes also have been added to different categories to explain how codes should be assigned. For example, under category Z01, Encounter for other special examination without complaint, suspected or reported diagnosis, is the following note: "Codes from category Z01 represent the reason for the encounter. A separate procedure code is required to identify any examination or procedure performed." Also, under category Z85, Personal history of malignant neoplasm, is the following note: "Code first any follow-up examination after treatment of malignant neoplasm (Z08)."

There are published chapter-specific guidelines for Chapter 21 of ICD-10-CM:

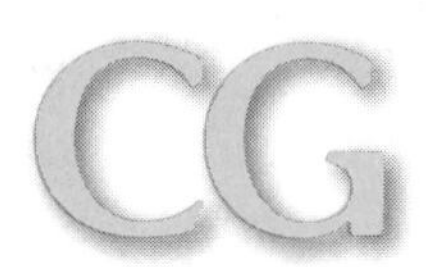

- Guideline I.C.21.a. Use of Z codes in any healthcare setting

Z codes are for use in any healthcare setting. Z codes may be used as either a **first-listed** (principal diagnosis code in the inpatient setting) or secondary code, depending on the circumstances of the encounter. Certain Z codes may only be used as **first-listed** or principal diagnosis

- Guideline I.C.21.b. Z codes indicate a reason for an encounter

Z codes are not procedure codes. A corresponding procedure code must accompany a Z code to describe any procedure performed.

- Guidelines I.C.21.c. Categories of Z codes

The guidelines describe the meaning or intent of the various types of Z codes available to describe factors influencing health status and contact with health services.

To gain an understanding of these rules, access the 2014 guidelines from NCHS website (http://www.cdc.gov/nchs/icd/icd10cm.htm) and read Chapter 21, Factors influencing health status and contact with health services guidelines I.C.21.a–I.C.21.c.

## Coding Overview for ICD-10-CM Chapter 21

ICD-10-CM's Chapter 21 contains similar reasons for visits as are included in ICD-9-CM's V codes, as well as some new situations that can be coded with Z codes. Listed next are the ranges of Z codes.

Z00–Z13 Persons encountering health services for examinations

**EXAMPLES:** Z00.00 Encounter for general adult medical examination without abnormal findings

Z00.01 Encounter for general adult medical examination with abnormal findings

Z14–Z15 Genetic carrier and genetic susceptibility to disease

**EXAMPLES:** Z14.01 Asymptomatic hemophilia A carrier
Z15.01 Genetic susceptibility to malignant neoplasm of breast

Z16 Resistance to antimicrobial drugs

Z17 Estrogen receptor status

Z20–Z28 Persons with potential health hazards related to communicable diseases

**EXAMPLES:** Z21 Asymptomatic human immunodeficiency virus (HIV) infection status
Z23 Encounter for immunization

Z30–Z39 Persons encountering health services in circumstances related to reproduction

**EXAMPLES:** Z30.011 Encounter for initial prescription of contraceptive pills
Z34.81 Encounter for supervision of other normal pregnancy, first trimester
Z37 Outcome of delivery
Z38 Liveborn infants according to place of birth and type of delivery

Z40–Z53 Encounters for other specific healthcare

**EXAMPLES:** Z48.22 Encounter for aftercare following kidney transplant
Z51.11 Encounter for antineoplastic chemotherapy

Z55–Z65 Persons with potential health hazards related to socioeconomic and psychosocial circumstances

**EXAMPLES:** Z59.5 Extreme poverty
Z62.0 Inadequate parental supervision and control

Z66 Do not resuscitate (DNR) status

Z67 Blood type

Z68 Body Mass Index

Z69–Z76 Persons encountering health services in other circumstances

**EXAMPLES:** Z71.42 Counseling for family member of alcoholic
Z72.0 Tobacco use

Z77–Z99 Persons with potential health hazards related to family and personal history and certain conditions influencing health status

**EXAMPLES:** Z79.4 Long-term (current) use of insulin
Z85.3 Personal history of malignant neoplasm of breast

Certain codes have been moved from other chapters in ICD-9-CM to Chapter 21 in ICD-10-CM. For example, elective, legal, or therapeutic abortions have been moved from ICD-9-CM Chapter 11, Complications of Pregnancy, Childbirth, and the Puerperium, to ICD-10-CM Chapter 21.

Several codes have been expanded in ICD-10-CM; for example, personal and family history codes have been expanded.

In addition, codes have been added for concepts that currently do not exist in ICD-9-CM; for example, category Z67 identifies the patient's blood type.

By contrast, there are also concepts that existed in ICD-9-CM that no longer exist in ICD-10-CM, for example, there is no comparable category in ICD-10-CM to ICD-9-CM category V57, Care involving use of rehabilitation procedures. For encounters for rehabilitative therapy, report the underlying condition for which therapy is being provided (such as an injury) with the appropriate seventh character indicating subsequent encounter. This change greatly impacts certain settings providing aftercare.

The note at the beginning of the chapter explains the use of the codes:

> Z codes represent reasons for encounters. A corresponding procedure code must accompany a Z code if a procedure is performed. Categories Z00–Z99 are provided for occasions when circumstances other than a disease, injury or external cause classifiable to categories A00–Y89 are recorded as "diagnoses" or "problems." This can arise in two main ways:
>
> 1. When a person who may or may not be sick encounters the health services for some specific purpose, such as to receive limited care or service for a current condition, to donate an organ or tissue, to receive prophylactic vaccination (immunization), or to discuss a problem which is in itself not a disease or injury.
> 2. When some circumstance or problem is present which influences the person's health status but is not in itself a current illness or injury.

Aftercare Z codes in ICD-10-CM should not be used for aftercare of fractures. For aftercare of a fracture, assign the acute fracture code with the seventh character for the subsequent encounter values such as initial encounter for closed or open fracture, subsequent encounter for routine healing, delayed healing, nonunion or for sequela. Some of the fracture codes have as few as six possible seventh characters, (for example, see S02, Fracture of skull and facial bones) or as many as 16 possible seventh characters for the long bone fractures (for example, see 52, Fracture of forearm).

Category Z68, BMI is divided into adult and pediatric codes. The BMI adult codes are for use for persons 21 years of age or older. BMI pediatric codes are for use for persons 2–20 years of age. The percentiles listed with the codes are based on the growth charts published by the CDC.

## ICD-10-CM Review Exercises: Chapter 23

Assign the correct ICD-10-CM diagnosis codes to the following exercises:

1. The patient was seen in his primary care physician's office for fracture aftercare concerning the traumatic fracture of the anterior wall of the acetabulum of the right pelvis. The patient was hit by a car, knocked down, and the car ran over his pelvis. The pelvic fracture is healing appropriately. What diagnosis codes are assigned?

2. Medical examination of four-year-old child prior to admission to preschool

3. Patient seen for fitting of right artificial leg after patient had below-knee amputation due to medical condition

4. This single newborn was born vaginally in the hospital. The baby is being treated for Rh incompatibility in a baby with documented type A+ blood and the mother's blood type documented as A-. What is the correct diagnosis code(s)?

5. This 59-year-old male had lateral wall STEMI and was brought by ambulance to the emergency room. He received tPA and was transferred to a tertiary care center for continued care. The patient was received with the tPA infusion continuing, and immediately taken to the cardiac cath lab. What codes are assigned at the receiving hospital?

6. The patient who had his bladder removed due to carcinoma without recurrence is scheduled for a radiology procedure to evaluate the patency of his ileal conduit (artificial opening for the urinary tract), including ureteropyelography using contrast media. The entire procedure is performed in the radiology suite with the radiologists' impression of "normal functioning ileal conduit." What is the correct diagnosis code(s)?

7. Postmenopausal osteoporosis in a 63-year-old female with a history of healed osteoporotic fracture of the ankle

8. The patient's reason for coming to the outpatient department at the hospital today is to undergo a screening colonoscopy. The patient is a 50-year-old male and he does not have any symptoms of intestinal disease. The doctor writes the post-procedure diagnosis as "screening for malignant neoplasm of colon, none found" with instructions to the patient to return in 10 years for repeat colonoscopy.

9. The patient is a 55-year-old female who comes to the hospital outpatient mammography department with an order including the reason for the mammogram as "Routine screening mammogram for breast malignancy. The patient has no signs or symptoms of breast disease. The mammogram was reported by the radiologist as a normal study.

10. A one-year-old child is brought to the pediatrician's office for a well-child visit with scheduled immunizations to be administered. During the visit, the parents decide not to have the immunization performed. The child is healthy with no abnormal findings found during the examination.

# Chapter 24

# Coding and Reimbursement

## Learning Objectives

At the conclusion of this chapter, you should be able to:

1. Define the terms *DRG* and *MS-DRG*
2. Briefly describe the hospital inpatient prospective payment system, including how base payment rates are determined and the formula for computing the hospital payment
3. Describe the purpose and activities of quality improvement organizations and recovery audit contractors
4. Define the term *medical necessity* and explain its relationship to ICD-9-CM diagnosis codes
5. Define the term *advance beneficiary notice* and explain its purpose

This textbook has included a thorough review of the characteristics and conventions of ICD-9-CM and an introduction to ICD-10-CM/PCS. While coding systems were originally established for statistical comparison and research purposes, in many cases the codes are used for reimbursement and other purposes. This chapter includes a brief discussion of some of the reimbursement purposes for coding: the hospital inpatient prospective payment system, recovery audit contractors, and medical necessity.

## Hospital Inpatient Prospective Payment System

The hospital IPPS is a method of payment undertaken by the Centers for Medicare and Medicaid Services (CMS) to control the cost of inpatient acute care hospital services to Medicare recipients. Title VI of the Social Security Amendments of 1983 established the prospective payment system (PPS) to provide payment to hospitals for each Medicare case at a set reimbursement rate, rather than on a fee-for-service or per-day basis. The payment rates to hospitals are established before services are rendered and are based on **diagnosis-related groups (DRGs)**.

For fiscal year 2008, Medicare adopted a severity-adjusted DRG system called **Medicare-Severity DRGs (MS-DRGs)**. This was the most drastic revision to the DRG system in 24 years. The goal of the new MS-DRG system was to significantly improve Medicare's ability to recognize severity of illness in its inpatient hospital payments. One of the goals of the new system was to increase payments to hospitals for services provided to the sicker patients and decrease payments for treating less severely ill patients.

MS-DRGs represent an inpatient classification system designed to categorize patients who are medically related with respect to diagnoses and treatment and who are statistically similar in their lengths of stay. Each DRG has a preset reimbursement amount that the hospital receives whenever the MS-DRG is assigned.

The base payment rates for each DRG are determined from two basic sources. First, each MS-DRG is assigned a relative weight. The relative weight represents the average resources required to care for cases in that particular DRG relative to the national average of resources used to treat all Medicare cases. The average Medicare case is assigned a relative weight of 1.0000. Thus, cases in a MS-DRG with a weight of 2.0000, on average, require twice as many resources as the average Medicare case; on the other hand, cases in a MS-DRG with a weight of 0.5000, on average, require half as many resources as the average Medicare case. Each year, the relative weights of the MS-DRGs are updated to reflect changes in treatment patterns, technology, and any other factors that may change the relative use of hospital resources.

The second source that determines MS-DRG payment rate is the individual hospital's payment rate per case. This payment rate is based on a regional or national adjusted standardized amount that considers the type of hospital; designation of the hospital as large urban, other urban, or rural; and a wage index for the geographic area in which the hospital is located.

Thus, the actual amount the hospital is reimbursed for each Medicare inpatient is determined by multiplying the hospital's individual payment rate by the relative weight of the DRG, less any applicable deductible amount.

The formula for computing the hospital payment for each MS-DRG is as follows:

*DRG Relative Weight × Hospital Base Rate = Hospital Payment*

For any given patient in an MS-DRG, the hospital knows, in advance, the amount of reimbursement it will receive from Medicare. It is the responsibility of the hospital to ensure that its resource use is in line with that payment.

In addition to the basic payment rate, Medicare provides for an additional payment for other factors related to a particular hospital's business. If the hospital treats a high percentage of low-income patients, it receives a percentage add-on payment applied to the MS-DRG-adjusted base payment rate. This add-on payment, known as the **disproportionate share hospital (DSH)** adjustment, provides for a percentage increase in Medicare payments to hospitals that qualify under either of two statutory formulas designed to identify hospitals that serve a disproportionate share of low-income patients.

If the hospital is an approved teaching hospital, it receives a percentage add-on payment for each Medicare discharge paid under IPPS, known as the indirect medical education (IME) adjustment. This percentage varies, depending on the ratio of residents to beds.

Additional payments may be made for Medicare beneficiaries that involve new technologies or medical services that have been approved for special add-on payments. To qualify, a new technology or medical service must demonstrate that it is a substantial improvement over technologies or services otherwise available, and that, absent an add-on payment, it would be inadequately paid under the regular DRG payment.

The costs incurred by a hospital for a Medicare beneficiary are evaluated to determine whether the hospital is eligible for an additional payment as an outlier case. This additional payment is designed to protect the hospital from large financial losses due to unusually expensive cases. Any outlier payment due is added to the DRG-adjusted base payment rate, plus any DSH, IME, and new technology or medical service add-on adjustments.

Some categories of hospitals are paid the higher of a hospital-specific rate based on their costs in a base year. For example, sole community hospitals (SCHs) are the sole source of care in their areas, and small rural, Medicare-dependent hospitals (MDHs) are a major source of care for Medicare beneficiaries in their areas. Both of these categories of hospitals are afforded this special payment protection in order to maintain access to services for beneficiaries.

MS-DRG assignment is based on information that includes:

- Diagnoses (principal and secondary)
- Surgical procedures (principal and secondary)
- Discharge disposition or status
- Presence of major or other complications and comorbidities (MCC or CC) as secondary diagnoses

CMS evaluates the Medicare IPPS annually. CMS's Notice of Proposed Rulemaking is published in the *Federal Register* in late April or early May each year. This notice, on which the public may comment, announces the final decisions on all ICD-9-CM code changes and proposed revisions to the DRG system. CMS's Final Rule announcing final revisions to the IPPS, including the DRG system, is published in the *Federal Register* in July or August, and the changes become effective October 1 each year.

Prior to October 1, 1995, hospitals were required to obtain the physician's signature on each Medicare and Civilian Health and Medical Program of Uniformed Services (CHAMPUS) health record, which attested to the diagnoses and procedures documented on the face sheet. Then, on July 11, 1995, the HHS and the White House announced that physician attestation was no longer required for Medicare discharges, effective October 1, 1995. Shortly thereafter, elimination of the physician attestation requirement for CHAMPUS discharges was announced. It was anticipated that these actions would decrease administrative costs and paperwork for hospitals. With the end of physician attestation requirements, all HIM professionals, but especially coders, have faced greater responsibility for ensuring the accurate and ethical coding of health records. AHIMA has developed several documents related to data quality as guides toward attaining and maintaining high-quality coding. The Standards of Ethical Coding and an AHIMA practice brief on data quality are contained in appendices G and H, respectively, on the website accompanying this text book.

## Medicare Coding Reviews: QIOs, FIs, MACs, and CERTs

CMS reviews acute IPPS and long-term care hospitals (LTCHs) hospital records for payment purposes. CMS contracts with Medicare Fiscal Intermediaries (FIs) and Medicare Administrative Contractors (MACs) to conduct medical and coding reviews to prevent improper payment of inpatient hospital claims. This review is done to ensure that billed items or services are covered and are reasonable and necessary as specified in section 1862(a)(1)(A) of the Social Security Act. In addition, the Comprehensive Error Rate Testing (CERT) contractors conduct medical review to measure inpatient hospital payment error rates.

Previously, each state's quality improvement organization (QIO), in addition to their focus on quality issues, was responsible for the following for acute IPPS and LTCHs:

- The Hospital Payment Monitoring Program (HPMP), which was performed on a post payment basis and consisted of two parts:
  1. Utilization review of randomly selected cases for payment purposes, and
  2. Measurement of the accuracy of the Medicare Fee-for-Service (FFS) payments to acute IPPS hospitals and LTCHS, that is, the error rate.

As of 2008, QIOs are no longer responsible for the functions previously included in the HPMP. Currently, the activities related to acute IPPS and LTCH claim reviews that are performed by the QIOs are:

- Quality of care reviews due to beneficiary complaints, complaints other than from beneficiaries, and quality of care reviews referred by CMS or CMS-designated entities (that is, FI, Carriers, MACs, SSAs, OIG)
- Utlization reviews for hospital-requested higher weighted DRG payments;
- Utilization reviews referred by CMS or CMS designated entities for cases involving issues such as transfers and readmissions;
- Review of Emergency Medical Treatment Active Labor Act (EMTALA) cases;
- Performance of Expedited Determinations; and
- Provider education on quality of care issues and other issues under their purview (that is, hospital-requested higher weighted DRG review, and such.)

The transition of responsibility for measuring and preventing improper payments to inpatient hospitals from the QIOs to the FIs, MACs, and the CERT contractors allows the QIOs to concentrate on improving patient quality of care.

FIs and MACs perform medical reviews of acute IPPS hospitals and LTCH claims to ensure that they are for covered, correctly coded, and reasonable and necessary services. These reviews are performed on either a prepayment or post-payment basis. The FI or MAC will conduct claim adjustments as needed. The FI or MAC conducts provider feedback, through their medical review departments, based on their review findings. They also conduct provider education through their provider outreach and education departments on issues related to submitting inpatient claims correctly as part of their goal to reduce the payment error rate.

The CERT contractor reviews claims for the purpose of measuring error rates for acute IPPS hospital and LTCH claims. The CERT contractor performs reviews on a post-payment basis in order to determine the degree to which Medicare FIs and MACs are paying acute IPPS hospitals and LTCHs claims appropriately, in accordance with coverage, coding, and medical necessity guidelines.

Each hospital is notified when a claim has been selected for review in slightly different ways, depending on the review entity. The CERT contractor notifies providers that a claim is selected for CERT review via letter or telephone contact. The hospital provides copies of the selected reviews by mail to the CERT contractor. For prepay review, the FIs and MACs suspend claims for review and send out a request for supporting documentation, usually a copy of the patient's health record, which is then sent back to the FI or MAC by the hospital. For postpayment review, the claim is already paid. An FI or MAC performing the review sends a request for health records to the provider. Hospitals submit a copy of the record as requested. The FI or MAC reviews the claim and makes any necessary payment adjustments based on the review.

Current information about the IPPS and LTCH hospital review programs are available on the Medicare website at http://www.cms.gov/QualityImprovementOrgs/09_Current.asp#TopOfPage and http://www.cms.gov/Outreach-and-Education/Medicare-Learning-Network-MLN/MLNProducts/downloads/AcutePaymtSysfctsht.pdf and http://www.cms.gov/AcuteInpatientPPS/Downloads/InpatientReviewFactSheet.pdf.

## Recovery Audit Contractors

Despite the efforts of QIOs and other initiatives that CMS has undertaken, there are concerns that the Medicare Trust Fund may not be adequately protected against improper payments. Congress passed the Medicare Prescription Drug, Improvement, and Modernization Act of 2003 (MMA), which was designed to enhance and support Medicare's current efforts. Congress directed the HHS to conduct a three-year demonstration project using **RACs** to detect and correct improper payments in the Medicare traditional FFS program. Section 302 of the Tax Relief and Health Care Act of 2006 made the RAC program permanent and required the program be expanded to all 50 states no later than 2010.

The demonstration project began in 2005 and ended in 2008 with three contractors focusing on healthcare claims in three states with large numbers of Medicare beneficiaries: New York, Florida, and California. The demonstration project allowed Medicare to evaluate the efficiency and effectiveness of the program in order to make improvements in the RAC program. The RACs performed reviews of medical records with the corresponding Medicare claims to:

- Detect improper Medicare payments, including both underpayments and overpayments
- Correct improper Medicare payments

Each Recovery Auditor is responsible for identifying overpayment and underpayments in approximately one-quarter of the country. The Recovery Audit Contractor in each jurisdiction is as follows:

Region A: Diversified Collection Services (DCS)

Region B: CGI

Region C: Connolly, Inc.

Region D: HealthDataInsights, Inc.

Current information about the RAC program can be found on the CMS website: http://www.cms.gov/Research-Statistics-Data-and-Systems/Monitoring-Programs/Medicare-FFS-Compliance-Programs/Recovery-Audit-Program/

The examination of the ICD-9-CM coding is a major area of focus for the RACs because the diagnosis and procedure codes create the MS-DRGs that are the basis of payment for acute care hospitals. ICD-9-CM and CPT coding in other healthcare organizations, such as rehabilitation hospitals and units, and physician offices, determine reimbursement to the providers and therefore are a focus of attention during these providers' reviews. Certified coders are employed by RACs to perform coding reviews.

## Coding for Medical Necessity

Three factors help define the **medical necessity** of a diagnostic test, procedure, or treatment:

1. The likelihood that a proposed healthcare service will have a reasonable beneficial effect on the patient's physical condition and quality of life at a specific point in his or her illness or lifetime.
2. Healthcare services and supplies that are proven or acknowledged to be effective in the diagnosis, treatment, cure, or relief of a health condition, illness, injury, disease, or its symptoms and to be consistent with the community's accepted standard of care. Under medical necessity, only those services, procedures, and patient care warranted by the patient's condition are provided.
3. The concept that procedures are only reimbursed as a covered benefit when they are performed for a specific diagnosis or specified frequency.

Accurate ICD-9-CM diagnosis coding is essential to establish the medical necessity of a particular service as required by Medicare's reasonable and necessary medical coverage policies. Other third-party payers also want to know the reason for the service before payment is determined. MACs that process Part A and Part B Medicare claims may develop local coverage decisions (LCDs), formerly known as local medical review policies (LMRPs). These policies ensure that claims submitted for certain services—typically outpatient services—have been deemed reasonable and necessary for the patient's condition. National coverage determinations (NCDs) also exist for other diagnostic and therapeutic services including many laboratory tests, for which Medicare payment is contingent on a particular condition being established as the reason the test was ordered. The coder must be certain that documentation contains all of the reasons why the physician ordered a diagnostic or therapeutic service. Then the coder must assign all of the appropriate ICD-9-CM diagnosis codes for the claim to be reviewed accurately for medical necessity and paid appropriately. The requirements for determining medical necessity have moved the coding personnel outside the traditional HIM department into hospitals' emergency departments, admitting/registration or access departments, central scheduling centers, and a variety of clinical departments performing many outpatient services, such as radiology and laboratory. The need to know if a patient's condition meets the medical necessity requirements of a particular service is essential prior to issuing an advance beneficiary notice (ABN). An ABN is a statement signed by the patient when he or she is notified by the provider, prior to a service or procedure being performed, that Medicare may not reimburse the provider for the service, whereupon the patient indicates that he or she will be responsible for any charges. Medical necessity processing has brought the coding function closer to the point of care and, in some institutions, improved the documentation related to the reasons for outpatient therapy and testing services.

## Review Exercises: Chapter 24

1. How does Medicare or other third-party payers determine whether the patient has medical necessity for the tests, procedures, or treatment billed on a claim form?

2. What is the basic formula for calculating each MS-DRG hospital payment?

3. What was the goal of the MS-DRG system that replaced the DRG system?

4. What additional factor is involved in the assignment of MS-DRGs besides principal and secondary diagnoses including the presence of MCCs or CCs, and discharge disposition or status?

5. What are possible add-on payments that a hospital could receive in addition to the basic Medicare MS-DRG payment?

6. What is the name of the program that functions to detect and correct improper payments in the Medicare traditional FFS programs?

7. What activities related to acute IPPS and LTCH claim reviews are performed by the QIOs?

8. What factors are taken into consideration to determine an individual hospital's payment rate per case?

9. During the demonstration project what were the two reasons that RACs performed reviews of health records?

10. What is an ABN?

# References and Bibliography


45 CFR 162. Final Rule 2009. HIPAA Administrative Simplification: Modifications to Medical Data Code Set Standards to Adopt ICD-10-CM and ICD-10-PCS. 2009 (January 16). http://edocket.access.gpo.gov/2009/pdf/E9-743.pdf.

American Academy of Orthopaedic Surgeons. 2007. Joint Revision Surgery - When Do I Need It? http://orthoinfo.aaos.org/topic.cfm?topic=A00510#A00510_R1_anchor

American Health Information Management Association. 2000. Where in the world is ICD-10? *Journal of AHIMA* 71(8).

American Health Information Management Association. 2009a. AHIMA home page for ICD-10. http://www.ahima.org/icd10.

American Health Information Management Association. 2012. ICD-9-CM Coordination and Maintenance Committee Meeting, Summary of September 2012. http://library.ahima.org/xpedio/groups/public/documents/ahima/bok1_049912.pdf

American Heart Association. 2014. Ejection Fraction Heart Failure Measurement. http://www.heart.org/HEARTORG/Conditions/HeartFailure/SymptomsDiagnosisofHeartFailure/Ejection-Fraction-Heart-Failure-Measurement_UCM_306339_Article.jsp

American Health Information Management Association and the American Hospital Association. 2003. ICD-10-CM Field Testing project: Report on findings. http://www.ahima.org/~/media/AHIMA/Files/HIM-Trends/FinalStudy_000.ashx

American Hospital Association. 1985–2014. *Coding Clinic for ICD-9-CM*. Chicago: American Hospital Association.

American Medical Association. 2003. *Complete Medical Encyclopedia.* New York: Random House Reference.

American Psychiatric Association. 2013. *Diagnostic and Statistical Manual of Mental Disorders,* Fifth ed. Arlington, VA.: American Psychiatric Press.

Barta, A. et al. 2008. ICD-10-CM primer. *Journal of AHIMA* 79(5):64–66.

Barta, A. and A. Zeisset. 2011. *Root Operations: Key to Procedure Coding in ICD-10-PCS.* Chicago: AHIMA.

Beers, M.H. and R. Berkow, eds. 2000. *The Merck Manual*, 17th ed. Rahway, N.J.: Merck & Co.

Bergeron, C. 2003. The 2001 Bethesda System. http://www.scielosp.org/pdf/spm/v45s3/v45s3a07

Braunwald, E., A. Fauci, D. Kasper, S. Hauser, D. Longo, and J. Jameson. 2001. *Harrison's Principles of Internal Medicine*. New York: McGraw-Hill.

Bowman, S. 2008a. Brushing up on ICD-10-PCS. *Journal of AHIMA* 78(9):108–112.

Bowman, S. 2008b. Why ICD-10 is worth the trouble. *Journal of AHIMA* 79(3):24–29.

Brown, F. 2010. *ICD-9-CM Coding Handbook, with Answers*. Chicago: American Hospital Association.

Canobbia, M.M. 1990. *Cardiovascular Disorders*. Mosby's Clinical Nursing Series. Vol. 1. St. Louis: Mosby-Year Book.

Centers for Disease Control and Prevention. 2014. National Center for Health Statistics and Centers for Medicare and Medicaid Services. *ICD-10-CM Official Guidelines for Coding and Reporting, 2014.* http://www.cdc.gov/nchs/icd/icd10cm.htm

Centers for Disease Control and Prevention. 2014. National Center for Health Statistics and Centers for Medicare and Medicaid Services. *ICD-9-CM Official Guidelines for Coding and Reporting, 2011.* http://www.cdc.gov/nchs/icd/icd9cm.htm

Centers for Disease Control and Prevention. 2014a. Centers for Disease Control and Prevention. www.cdc.gov

Centers for Disease Control and Prevention. 2014b. Infant mortality: http://www.cdc.gov/reproductivehealth/MaternalInfantHealth/InfantMortality.htm)

Centers for Disease Control and Prevention. 2014c. Concussion. MedlinePlus. http://www.nlm.nih.gov/medlineplus/concussion.html

Centers for Disease Control and Prevention. 2013. Highly Pathogenic Avian Influenza A (H5N1) in People. http://www.cdc.gov/flu/avianflu/h5n1-people.htm.

Centers for Medicare and Medicaid Services. 2015. *ICD-10-PCS Reference Manual*. http://www.cms.gov/Medicare/Coding/ICD10/Downloads/2015-Reference-Manual.zip

Centers for Medicare and Medicaid Services and the National Center for Health Statistics. 2014. *ICD-10-PCS Official Guidelines for Coding and Reporting*. http://www.cms.gov/Medicare/Coding/ICD10/Downloads/2015-PCS-guidelines.pdf

Centers for Medicare and Medicaid Services. 2010 (March 5). *MLN Matters* number MM6851: Additional ICD-9 Codes Analysis and Processing Direction (Institutional Claims Only). http://www.cms.gov/MLNMattersArticles/downloads/MM6851.pdf.

Centers for Medicare and Medicaid Services. 2008. ICD-10 Overview. *Coordination and Maintenance Committee Meeting* (Baltimore, MD, September 24–25). http://www.cdc.gov/nchs/icd/icd9cm_maintenance.htm

Chen, H. 2014. Down Syndrome. MedScape. http://emedicine.medscape.com/article/943216-overview#aw2aab6b2b2aa

Davis, N.M. 2014. *Medical Abbreviations: 32,000 Conveniences at the Expense of Communication and Safety*, 15th ed. Warminster, PA: Neil M. Davis Associates.

Department of Health and Human Services. 1994. *Living with Heart Disease: Is It Heart Failure?* Consumer Version, Clinical Practice Guideline, Number 11. Rockville, MD: Agency for Health Care Policy and Research.

Department of Health and Human Services. 2010. *International Classification of Diseases, 9th Revision, Clinical Modification*. Washington, D.C.: U.S. Government Printing Office.

Dorland, W.A.N., ed. 2012. *Dorland's Illustrated Medical Dictionary,* 32nd. Philadelphia: W. B. Saunders. (s.v. "debridement")

Ertl, L. 1992. Clinical notes: Intestinal ostomies. *Journal of AHIMA* 63(6):18–22.

Food and Drug Administration. 2010. Fatalities Reported to FDA Following Blood Collection and Transfusion: Annual Summary for Fiscal Year 2009. http://www.fda.gov/BiologicsBloodVaccines/SafetyAvailability/ReportaProblem/TransfusionDonationFatalities/ucm204763.htm#overall.

Graham, L.L. 1999. *Understanding Clinical Disease Processes for ICD-9-CM Coding.* Chicago: AHIMA.

Grimes, D. et al. 1990. *Infectious Diseases.* Mosby's Clinical Nursing Series. Vol. 3. St. Louis: Mosby-Year Book.

Harman, .B. 2006. *Ethical Challenges in the Management of Health Information.* Sudbury, MA: Jones and Bartlett Publishers.

Hazelwood, A.C. and C.A. Venable. 2009. *ICD-10-CM and ICD-10-PCS Preview,* 2nd ed. Chicago: AHIMA.

Heller, J.L. 2014. Concussion. A.D.A.M Medical Encyclopedia. PubMed Health. http://www.ncbi.nlm.nih.gov/pubmedhealth/PMH0001802/

ICD-9-CM Coordination and Maintenance Committee. 1999–2014. Excerpts (agendas, proposals, and background materials) from the "Diagnoses and Procedures" portion of meeting minutes. http://www.cdc.gov/nchs/icd/icd9cm_maintenance.htm.

Illinois Department of Public Health. 2012. *Trends in the Prevalence of Birth Defects in Illinois and Chicago 1989-2009.* Epidemiologic Report Series 12:04. Springfield, IL: Illinois Department of Health, Division of Epidemiologic Studies.

Infertility reference, http://emedicine.medscape.com/article/274143-overview#aw2aab6b4

Innes, K.K. and R. Roberts. 2000. Ten down under: Implementing ICD-10 in Australia. *Journal of AHIMA* 71(1):52–56.

Johnson, P. et al. 1999. Cardiac Troponin T as a marker for myocardial ischemia in patients seen at the emergency department for acute chest pain. *American Heart Journal* 137(6):1137–44.

Kim, E.D. 2014. Erectile Dysfunction. Medscape. http://emedicine.medscape.com/article/444220-overview.

Li, H.H and M.A. Kaliner. 2006. Allergic Asthma: Symptoms and Treatment. http://www.worldallergy.org/professional/allergic_diseases_center/allergic_asthma/

Madhur, M.S. 2014. Hypertension. http://emedicine.medscape.com/article/241381-overview.

Mayo Clinic Staff. 2009. Mitral valve stenosis: definition. http://www.mayoclinic.com/health/mitral-valve-stenosis/DS00420

MedLinePlus. 2013. Neurologic Diseases. http://www.nlm.nih.gov/medlineplus/neurologicdiseases.html

MedLinePlus. 2014. Concussion. http://www.nlm.nih.gov/medlineplus/concussion.html

Melloni, J. 2001. *Melloni's Illustrated Medical Dictionary*, 4th ed. Pearl River, N.Y.: The Parthenon Publishing Group.

Merck Manual. 2104. Rheumatic Fever. http://www.merckmanuals.com/home/childrens_health_issues/bacterial_infections_in_infants_and_children/rheumatic_fever.html

National Center for Health Statistics. 2014. About the International Classification of Diseases, Tenth Revision, Clinical Modification (ICD-10-CM). http://www.cdc.gov/nchs/icd/icd10cm.htm.

National Heart Lung and Blood Institute. 2014. What is Heart Failure? http://www.nhlbi.nih.gov/health/health-topics/topics/hf/

NLM. 2014. Concussion. PubMed Health. http://www.ncbi.nlm.nih.gov/pubmedhealth/PMH0001802/

Nicholas, T. 1992. Clinical notes: Cardiac catheterization. *Journal of AHIMA* 63(3):25–26.

Office of the Inspector General. 1985. UHDDS Definitions. *Federal Register*. 50(147):31038-40

Optum. 2014a. *ICD-10-CM: The Complete Official Draft Code Set* (2014 Draft). Salt Lake City: Ingenix.

Optum. 2014b. *ICD-10-PCS: The Complete Official Draft Code Set* ( 2014 Draft). Salt Lake City: Ingenix.

National Pressure Ulcer Advisory Panel. 2014. NPUAP Pressure Ulcer Stages/Categories. http://www.npuap.org/resources/educational-and-clinical-resources/npuap-pressure-ulcer-stagescategories/

Paprosky W.G., N.V. Greidanus, J. Antonius. 2007. Minimum 10-year results of extensively-porous-coated stems in revision hip arthroplasty. Clin Orthop 1999;369:230-242 and http://orthoinfo.aaos.org/topic.cfm?topic=A00510#A00510_R1_anchor

Prophet, S. 2002a. ICD-10 on the horizon. *Journal of AHIMA* 73(7):36–41.

PubMed Health. 2012. Mitral stenosis. http://www.ncbi.nlm.nih.gov/pubmedhealth/PMH0001227.

Puckett, C.D. 1998. *The Educational Annotation of ICD-9-CM,* 5th ed. Reno: Channel Publishing.

Puscheck, E.E. 2013. Infertility. Medscape. http://emedicine.medscape.com/article/274143-overview#aw2aab6b4.

RAND Corporation. 2004. The Costs and Benefits of Moving to the ICD-10 Code Sets. http://www.rand.org/pubs/technical_reports/2004/RAND_TR132.pdf.

Reuters. 2014. Canadian Dies From H5N1 Avian Influenza on Return From China. Medscape. http://www.medscape.com/viewarticle/818927

Rice, M. and D. MacDonald. 1999. Appropriate roles of cardiac Troponins in evaluating patients with chest pain. *Journal of the American Board of Family Practice* 12(3):214–18.

Rogers, V. and A. Zeisset. 2004. *Applying Inpatient Coding Skills under Prospective Payment.* Chicago: AHIMA.

Segan, J. 2006. *Concise Dictionary of Modern Medicine.* New York: McGraw-Hill.

Sepilian, V.P. 2014. Ectopic Pregnancy. Medscape. http://emedicine.medscape.com/article/2041923-overview#aw2aab6b2b2

Skidmore-Roth, L. 2004. *Mosby's Nursing Drug Reference*. St. Louis: Mosby.

Stedman, T. 2000. *Stedman's Medical Dictionary*, 27th ed. Baltimore: Williams & Wilkins.

WebMD. 2013. Spina Bifida. http://www.webmd.com/parenting/baby/tc/spina-bifida-topic-overview

Way, L.W. 1996. *Current Surgical Diagnosis & Treatment,* 10th ed. New York: McGraw-Hill Professional Publishing Group.

Weinberg, G.A. 2006. Rheumatic Fever. Whitehouse Station, NJ: Merck. http://www.merckmanuals.com/home/childrens_health_issues/bacterial_infections_in_infants_and_children/rheumatic_fever.html

# Coding Self-Test for ICD-9-CM or ICD-10-CM and ICD-10-PCS

INSTRUCTIONS: Assign the appropriate ICD-9-CM codes (include procedure codes, M codes, E codes, and V codes, where applicable) and/or assign the appropriate ICD-10-CM diagnosis codes and the ICD-10-PCS procedure codes to the following:

1. Encounter for complete induced elective abortion due to maternal rubella, suspected damage to fetus, 10 weeks of gestation. The patient does not have rubella now; it was during week four (before she knew she was pregnant) that she contracted it. Procedure: uterine aspiration curettage via vagina to terminate the pregnancy.

2. Postpartum abscess, purulent mastitis of breast; patient discharged five days ago following spontaneous delivery of live triplets

3. Adenocarcinoma of descending colon with extension to mesenteric lymph nodes. Procedure: open permanent sigmoid colostomy to lower abdominal wall (cutaneous).

4. Paranoid schizophrenic patient in remission

5. Obstructive hydrocephalus. Procedure: open ventriculoatrial (circulatory system, atrium) shunt using synthetic catheter, tubing and valves.

6. Parkinsonism secondary to haloperidol (neuroleptic) drug therapy, subsequent encounter visit

7. Gangrene of lower leg due to uncontrolled Type I diabetes

8. Newborn twin, male, delivered by cesarean delivery (in hospital) with hypoglycemia due to maternal diabetes; newborn's mate twin was stillborn.

9. History of allergic reaction to sulfonamides

10. Scheduled renal dialysis session for a patient who requires (is dependent on) dialysis for end-stage renal disease. Procedure: hemodialysis, single filtration.

11. Chronic obstructive asthma with chronic obstructive pulmonary disease

12. Unstable angina

13. Unexplained dizziness

14. Hypertensive heart and kidney (cardiorenal) disease with chronic kidney disease, stage III

15. Iron deficiency anemia due to chronic blood loss

16. Cystic pancreatitis with cyst of pancreas

17. Reye's syndrome

18. Third-degree burn of chest wall and third-degree burn of right leg, initial visit to emergency department (Do not assign external cause of injury code)

19. Organic brain syndrome due to underlying physiologic condition, cerebral arteriosclerosis

20. Traumatic fracture of frontal bone with subarachnoid hemorrhage without loss of consciousness, due to motor vehicle accident. Patient was the driver of a car injured in a collision with an other type of car in traffic. This is an admission to the hospital following emergency room evaluation.

21. Infiltrative tuberculosis of both lungs, confirmed by bacterial culture; tuberculous spondylitis, bacterial and histological examinations not done at this time

22. Ovarian retention cyst, left side. Procedure: laparoscopic partial oophorectomy, left ovary

23. Lyme disease with associated arthritis

24. Abnormal prothrombin time, cause to be determined

25. Newborn born in community hospital transferred to university medical center. Code for the infant at the university medical center treated for hypoplastic left heart syndrome.

26. Ingestion of 30 doxepin (Sinequan) tablets resulting in an overdose, determined to be a suicide attempt; tachycardia (Doxepin is a tricyclic antidepressant drug), with hospital admission following initial evaluation in the emergency department.

27. Emergency department evaluation of a male patient diagnosed with a traumatic fracture of the right humerus, upper end (head), as the result of a fall from a ladder. Occurred at a private residence in the garage of his single-family residence. Procedure: closed reduction, humeral head, upper end, with immobilization, right upper arm.

28. Multiple inflamed seborrheic keratoses of right side of face. Procedure: cryotherapy of lesions on right side of face.

29. Moderate mental retardation as the result of acute bacterial meningitis 10 years ago

30. Chlamydial vaginitis

31. Female patient, age 57 with left-sided infiltrating duct carcinoma, upper outer quadrant, with metastases to bone

32. Diabetic hypoglycemic coma in a patient with Type I diabetes

33. Secondary thrombocytopenia due to hypersplenism. Procedure: total open splenectomy.

34. Pneumonia due to coagulase-positive *Staphylococcus aureus.* Procedure: fiberoptic bronchoscopy.

35. Peptic ulcer of the lesser curvature of the stomach, acute, with hemorrhage. Procedure: esophagogastroduodenoscopy with closed excision type biopsy of stomach.

36. Rapidly progressive glomerulonephritis. Procedure: percutaneous renal biopsy, right kidney.

37. Coronary artery disease in previous vein bypass grafts in the left anterior descending, left circumflex, and right posterior descending arteries. Procedures: coronary artery bypass grafts with double internal mammary bypass, that is, left internal mammary graft to the left anterior descending and right internal mammary graft to the circumflex. The internal mammary arteries were loosened and stretched to perform the bypass. A single aortocoronary bypass to the right posterior descending artery using greater saphenous vein excised from the right leg with an open approach, with extracorporeal circulation (cardiopulmonary bypass).

38. Patient with a history of bladder carcinoma seen for a follow-up examination related to his past partial cystectomy treatment; no recurrence found. Procedure: cystourethroscopy with excision type biopsy of bladder.

39. Degenerative joint disease, primary, localized in both knees. Procedure: total knee replacement, left knee, using artificial joint cemented into joint.

40. Malignant lymphoma, undifferentiated Burkitt's type, found in lymph nodes of the neck. Procedure: percutaneous bone marrow biopsy from iliac crest.

41. Postcatheterization stricture of urethra with urinary incontinence in a male patient. Procedure: release of urethral stricture by cystoscopy.

42. Chronic hidradenitis suppurativa, right axilla. Procedure: open local excision of hidradenitis of right axilla (procedure performed in the anatomic region of the upper extremity).

43. Initial emergency department visit for male patient with a heroin poisoning, accidental overdose; coma; drug dependence including heroin and barbiturates

44. Positive tuberculosis skin test

45. Gunshot wound of anterior chest with massive lacerations to both lungs with multiple retained bullets; shot by another person with a handgun who was charged with attempted homicide; injury occurred on a local residential/public street; after being transferred from the emergency department, the patient died in surgery before any therapeutic procedure could be done. Procedure: an emergency exploratory thoracotomy to inspect the respiratory tract.

46. Patient admitted for her first round of antineoplastic chemotherapy after a total abdominal hysterectomy and salpingo-oophorectomy for left ovarian carcinoma with known metastases to intrapelvic lymph nodes. Procedure: administration of antineoplastic chemotherapy via central vein.

47. Congenital hypertrophic pyloric stenosis. Procedure: open pyloromyotomy to dilate the pylorus of the stomach in a four-week-old infant

48. Internal derangement of lateral meniscus, posterior horn, right knee due to past sports injury tear. Procedure: arthroscopy, right knee with partial meniscectomy

49. Traumatic arthritis of left wrist, late effect of old fracture of wrist, which was the result of a fall

50. Pregnancy, delivered at 35 weeks (third trimester) following onset of preterm labor, single liveborn infant; postpartum fever of unknown origin; patient with known continuous marijuana drug dependence still present at the time of delivery. Procedure: manually assisted vaginal delivery.

# Index

D

## E

## F

I

O



P

T

W



Z